CW00940904

THE P:E DIET

LEVERAGE YOUR BIOLOGY TO ACHIEVE OPTIMAL HEALTH.

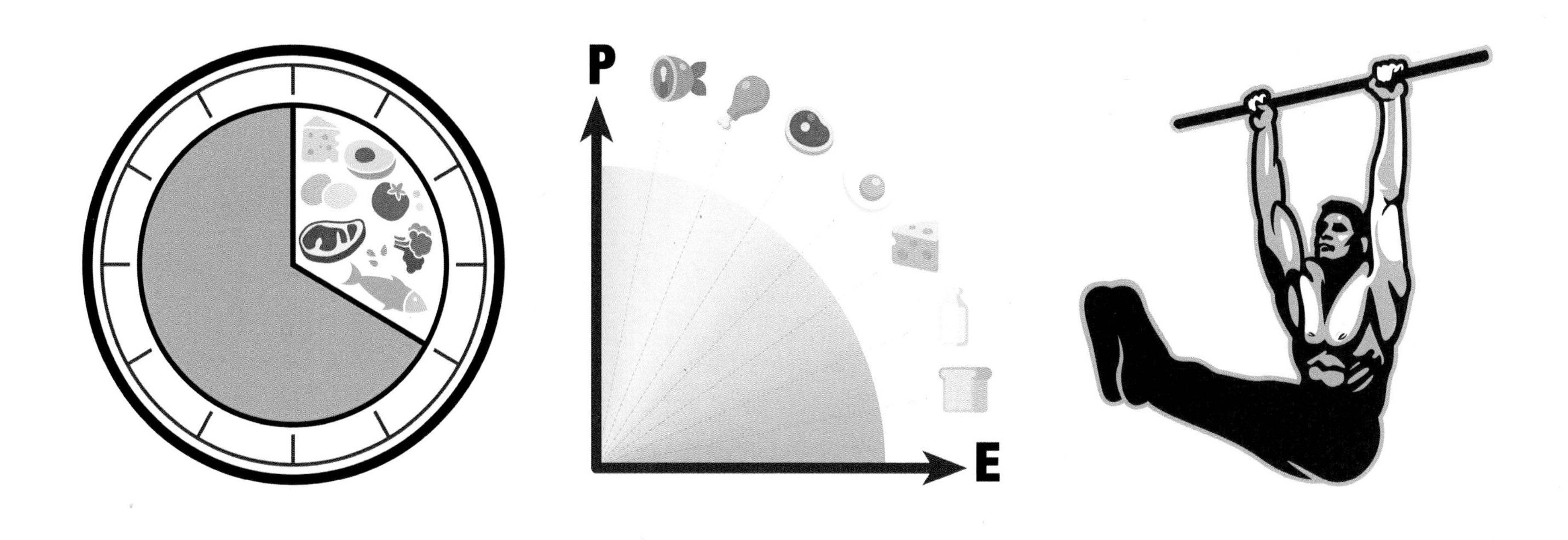

THE P:E DIET

TED NAIMAN M.D.

WILLIAM SHEWFELT

The material in this book is for informational purposes only. It is not intended or implied to be a substitute for professional medical advice. Reading the information in this book does not constitute a physician-patient relationship. The reader should always consult his or her healthcare provider to determine the appropriateness of this information for his or her own situation or if he or she has any questions regarding a medical condition or treatment plan. As with any new or changed diet or exercise regimen, the programs described in this book should be considered only after consulting with your physician to determine which might be appropriate for your individual circumstances and the current state of your health. Certain individuals, especially those with any medical conditions and those on any diabetes and blood pressure medications, are at increased risk and must consult their physician prior to making any changes to their current diet and exercise protocols. The intensive nature of some of the protocols in this book may involve a higher degree of risk for certain individuals, and your physician should help you determine if that risk is appropriate for you. The authors expressly disclaim responsibility for any adverse effects that may result from the use or application of the information contained in this book.

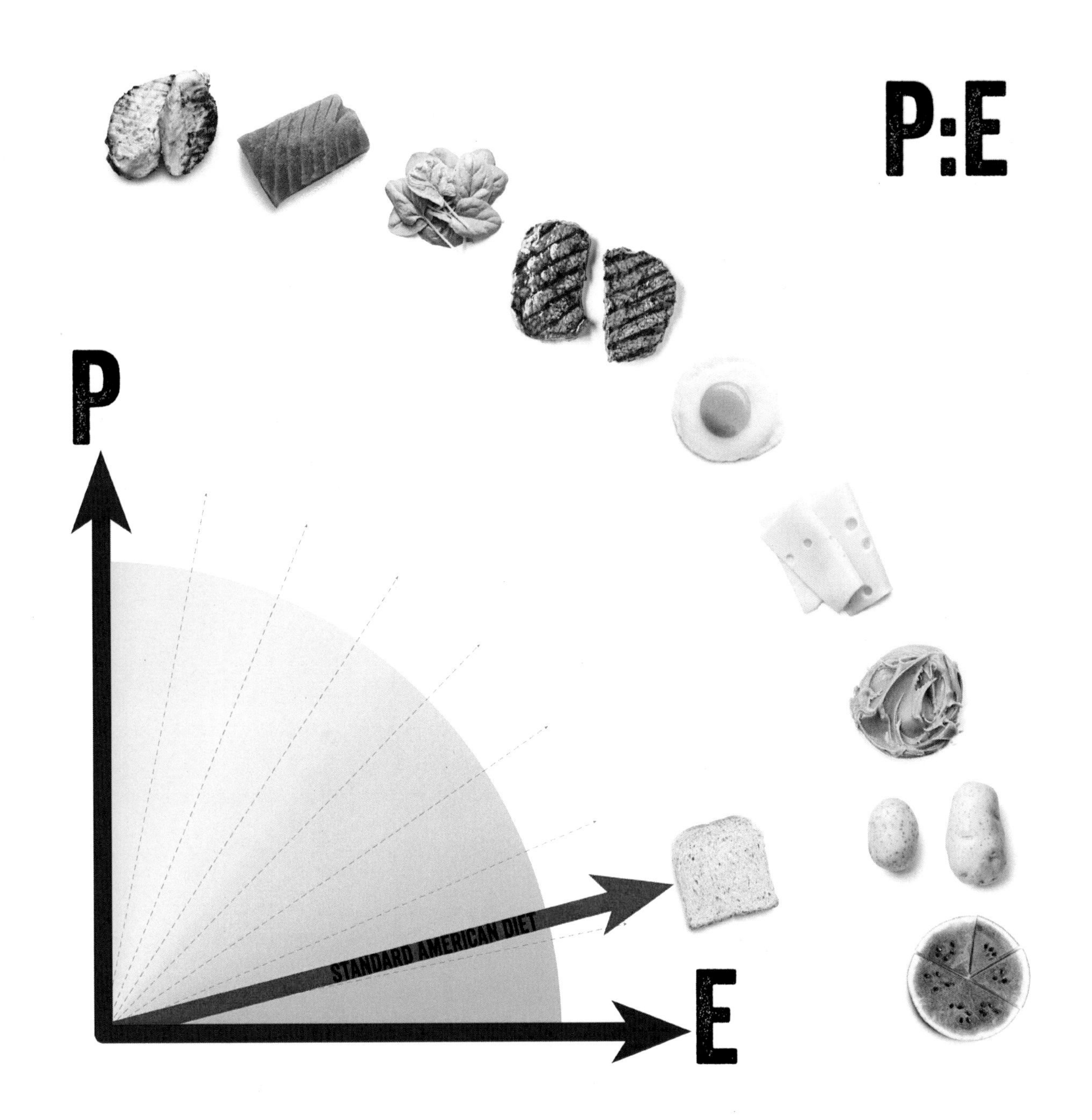
P:E
P
E
STANDARD AMERICAN DIET

ABOUT THE AUTHORS

TED NAIMAN M.D.

Ted Naiman is a board-certified Family Medicine physician in the department of Primary Care at a leading major medical center in Seattle. His research and medical practice are focused on the practical implementation of diet and exercise for health optimization. He has an undergraduate degree in mechanical engineering and an addiction to Ultimate Frisbee. He is a pro-level bassist in his spare time.

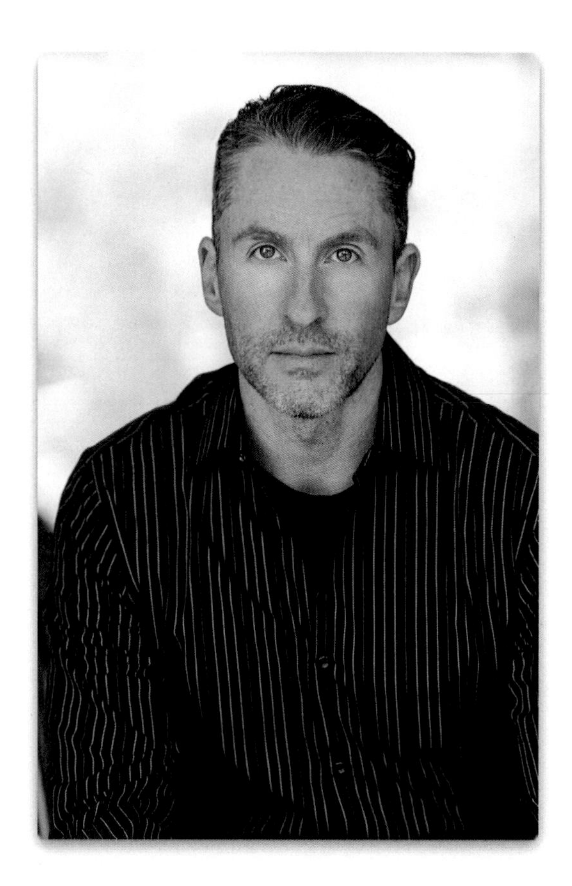

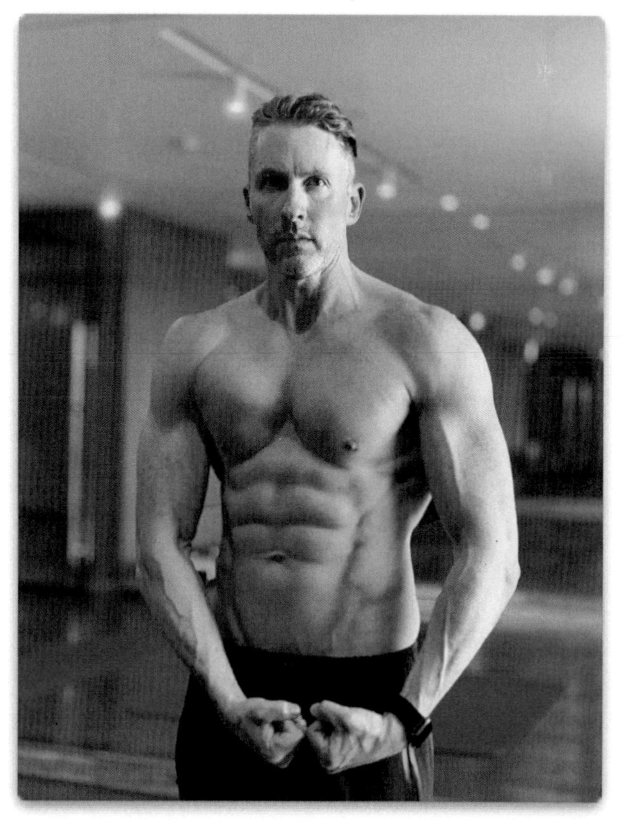

WILLIAM SHEWFELT

William Shewfelt is an actor, host of the *Will to Win* Podcast and the http://PrimalBody.co coaching community. He is known for his portrayal of Brody the Red Power Ranger on *Power Rangers Ninja Steel* (2017-2018). He was nominated for Favorite TV Actor at the 2018 Kids Choice Awards.

By combining carnivore-style eating, a strategic blend of cardio and explosive strength workouts, and focused goal setting, he has been celebrated for achieving a 5% body fat physique, and for guiding many others to breakthrough success on low carb diets.

William has modeled for a number of fitness apparel and mens' apparel brands. He is a regular feature on health podcasts and co-hosts the *Better Stronger Faster* Podcast with Chris Bell.

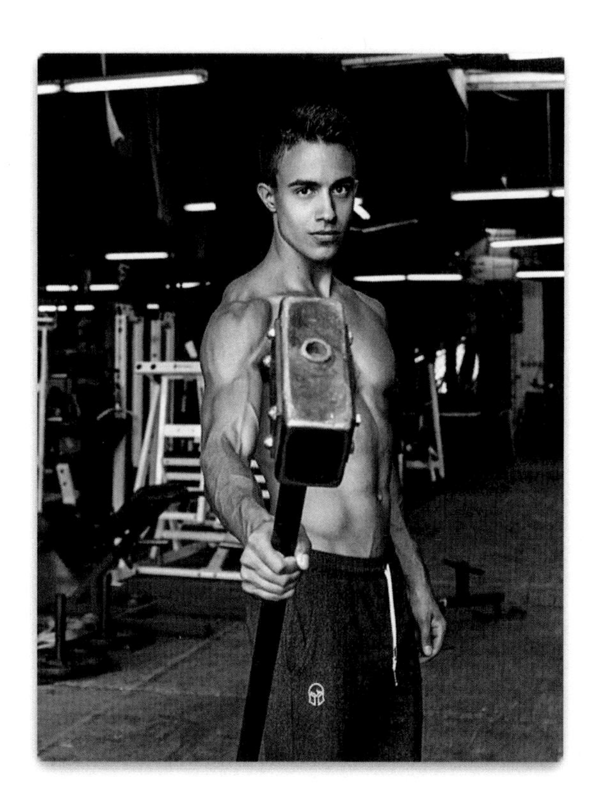

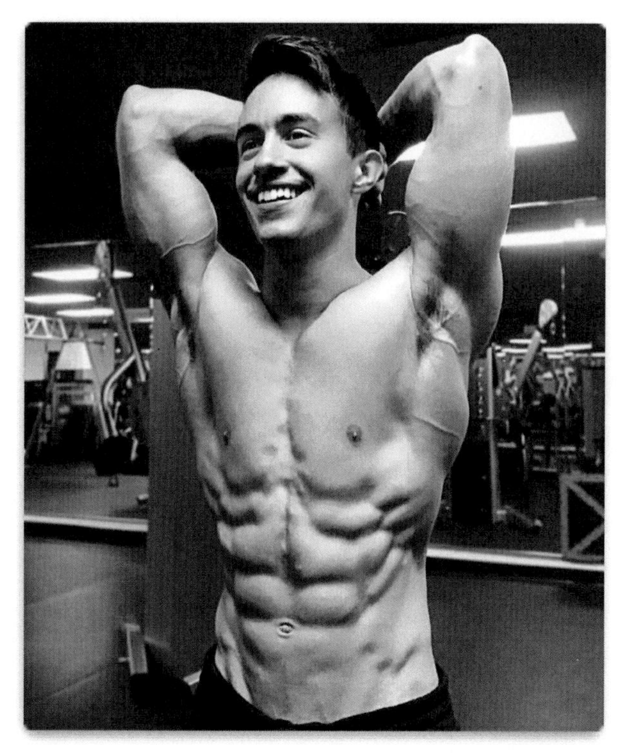

PROLOGUE

One hundred patient encounters a week, fifty weeks a year, for twenty years. About 100,000 physician/patient interactions. And I never cease to be amazed at the radical gradients in health. One moment I could be examining the healthiest professional CrossFitter you have ever seen, with a chiseled-from-granite body and absolute perfection for labwork. The next minute? A frail and weak shell of a human, struggling just to walk, with a problem list a mile long and failure of half a dozen different organ systems. It didn't dawn on me all at once, but somewhere in there I came to a shocking realization. Most of the time, the only difference between the fittest people on earth and the most decrepit really did just come down to two things: diet, and exercise.

I started paying extremely close attention. What EXACTLY were the differences between the diet and exercise of these healthy elites versus those plagued by chronic disease? Gradually I came to the realization that the principles at work were unbelievably simple, and equally simple to implement. The rules for diet were so basic that I couldn't believe I hadn't realized them earlier. Target nutrient density—mostly just protein and minerals—while minimizing toxins, including the energy toxicity of exceeding your carbohydrate and fat storage. Exercise? Generate the highest tension possible in all of your muscles, for as long as possible, on a regular basis.

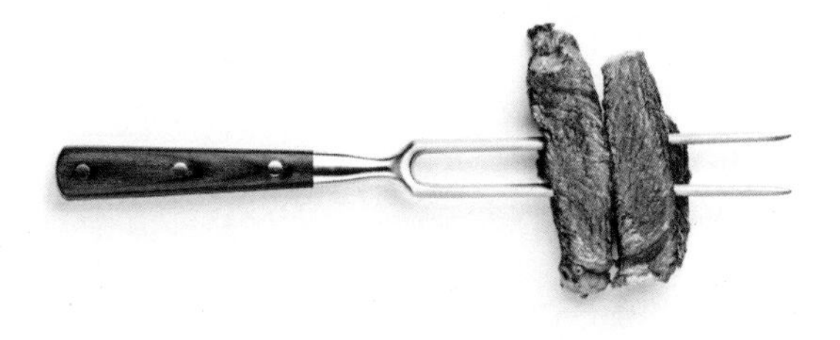

The only reason people aren't already doing these things? Lack of knowledge or awareness for most. For the rest, an unwillingness to experience the transient discomforts that come along with high-intensity exercise and eating a species-appropriate diet. But for those who are willing to expend a small amount of effort, this book will help provide the basic knowledge you will need on your path to optimum health.

In the end, health is everything. If you don't have your health, literally nothing else on earth matters. For this reason, it should be of the utmost importance to every single person to maximize their health potential. Fortunately, it is easy to achieve optimum health once you understand a few very basic principles. The object of this book is to explain these principles as simply as possible.

KNOWLEDGE IS POWER. Read on, and I wish you the best health possible.

TED NAIMAN MD 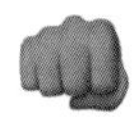

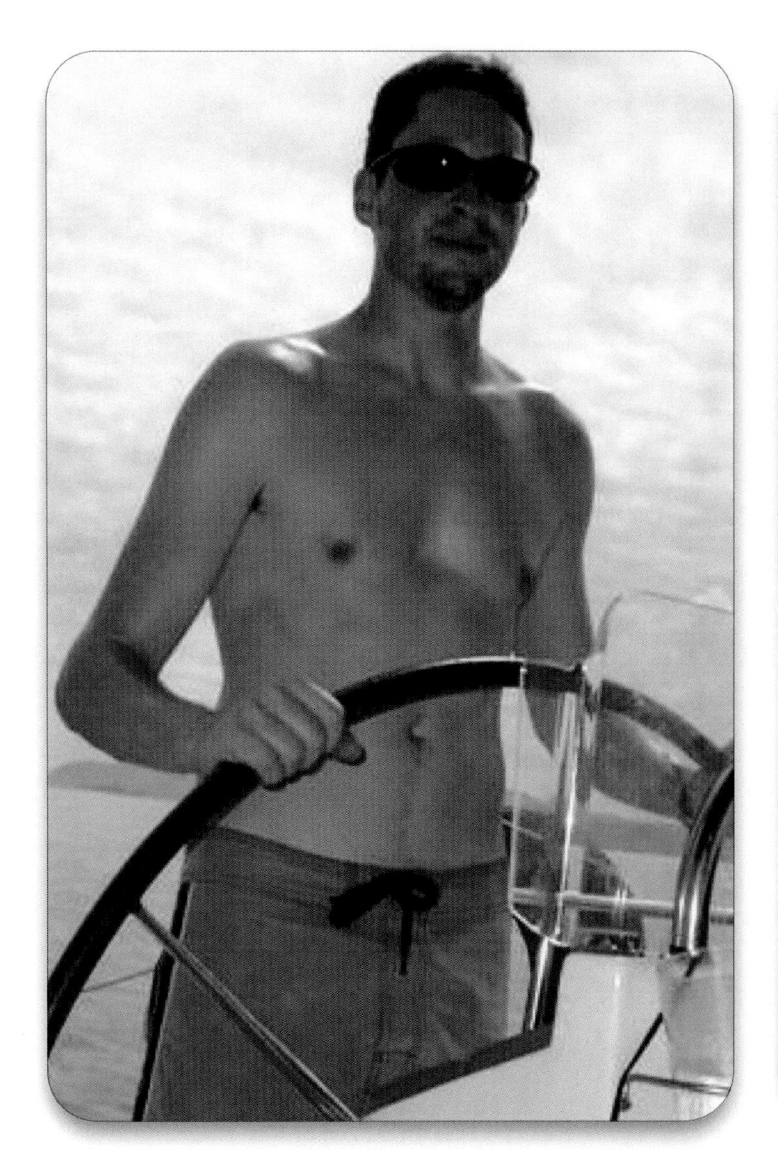
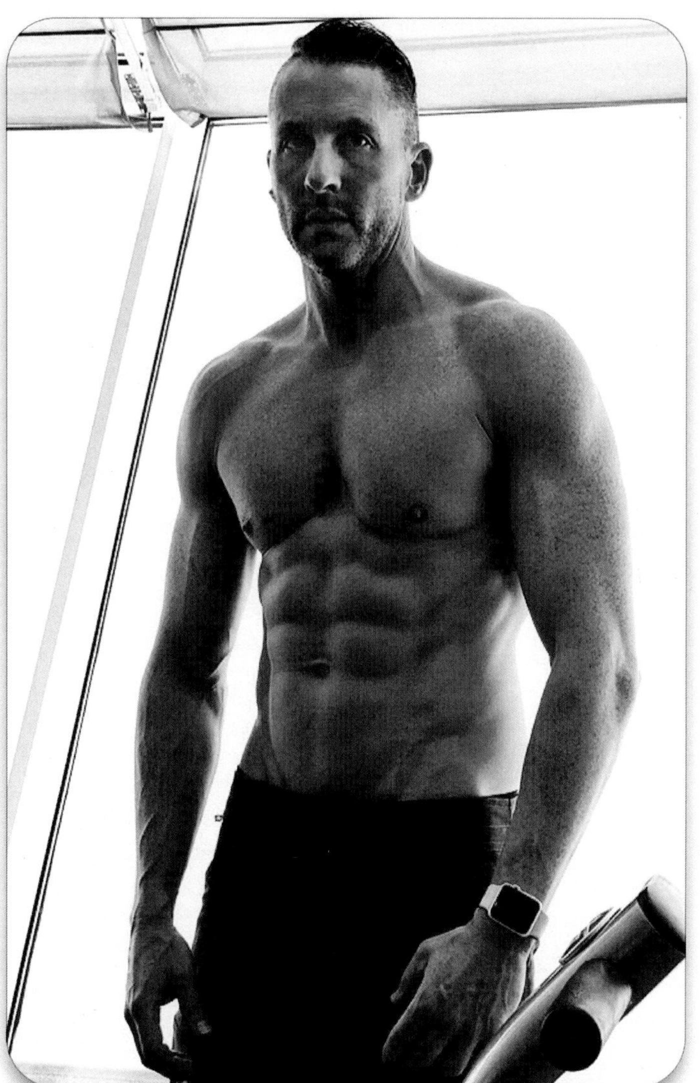

Ted Naiman, before and after using the principles of The P:E Diet.

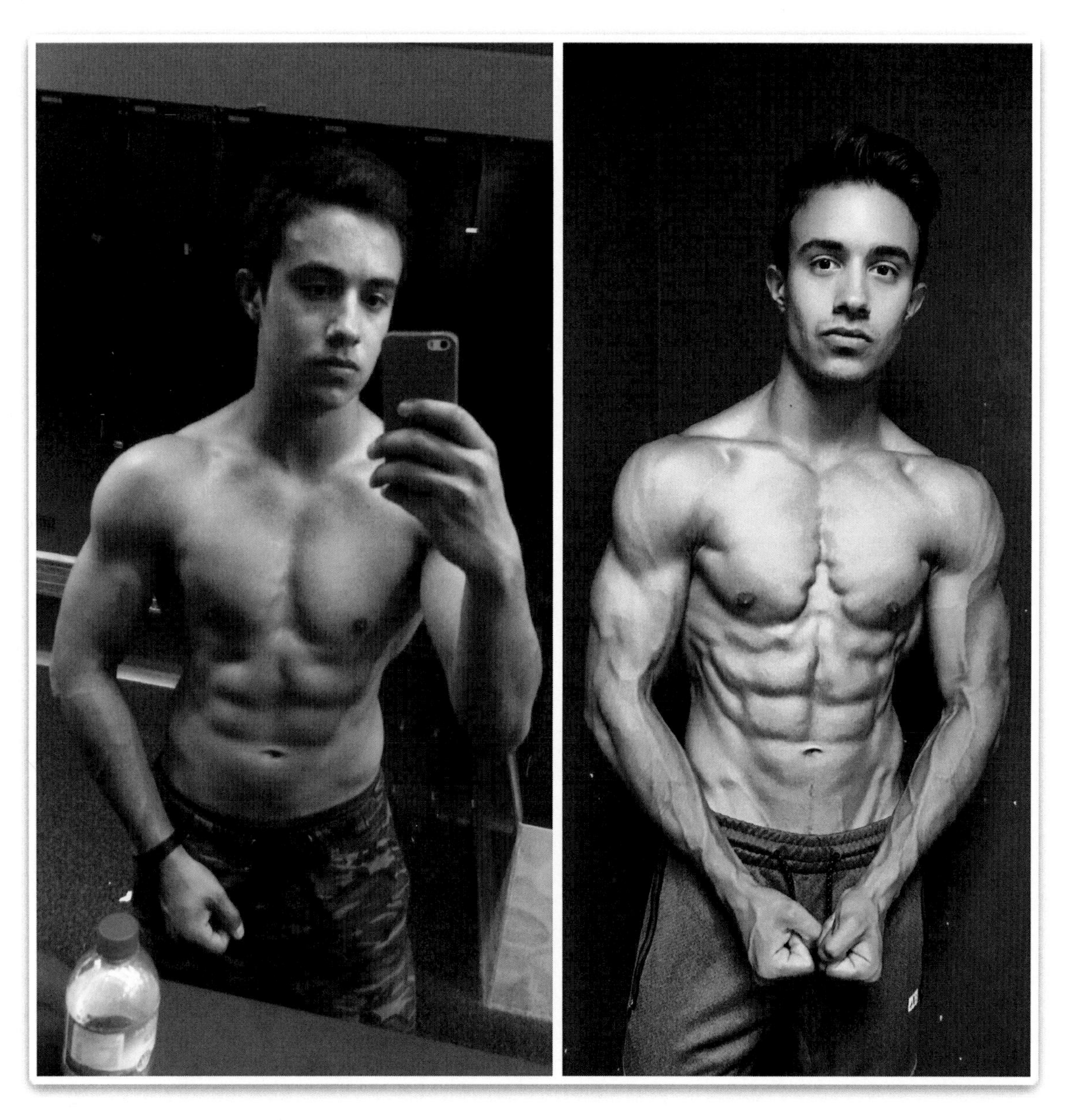

William Shewfelt, before and after using the principles of The P:E Diet.

INTRODUCTION

WE SHOULD NOT BE THIS FAT AND THIS SICK.

It happened just slowly enough that we all got used to it. Hell, now we are conditioned to expect it. Like death and taxes, or your dropped piece of toast landing butter side down. Everyone expects to slowly and inexorably gain weight their entire adult life. We just naturally assume that you will have a 'dad bod' or be 'full-figured' in your young adulthood, and a few decades and a few dozen pounds later you inevitably end up as a 'bigger' man or woman. Sure, we cover it up fairly well—with larger clothes, larger chairs, larger everything. In fact, we blend in so well with the landscape that practically nobody even knows they are morbidly obese unless their doctor highlights it at a depressingly demotivating less-than-yearly 'physical'. Yet, even if your doctor happens to point out that your BMI, or Body Mass Index, is out of range, the notification feels blasé. After all, what could you possibly do about this? Sure, there is the perfunctory "Eat less and move more", or perhaps the even more vague and impotent hand-wave of "Watch your calories". But hey, it's not like you aren't trying. This is just the way it works.

Even if you are one of the rare lucky ones who seem to stay thinner, through no apparent fault of your own (excepting some fortuitous genetics), we just wait for the chronic diseases. You are supposed to watch your grandparents slowly decline right before your eyes, accumulating frailty and dental disease and so many orthopedic problems that eventually it seems that they have nothing else to talk about. Until cognitive decline sets in. Then they start telling you the same thing they told you yesterday, every day. This is just the way it goes. Fifty percent of 80-year-olds have enough cognitive decline to be formally diagnosed with Alzheimer's disease. We know this instinctively, and we see so much memory impairment in the elderly around us that ending up in a skilled nursing facility seems inevitable.

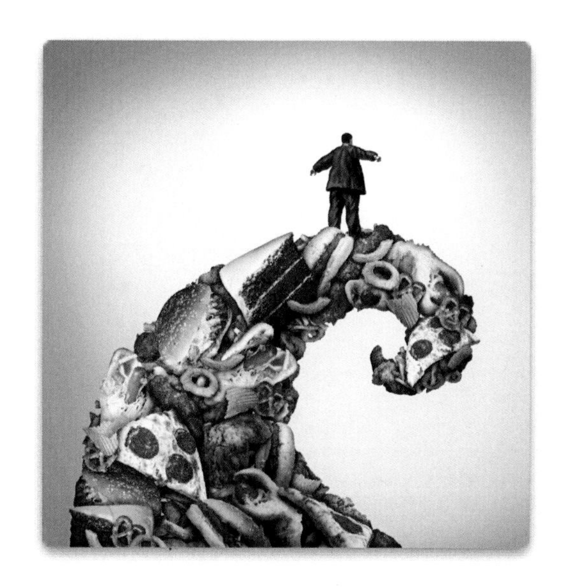

That is, if we are lucky enough to live that long, without succumbing to cardiovascular disease or, even more terrifying, cancer. Almost half of us in the modern world are eventually diagnosed with some sort of cancer, and the subsequent sensation of inevitability and randomness is pretty much identical to what you would expect from the love child of Russian Roulette meets Sword of Damocles. Every time you hear that a food causes cancer, your anxiety ratchets up one more notch, and you make a quick mental note to avoid this terrible poison. That is, until you eventually hear that pretty much everything causes cancer, once you've sifted through enough epidemiological data. After that, you just try not to think about it, which works about as well as your weight loss attempts so far.

Everyone knows someone with at least one chronic degenerative disease, maybe even having one themselves. This is just how it works. Your acid reflux is bad, but hey that is just what you should expect when you get older, right? We have pills for that. And thankfully your sleep apnea has a treatment, or at least that's what they told you when they gave you that disconcertingly unsexy breathing contraption. Of course your knees should hurt at your age—after all, when was the last time you saw any old person running anywhere? Yeah, that's what we thought. We are usually impressed if they can slowly get up out of a chair without using both arms like a drowning victim, or walk across the room without shuffling, hunched over a walker, like some sort of extra in that bad zombie apocalypse movie you saw one late night on SciFi.

We expect to slowly get fatter, then sicker, then physically weaker, until we eventually succumb to cognitive decline and a nursing home—that is, if a massive heart attack, crippling stroke, or terrifying incurable cancer doesn't take us first. We watch this happen all around us every day, and we just wait for it, like a frog in tepid water placed on the boil.

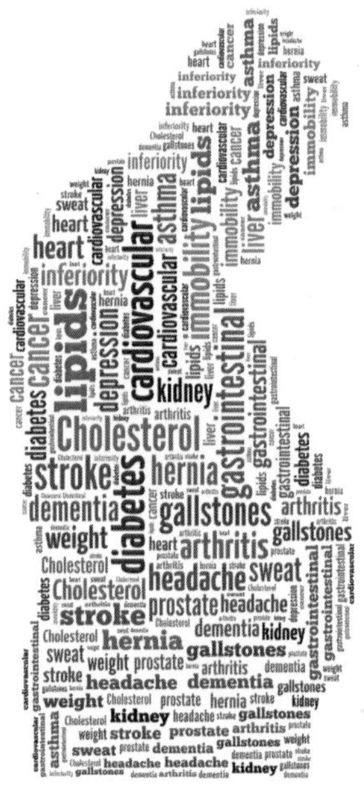

An elite few seem to have somehow transcended all of this. We see them on TV or movies, or maybe, vanishingly rare, we know someone like this in real life. You see their toned, muscular physique, and you can almost feel an aura of health, as if it was exuding from their pores. Just watching them walk around feels like viewing an entirely different species at the zoo. Even at ease, they are standing impossibly straight and tall, shoulder blades firmly retracted, with so much tension in their spinal erectors that they perpetually look ready to lift an absurdly heavy object with no more effort than you might expend lifting a large bag of cool ranch Doritos. Comparing their bodies—with six-pack abs carved from solid granite—to your own decidedly fluffier corporeal vessel would be painful indeed without the usual coping strategies. "I wish I had that much time to work out", you bitterly tell yourself. Of course these people spend almost all day in the gym, with short breaks to eat small, perfectly formulated gourmet meals six times a day, crafted by the sort of personal chef that only extravagant wealth can afford. Oh, and don't forget the large-animal-veterinary-sized injection of testosterone daily, right? Yeah, if you were as genetically and financially lucky as these privileged people, you would look pretty good too. Or so you tell yourself, and this does make you feel 1% better, just long enough to stop thinking about it.

Nobody can say you aren't trying. In fact, losing weight and getting healthy have topped your priority list for as long as you can remember. You start the day out right with a light smoothie, so far so good. A few hours later, you fight off the hunger with a healthy snack or two, maybe some fruit and nuts—what could be healthier than that? Lunch is a salad with light dressing or a sandwich on whole wheat—hold the mayo—and you always opt for the baked chips instead of fried. When afternoon hunger strikes, you are ready with some healthy granola bars and trail mix. Dinner of pasta or rice, with a perfectly palm-sized serving of protein, usually chicken or fish because, hey, you are trying to be as healthy as possible. You are always mindful of quantity, and your meager portion does sort of look larger on those extra small dinner plates you bought recently. On paper, your whole day of eating seems perfect, except for this lingering hunger at the end of the day that inevitably leads to you standing in your pantry at 9:00 p.m. with an empty box of wheat thins, hunger pangs replaced with pangs of guilt. But hey, at least they were cholesterol-free and had plenty of whole grains, right? It's not like you are binging on cake and candy over here.

You bust your ass at the gym as well, staying on that treadmill for an entire hour no matter what. The dozens of TVs on the walls make this somewhat bearable. Sometimes you take a class, jumping around to the dance version of a pop song sped up to approximately the same beats per minute as your heart rate—hoping you don't look like you are flailing quite as much as you suspect. The logistics of getting back and forth to the gym turn exercise into a massive time burden, and what starts out as a daily regimen slowly erodes into a couple of times a week. But that's ok, because you still have your fitness tracker, and you have been hitting 10,000 steps a day all over the place. A standing desk, taking the stairs, these are all built into your routine.

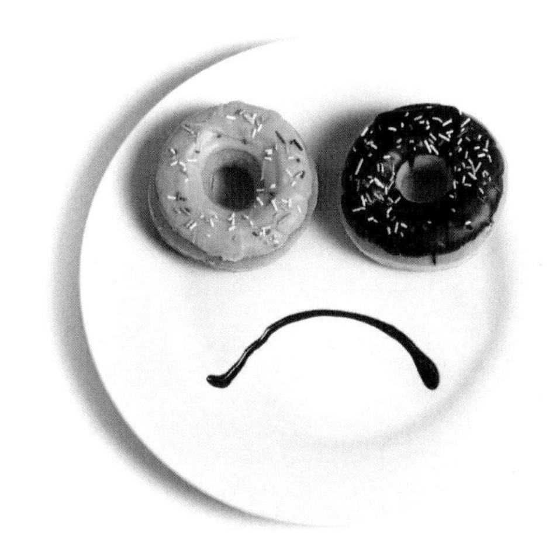

And yet, you can feel yourself getting fatter. What started out as a corner of your closet dedicated to the clothes that you would someday shed enough pounds to fit back into has now engulfed half of your wardrobe. Looking in a full-length mirror just lowers your self-esteem even further, and you haven't stepped on the scale for months because deep inside you are more than a little afraid to see what will almost certainly be the highest number you have ever seen there before. You take some solace in those around you who are struggling even more than you are. They aren't hard to find—try the grocery store or the food court at the mall, or now that we think about it, almost any public place. Seeing someone larger than yourself is a daily occurrence, and one that gives you a momentary feeling of relief, with a side order of pity. At least you aren't THAT bad. Those people should probably be trying harder.

YOU are the reason we wrote this book. That's right. You have the drive to make it happen. You really want it, and you can do what it takes. In fact, the only thing you are missing is a laser focused direction for your efforts. If you took all of your existing time and energy and dedication and melded it into a tight purposeful beam of pure intensity at exactly the right angle, you would slice through the obesity epidemic like a hot nanowire through butter. The goal of this book is to forge down all of your existing resources into the deadly fine-tipped spear that will pierce the soft underbelly of obesity and chronic disease once and for all, allowing you to break free and achieve the complete mastery of your body composition that you have always wanted.

The strategies we will present here are so damn simple and common-sense that you will be asking yourself why you didn't think of them yourself and write your own book about it. But as a necessary part of the process, you have to understand exactly why and how these strategies work. And that is going to require a pretty good-sized chunk of knowledge. And to get there, we are going to have to alternate between focusing in on some sub-micron minutiae of human physiology and zooming way way back out again to look at the entire landscape from the 50,000 foot level. But if you hang in there, you should take away from this book some extremely powerful weaponry in the war to achieve and maintain perfect body composition and health. And, almost as importantly, you will understand why it works.

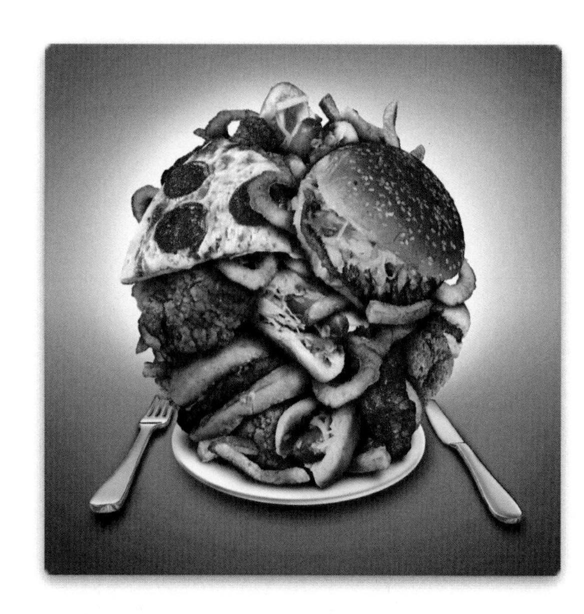

Strap in and read on.

Nutrition has often been the subject of conjectures and ingenious hypotheses—but our actual knowledge is so insufficient that their only use is to try to satisfy our imagination. If we could arrive at some more exact facts they could well have applications in medicine.

—François Magendie (1783–1855)

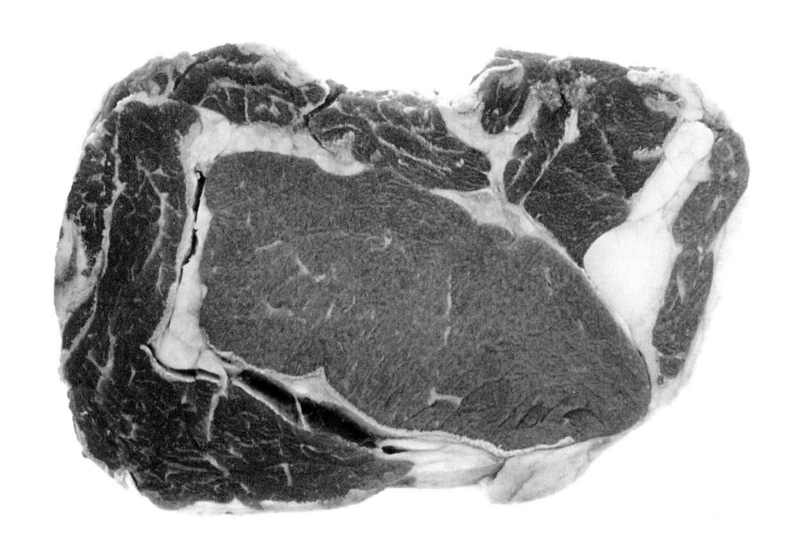

SIMPLE AND PRACTICAL

This book is designed to be as simple and practical as possible. No, it is not designed to be some sort of unabridged encyclopedia that deals with 100% of all edge cases for everyone on earth. Instead, this is going to provide the majority of diet and exercise information necessary for the majority of people. We are intentionally skipping the references and minutiae and instead providing the basic concepts you need to know in order to implement the best diet and exercise plan for yourself. Everyone is different and there will be plenty of individual customization, but the basic template is more or less the same for everyone. Our goal is to provide a book that absolutely anyone can pick up, read in an hour, and walk away with a double-barreled blast of extremely easy to comprehend yet life-changing and actionable knowledge.

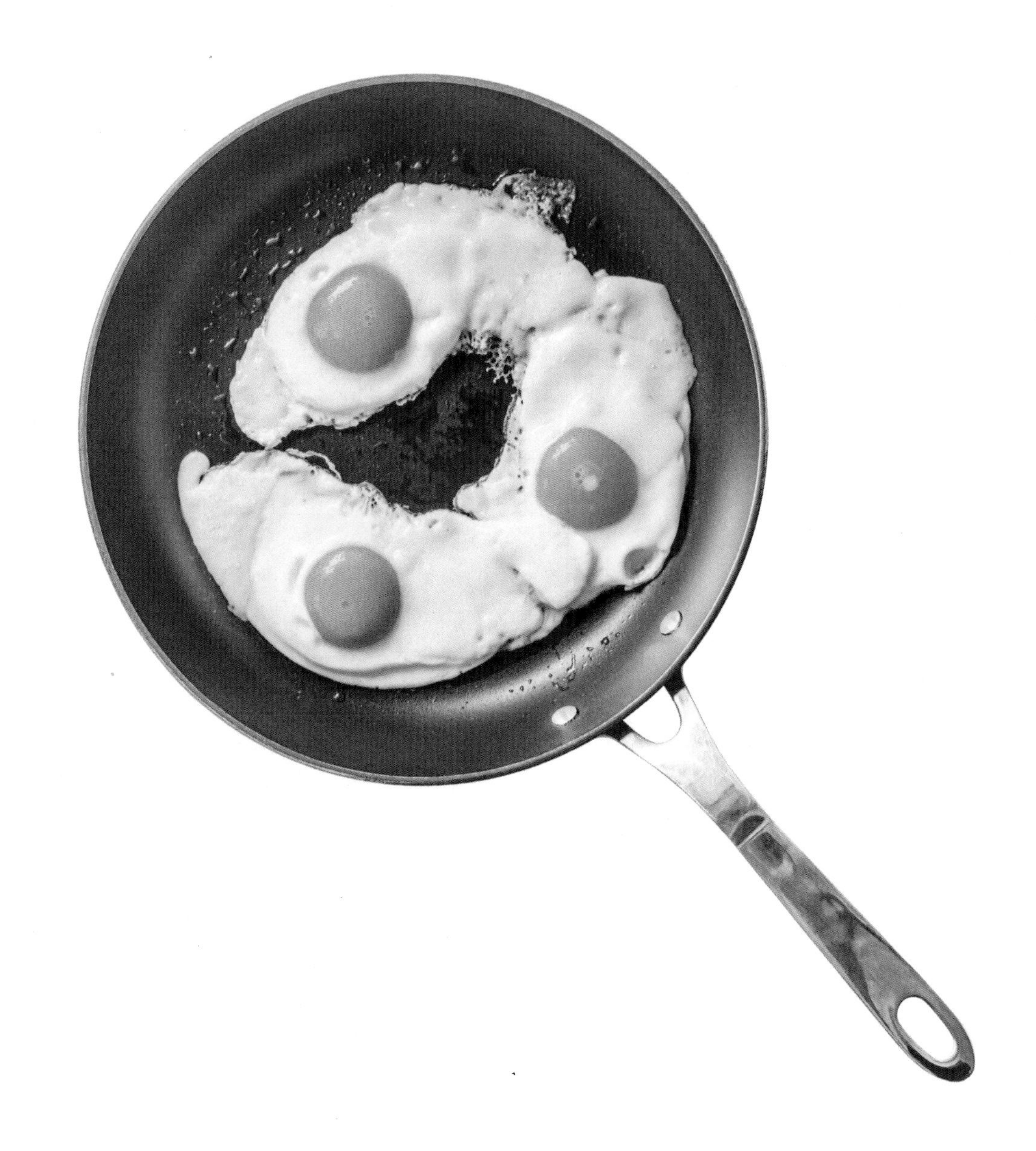

PARETO PRINCIPLE ("80/20% RULE")

Also known as the '80/20' principle. 20% of knowledge will get you 80% of what you are looking for. 20% of effort will give you 80% of your results. Think of this book, and the things recommended in this book, as the 20% of knowledge you need to get 80% of health improvements. The diet and exercise principles outlined here will require 20% of the effort it will take to get 80% of your desired results. This kind of efficiency is really what this entire book is based upon, and you will see this approach over and over here.

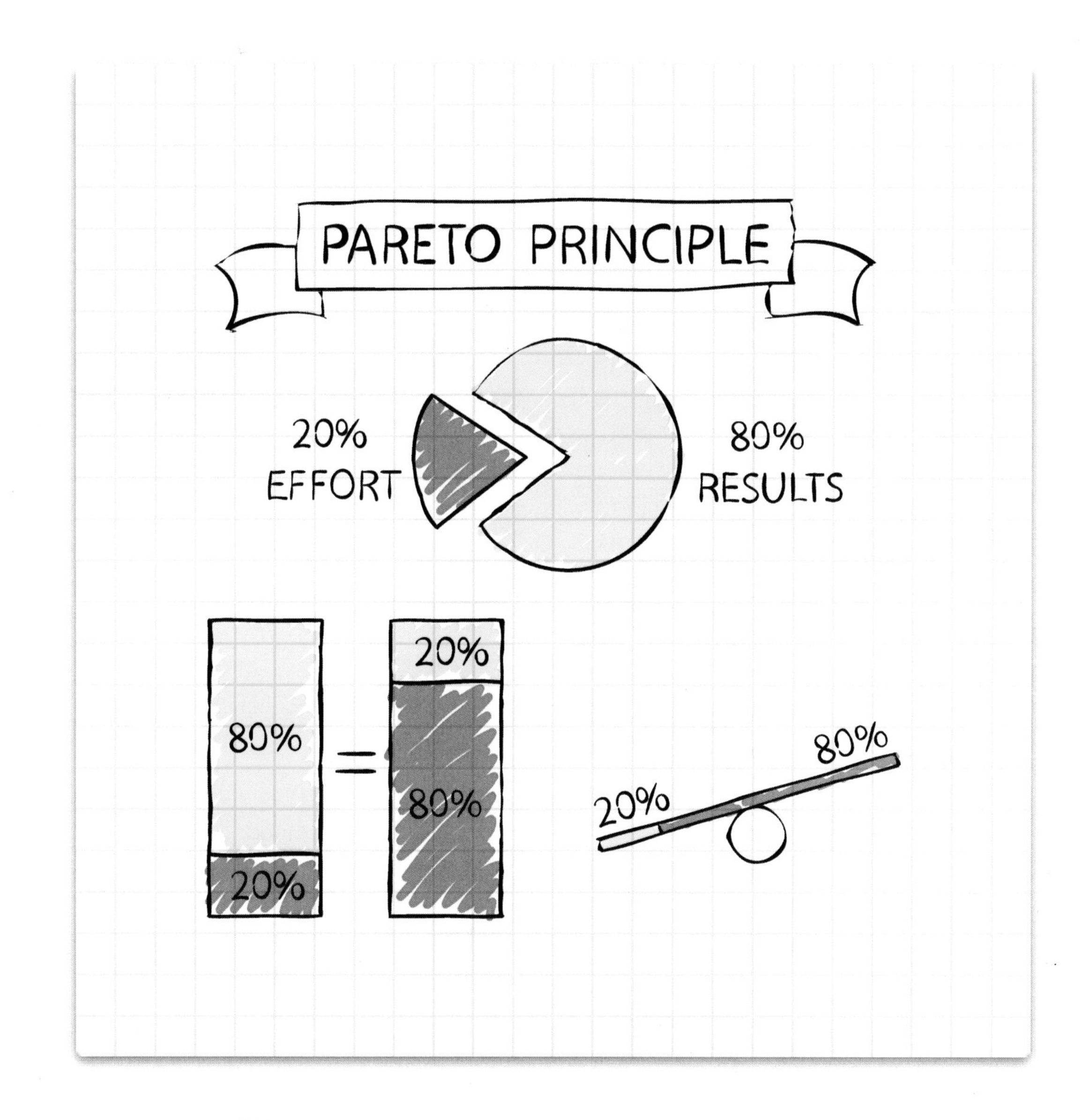

PROGRESSION PRINCIPLE

Progression is a crucial concept. It is probably easiest for people to understand the principle of progression when it comes to resistance exercise. In order to progress, you have to constantly and continually increase the challenge to your muscles. We will explore exactly how and why you do this later in this book. The idea of progression when it comes to diet is probably more difficult to grasp, but the Protein to Energy ratio concept introduced in this book will give you an easy framework for incrementally improving your existing diet. Optimizing diet and exercise is a life-long marathon, not a sprint. The idea here is to steadily improve yourself, little by little, in a gradual and progressive fashion. This is not a crash diet or a short-term fix. Instead, the idea is to slowly and continually improve, using small and sustainable changes as you incrementally maneuver towards your goal.

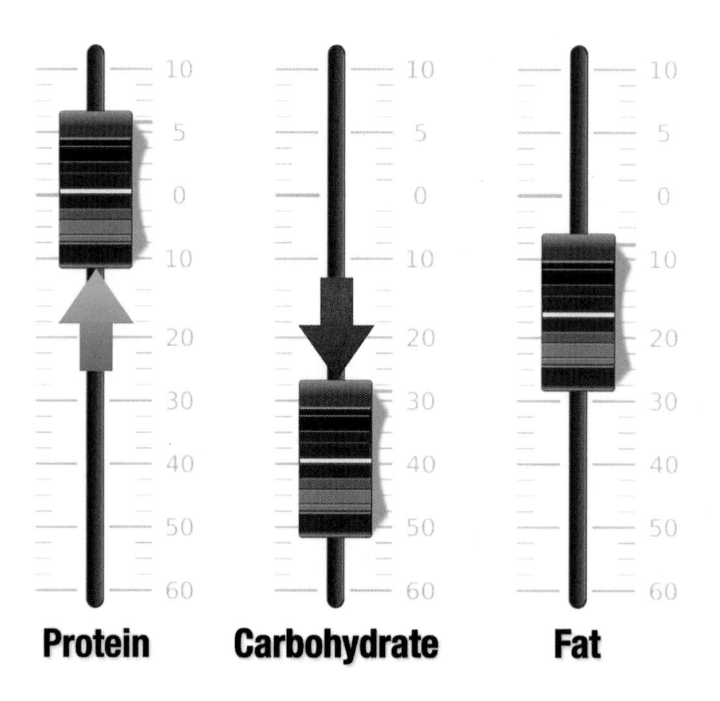

We don't like any diet or exercise program with a 'stop' date. There will be no '30 day cleanse' here. No ten day 'boot camp'. The very most important thing is SUSTAINABILITY. You want to aim towards eating and exercising now the way you are going to eat and exercise forever. And that is going to take a slow series of small incremental positive changes—PROGRESSION—to both your diet and your exercise.

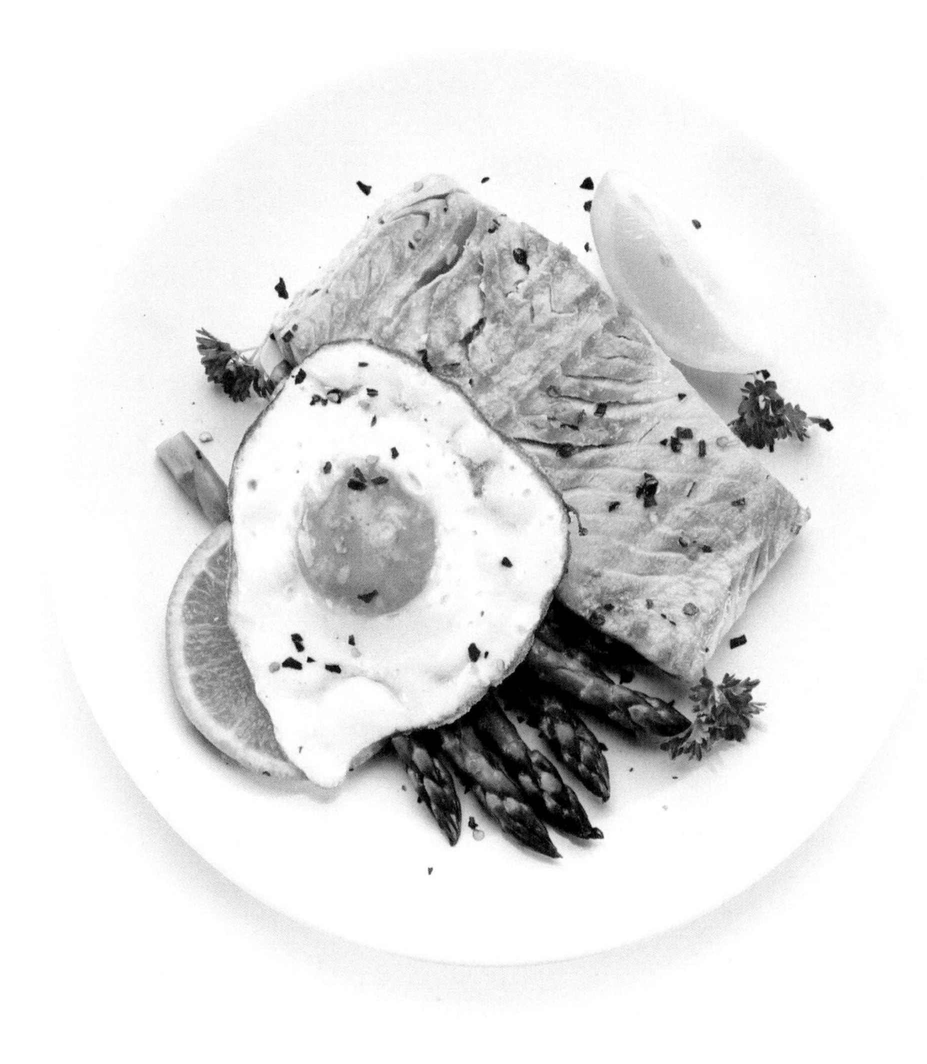

S.A.I.D. PRINCIPLE

Specific Adaptation to Imposed Demand. We will be utilizing the S.A.I.D. Principle throughout this book. Want to get better at burning fat instead of glucose? Eat fewer carbs, and your body will have to adapt to this demand. Want to add muscle? You have to communicate to your body that it has no choice but to add muscle—adapt or die. Humans are amazingly adaptable and we can live in any environment, on any sort of diet. Take advantage of this adaptability—this is how we improve our physical health. This usually involves some level of discomfort, so get used to pushing yourself way out of your comfort zone. Trust us, the transient discomforts you experience when you implement these changes is nothing compared to the lifelong suffering from the chronic diseases you will avoid.

SPECIFIC ADAPTATION TO IMPOSED DEMAND

Adaptability. Humans are amazing survival machines, which is why we live in all climates, eating all diets. Your body will always adapt to meet the demands you impose upon it.

If you want your body to be better at burning fat, you only have to do one thing:

Eat fewer carbohydrates.

If you want your body to be better at burning its own stored body fat, you only have to do two things:

Eat fewer carbohydrates, and then eat less fat.

THE THREE PILLARS OF THE P:E DIET APPROACH

There are three basic strategies for dietary improvement that underlie all of the advice in the diet section of this book. In the following chapters, we will explore all of these in depth, but we want to call attention to these at the very beginning, so you can see where we are headed.

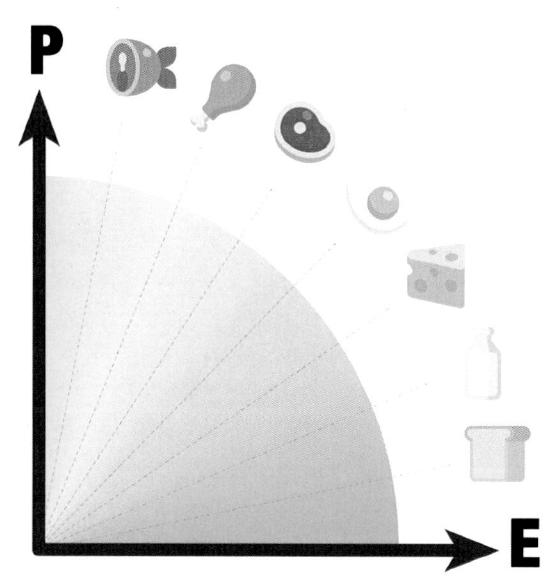

1. Increase protein percentage.

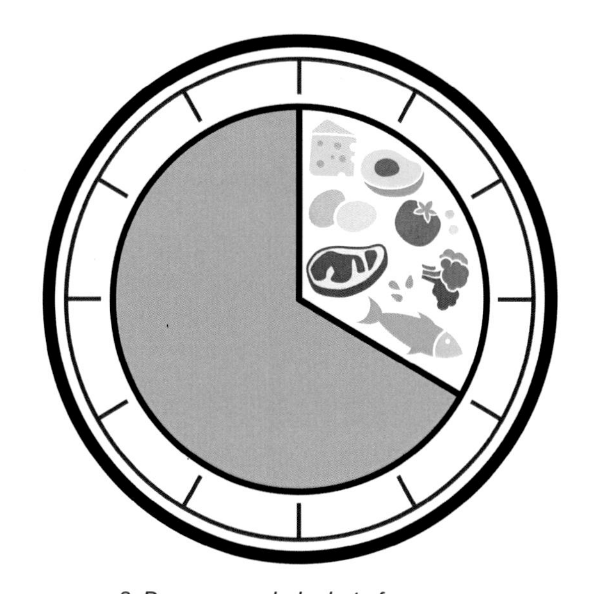

2. Decrease carbohydrate frequency.

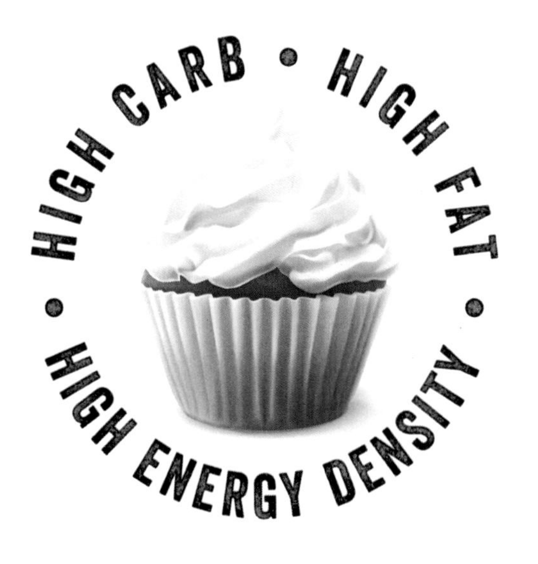

3. Avoid high carb + high fat.

1. INCREASE PROTEIN PERCENTAGE.

As you will learn in the near future, HOW MUCH you eat is completely dependent on WHAT you eat. By focusing on food choice and food selection, and intentionally eating higher protein foods, you will automatically tend to eat less.

It is ok if you don't know what we mean by this because we will be exploring all of this in depth in just a few minutes! But we want to establish this concept first so you have it in mind going forward.

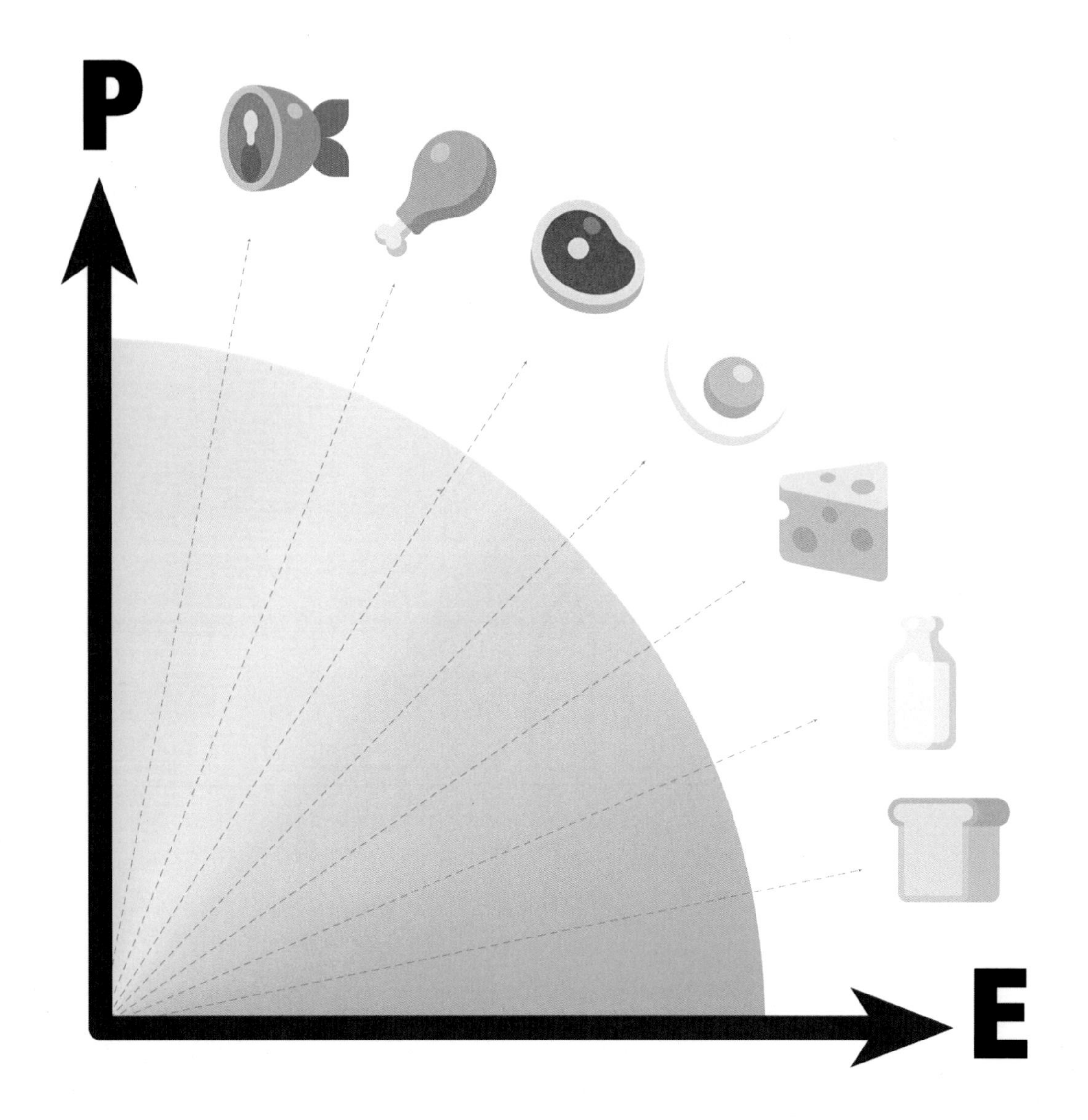

2. DECREASE CARBOHYDRATE FREQUENCY.

Reducing the frequency with which you eat carbohydrates forces your body to become more "fat adapted", or able to function using only stored body fat, without a constant influx of dietary carbohydrates. The fact that this is initially quite difficult further underscores the reality that this is a form of METABOLIC EXERCISE, almost like weight lifting for your metabolism. If you strengthen this, you will reap the rewards of being much less tied to frequent eating. The stability of blood sugar and mood, as well as the ability to live your life without being a slave to mealtimes and snack times, is well worth the transient discomfort of the fat adaptation process. We will cover all of this in depth just ahead!

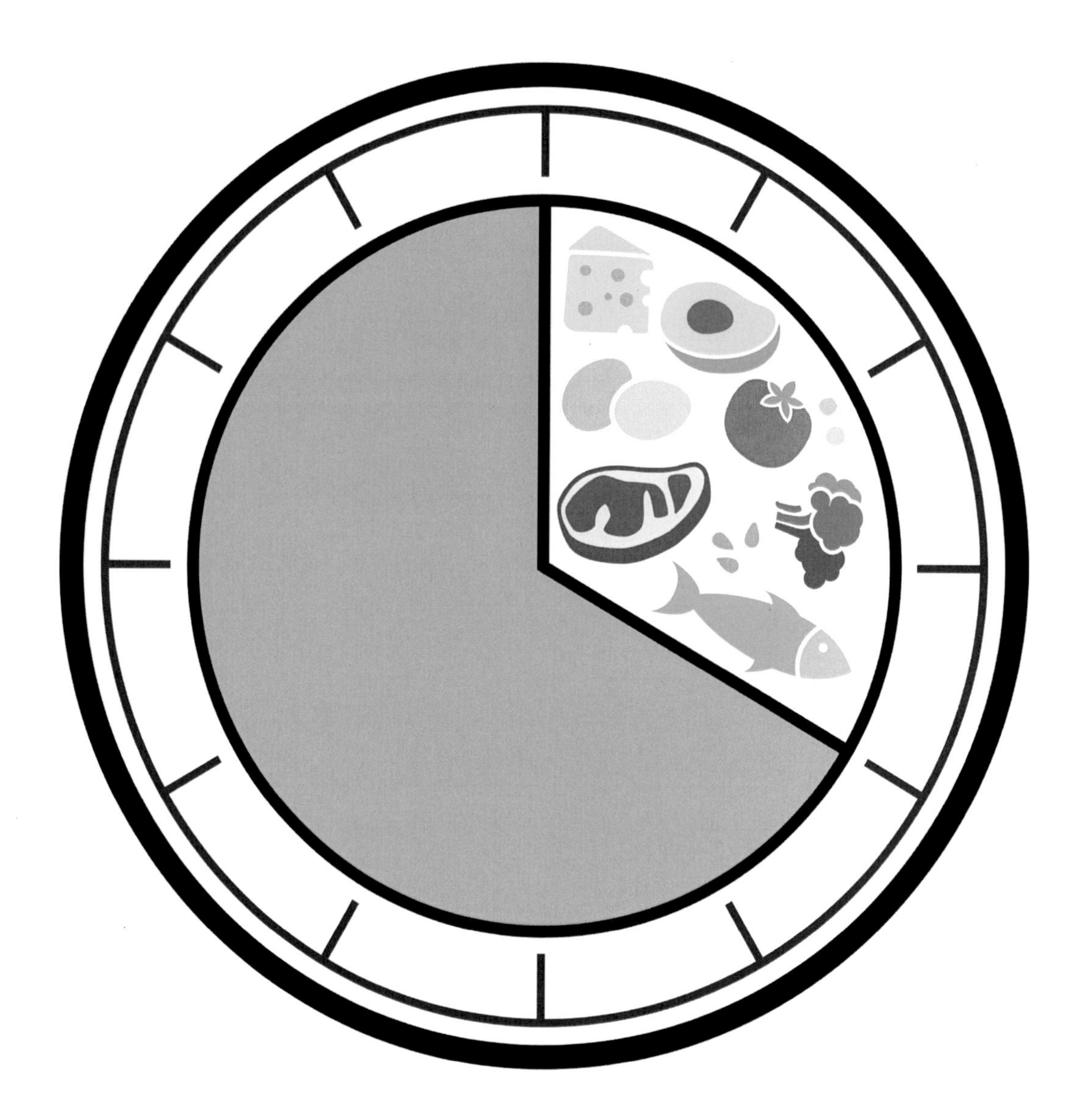

3. AVOID HIGH CARB + HIGH FAT.

Foods that are simultaneously high in carbohydrates and fat, with a high energy density, are rarely found in nature and they are highly palatable and addictive. These foods completely hijack our satiety and mercilessly drive overeating. We will explore how this works and go in depth on which foods to minimize and why! Read on.

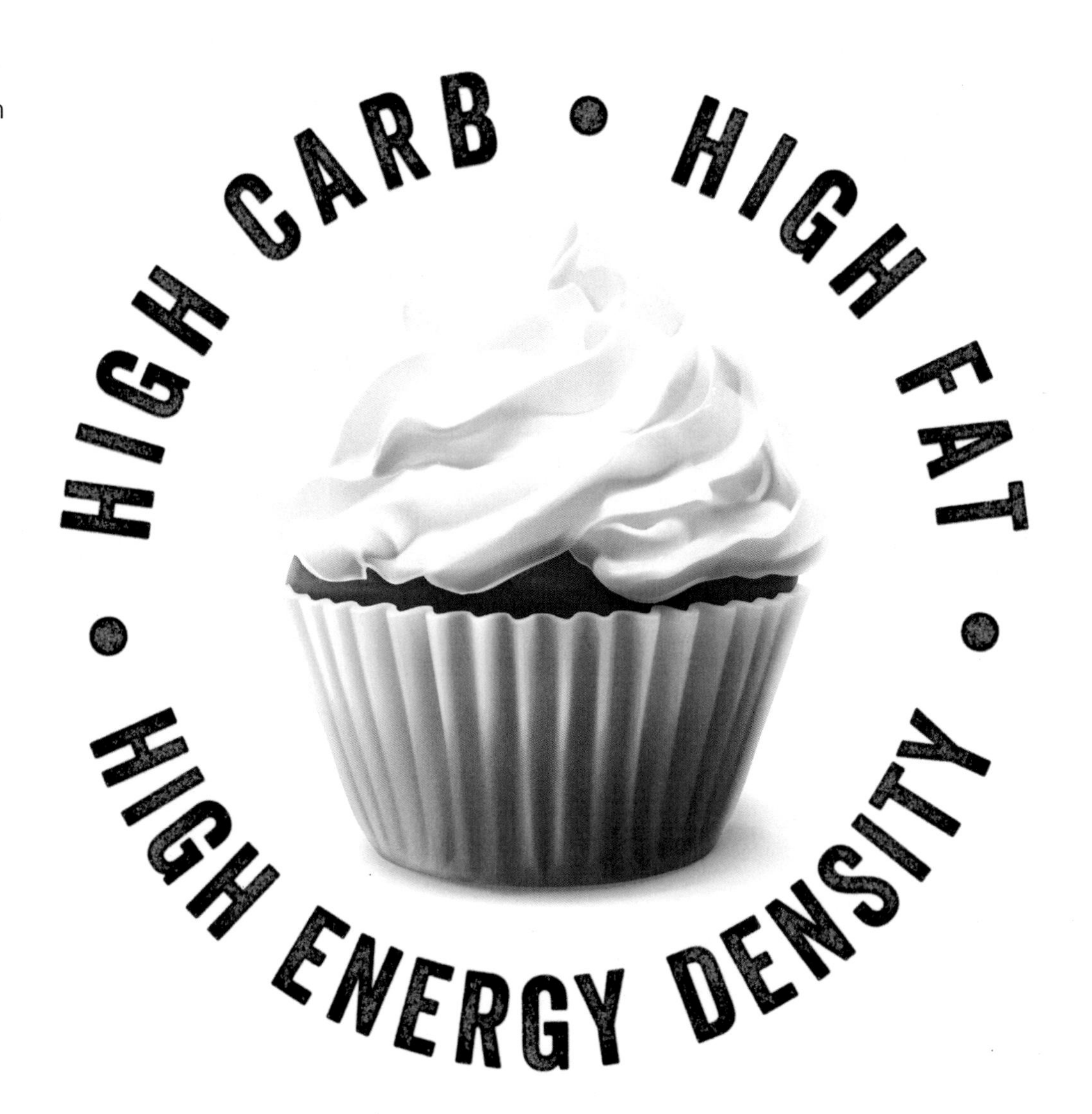

THIS ENTIRE BOOK ON ONE SHEET OF PAPER:

Plants store solar energy as the high energy carbon bonds in carbs and fats.

Plants absorb nitrogen for protein, as well as other minerals, from soil.

Animals have to ingest other living organisms in order to receive both this chemical energy and these proteins and minerals.

Problems arise when we extract pure energy from plants; this is most egregious in the form of refined carbs and fats such as sugar, flour, and oil.

First of all, this energy is now cheap and profitable. This dilutes protein and minerals throughout the human food supply, leading to a protein and mineral nutrient hunger—we literally HAVE to eat more energy just to satisfy our nutrient needs.

Second, we really enjoy eating pure concentrated fat and carb energy, because doing so produces a drug-like reward in our brains—this kept us alive back when energy was scarce. High energy density carbs and fats together, a combination rarely found in nature, produces the greatest brain reward of all and can be quite addictive—so we WANT to eat more.

As a result of all of this, we now have a global epidemic of energy toxicity. Almost 90% of us have ingested too much energy and we are no longer metabolically healthy. This puts us at risk for obesity and chronic disease.

You can combat energy toxicity by going out of your way to target protein and minerals, allowing yourself to reach nutrient satiety at a lower energy intake. You can also use caution with the highly addictive trifecta of foods that are high carb, high fat, and high energy density all at the same time. In addition, a lowered carbohydrate frequency can improve fat adaptation, allowing you to function properly in lower energy food environments.

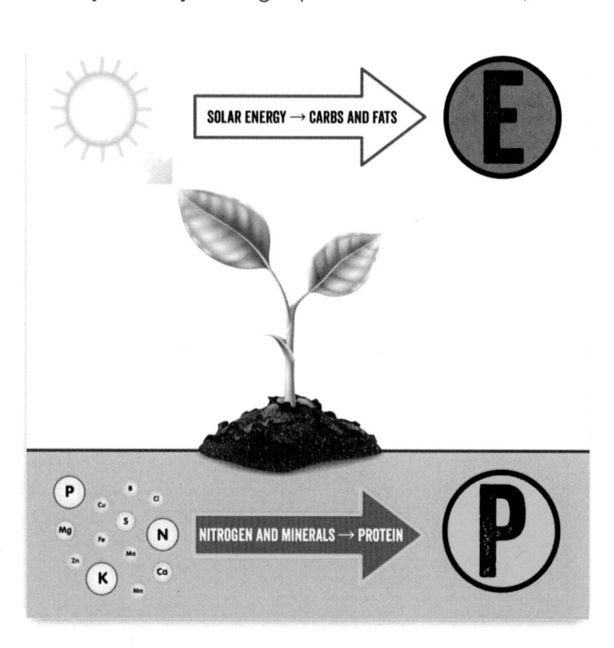

Finally, for optimum healthspan, your goal should be achieving the highest lean mass (muscle and bone) at the lowest fat mass—this allows for the greatest insulin sensitivity and metabolic flexibility. However you will only maximize lean mass if you DEMAND it of your body—by placing the highest amount of tension in your muscles possible, for the longest amount of time possible. Luckily this can be accomplished with only three basic human movements: pushing, pulling, and using the legs against gravity. By targeting these three movements in a specific fashion on a regular basis, and by placing maximum tension in the involved muscles for a maximum amount of time, you can achieve optimum lean mass in the most efficient manner possible.

THE P:E DIET

PROTEIN VERSUS ENERGY

The title of this book, **The P:E Diet**, refers to the amount of protein in your diet versus the amount of non-protein energy: carbs and fat. We know this is a foreign concept to almost everyone on the planet, so we will start out with some background on what the heck we are talking about here!

Time to introduce you to the dietary concept of Protein versus Non-Protein Energy. In order to set the stage, we are going to have to zoom out a little and start at the very beginning. We are going to assume that most everyone is at least a little familiar with the three basic macronutrients: protein, fat, and carbohydrates. But if you aren't totally familiar, don't worry—you will get up to speed pretty fast.

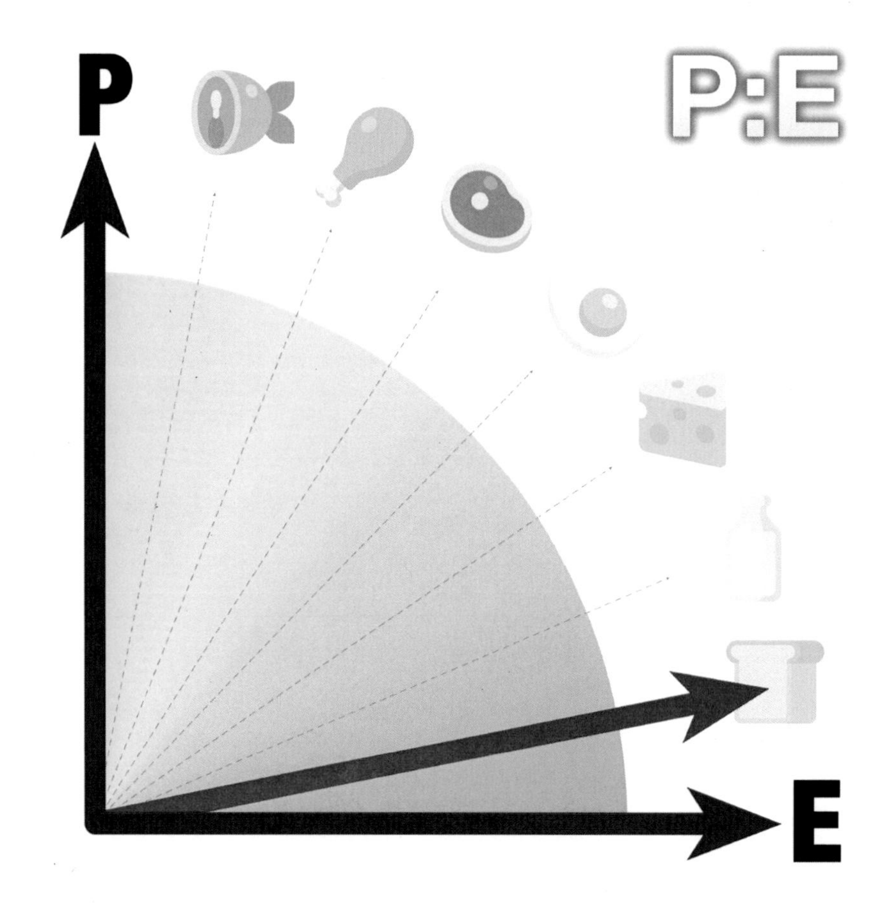

WHAT IS EATING?

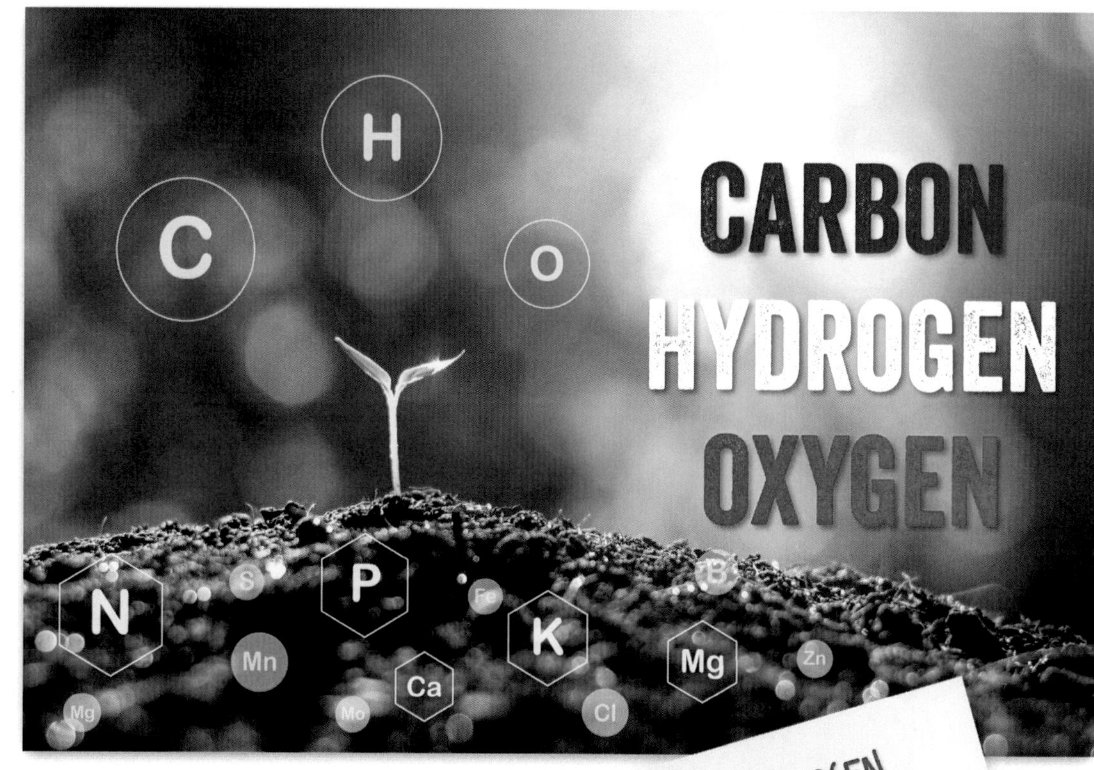

Let's start as basic as it gets. Plants are 'autotrophs'. That means they make their own food. They use carbon, hydrogen, and oxygen, the three major elements of all life on earth (from air and water), plus the energy from sunlight, to make all of the food they need. They get nitrogen, required for protein—along with a few dozen other necessary elements—from the soil (in mineral form).

Animals, on the other hand, are 'heterotrophs'. That means that all animals on earth are only alive because they constantly eat other living organisms. Humans, of course, are animals—like all animals, we are also only alive because we eat other living things. This is just the way the system works, and if you were hoping to get by without constantly killing other living organisms to survive, well then we would suggest looking into Breatharianism (Google it). We didn't create the system, so don't blame us!

Because they can make food, plants are at the base of all animal nutrition on earth. Make no mistake—they don't want to be. Plants want to live as much as any of us, and in fact they have a host of complicated chemical defense systems to avoid being eaten. But herbivores are essentially predators of plants, and carnivores are predators of herbivores. Plants just so happen to be

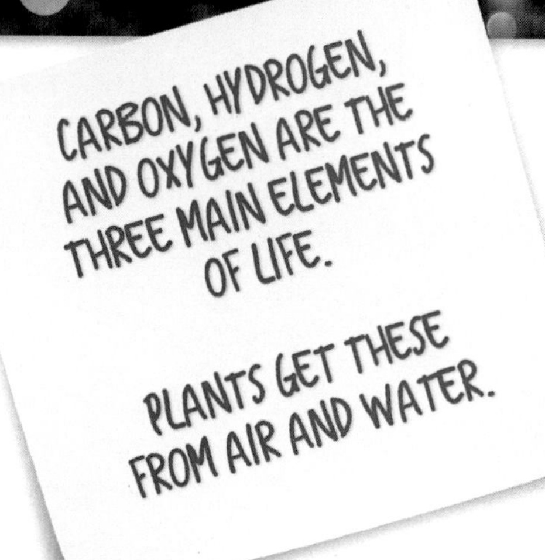

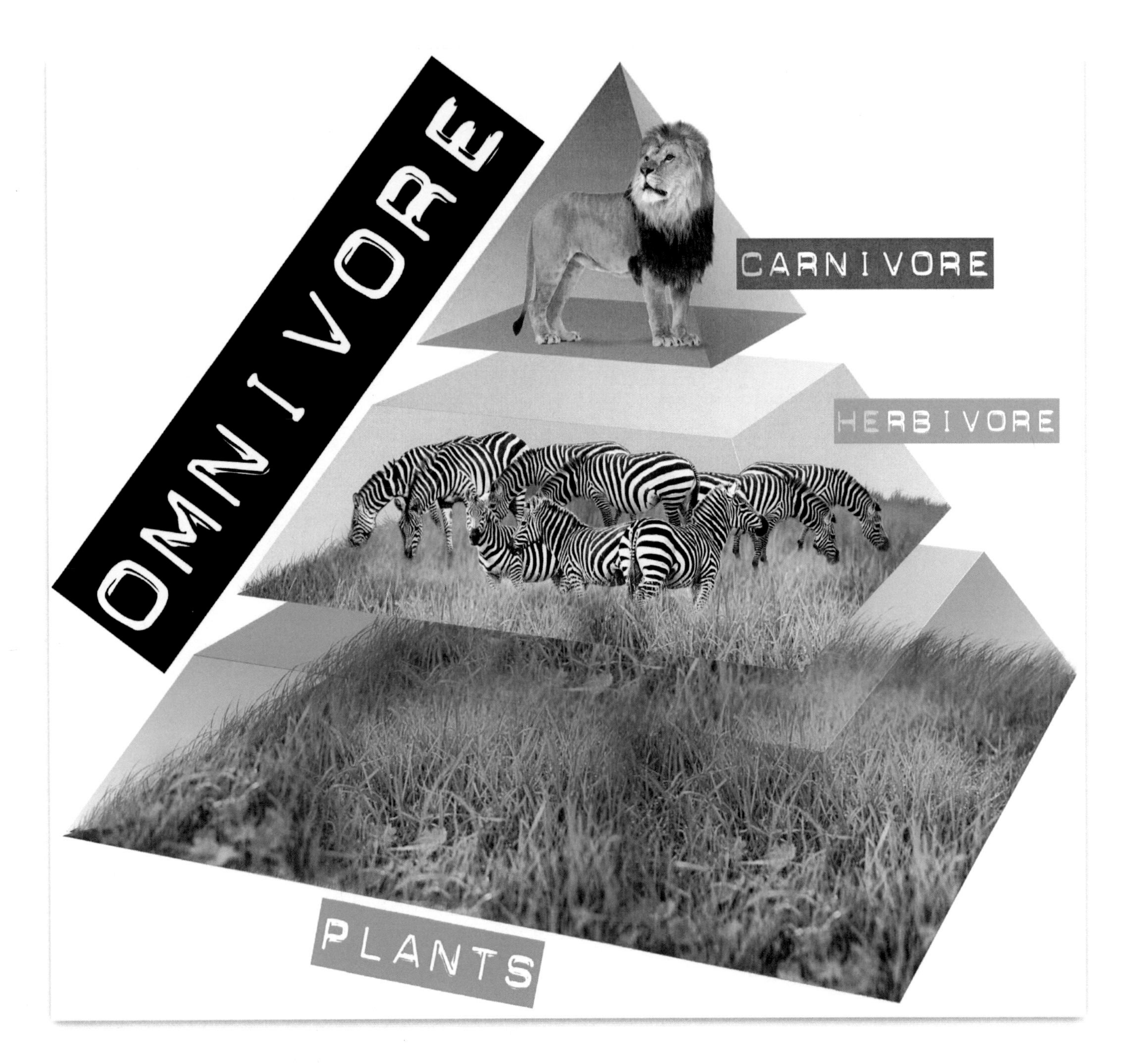

at the bottom rung of the ladder.

Animals are divided into herbivores (eating plants), carnivores (eating animals), and omnivores (eating everything). The reality is that all animals are omnivores if they are hungry enough —they just have a preference for one thing or the other. All carnivores will eventually eat some plant matter and all herbivores will eventually eat some animal matter—they just have a stronger preference for one or the other. This is in contrast to a true omnivore, like a human, who will happily eat plants AND animals. In all scenarios, plants are at the base of the food pyramid, and all animals are eating other living things to survive.

Plants store energy. They use carbon—from the carbon dioxide in air—to store solar energy as high-energy bonds between carbon molecules. These chains of carbons, with high-energy carbon-carbon (and carbon-hydrogen) bonds, are either CARBOHYDRATES or HYDROCARBONS (also known as fats). Carbohydrates would include things like glucose, and they are water-soluble (dissolves in water). Hydrocarbons are really just fats, and fats are NOT water-soluble (sort of how oil and water don't mix).

Anything on earth that is capable of 'burning' is, at some very basic level, either a carbohydrate or a hydrocarbon, which has been created by a plant. 'Burning' is just another term for oxidation

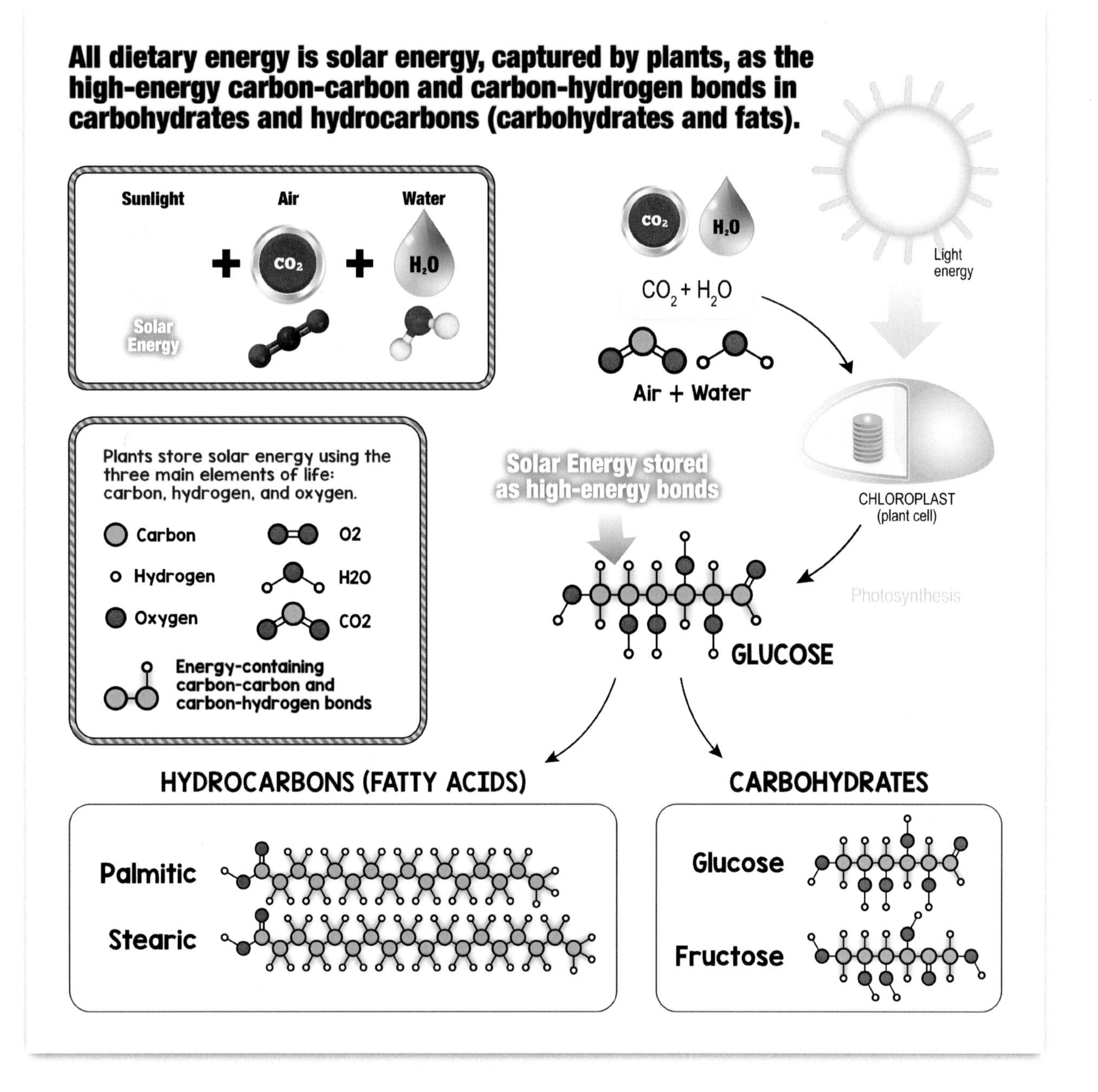

—you add oxygen to any carbohydrate or hydrocarbon and you release energy from the carbon-carbon bonds, and the byproducts are carbon dioxide and water. So all dietary energy on earth is either a carbohydrate or a fat that contains chains of carbons with high-energy bonds, made by plants, using sunlight plus air and water (for the carbons and hydrogens). And all animals break apart these bonds in our mitochondria—the little energy power plants in all your cells—using oxygen to 'oxidize' or 'burn' the carbs and fats to release energy (plus leftover carbon dioxide and water). You eat carbs and fats, then break apart the carbon-carbon bonds in your mitochondria (using oxygen that you breathe in)—this gives you energy, plus the leftover carbon dioxide and water (which you exhale).

So this is what carbs and fats actually are. Carbon-carbon

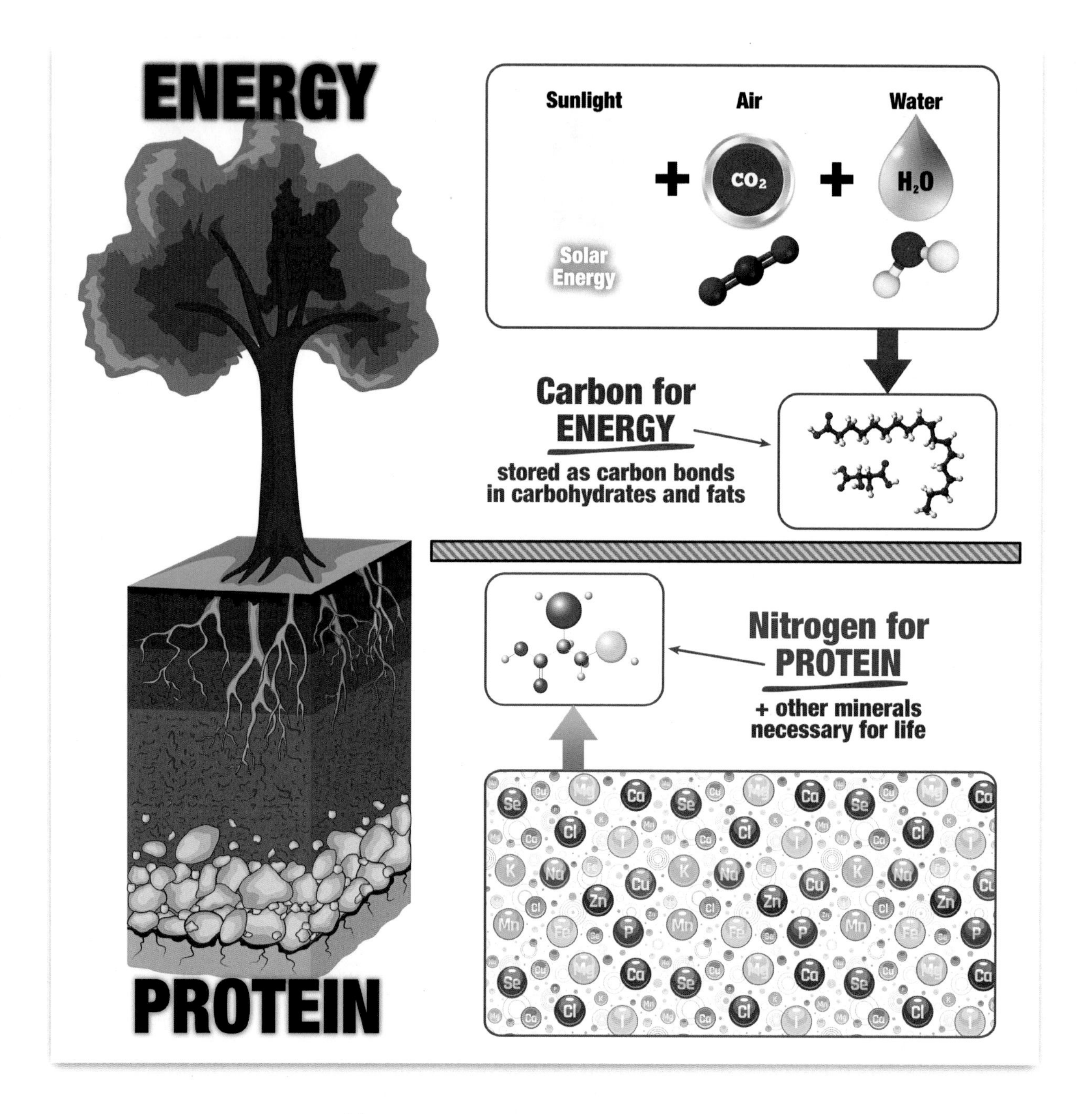

energy bonds, created by plants as a way to store solar energy. We 'burn' these in our cells to run our entire bodies, 100% of the time. All animal life on earth is constantly burning carbs and fats created by plants.

But it takes more than just energy to build an animal—you need a ton of protein, plus some minerals. Once again, plants provide the building blocks for all of these. But this time, plants are getting nitrogen—essential for all amino acids, the building blocks of protein—from soil. Plants absorb nitrogen in mineral form from the soil, along with a few dozen other minerals that are essential for plant and animal life. Plants then build amino acids out of nitrogen and use these to create all the protein in their structures.

Plants draw nitrogen and other minerals up from the nitrogen and mineral nutrient pool in topsoil, and they are also storing solar energy as the carbon-carbon bonds in carbs and fats.

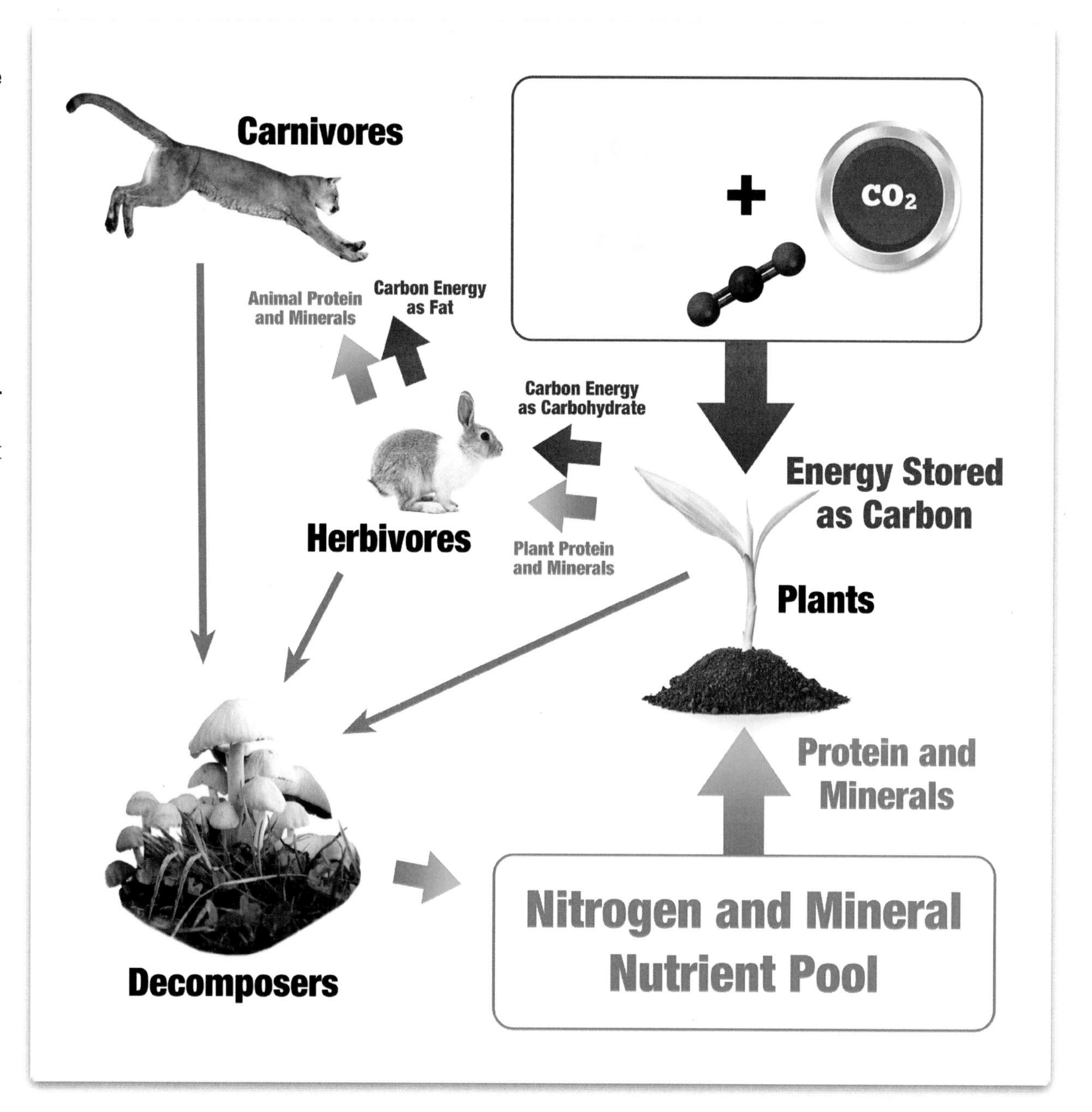

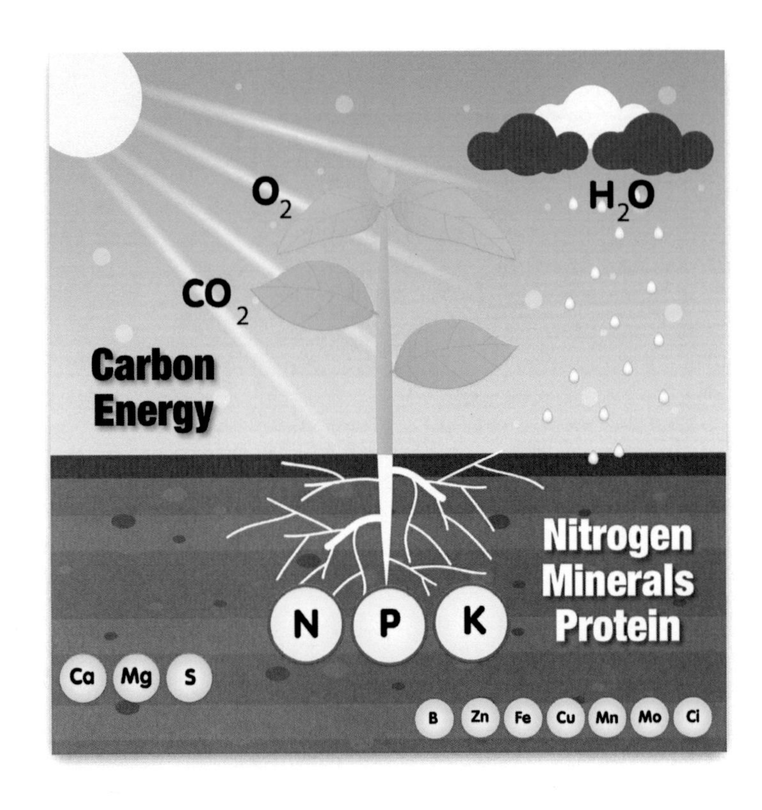

Herbivores come along and eat the plants, and all of these carbs, fats, and proteins get passed up to the herbivores. Then carnivores eat the herbivores, and everything is passed up one more rung of the food chain. Finally, when anything dies—plant or animal—it is decomposed by the fungi and bacteria in the topsoil and all of the nitrogen and minerals go back into the nutrient pool of topsoil. Pretty neat system, eh?

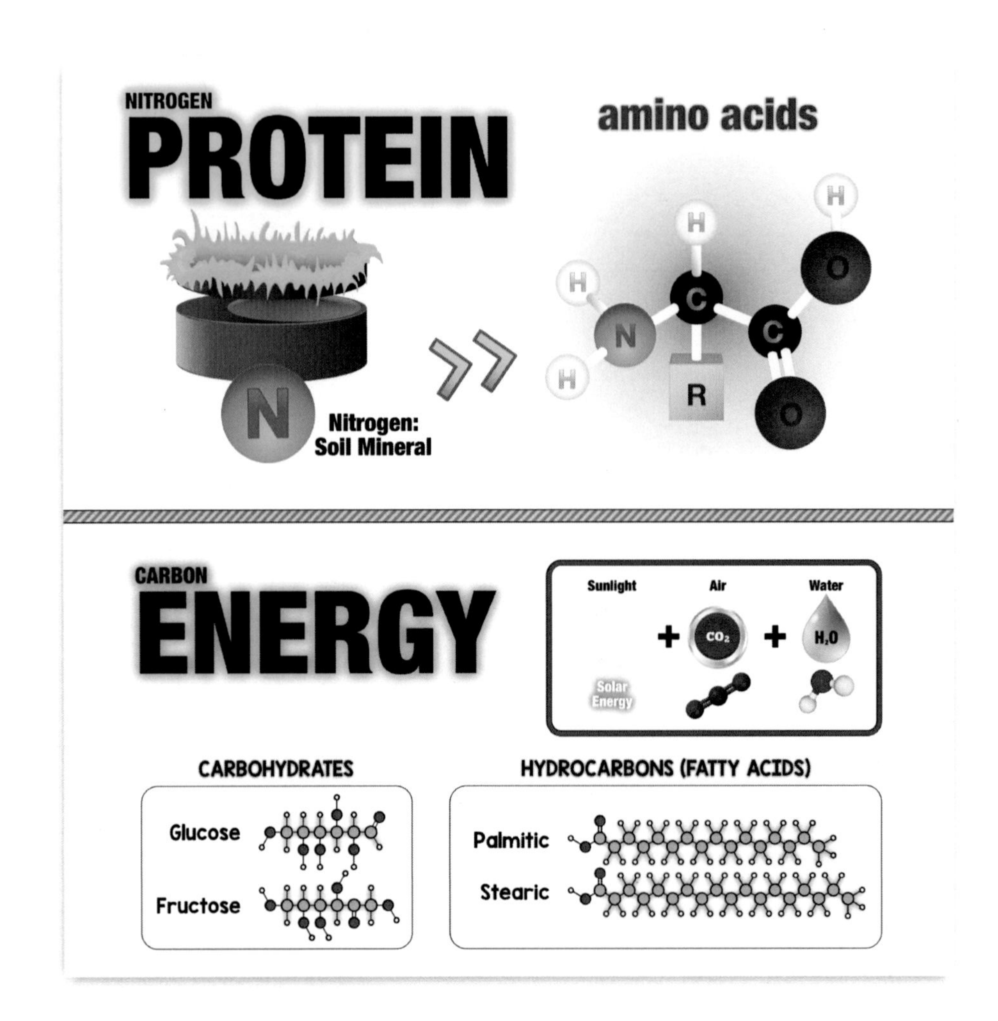

So plants have a certain amount of PROTEIN (nitrogen), and a certain amount of non-protein ENERGY (carbon). Similarly, animals also have a certain amount of PROTEIN and a certain amount of non-protein ENERGY. Your body, as well, has a protein quantity and an energy quantity. Your basic body composition goal should be to achieve the HIGHEST lean mass at the LOWEST fat mass, so the protein to energy ratio of your body is going to be an important concept going forward.

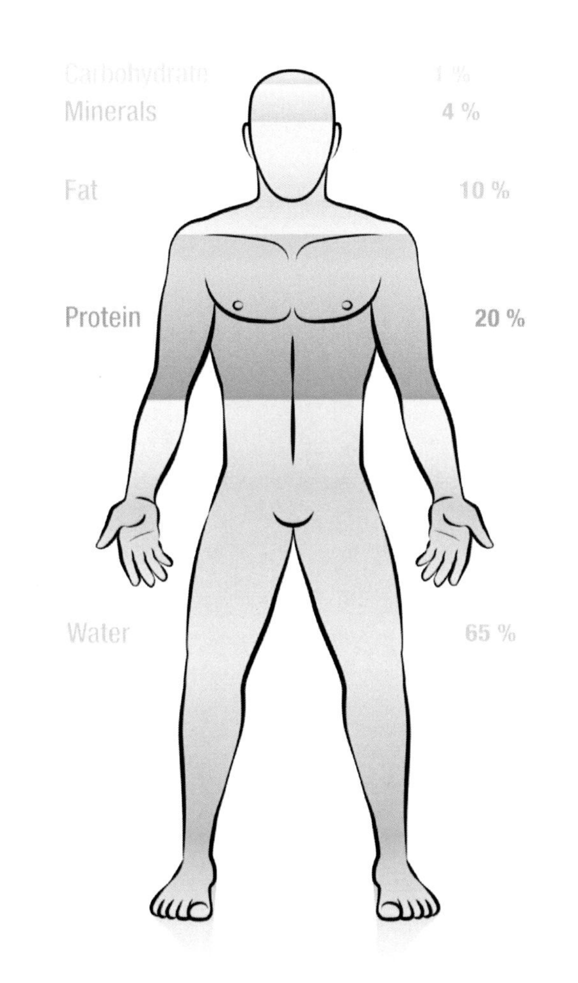

ENERGY 10%
PROTEIN 20%

MUCH LIKE YOUR DIET, YOUR BODY HAS A PROTEIN TO ENERGY RATIO AS WELL— HIGHER IS BETTER.

[WILL BE LOW IF YOU ARE OVERWEIGHT OR UNDER-MUSCLED]

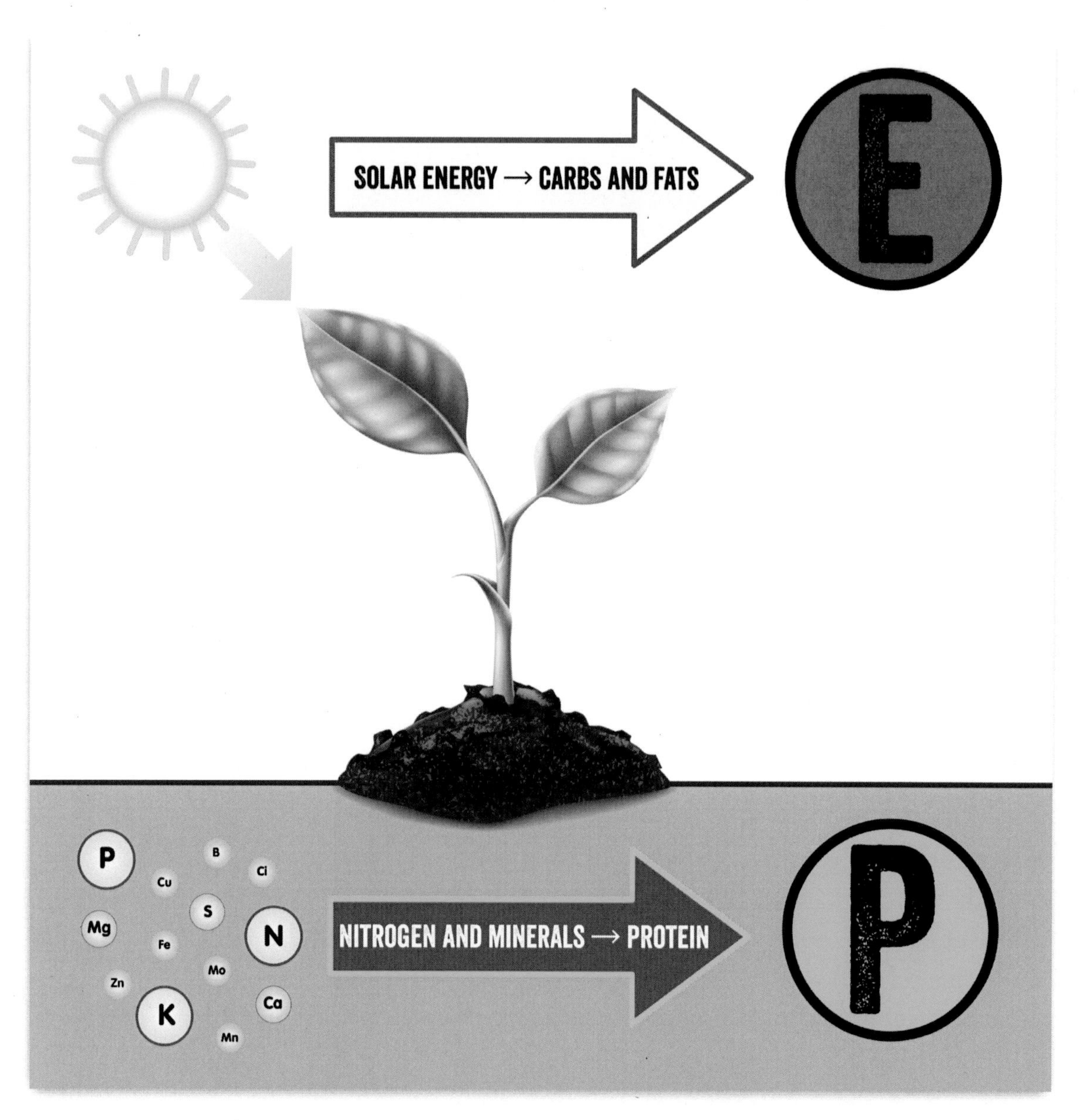

In very simple terms, all of your carb and fat ENERGY comes from the SUN, while all of your nitrogen and minerals for PROTEIN comes from the EARTH.

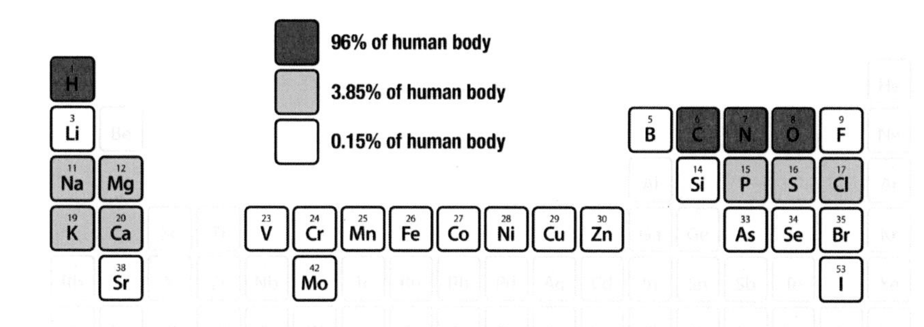

YOUR BODY IS MOSTLY OXYGEN, CARBON, HYDROGEN, AND NITROGEN.

OXYGEN COMES FROM AIR.

HYDROGEN COMES FROM WATER.

CARBON COMES FROM DIETARY

ENERGY

CARBOHYDRATES AND FATS

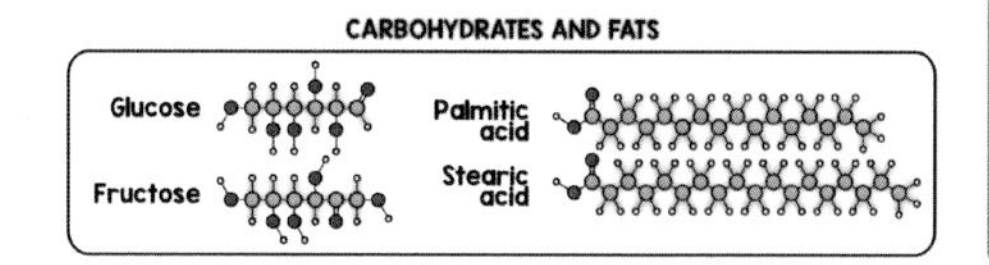

NITROGEN COMES FROM DIETARY

PROTEIN

AMINO ACIDS

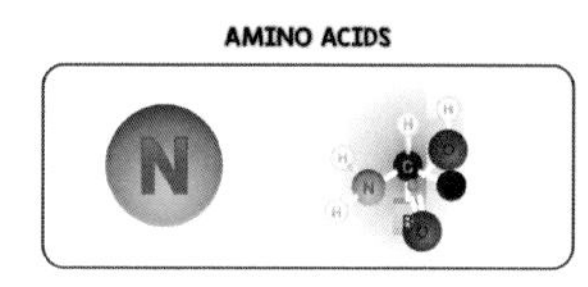

Carbon, hydrogen, oxygen, and all of the ENERGY they contain comes from AIR, WATER, and SUNLIGHT. All of your nitrogen and other elements, necessary for PROTEIN, come from soil and the EARTH.

EVOLUTIONARY LENS

Humans have been hunter-gatherers for at least 2.5 million years, but believe it or not, agriculture was only invented about 10,000 years ago. The potato only hit Europe about 400 years ago and kale arrived on our continent maybe 200 years ago. So domesticating plants and animals for food is pretty much a hypermodern technology in the scope of the evolution of homo sapiens. Prior to the domestication of plants and animals, we only ate that which we could hunt and gather.

Imagine we dump you off at a random location on the globe, at a random time of year, with nothing but a spear and a loincloth. Believe it or not, more than 98% of all plants on earth are inedible and toxic to humans. If you don't believe us, just go outside right now and try to eat some of the landscaping. We'll wait. So needless to say, pre-agricultural humans were eating mostly animals. As a result, we had a VERY high protein diet. The average animal carcass yields more protein than energy

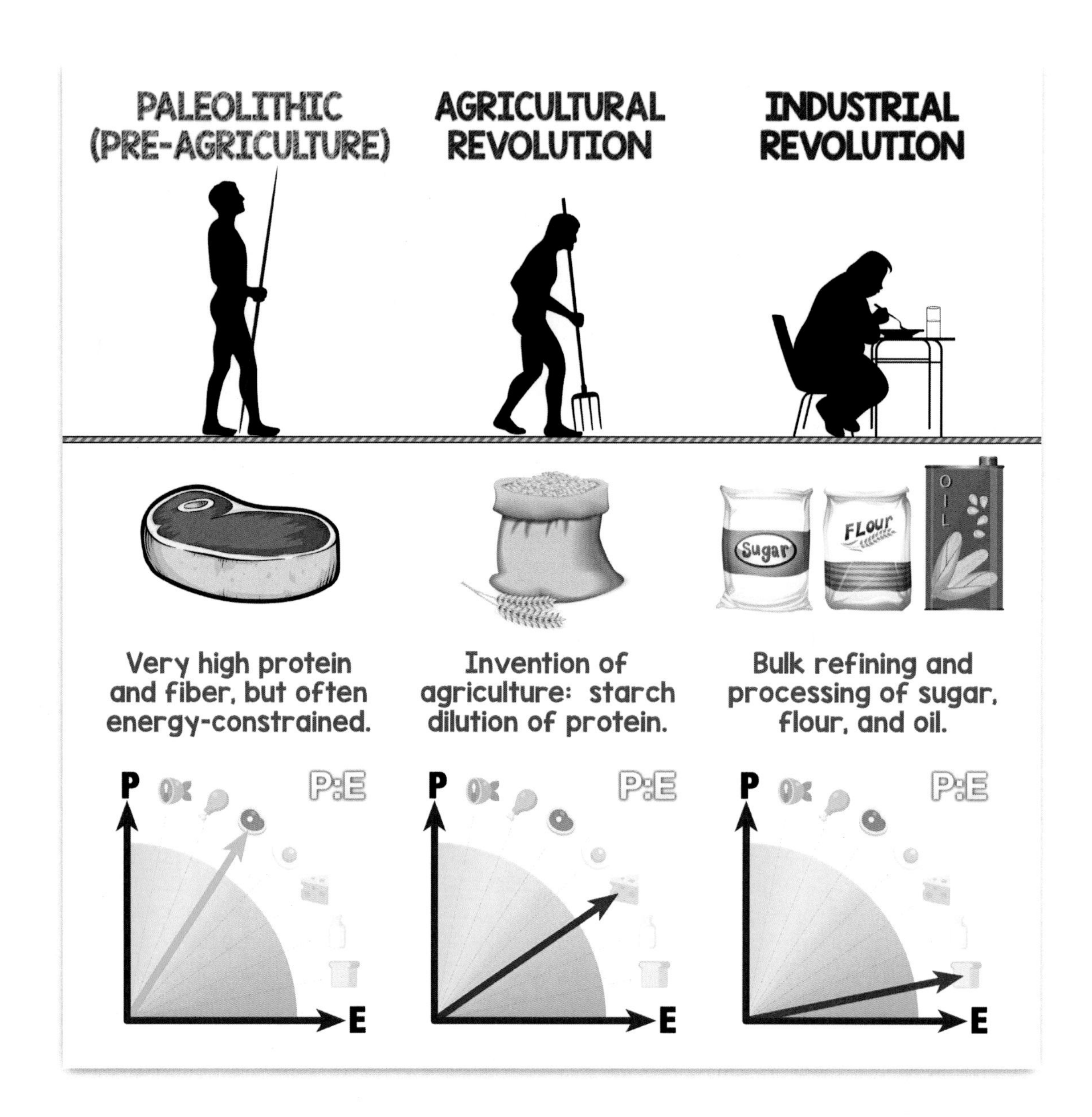

(fat). So hunter-gatherers in the Paleolithic (time-period just prior to the invention of agriculture) had plenty of protein but were often energy-constrained, or limited by dietary energy availability.

Humans have always used technology to feed ourselves—this is our superpower. We don't have particularly powerful teeth or jaws. We aren't particularly good at outrunning animals or out-climbing them. We don't have specialized body parts to directly hunt or kill anything. We can't digest cellulose like a herbivore, or dig up tubers like some omnivores. But what we DO have is intelligence, the ability to plan and work in groups cooperatively, and the ability to make tools. We also excel at throwing things—including weapons—with better strength and accuracy than any animal on earth.

We invented spears and other weapons to allow us to kill animals for food. We invented stone tools so we could eat fatter parts of animals, such as bone marrow and brains. We also sought out energy anywhere possible, even if it meant digging up tubers for starch, or braving bee stings to collect honey. Eventually we invented agriculture and the domestication of plants and animals for food.

With the invention of agriculture, we figured out how to grow starch, in the form of things like grains. These foods are very low in protein and very high in carbohydrate—starch is just chains of

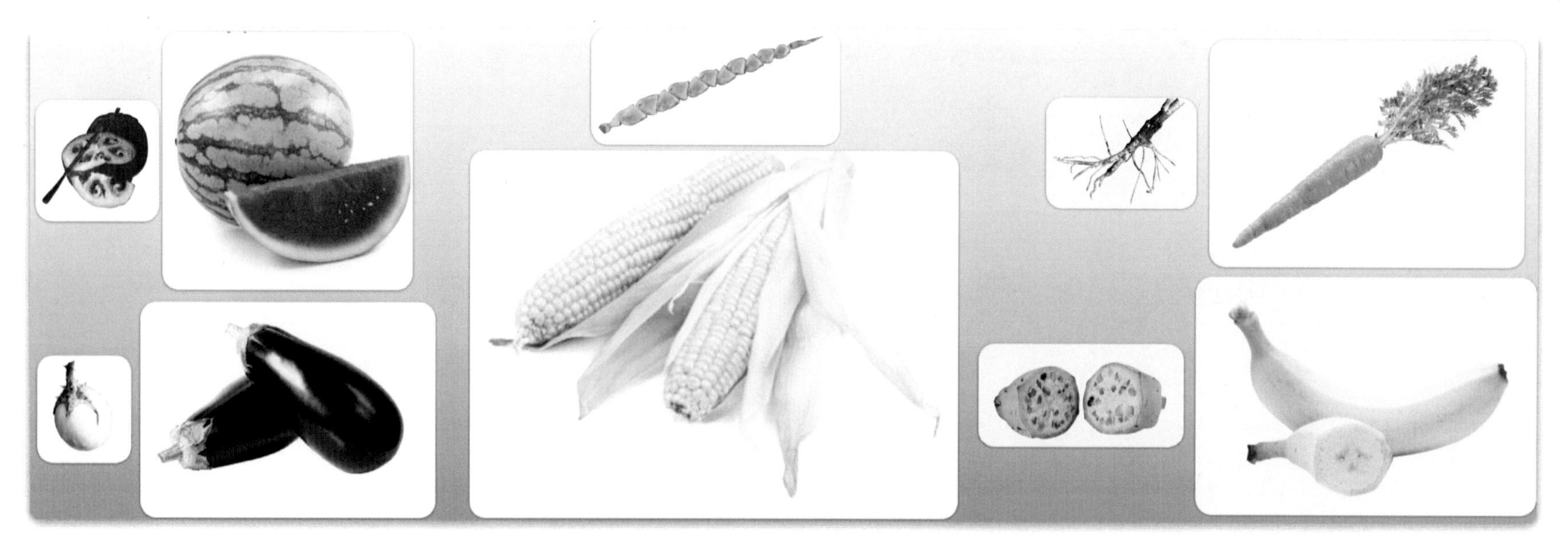

All modern agricultural foods have been bred for maximum energy yield, and are almost unrecognizable from their pre-agricultural ancestors.

glucose molecules. Agriculture significantly diluted the protein in our diets, and the result was a decline in the health of our species. Anthropologists can immediately tell if human remains came from Paleolithic hunter-gatherers (more than 10,000 years ago) or more modern humans. Post-agricultural humans had shorter stature, smaller brains, and poorer bone and dental health compared to hunter-gatherers. This was a direct result of the drop in dietary quality with the advent of agriculture: more energy, but less protein and minerals.

One of the problems with agriculture is that we humans like to eat the parts of plants that have the very most energy. Things like fruit, tubers, nuts, and seeds. These are the places where plants store energy, and we have carefully cultivated all our plants to have the very highest energy yield possible. Take

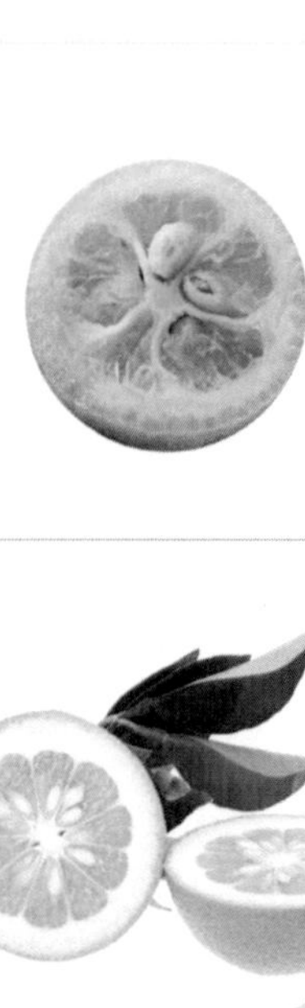

Plants store energy.

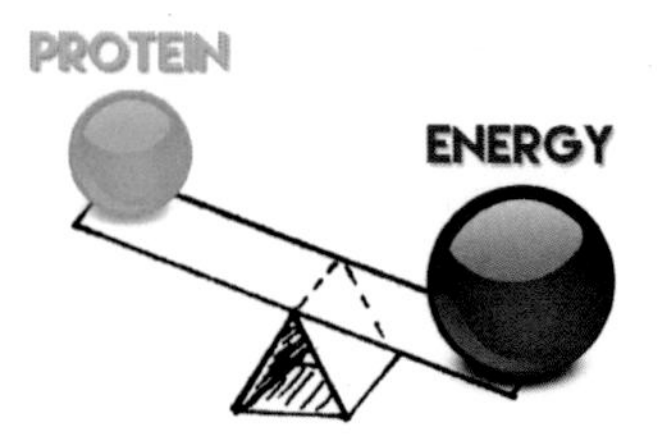

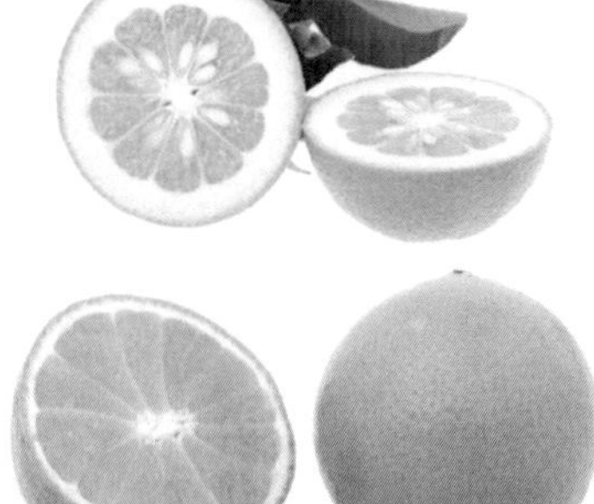

Cultivation increases energy.

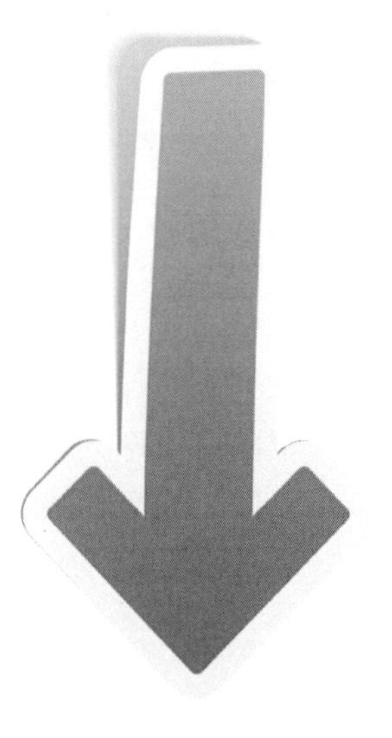

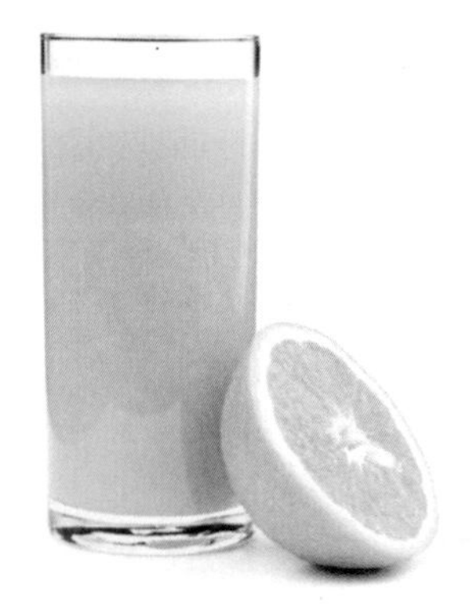

Refining increases energy even more.

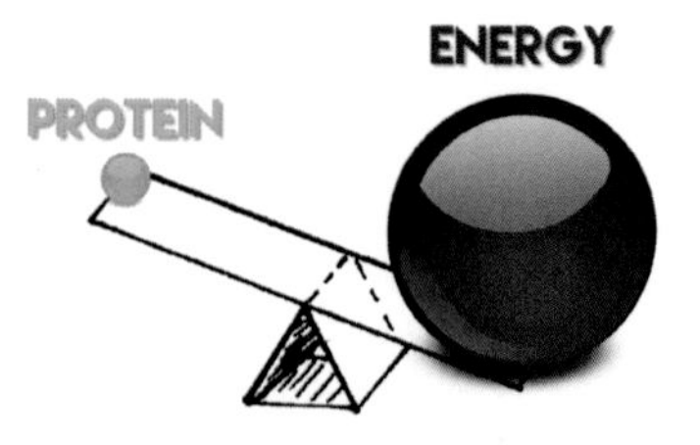

Protein Dilution

corn for example. Corn used to be the tiny seed head of grasses, maybe the size of modern wheat today. We crossbred this until corn is a huge carbon-laden monstrosity—such a high-energy food that you can simply squeeze it and make both corn syrup and corn oil.

Eventually, we humans took things one step too far. We invented the Industrial Revolution, with the bulk refining and transport of SUGAR, FLOUR, and OIL. Dumping these foods into the food supply resulted in a HUGE amount of protein dilution. The protein to energy ratio of our diets dropped enormously. As a result, the protein to energy ratios of our bodies has also dropped by an enormous amount.

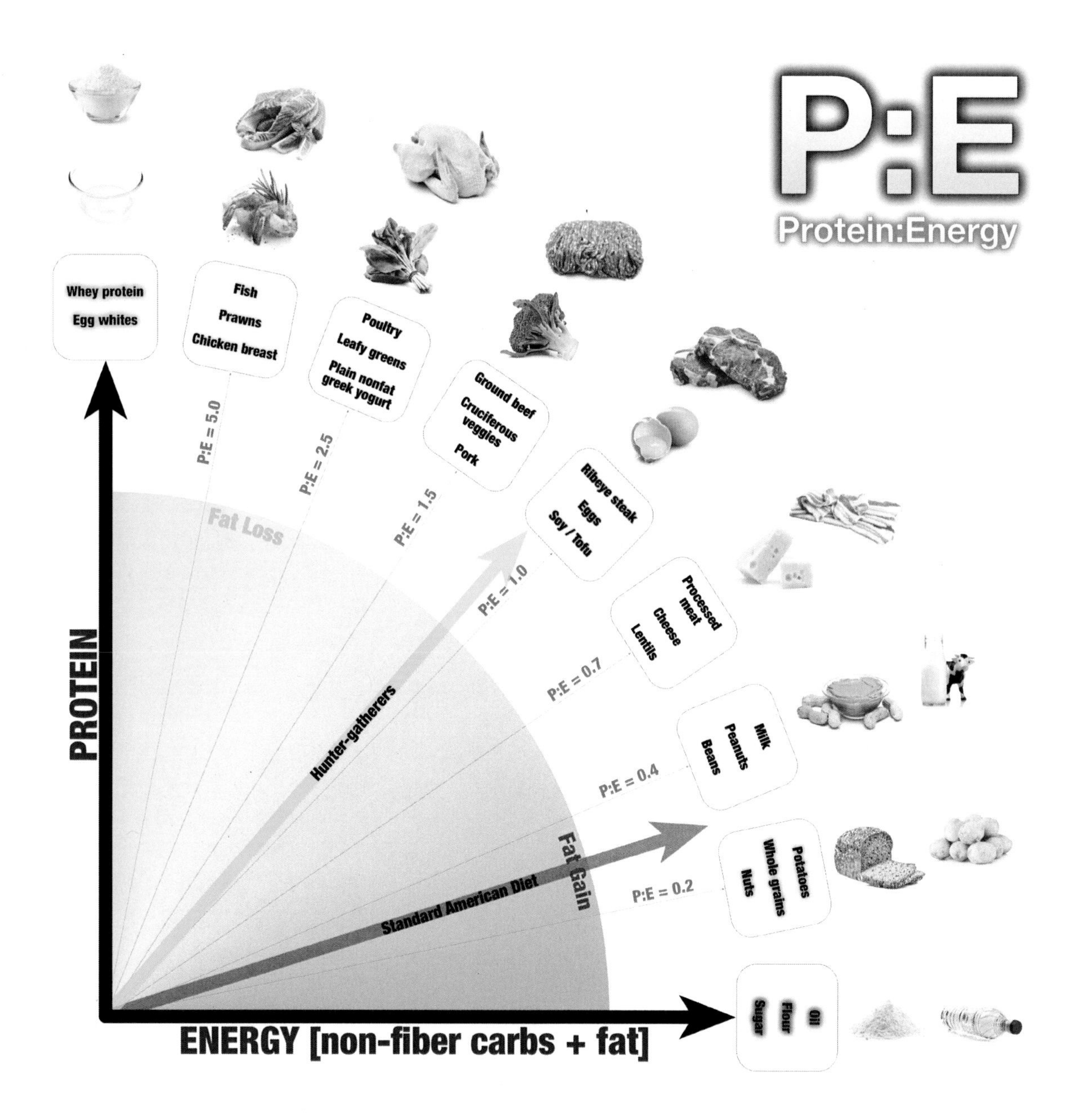

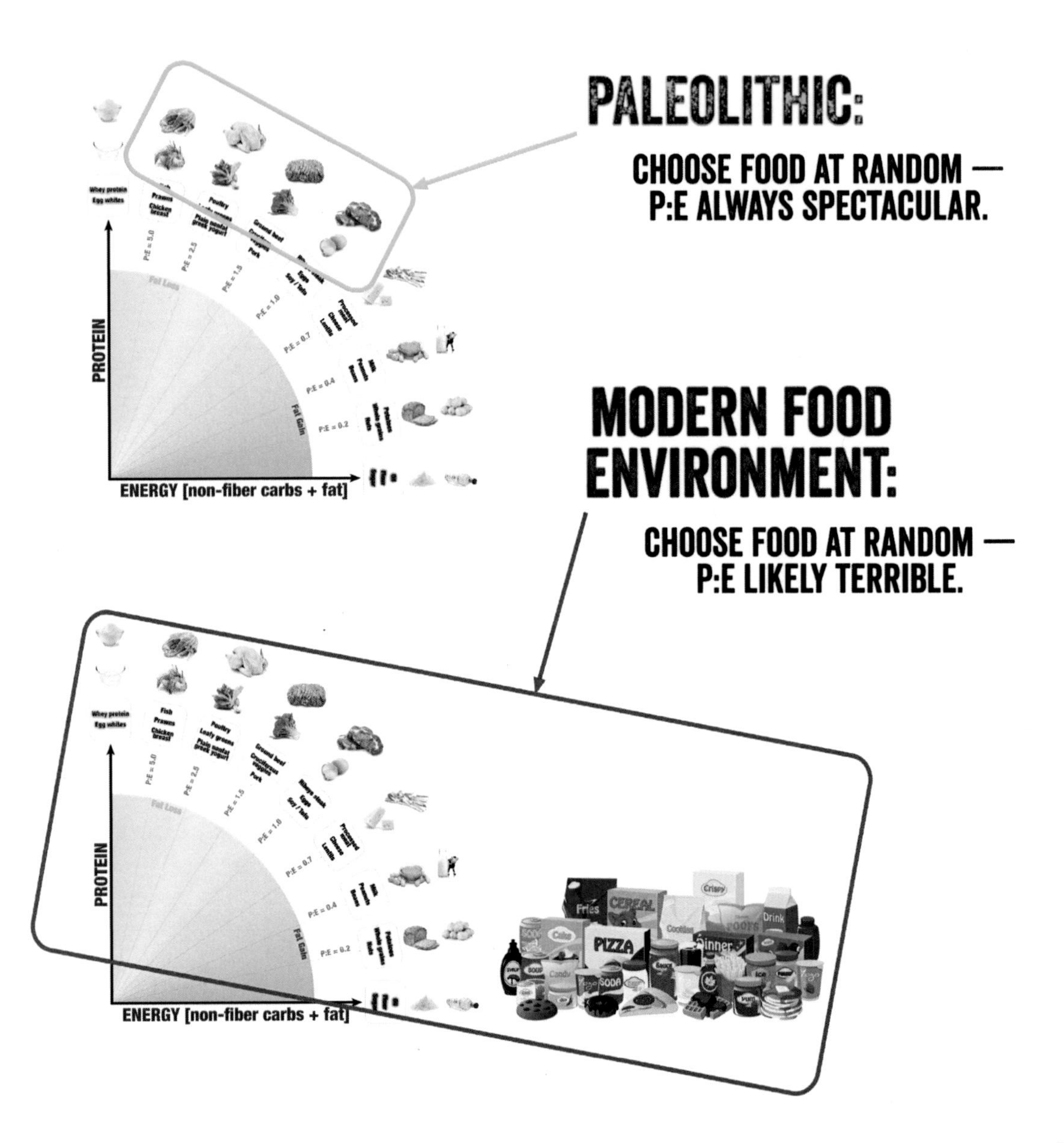

If you simply choose foods at random in today's modern food environment, they are extremely likely to have a horribly low P:E ratio. Contrast this with the Paleolithic pre-agricultural era, during which most of your foods had an excellent P:E ratio.

TOO MUCH OF A GOOD THING

If you look at a graph of obesity over the past fifty years of the obesity epidemic, you can see that somewhere in the 70's, something happened—and obesity took off. If we zoom in on the macronutrients that Americans have been eating, it is quite obvious what happened. Carbs and fats both went up equally and significantly—but not protein. Absolute protein rose slightly, but protein PERCENTAGE actually dropped—from around 14% of calories, which is pretty close to global average, down to a current 12.5% in America. Talk about protein dilution! What happens when the food you eat drops in protein percentage? You have to eat significantly more non-protein energy (carbs and fats) in order to get the amount of protein you absolutely have to eat. This protein dilution fully explains much of our modern obesity epidemic.

It turns out that humans and many other animal species exhibit protein prioritization, meaning that they will eat and eat until they have eaten an adequate absolute quantity of protein—even if they have to significantly overeat

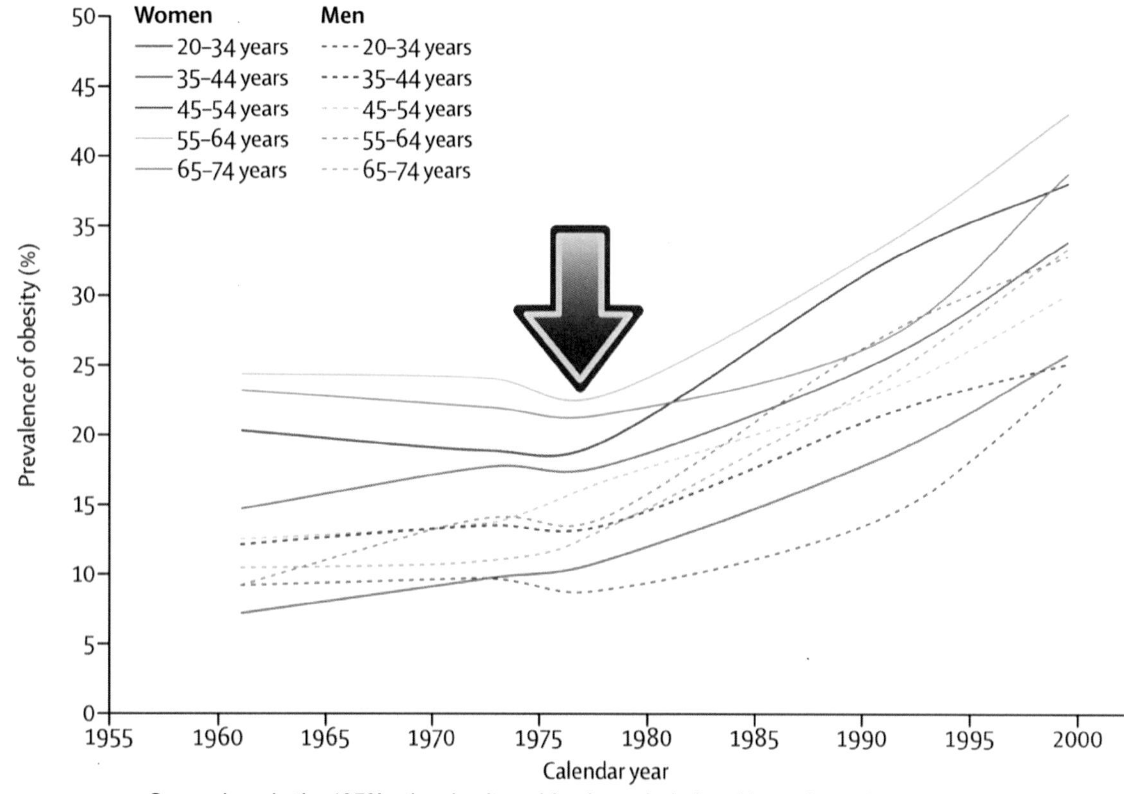

Somewhere in the 1970's, the obesity epidemic exploded—with no signs of slowing down to date.

carb and fat non-protein energy in order to get there. Meta-analysis of human feeding studies have shown that humans tightly prioritize protein, and the lower the protein percentage of their food, the more energy they will eat in order to get adequate protein. The opposite is also true, and the higher the protein percentage of the diet, the less energy humans will consistently eat. This is the very first—and most important—rule of our book: prioritize protein, and keep the protein percentage of your diet high. If the protein percentage of your diet is high, you will tend to automatically eat less energy.

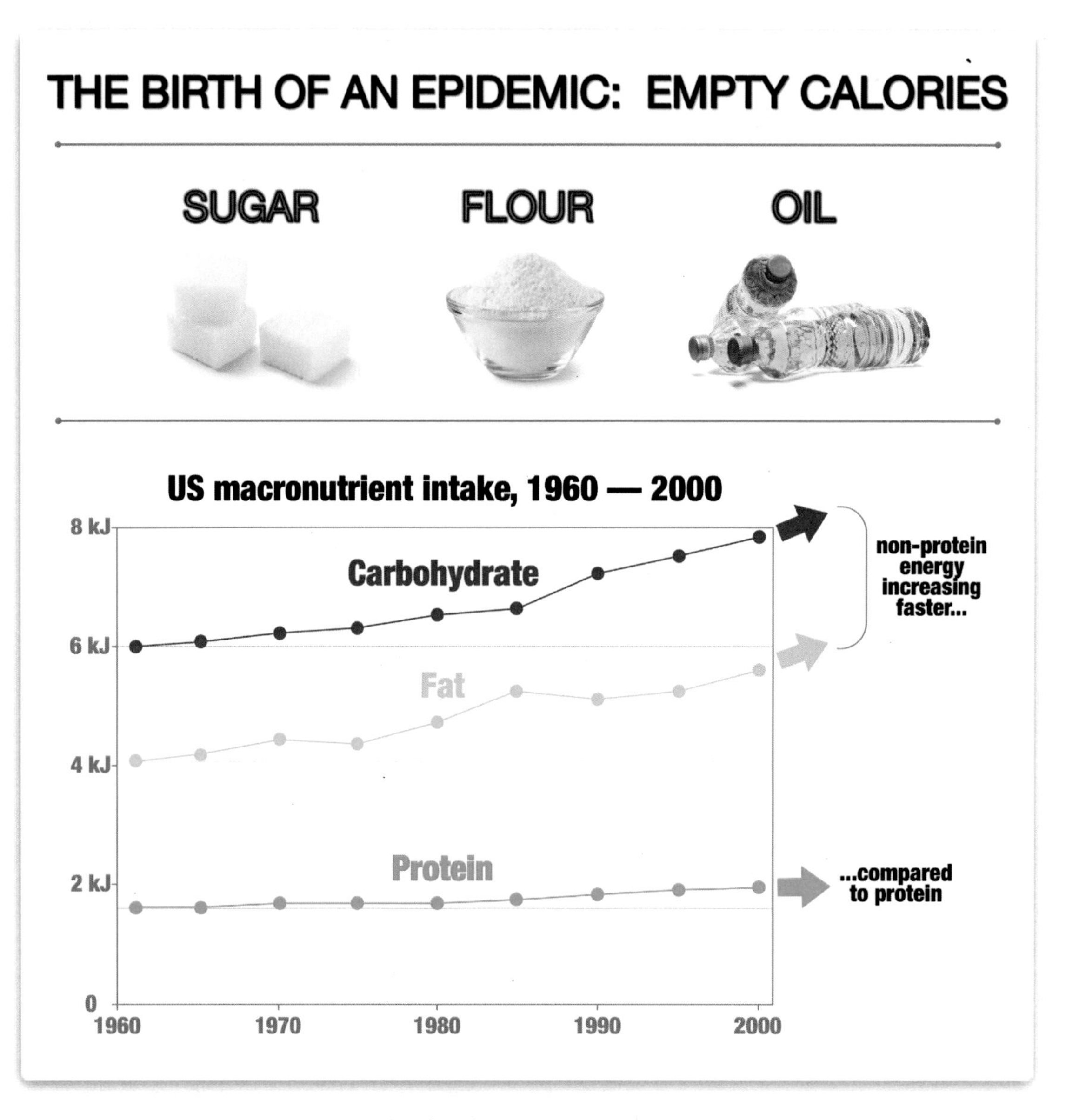

The real cause of obesity is EMPTY CALORIES — which by definition are carbs and fats with little to no protein or minerals.

INTRODUCTION TO P:E RATIO [PROTEIN TO ENERGY RATIO]

All free-living animals on earth have to combine foods in a complementary fashion in order to achieve optimum function. Nutritional ecology is the science that looks at what animals NEED to eat versus what they actually GET to eat. Imagine that an animal has access to two foods, one that is higher in protein, and one that is higher in energy. The animal is going to have a fitness target where it functions optimally and is best able to thrive and reproduce. The fitness target could be variable depending on the animal's activity level and a bunch of other factors. This animal will have to combine these two foods in a complementary fashion in order to get as close to its fitness target as possible.

fitness target

protein

energy

Now imagine that the animal only has access to the low protein high energy food. This poor animal will have to make a choice. It could overeat energy in order to get enough protein—likely leading to obesity. Or it could eat a normal amount of energy but insufficient protein, risking its ability to function properly. Not a great place to be, but that is where Americans find themselves in the current food environment. All species are somewhat different as to their 'rule of compromise', or how they deal with suboptimal food environments. But in the case of humans, it is quite clear that we will overeat energy in order to get enough protein—every single time.

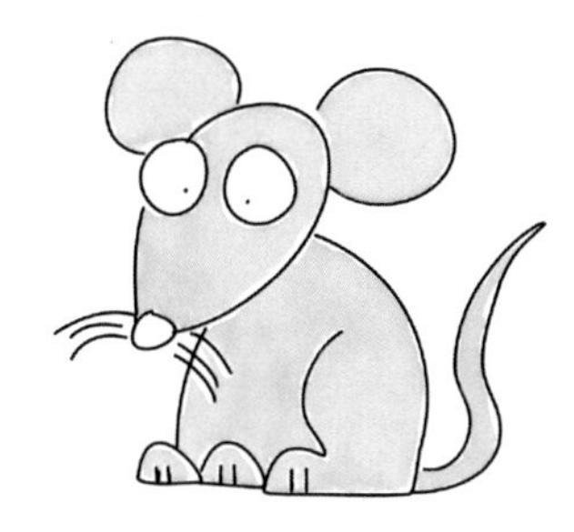

We are going to use the concept of nutritional ecology and dietary protein to energy ratios to evaluate individual foods and our overall diets a little bit later on—this is just background information so you will understand where this Protein to Energy approach comes from!

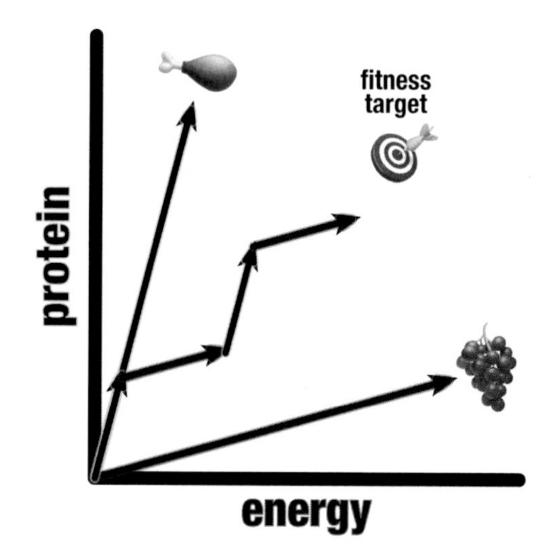

You are already eating enough protein.

Everyone is eating enough protein.

THAT IS NOT THE POINT.

The point is—

HOW MUCH ENERGY DID YOU HAVE TO EAT TO GET THAT PROTEIN?

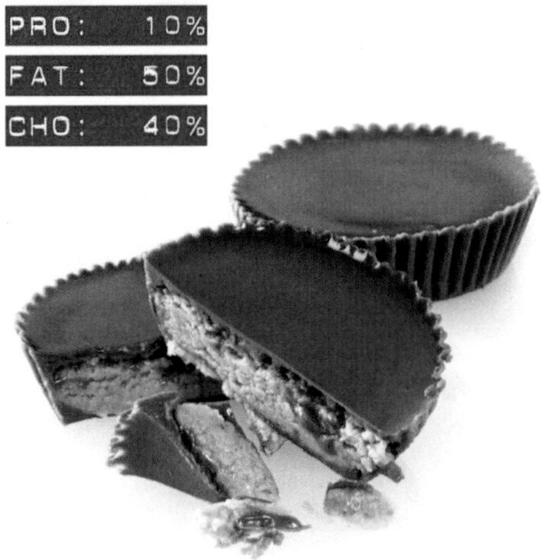

PRO: 10%

FAT: 50%

CHO: 40%

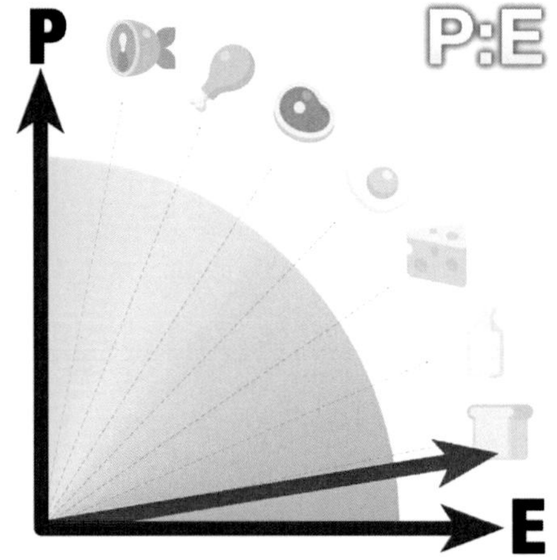

P

P:E

E

When you eat a low protein food, you have to radically overeat non-protein energy (carbs and/or fats) to get adequate protein.

ENERGY STORAGE AND METABOLISM

So far, we have lumped all carbs and fats together as just 'non-protein energy'. In a way, this is perfectly fair: both are simply chains of high-energy carbon bonds, made by plants as a way to store solar energy as chemical energy. But carbs and fats are radically different, and are treated in radically different ways by your body. It is ABSOLUTELY CRUCIAL to understand the basic differences between these two, so let's dive in!

First of all, carbohydrates are water-soluble. Think of a spoonful of sugar in your coffee. Fats, on the other hand, are absolutely NOT water-soluble—oil and water don't mix. So your body absorbs and transports and stores these two different energy sources in COMPLETELY different ways—and they have completely different effects on your metabolism.

All food is broken down into smaller units in your digestive tract before it is even absorbed in your small intestine. Proteins are broken down into amino acids, the building blocks of proteins, prior to absorption. Non-fiber carbohydrates are all broken down into simple sugars like glucose and fructose before they are absorbed (fiber carbs are not absorbed at all and continue their way through the digestive tract, exiting out the other side). Dietary fats are eaten as triglycerides (three fatty acids packaged together) and are broken down into individual fatty acids prior to being absorbed.

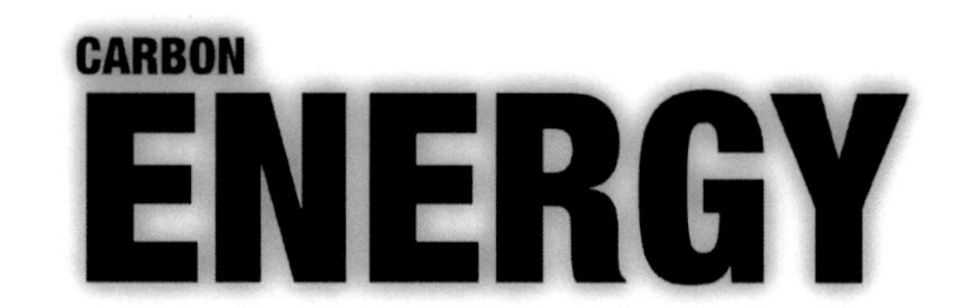

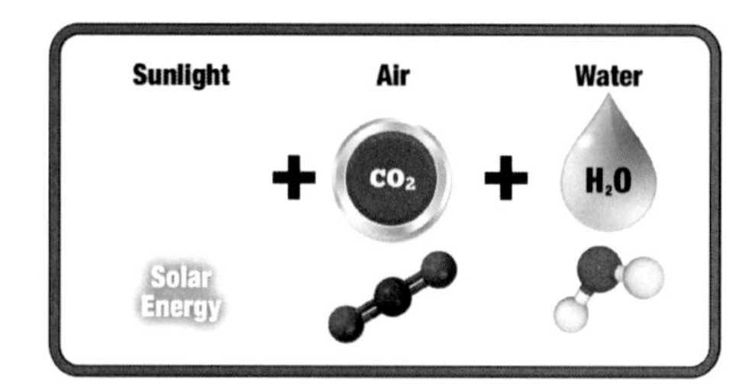

CARBOHYDRATES

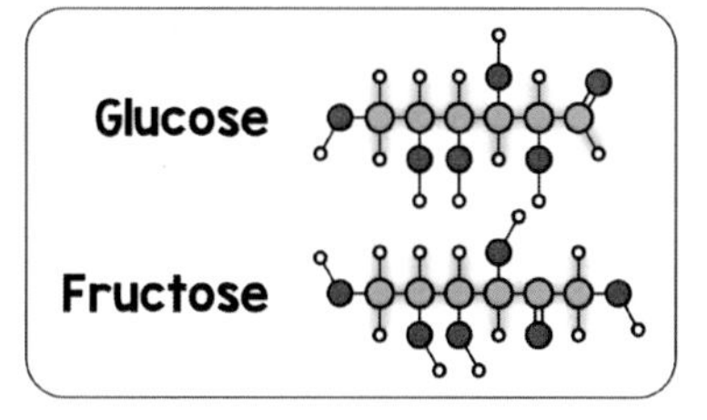

HYDROCARBONS (FATTY ACIDS)

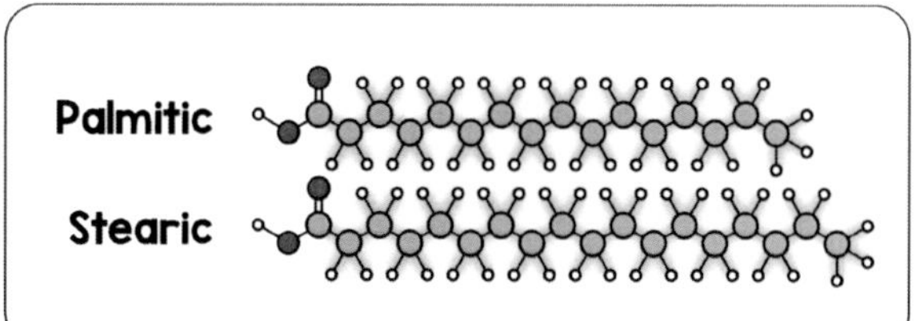

All dietary energy is chains of carbons with high-energy carbon-carbon bonds — carbs and fats. We break apart these bonds in our mitochondria to release energy.

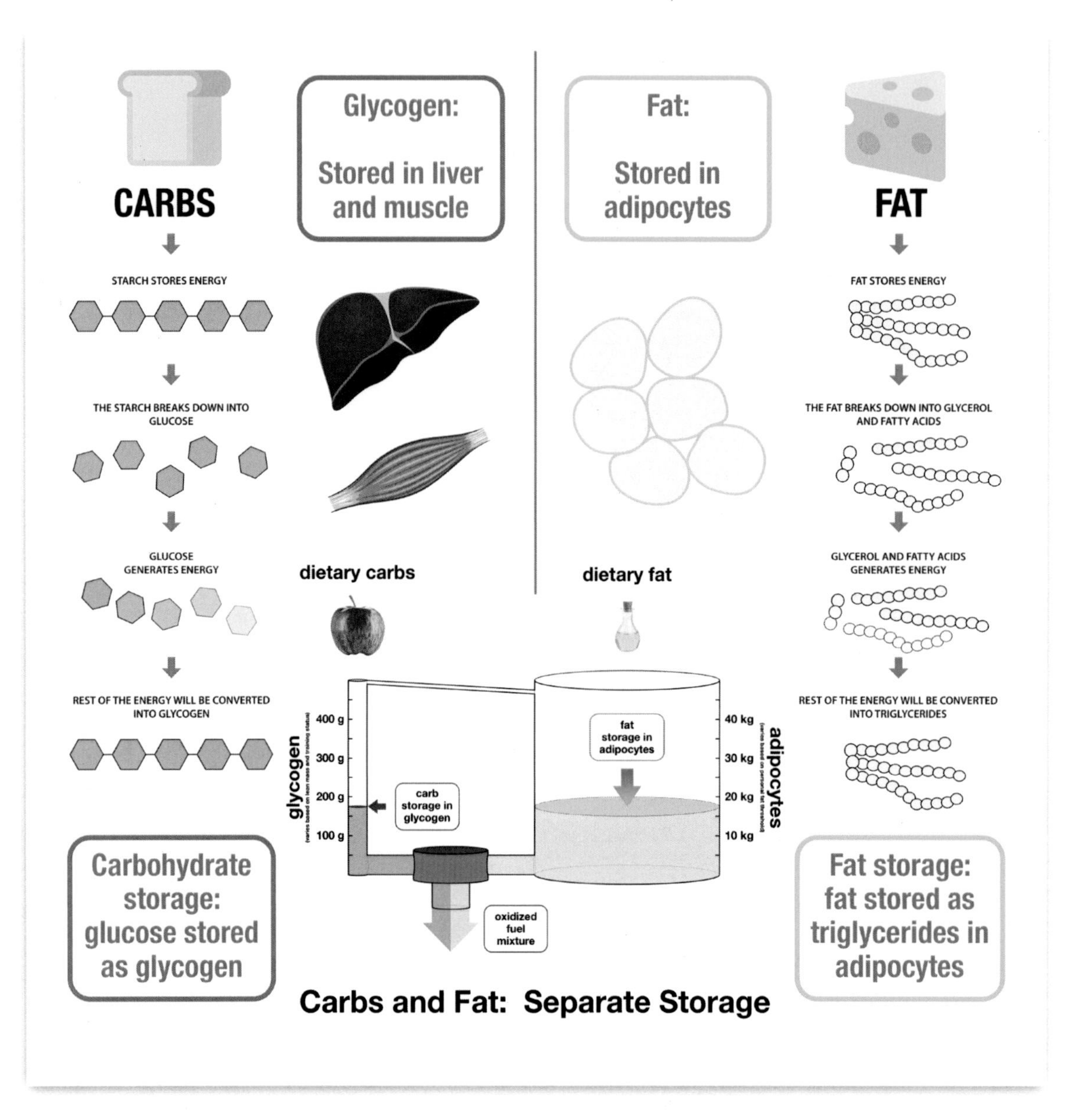

All non-fiber carbs are broken down into simple sugars like glucose and stored as glycogen. All fats are broken down into fatty acids, then stored as triglycerides in fat cells (adipocytes).

TWO COMPARTMENT SYSTEM

So you have two completely separate energy storage compartments in your body. Glucose (carbohydrate), which is water-soluble, is stored as glycogen (just chains of glucose) in your liver and your muscles. Fat, which is NOT water-soluble, is stored in your adipocytes. Fat storage is MUCH larger, and your body prefers to carry only about 1% of your energy as glycogen. What gives?

It turns out that glucose, from glycogen, is FAST. You can convert glucose into energy SIX TIMES faster compared to fat. So why don't we only use glycogen to store energy? Because glycogen is HEAVY! Glycogen is 'fully hydrated' (this is why we call them carboHYDRATES), which means it has a lot of water attached to it. And that water weighs a lot! So glycogen is about six times heavier than the same amount of energy stored as fat.

Glycogen, which is just chains of glucose molecules, is a sort of 'human starch' and is identical to the starch in potatoes. The fat in the lipid droplets of your adipocytes is very similar to olive oil. Note the photo below of the same amount of stored energy as olive oil versus potatoes. At six times the size and

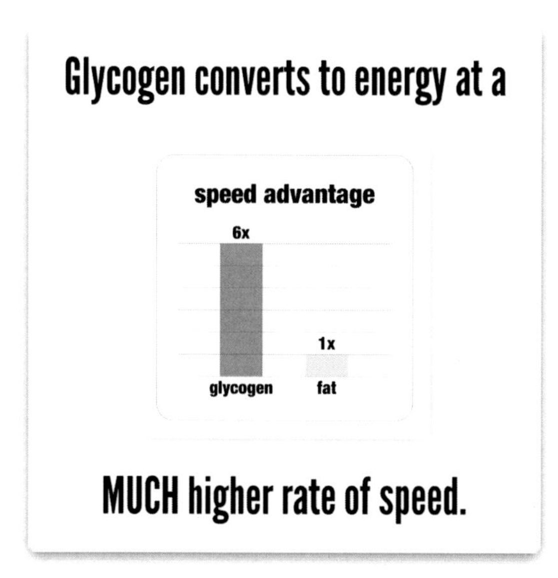

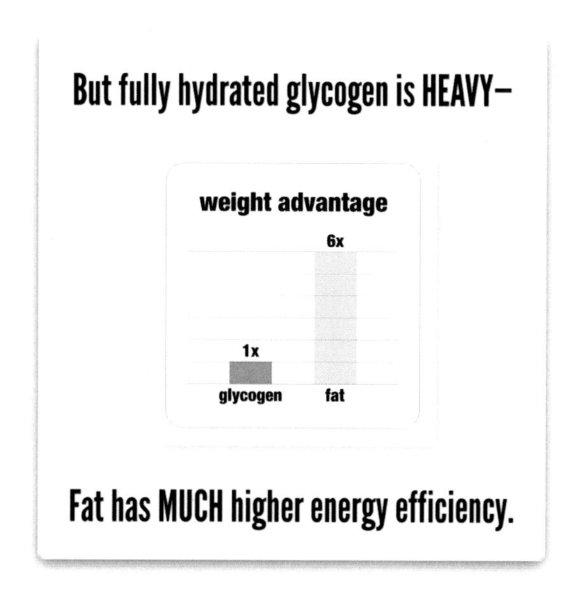

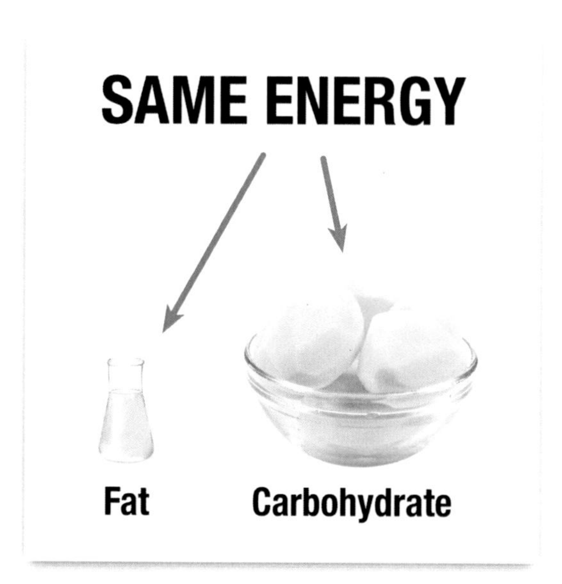

weight, you can see why your body doesn't want to carry around all your energy as glycogen. In fact, because of the weight efficiency, your body carries 100 times more fat than glycogen.

But you always HAVE to have glycogen around for emergency use. In a fasted state, when we are sedentary or only lightly exercising, like walking, we are burning mostly fat. But at high intensities of exercise, we are burning mostly glucose. And in fact, at the VERY highest intensity, like sprinting for your life, you are always burning 100% pure glucose. Because it is so helpful for emergency use, your body will ALWAYS keep glycogen in your muscles, so you can run for your life at a moment's notice. This is an essential safety feature!

Glycogen storage is quite tiny. You can only hold about 4 grams of glucose in your bloodstream, and maybe 100 grams of glucose in your liver. Your muscles can hold around 300 grams of glucose on average, but this glucose is only for emergency use and remains untouched UNLESS you are doing very high intensity exercise—in which case you can actually burn a ton of glucose quite rapidly, if you get the intensity all the way up to maximum. This is why people who are doing a ton of super high intensity exercise can pretty much get away with carbs. But the average American is doing

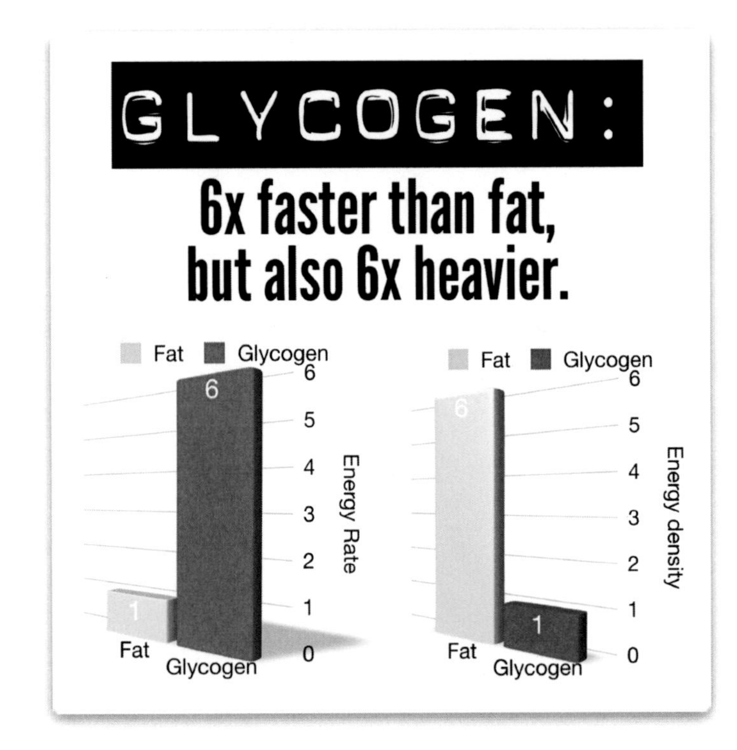

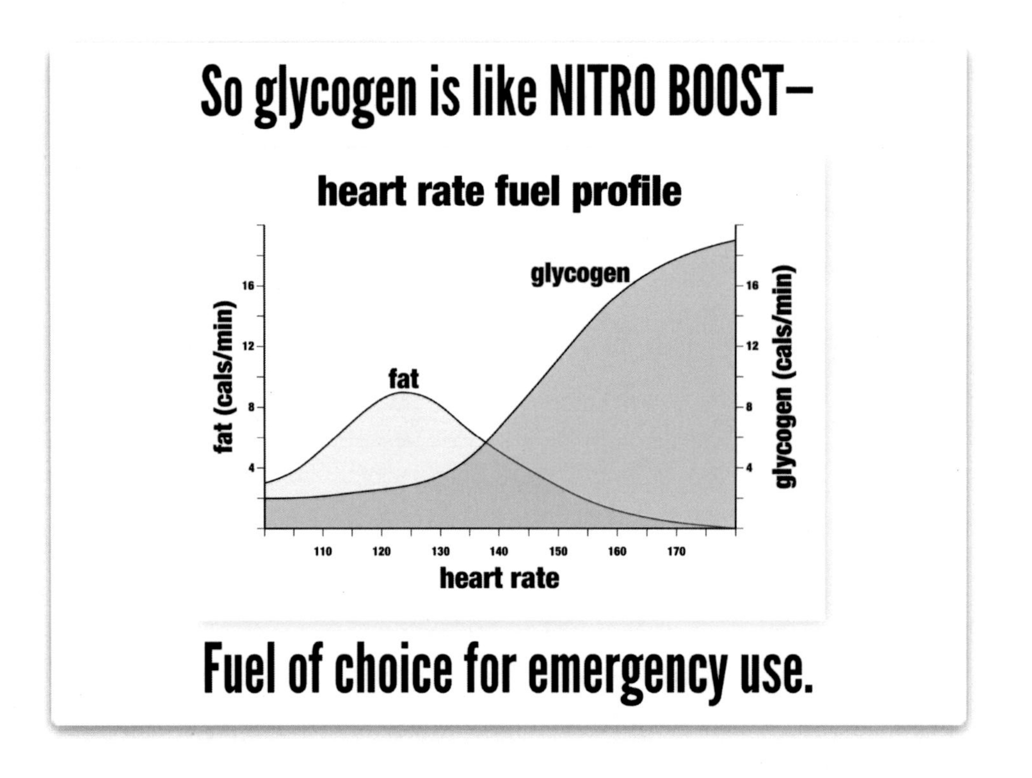

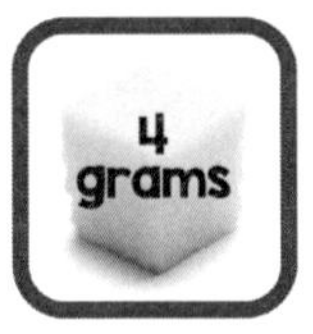

Your bloodstream can only hold 4 grams of glucose.

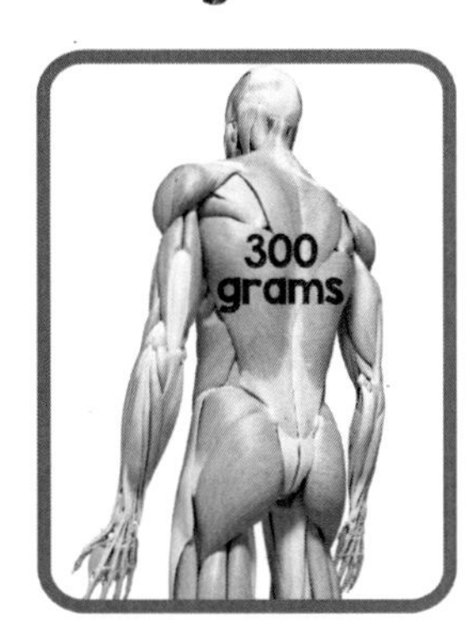

Your muscles can hold about 300 grams, but this is only used in very high intensity exercise.*

*About 90 minutes at high intensity to deplete.

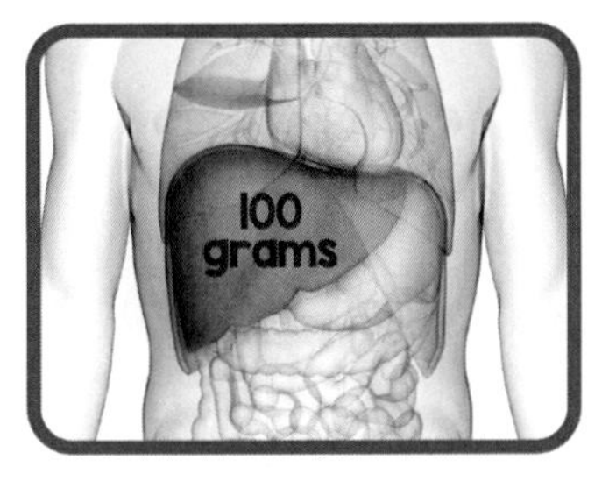

Your liver can hold around 100 grams of glucose, but it takes about 24 hours of fasting to deplete this.

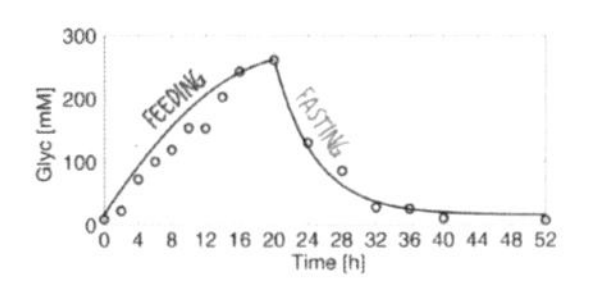

So unless you are engaging in high intensity exercise, you might want to limit yourself to 100 grams of net carbohydrates per day.

Which is roughly equivalent to four apples.

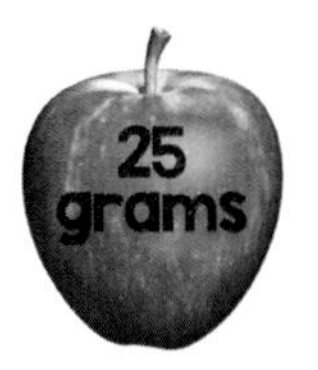

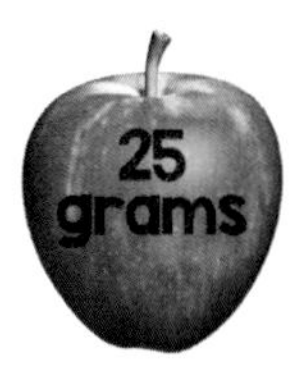

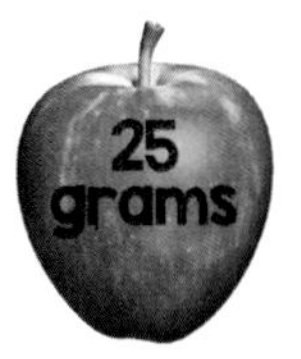

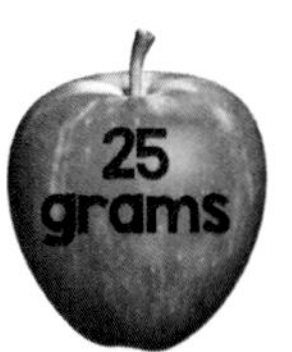

Glycogen storage is quite small and, without high-intensity exercise, most people only have room for about 100 grams of dietary glucose (stored as liver glycogen) per 24 hours.

an average of zero minutes per day of high intensity exercise (seriously), so for most of us, we should probably stay under 100 grams. More about this later!

Time for a super important concept: CARBS AND FATS ARE OXIDIZED RECIPROCALLY! And it is GLUCOSE, not fat, that controls which fuel is oxidized at all times. This is an absolute requirement because glucose storage (glycogen) is so tiny. We have very little space for glucose storage as glycogen, so the minute we start eating more glucose we immediately have to burn more glucose. Conversely, as soon as we stop eating glucose, we immediately start burning more fat. Understanding this interplay between carbs and fats is absolutely essential if you want to understand what is required to increase fat oxidation.

Fat and glucose are metabolized reciprocally in your body.

The availability of GLUCOSE, not fat, controls the fuel that is burned for energy at all times.

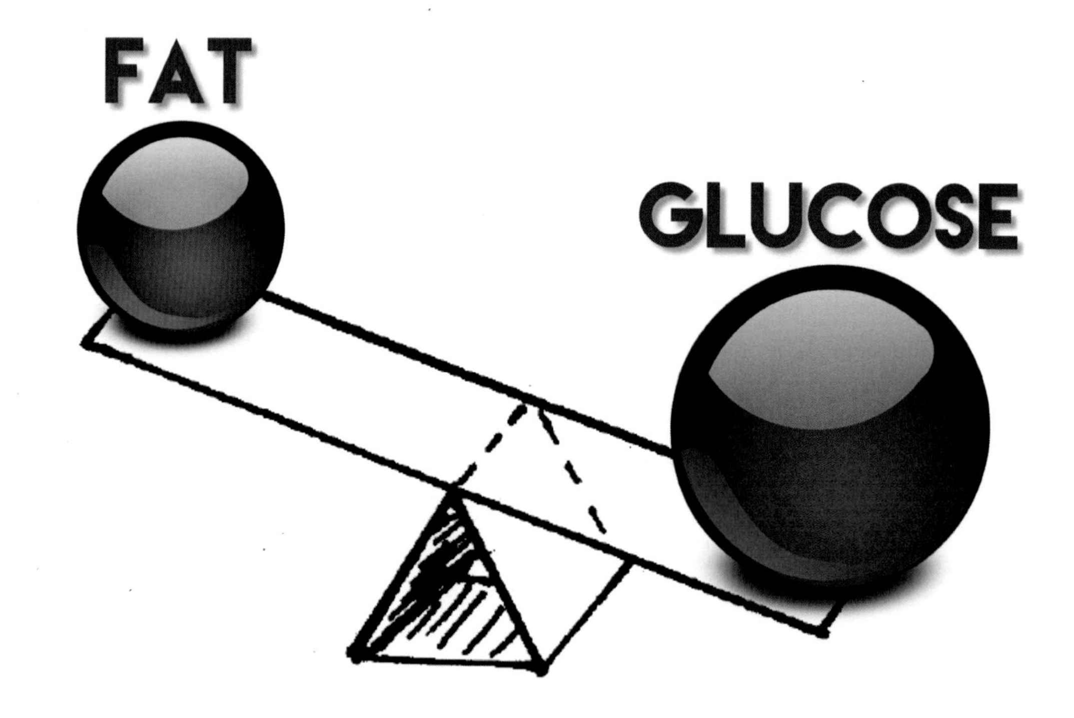

High carb diets can increase carbohydrate oxidation 10x and decrease fat oxidation 10x at the same time. If you want to get better at burning fat for fuel, the simplest and most direct strategy is to eat fewer carbohydrates. Here we are going to invoke the S.A.I.D. Principle —Specific Adaptation To Imposed Demand—for the first time. If you want your body to be better at burning fat, you only have to do one thing: eat fewer carbohydrates. More on this later!

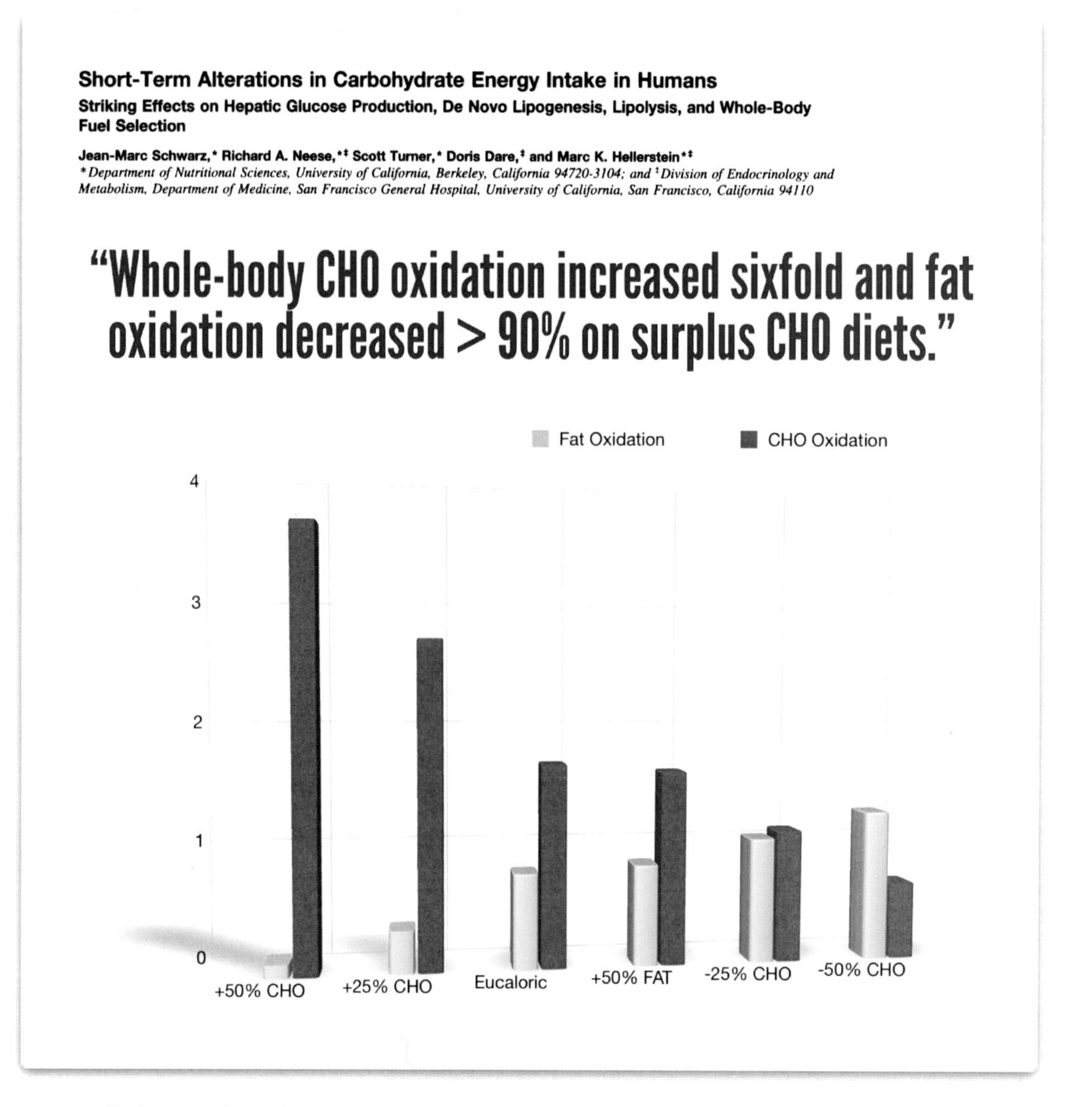

Carbs control metabolism: as carbohydrate intake increases, carbohydrate oxidation increases exponentially, while fat oxidation decreases exponentially at the same time.

Back to the two compartment storage system for energy in your body. There are really four basic permutations for dietary energy. Let's list them all here, on the following pages:

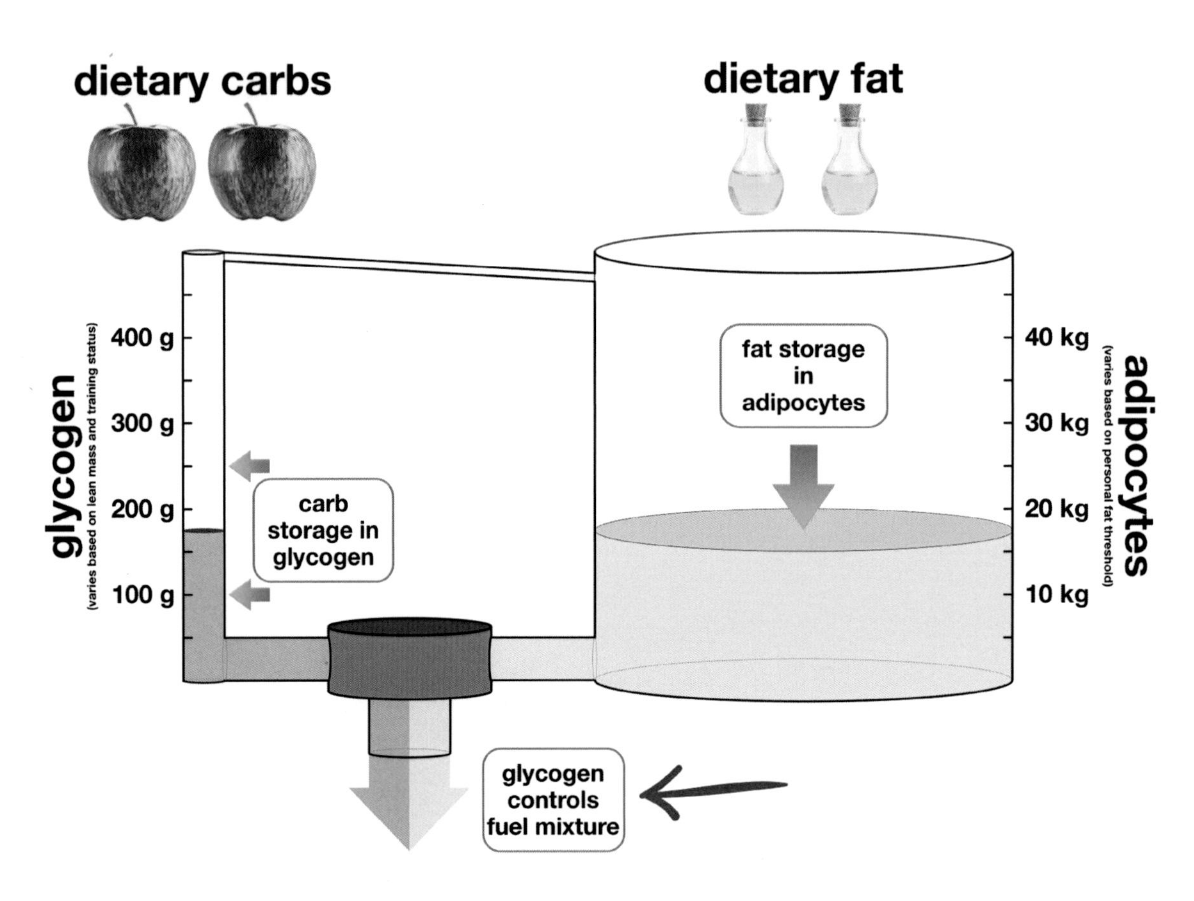

High Carb Low Fat.

This is your typical weight loss diet. Fat has the most "calories", so from a caloric point of view it made the most sense to eliminate those. Plus we used to think that dietary fat immediately clogged your arteries, just like bacon grease in your sink drain. Turns out that calories aren't the best way of thinking about your diet, and eating fat doesn't clog your arteries after all. More on all of that later. But in any case, if you are eating a high carb low fat diet, you will be burning a higher amount of glucose for energy, and less fat. A person on this diet can be lean and healthy, but you probably have to eat more frequently as you will be less 'fat-adapted', or able to run your whole metabolism from stored body fat. Frequently somewhat 'glucose-dependent', with blood sugar highs and lows. As liver glycogen falls, blood sugar falls as well, and falling blood sugar equals hunger. More on this later!

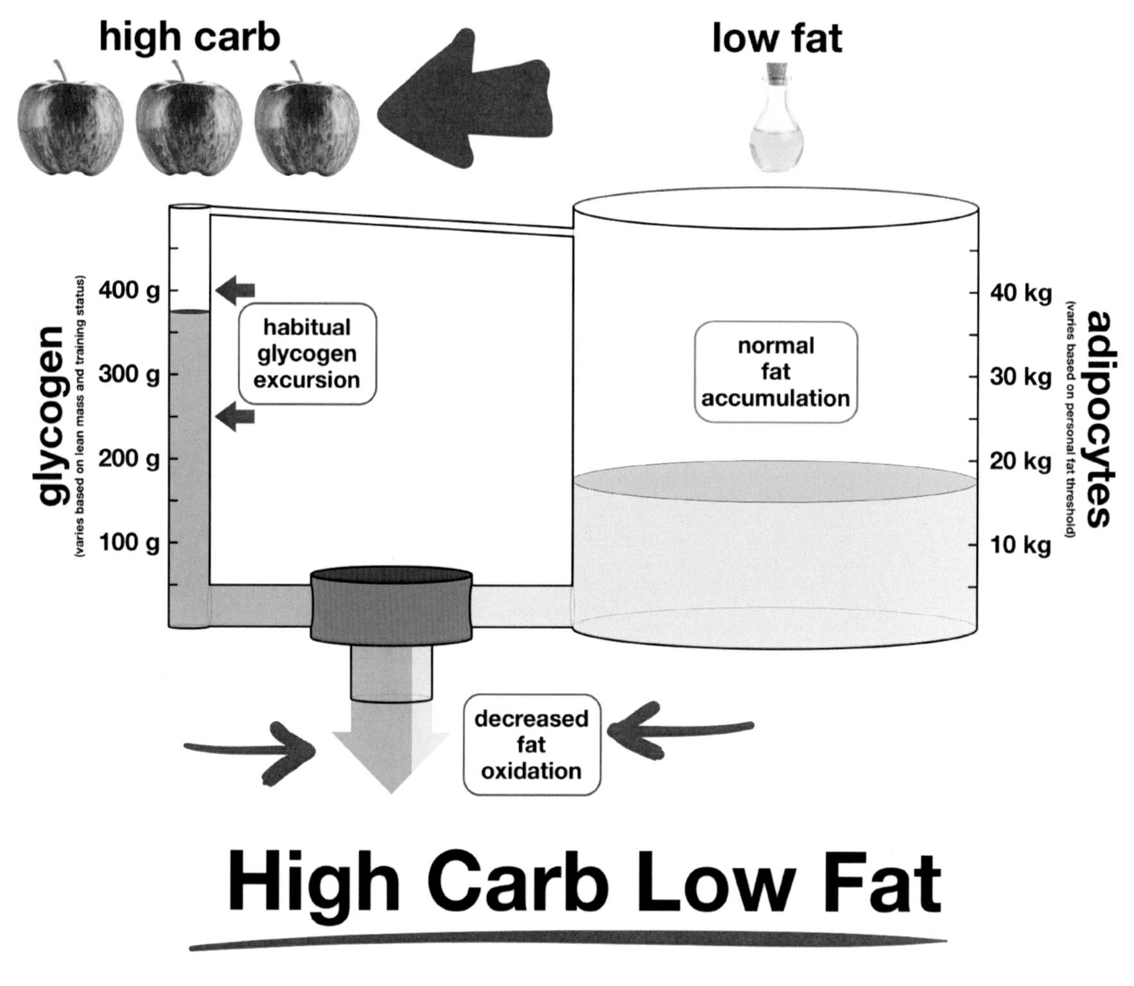

Low Carb High Fat.

This would be your standard Atkins-type diet. You are eating a lot of fat, but that's ok because carbs and glucose and glycogen are low, so you are reciprocally burning a lot of fat. Very good for 'fat-adaptation', or the ability to run your entire metabolism from stored body fat. Definitely superior to high carb low fat for overweight and obese people, and in fact there are dozens of studies comparing low fat to low carb and low carb is simply more effective for losing weight. Low carb haters will argue that low fat and low carb are the same "when calories are matched", meaning studies where participants were given a fixed amount of calories to eat. This is true—but in the real world, low carb is better for overweight persons.

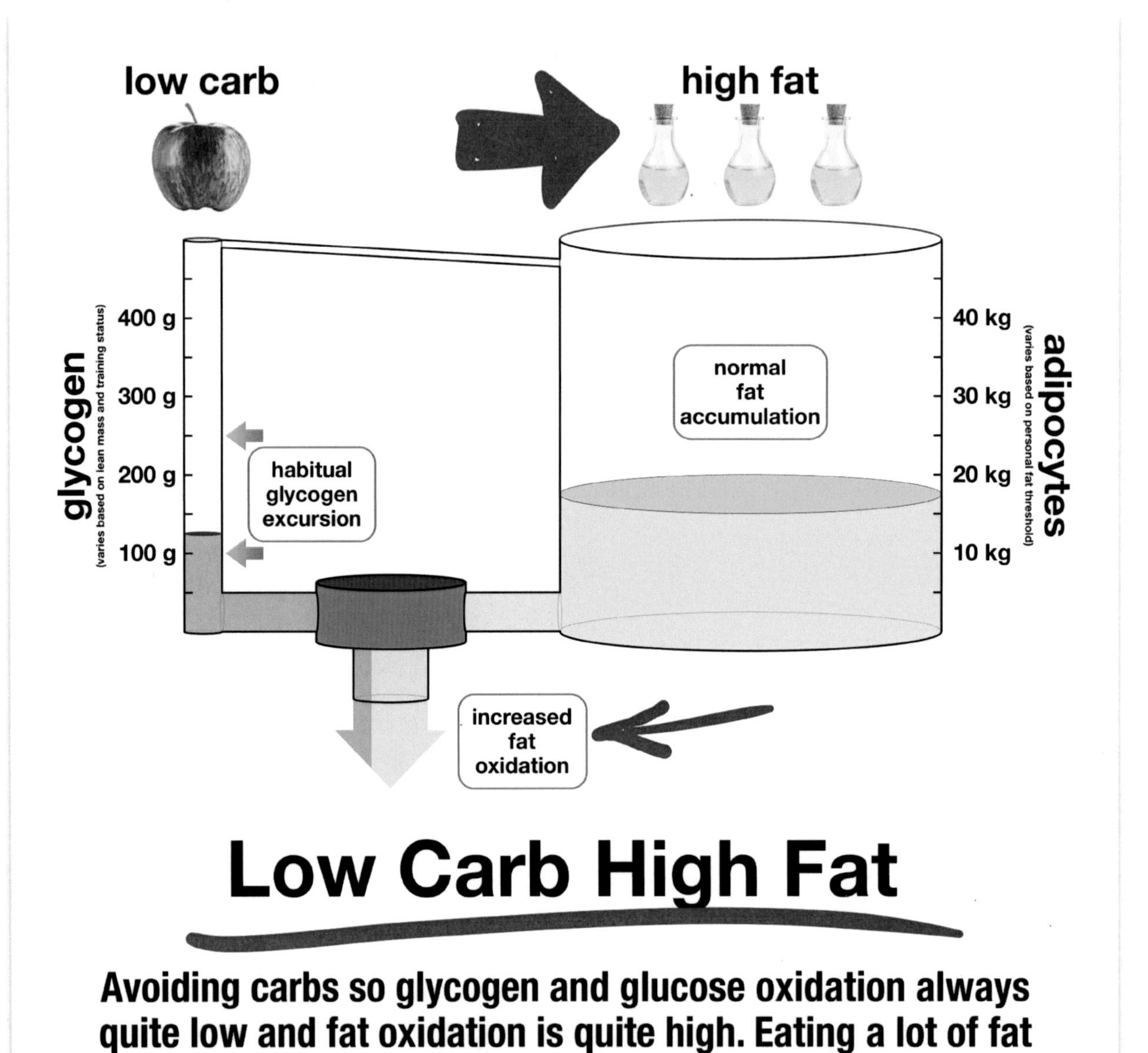

Low Carb Low Fat.

What is left to eat? Pretty much just protein and fiber. This is the diet of your typical bodybuilder or figure competitor. Extremely restrictive but gets you the very best results. These people have the lowest fat mass and unfortunately the highest HUNGER. Probably not sustainable long-term. This is however the ultimate fat loss diet, and we will talk about this in upcoming chapters! Eating less non-fiber carbs (carbs that break down to glucose) and less added fat is pretty much the general idea behind the Protein to Energy strategy in this book. Extremely basic concept, once you get the idea!

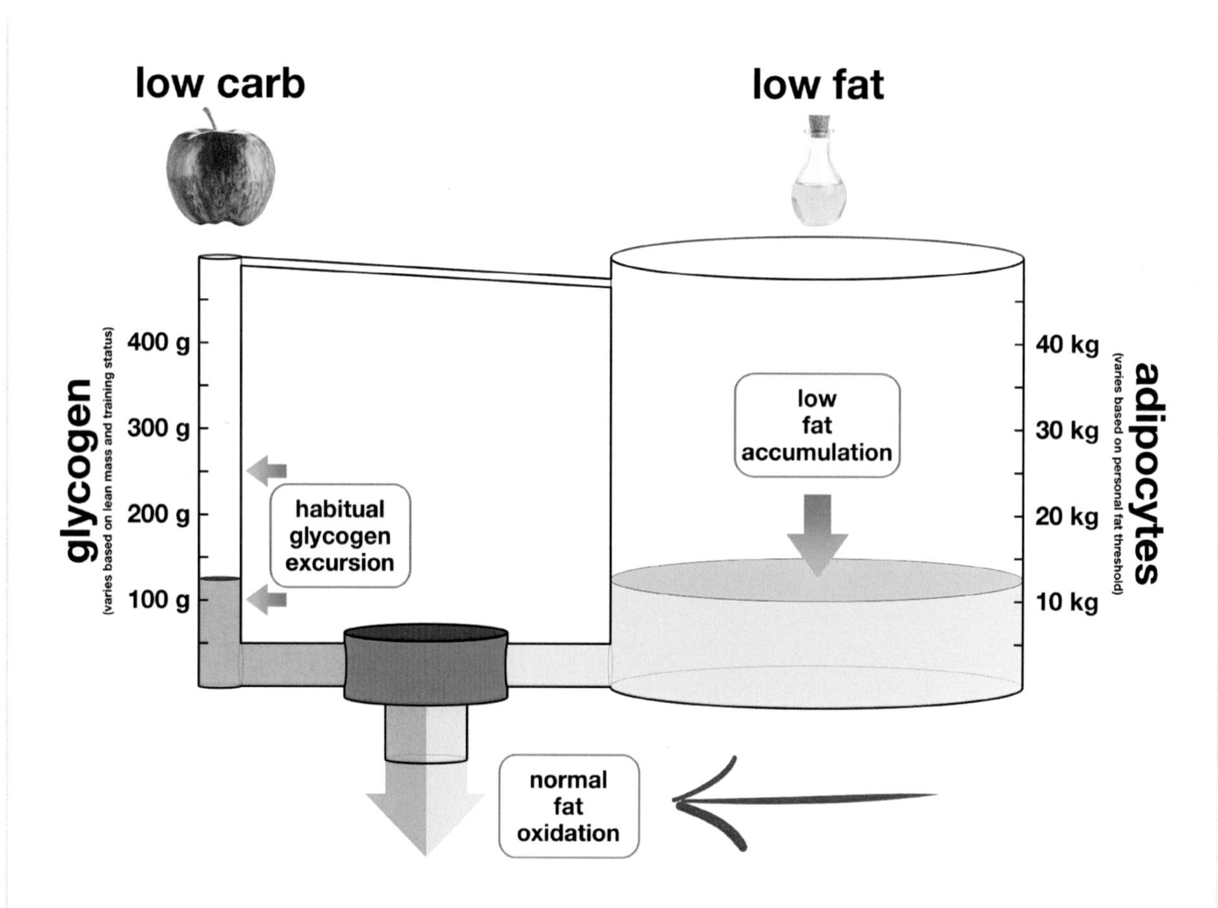

Low Carb Low Fat

Low carb and low fat. Glycogen low and fat oxidation is normal. Typical for bodybuilder or asthetic athlete, eating mostly protein and fiber. Very insulin sensitive, but hungry.

High Carb High Fat.

This is the "Standard American Diet", or highly appropriate acronym: S.A.D. This is the worst. This is also the way everyone around you is eating. Carbs and glucose and glycogen are high, and fat oxidation is lower as a result. Because you are displacing fat oxidation with glucose, all the fat you eat gets stored and not burned. You would probably be fine if you were eating less of either carbs OR fat, but because both are high, the result is a slow and gradual weight accumulation. On average, Americans are currently gaining three pounds of fat per year. And as a result, everyone is just slowly and inexorably getting fatter and fatter until we are all obese.

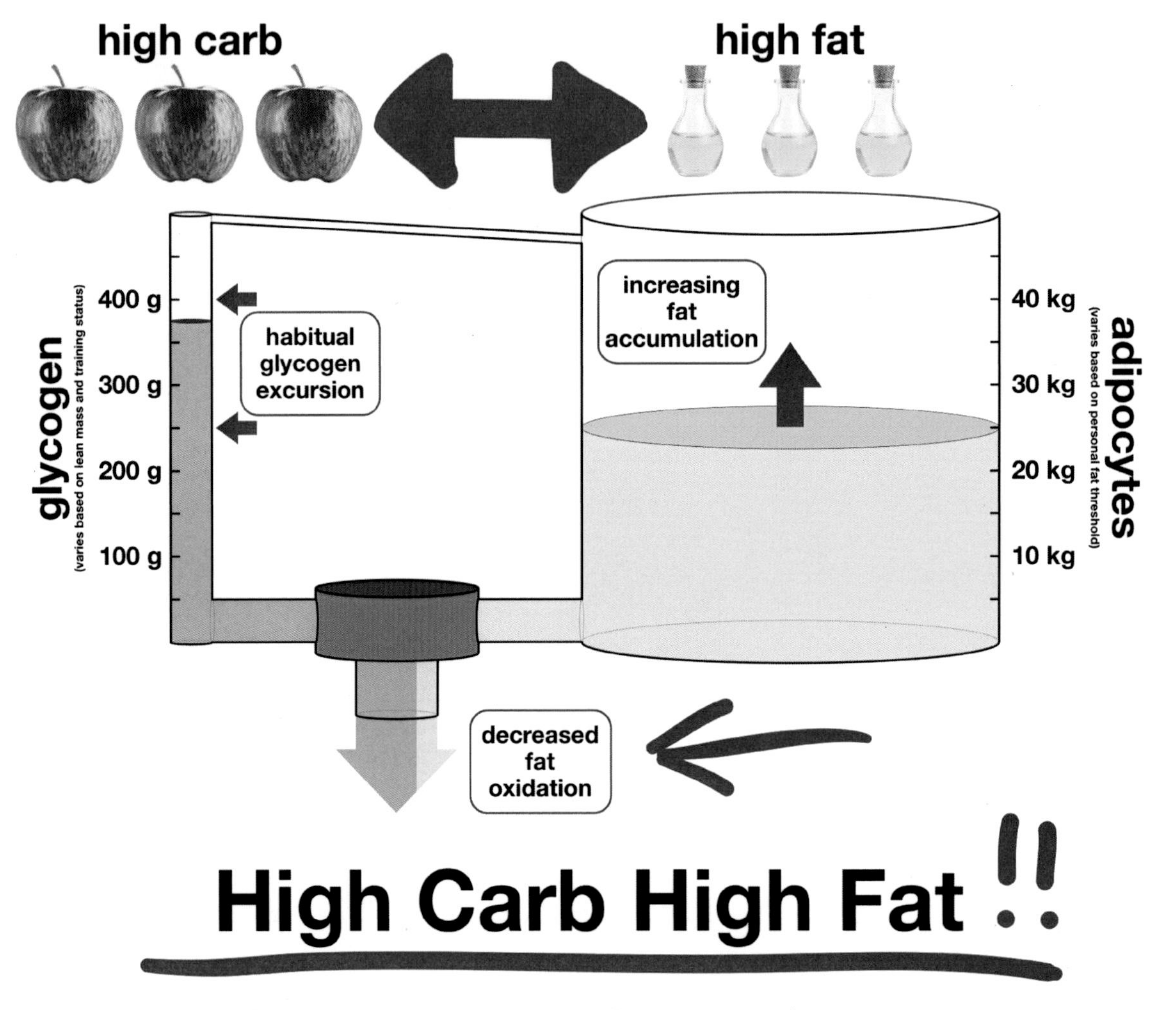

The worst. Standard American Diet. Lots of carbs so glycogen is always high and fat oxidation is low. Also eating fat, so gaining like one pound a year forever.

OBESITY: A 'SETTLING POINT'

Obesity is currently a massive out-of-control global epidemic, with no signs of slowing down. As it turns out, obesity is a 'settling point' where your fat oxidation finally equals your fat intake, despite your chronically high carbohydrate diet. You can reverse obesity with either a low carb or a low fat diet, and of course the most powerful strategy is to reduce BOTH carbs and fats, while increasing the percentage of protein in the diet for satiety.

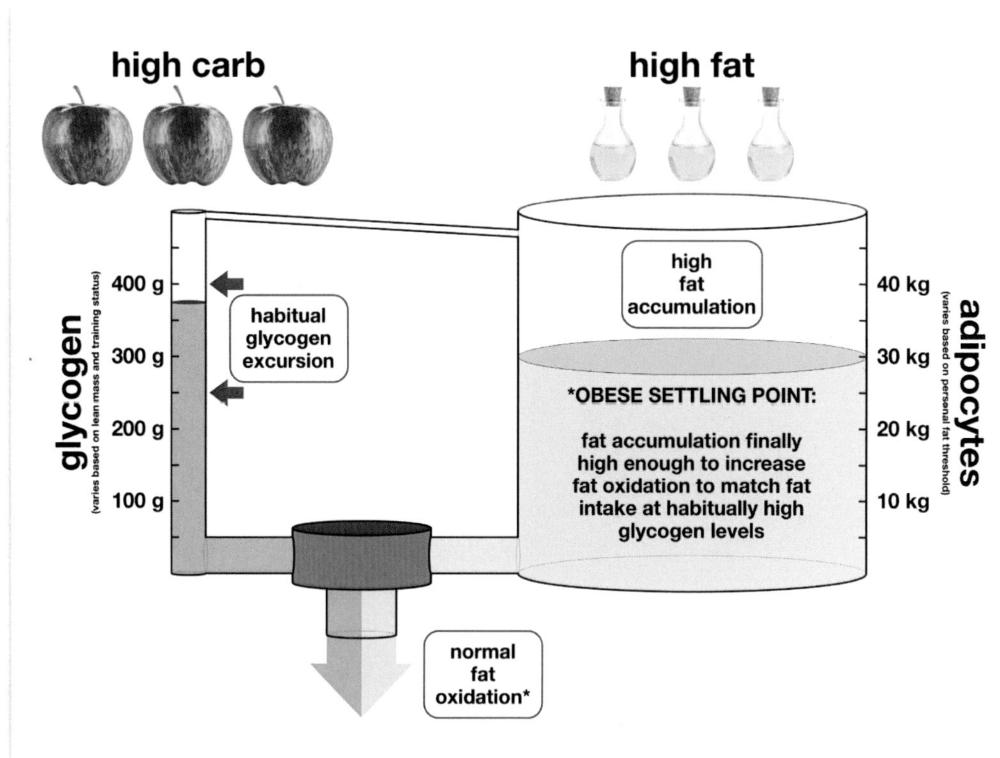

Obesity: Settling Point

As you get fatter, the pressure to oxidize fat goes up and finally at some point you reach the point where your fat oxidation equals your fat intake despite your high glycogen.

Obesity Prevalence, U.S. Adults

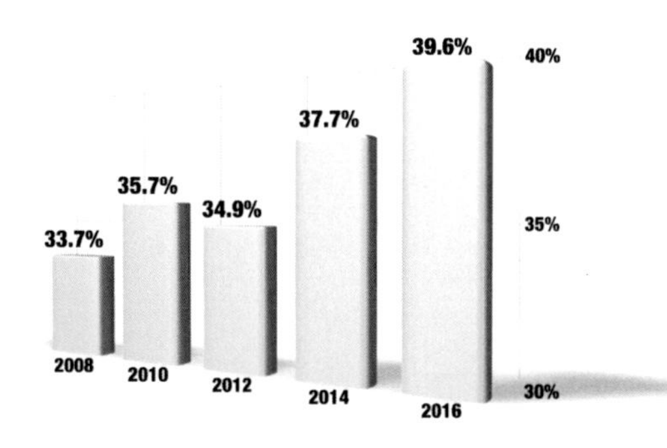

ENERGY TOXICITY

Alzheimer's disease. Asthma. Osteoarthritis. Rheumatoid arthritis. Cancer (especially breast, colorectal, esophageal, uterine, renal, prostate, and pancreatic cancers). Depression. Type 2 diabetes. Fatty liver. Acid reflux. Fibromyalgia. Gout. Sleep apnea. High cholesterol. High blood pressure. Osteoporosis. Stroke. Coronary artery disease and atherosclerosis. Heart failure. Erectile dysfunction. Polycystic ovarian syndrome. Acne. Low testosterone. Enlarged prostate. Gynecomastia. Baldness. Psoriasis. Lupus. Peripheral neuropathy. Glaucoma. Near-sightedness. Vertigo. Tinnitus. Inflammatory bowel disease. Sarcopenia. Tendinopathy. Carpal tunnel syndrome. Hearing loss. Macular degeneration.

We are facing an epidemic of chronic disease. And believe it or not, every one of the chronic ailments mentioned above are associated with one thing: chronically high insulin levels—also known as 'insulin resistance', or 'hyperinsulinemia'.

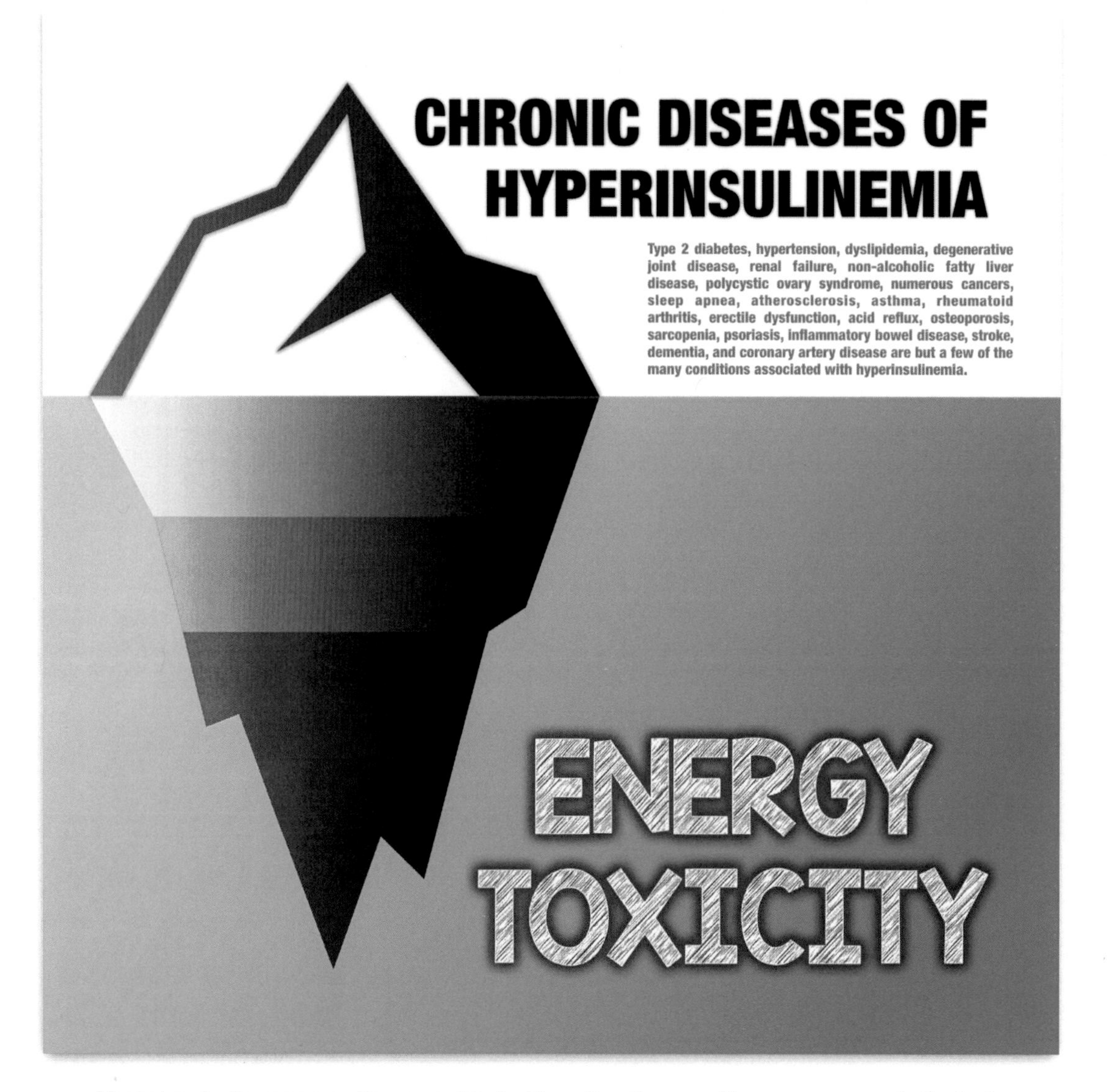

Most chronic diseases are either associated with or directly caused by excess energy in the body.

You may have heard of 'Metabolic Syndrome', another name for insulin resistance—defined by the five following things:

1. **<u>Abdominal obesity (abdominal fat storage, or increased waist circumference).</u>**
2. **<u>High triglycerides.</u>**
3. **<u>Low HDL (or "good") cholesterol.</u>**
4. **<u>High blood pressure.</u>**
5. **<u>High fasting glucose.</u>**

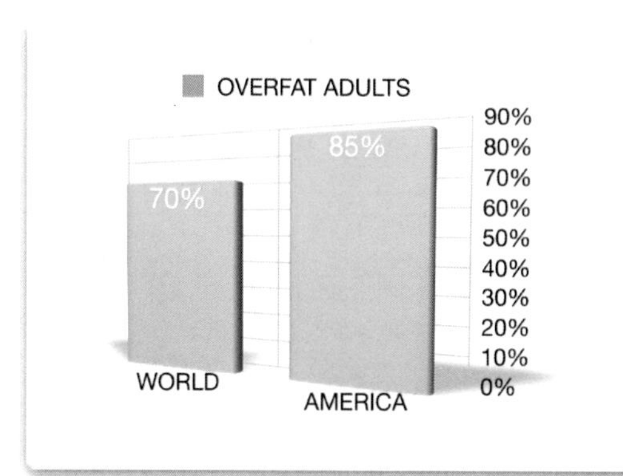

At the moment, over 80% of adult Americans have one or more of these findings. In fact, a recent study showed that only 12% of adult Americans are metabolically healthy (with no sign of insulin resistance). Persons with hyperinsulinemia have abnormally high fasting insulin levels, and also abnormally high insulin secretion after eating.

What is the cause of Metabolic Syndrome? The answer is simple. Overfilling your energy storage capacity. As the adipocytes fill up with fat, they start refusing glucose and triglycerides (fat in the bloodstream). If you continue to eat more energy, it builds up in the circulation. Then insulin—which is a storage hormone—attempts to signal cells to take up more energy but this signal is in vain, since the cells are already full. The result? High insulin all the time, and overflowing energy stores.

Fat cells can expand dramatically in size—but they all have a maximum size limit. Your body first stores fat as harmless subcutaneous fat, just under your skin. Some of this is perfectly great, and not a problem. Some people have the ability to grow new fat cells, and as long as they can sprout new fat cells that have plenty of room for fat storage, then they will remain insulin sensitive and metabolically healthy.

The average human has 30 billion adipocytes, with an average diameter of 0.1 mm each.

As adipocytes approach their maximum size, they become more and more insulin resistant.

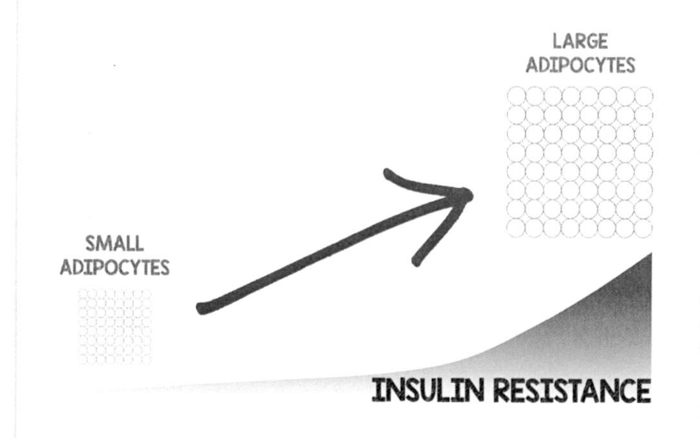

The trouble starts when your subcutaneous cells have reached their maximum size, and you have exceeded your genetically inherited capacity for growing new cells. Once this happens, excess energy "spills over" into your visceral, or abdominal, fat. This increases your waist size and contributes to the dreaded 'apple' body shape that we all know is a killer. As you gain more and more visceral fat, often evidenced by increasing abdominal circumference, you get more and more insulin resistant. Eventually even these visceral fat cells fill up entirely and then your body starts shoving fat anywhere it can, including your organs (fatty liver, for example), and even your blood vessels (not good). By this point, you have reached your personal fat threshold, which is the genetic ceiling for how fat you are capable of getting. Once you have exceeded this, the result is full-blown type 2 diabetes—a condition where the bloodstream is flooded with energy at all times (both glucose and also fat energy in the form of triglycerides).

OVERFILLING YOUR ADIPOCYTES CAUSES INSULIN RESISTANCE.

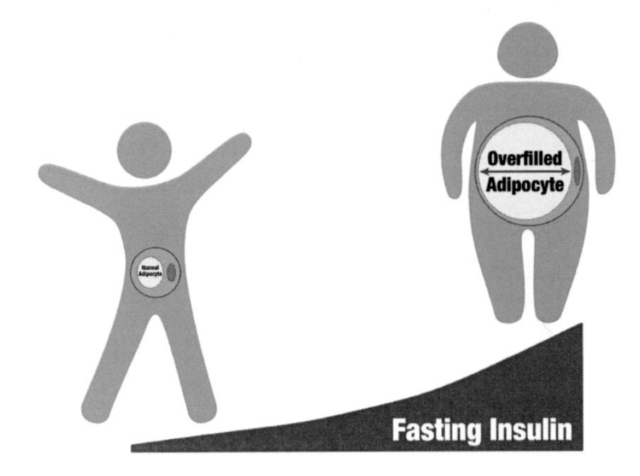

Once you have reached your 'Personal Fat Threshold' and become the most insulin resistant, you really can't get any fatter.

Waist Circumference and Insulin Resistance

Waist circumference is an excellent proxy for overfilled adipocytes, and waist-to-height ratio predicts insulin resistance.

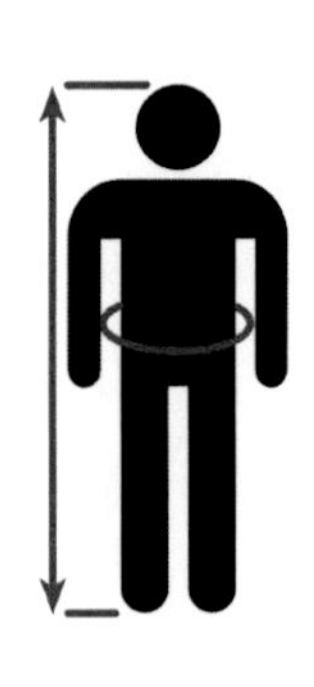

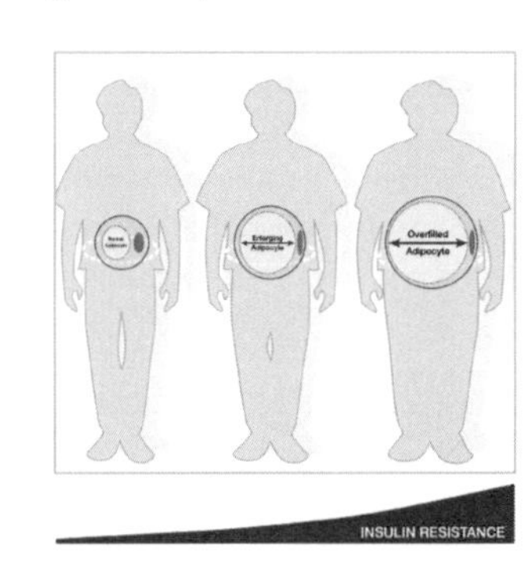

CALCULATING WAIST-TO-HEIGHT RATIO

- Measure height (any units—inches or centimeters).
- Measure waist circumference (using the same units). THIS IS NOT YOUR PANTS SIZE! Must be at the belly button, with abdomen fully relaxed.
- Divide waist by height to get ratio.
- Goal is 0.5 or lower!

Your ability to grow new fat cells and get fatter prior to developing insulin resistance is a genetically determined trait, just like height or eye color. Some people are capable of gaining hundreds of pounds prior to becoming significantly insulin resistant and diabetic. Others, however, might have an incredibly low personal fat threshold, and certain genetic groups of people might develop severe insulin resistance and even type 2 diabetes after only gaining a few pounds of abdominal fat. These people are often 'skinny fat': they look rather lean, maybe with almost no subcutaneous fat, and you might not even notice the abdominal fat storage unless you look very carefully at the waist circumference right at the belly button.

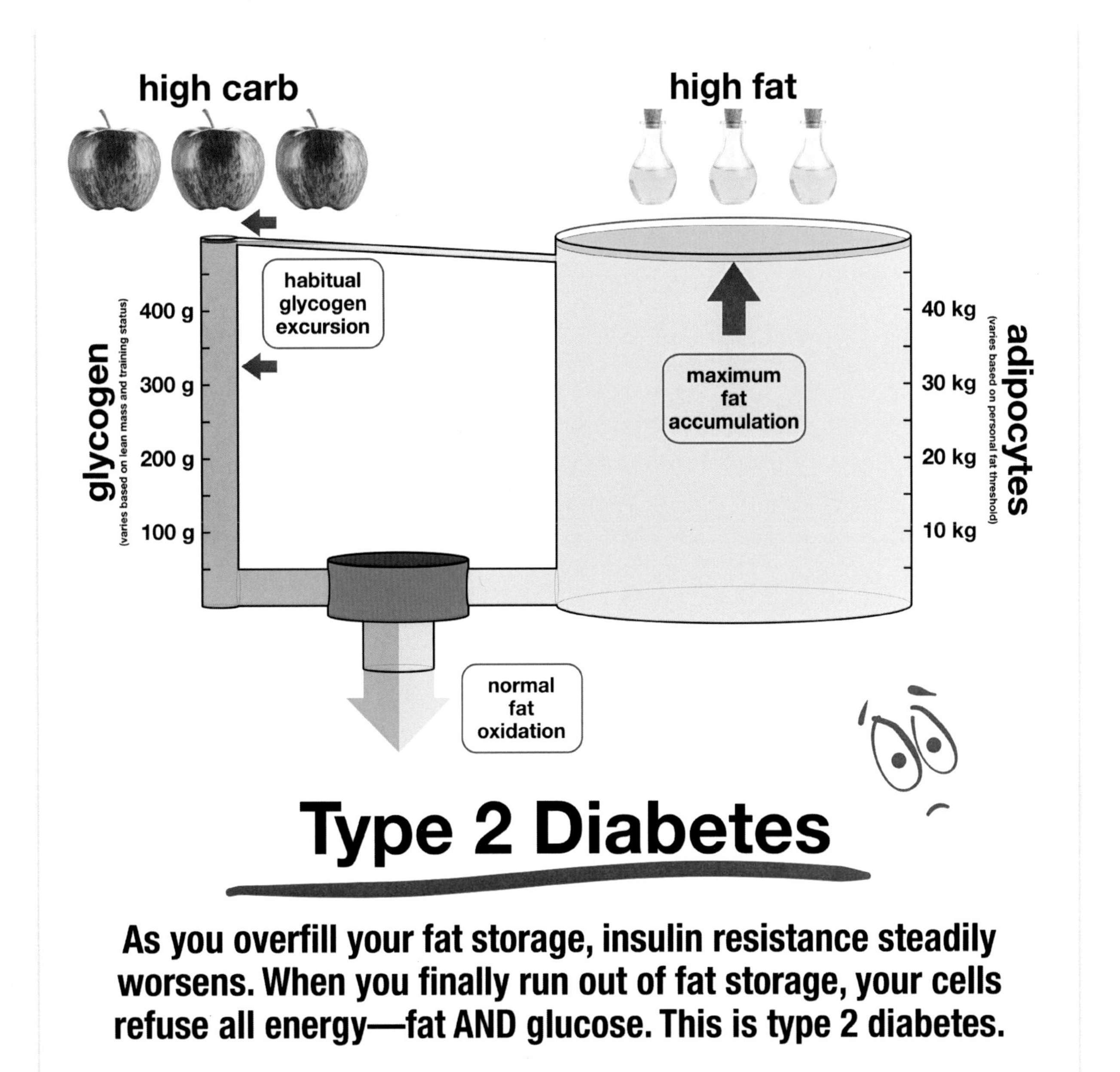

How do you know if you have insulin resistance? Well, waist circumference is an excellent proxy for overfilled abdominal fat cells. Therefore we can use waist circumference as a low-budget estimate of what is going on inside. The easiest way to evaluate your status is measuring your waist-to-height ratio. Divide your waist circumference (measured at the belly button) by your height. Anything under 0.5 is probably fine—and the lower the better. As this number increases, so does the likelihood that you have hyperinsulinemia.

It is also helpful to look for the other markers of Metabolic Syndrome by checking blood pressure plus a fasting lipid panel as well as fasting glucose. Blood pressure should be less than 120/80. Normal fasting glucose is under 100, and 100 or higher is a problem (we diagnose diabetes if it hits 126). Fasting triglycerides should be less than 150 (ideally well under 100, and elite is under 70). HDL ('H' for 'healthy')

Top 3 basic lab tests:

Test	Aim for			
A1C	**Aim for: 5.5% or lower**	**Amazing: < 5.0%**	**Ok: 5.0 — 5.6%**	**Prediabetes: > 5.6%**
TRIGLYCERIDES*	**Aim for: Under 100**	**Elite: <70 mg/dL**	**Ok: 70 — 150 mg/dL**	**High: >150 mg/dL**
HDL	**Aim for: Over 50**	**Too Low: <40 mg/dL**	**Ok: 40—60 mg/dL**	**Superb: >60 mg/dL**

*This is for FASTING triglycerides. Draw blood after consuming no calories for 9–12 hours.

cholesterol should be 40 or higher in men and 50 or higher in women—the higher the better. Typically, your goal is to have the LOWEST triglycerides and the HIGHEST HDL. Both of them are excellent predictors of insulin sensitivity, and in fact you can combine the two together in a 'triglyceride/HDL ratio', which dramatically increases their predictive value. You really want triglycerides divided by HDL (triglyceride/HDL ratio) to be 2.0 or lower, and elite would be 1.0 or lower—the lower the better. Anything over 3.0 is a huge problem, and the amount of concern should go up proportionately with this number!

Type 2 diabetes is the end stage of insulin resistance, which is the end stage of being 'overfat'—exceeding your fat storage capabilities. Along this entire spectrum, the primary problem is storing too much energy in your body.

Type 2 diabetes is 100% preventable.

How?

Increase the nutrient to energy ratio of your diet.

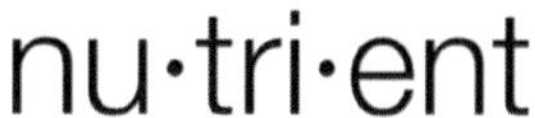

/ˈn(y)o͞otrēənt/

a substance that provides nourishment essential for growth and the maintenance of life.
"fish is a source of many important nutrients, including protein, vitamins, and minerals"

noun: **nutrient**; plural noun: **nutrients**

Origin LATIN nutrire

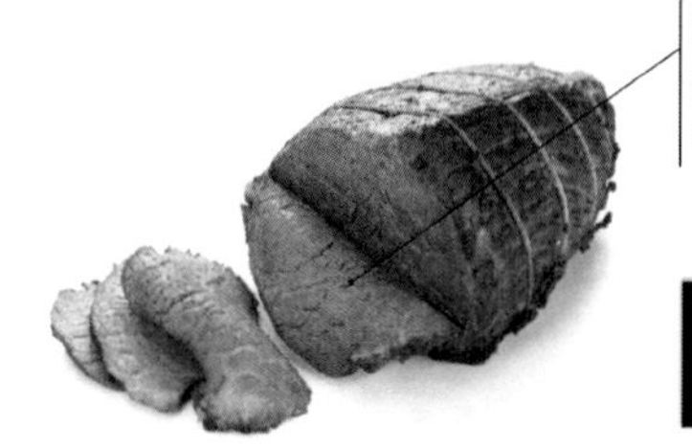

Protein is the most essential nutrient.

Whole food fat is an essential nutrient.

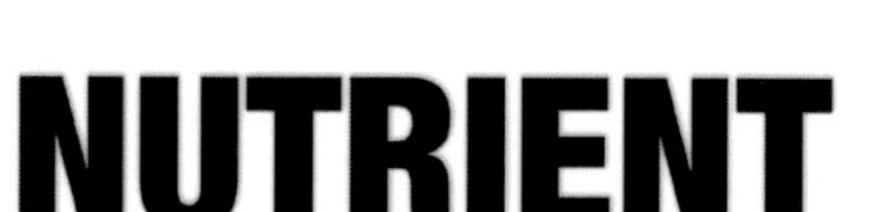

ENERGY

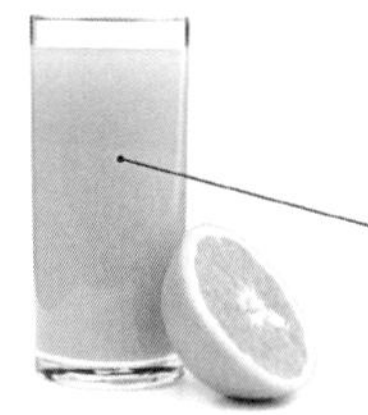

Carbohydrates exist ONLY to provide energy.

Added fat only provides extra energy.

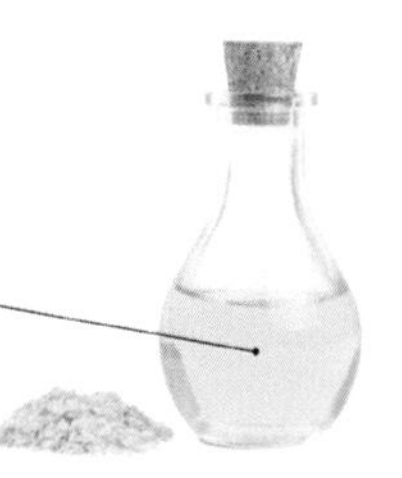

And how does this occur? You guessed it: eating too much energy.

Type 2 diabetes is entirely preventable. Protein is an essential nutrient. Minerals are an essential nutrient, and they tend to follow protein. Certain fats are essential, and these follow protein as well. But there are two things that are completely non-essential in the human diet: refined carbs and refined fats. These exist only to provide extra—and perhaps excessive—ENERGY to your diet. So how do you prevent the entire spectrum of diseases downstream of being 'overfat'? Target protein and avoid added energy. On a practical level, this looks like constantly being either low carb, low fat, high protein, or some combination of all three. More on this later!

BEING INSULIN RESISTANT DOES NOT MAKE YOU FAT—

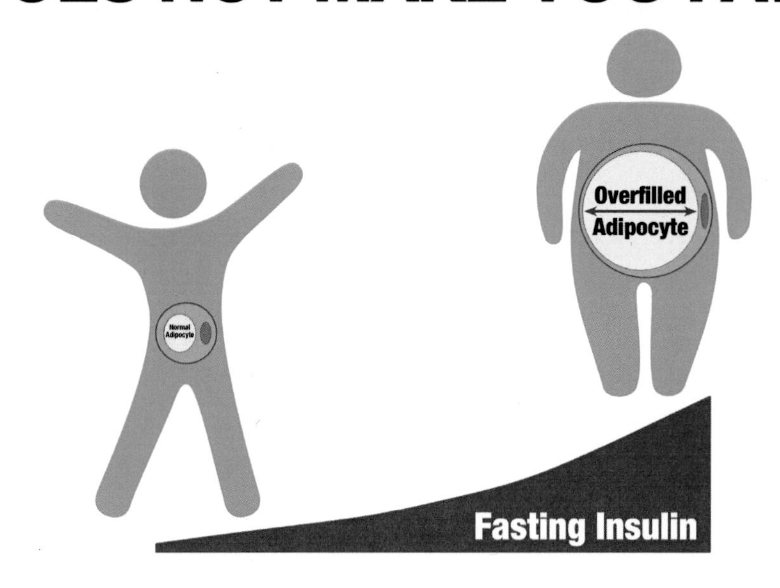

—BEING FAT MAKES YOU INSULIN RESISTANT.

In fact, once you have reached your 'Personal Fat Threshold' and become the most insulin resistant, you really can't get any fatter.

A lot of people mistakenly believe that they are overweight because they are insulin resistant, when it is always the other way around: chronically exceeding your energy tolerance leads to excessive fat storage in the adipocytes — the actual cause of insulin resistance ('metabolic syndrome'). Anything that leads to weight loss will improve insulin resistance.

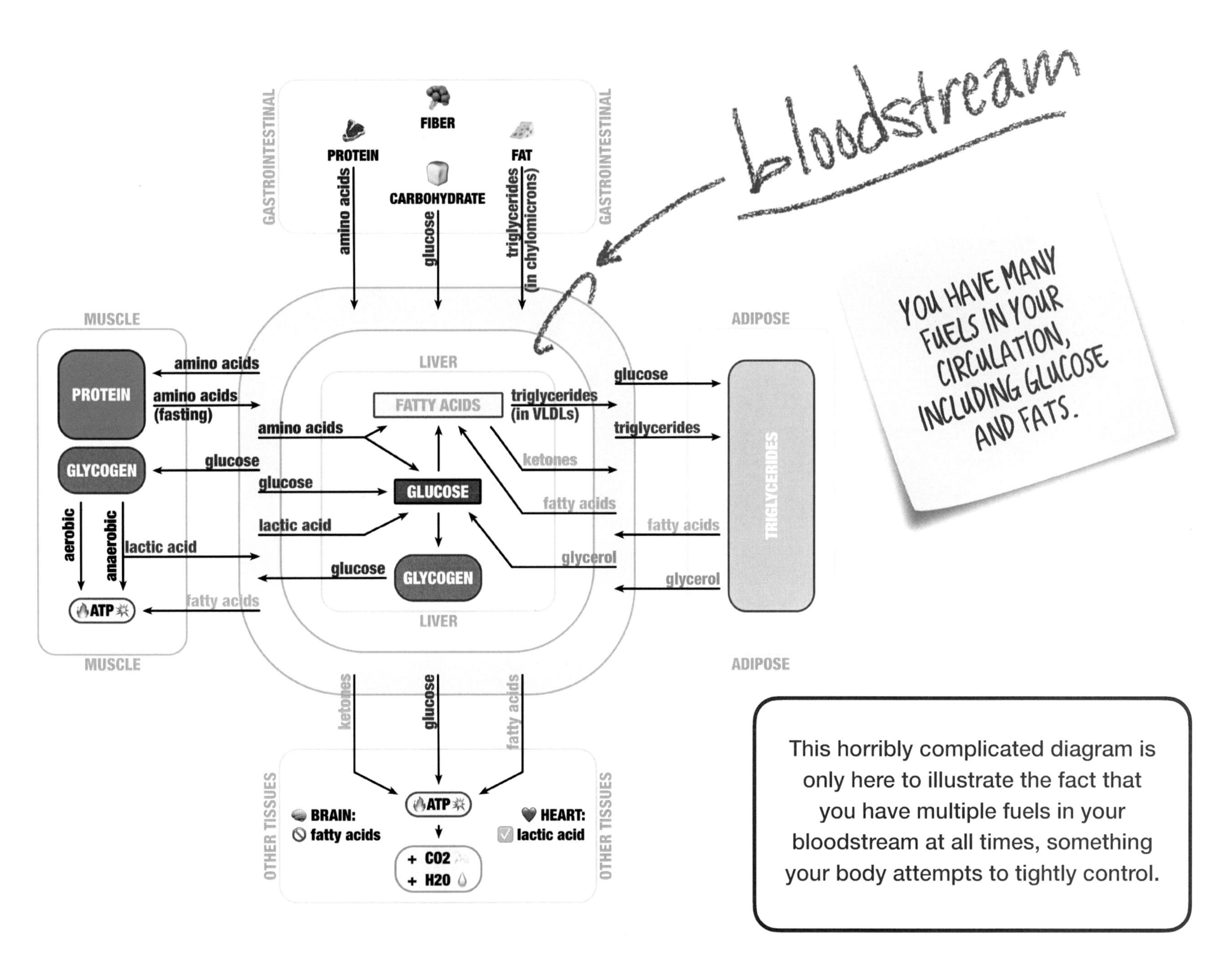

This horribly complicated diagram is only here to illustrate the fact that you have multiple fuels in your bloodstream at all times, something your body attempts to tightly control.

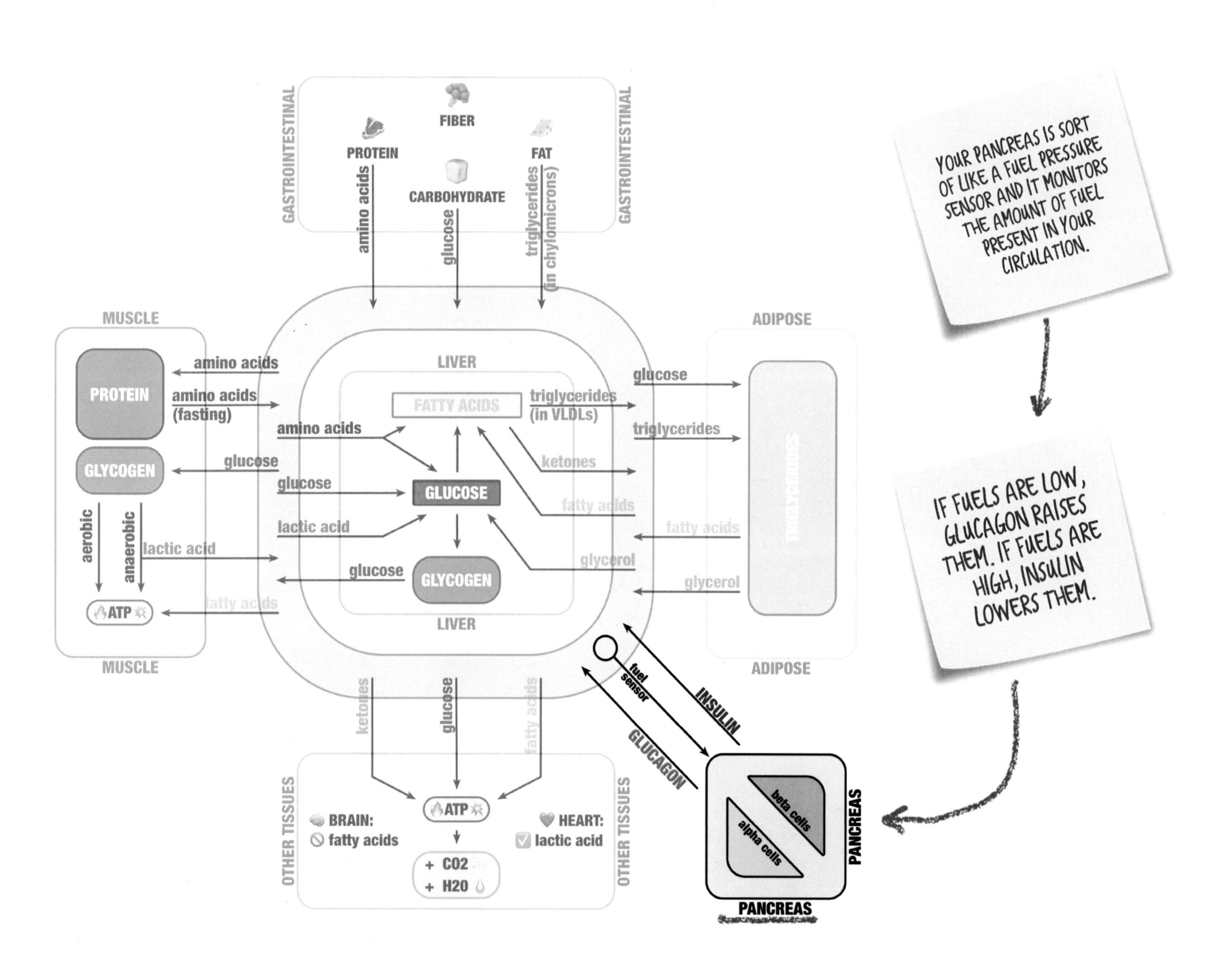
GASTROINTESTINAL
FIBER
PROTEIN
FAT
CARBOHYDRATE
amino acids
glucose
triglycerides (in chylomicrons)
MUSCLE
PROTEIN
amino acids
amino acids (fasting)
GLYCOGEN
glucose
aerobic
anaerobic
lactic acid
ATP
fatty acids
LIVER
FATTY ACIDS
amino acids
glucose
GLUCOSE
lactic acid
glucose
GLYCOGEN
triglycerides (in VLDLs)
ketones
fatty acids
glycerol
ADIPOSE
glucose
triglycerides
TRIGLYCERIDES
fatty acids
glycerol
ketones
glucose
fatty acids
OTHER TISSUES
BRAIN:
fatty acids
ATP
+ CO2
+ H20
HEART:
lactic acid
fuel sensor
INSULIN
GLUCAGON
beta cells
alpha cells
PANCREAS
YOUR PANCREAS IS SORT OF LIKE A FUEL PRESSURE SENSOR AND IT MONITORS THE AMOUNT OF FUEL PRESENT IN YOUR CIRCULATION.
IF FUELS ARE LOW, GLUCAGON RAISES THEM. IF FUELS ARE HIGH, INSULIN LOWERS THEM.

Insulin Resistance

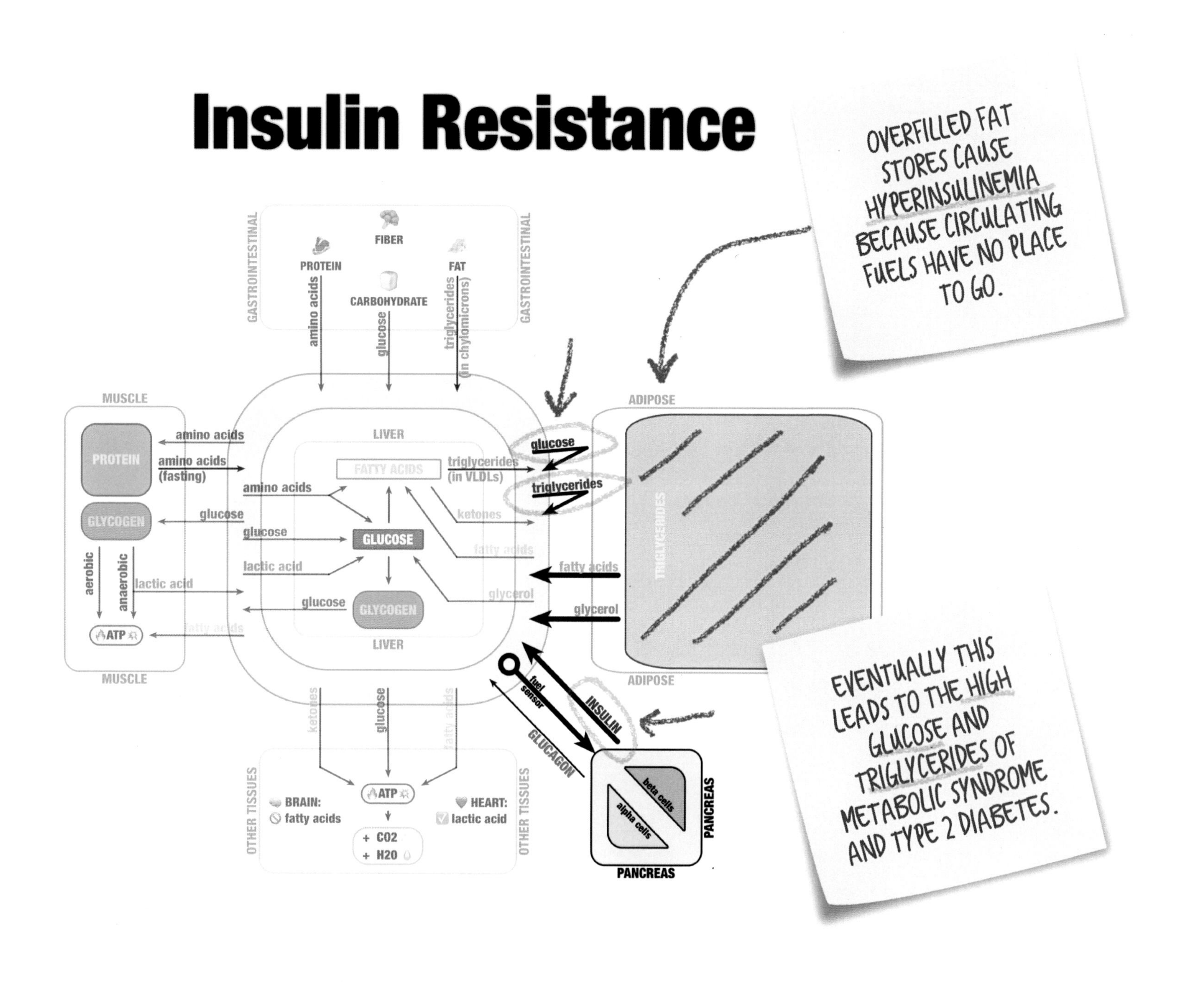

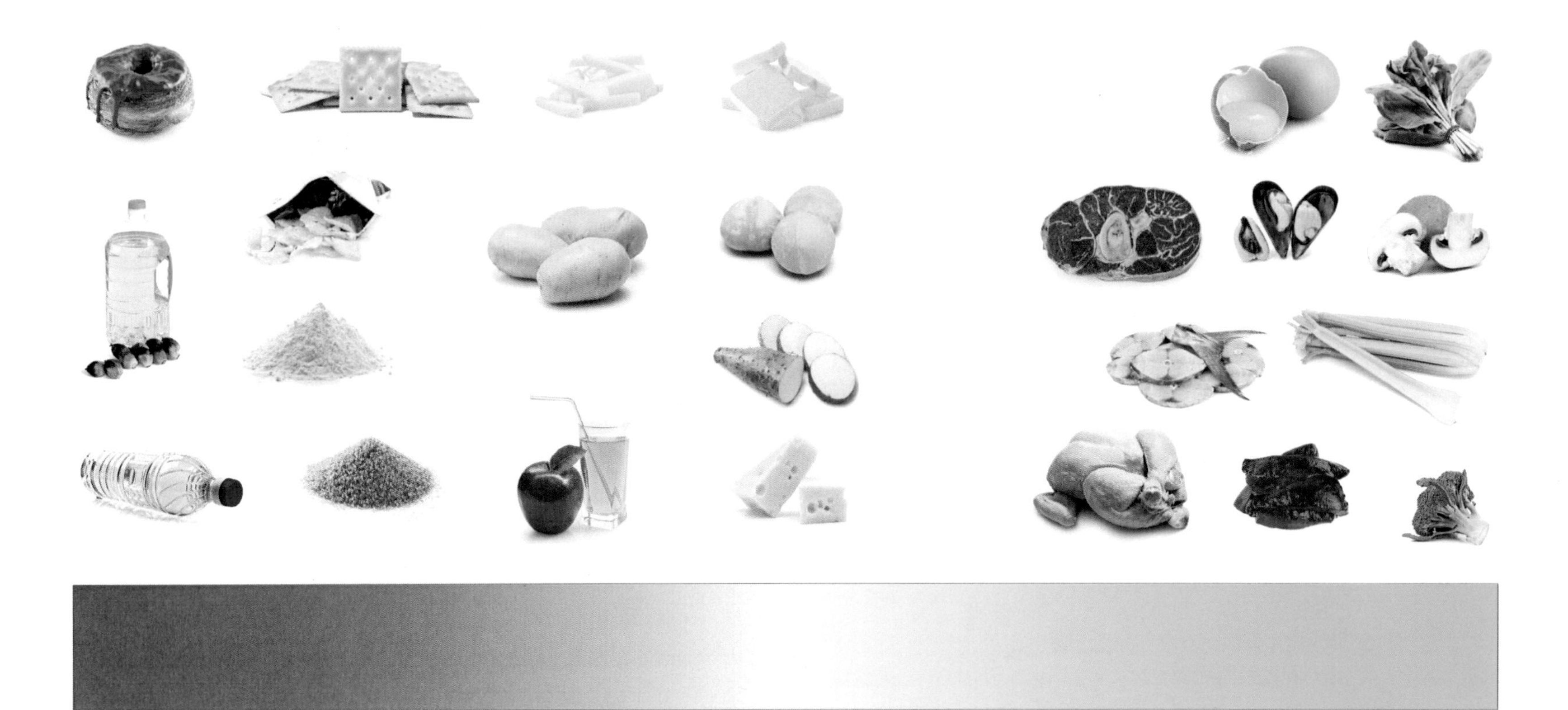

PURE ENERGY
Minimum Nutrient Density

PURE NUTRITION
Maximum Nutrient Density

Beware of processing that separates food ENERGY from its NUTRITION, leaving you with nutrient-devoid "edible products" — devitalized dead food which provides dangerously high energy with no micronutrient satiety.

THIS IS THE CAUSE OF INSULIN RESISTANCE AND OBESITY

CARBS + FAT

Ok, so far we have established that we are eating way more energy than we should. And we have established that a big driver of this phenomenon is the dilution of protein in our food supply due to a massive influx of sugar, flour, and oil —the cheap and plentiful agricultural energy sources that comprise the majority of the modern diet. But there is more to this story than pure protein dilution with carbs and fat.

We humans are hard-wired to seek out nutrients. We have a hunger for protein and minerals. Studies show that humans on a low protein diet have an increased craving for savory snacks, and salt restriction increases a craving for salty foods. Our nutrient hunger will drive us to eat and eat until we get the protein and minerals that we need to survive. Similarly, we are driven to seek out energy in our diets as well.

If eating wasn't somewhat pleasurable, it would be a huge chore. Like brushing your teeth. We would all forget to eat or

CARBS + FAT

This combination is rarely found in nature.

These foods produce drug-like dopamine reward in the brain and are highly addictive.

You can create obesity in any omnivore mammal with these junk foods.

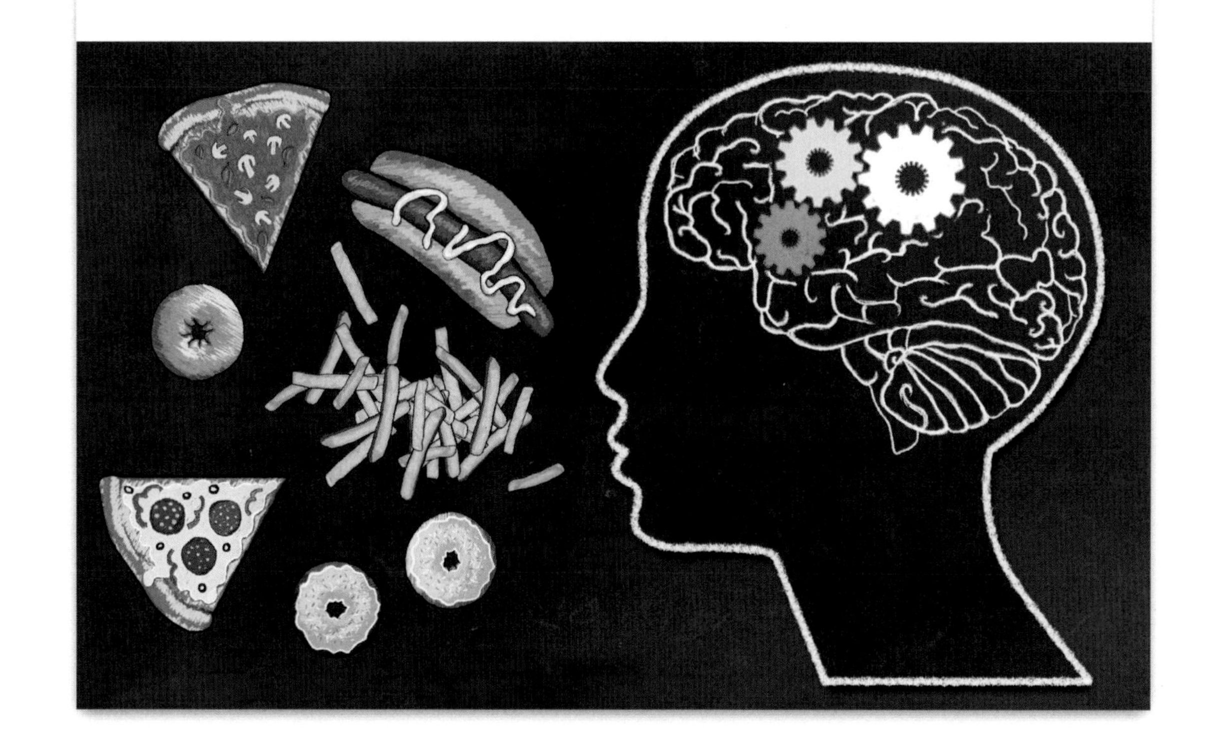

just procrastinate to the point of almost dying from starvation. Mother Nature understands this. As a result, everything we have evolved to require for success as a species brings some intrinsic reward along with it. Most would agree that the act of procreation, for example, can be quite rewarding—this reward helps to perpetuate our species. Similarly, we have a certain amount of reward when we eat energy. Carbs can be rewarding. Fat can be rewarding. But the most rewarding? Carbs and fats together. And the most rewarding food on earth? High carb, high fat, AND high energy density. These foods are EXTREMELY rewarding! And by rewarding, we are talking about the pure addictive chemistry of spiking dopamine in your brain, not unlike a drug.

Studies show that you can feed a high carb, high fat, and high energy density diet (picture a candy bar) to any omnivore mammal (human, rat, etc) and the majority of them will immediately overeat by around 30-40% of calories. A small number of humans and animals will spontaneously increase energy expenditure to successfully avoid weight gain, but the majority will immediately become overfat.

The combination of carbs and fats together is uniquely addictive, and drives overeating like nothing else. If you ask people which foods they find problematic when it comes to overeating, the responses are all foods that are high in carbs and fat and energy density. You

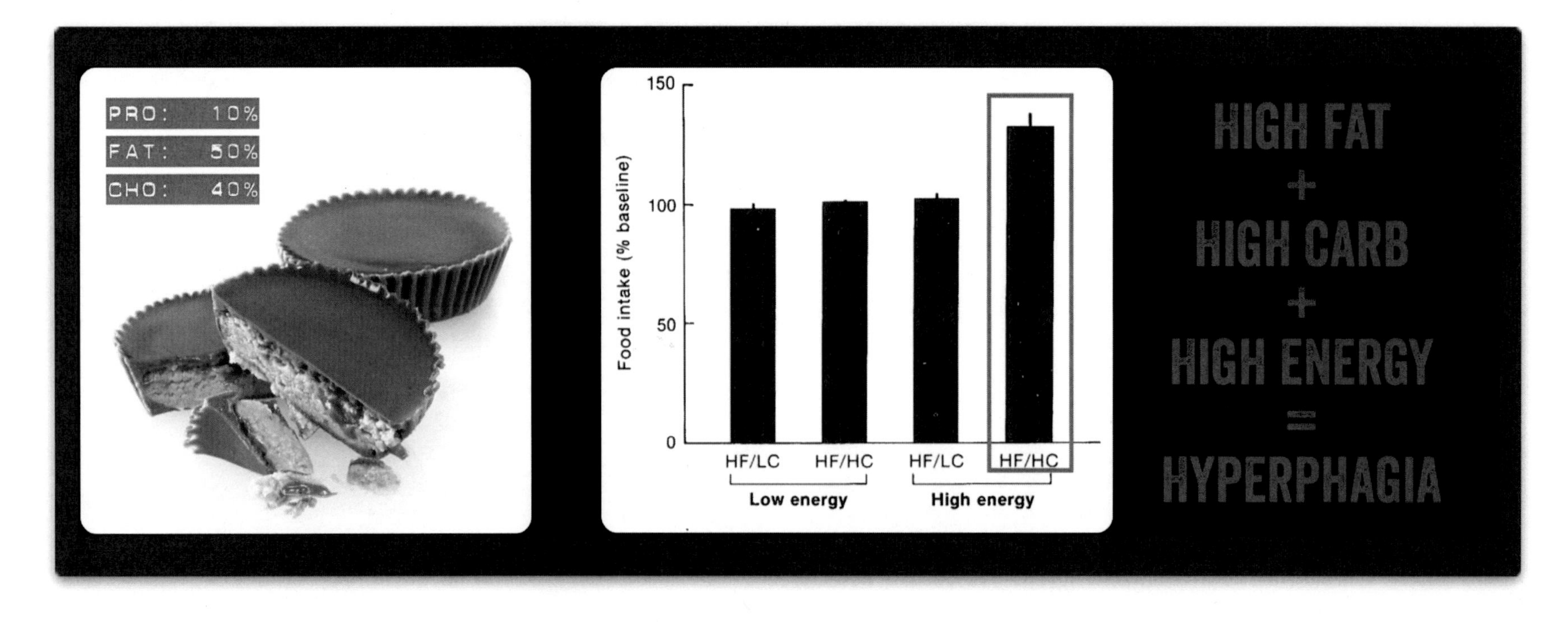

know the list. Doughnuts. Pizza. Ice cream. Chocolate. Cake. French fries. Potato chips. Candy bars. Few people would just crave a stick of butter by itself. And we don't know anyone who would just eat a pound of flour and then a pound of sugar. But combine sugar, flour, and butter together and you have SHORTBREAD, which is so amazingly rewarding that we're pretty sure you could eat your body weight in shortbread right now. No matter how full you are, there is always more room for these foods. Imagine you just ate a large and satisfying meal with a huge delicious ribeye and a salad. You are completely full and feeling good. At this point, you have certainly achieved NUTRITIONAL

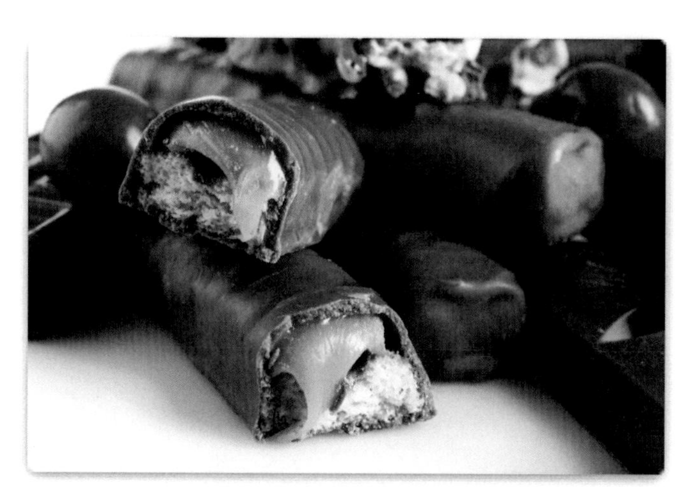

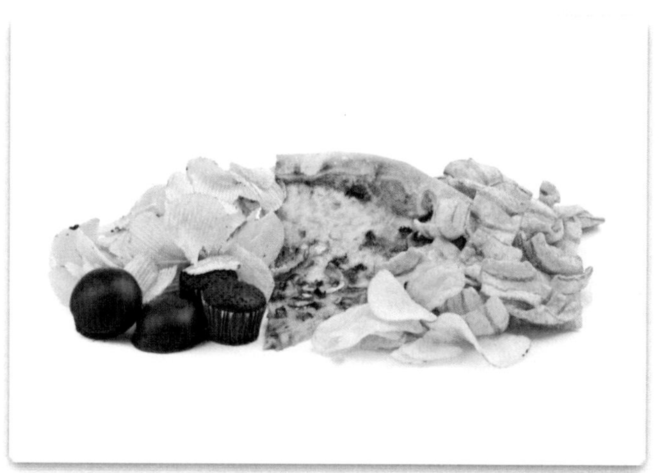

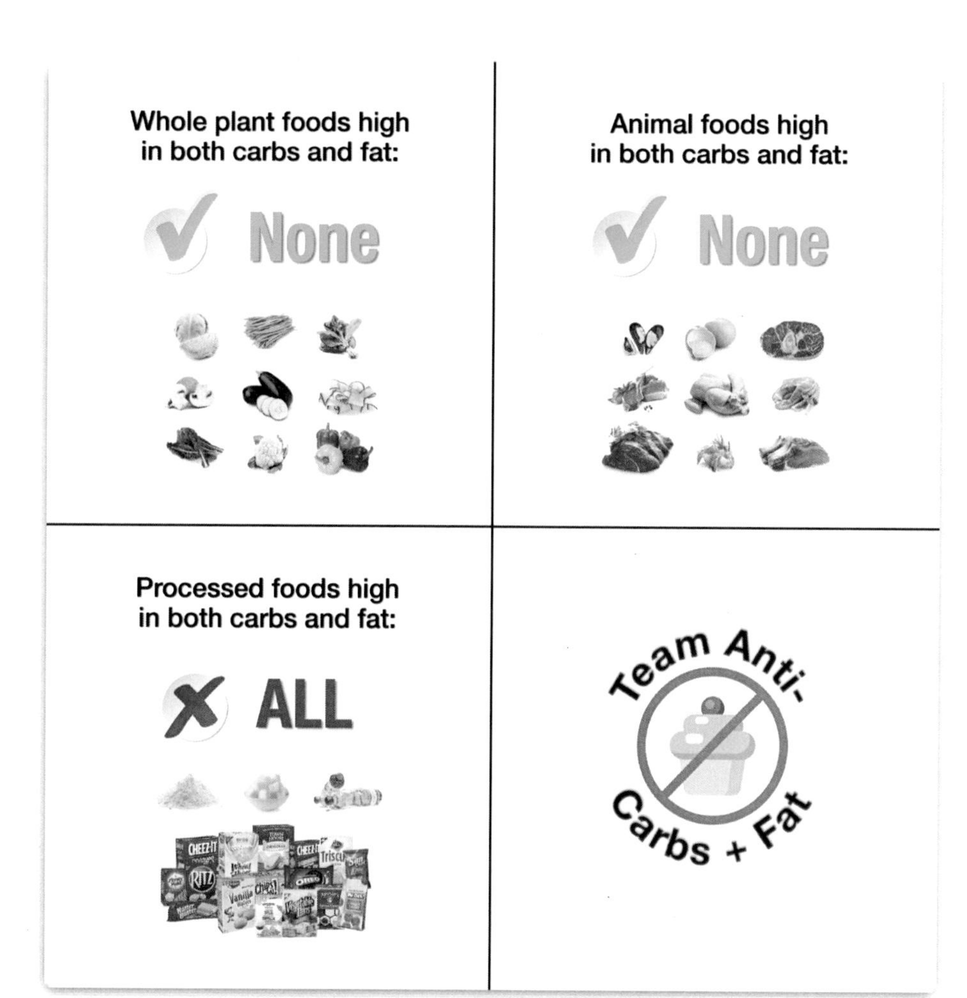

satiety. But then out comes some ice cream. Pure energy in the form of pure carbs and fats together, with an incredibly high energy density. Are you going to eat this too, even though you are 'full'? Because you have experienced the reward this food has to offer, the answer is frequently 'HELL YES'!

The combination of carbs and fats together is unique in how incredibly rewarding it can be. But it is also unique in one other way: this combination rarely occurs in nature! Wait, what?? Yup. Think about it. What foods in nature are high in both carbs AND fat at the same time? Plenty of foods are high in carbs. And plenty of foods are high in fat. But very few are high in both at the same time. There are two notable exceptions. The first one is mammalian milk. Milk is VERY high in energy—both carbs, in the form of lactose, and milkfat. All mammalian milk is high in both carb and fat energy for very good reasons. This food is designed to drive as much overeating as possible, because you really want to turn a small baby mammal into a larger mammal as fast as possible to ensure its viability. The second food in nature that is high in carbs and fat at the same time? Certain nuts, like acorns. Yup. This autumnal food (which is sort of the plant version of milk, now that we think about it) helps drive fat storage in squirrels and bears and other animals that need to store enough fat to survive the wintertime.

Because all food energy—carbs and fats—is solar energy which has been converted to chemical energy by plants, we see the very highest levels of dietary energy at the end of summertime. Plant carbohydrates are at their peak, and animals

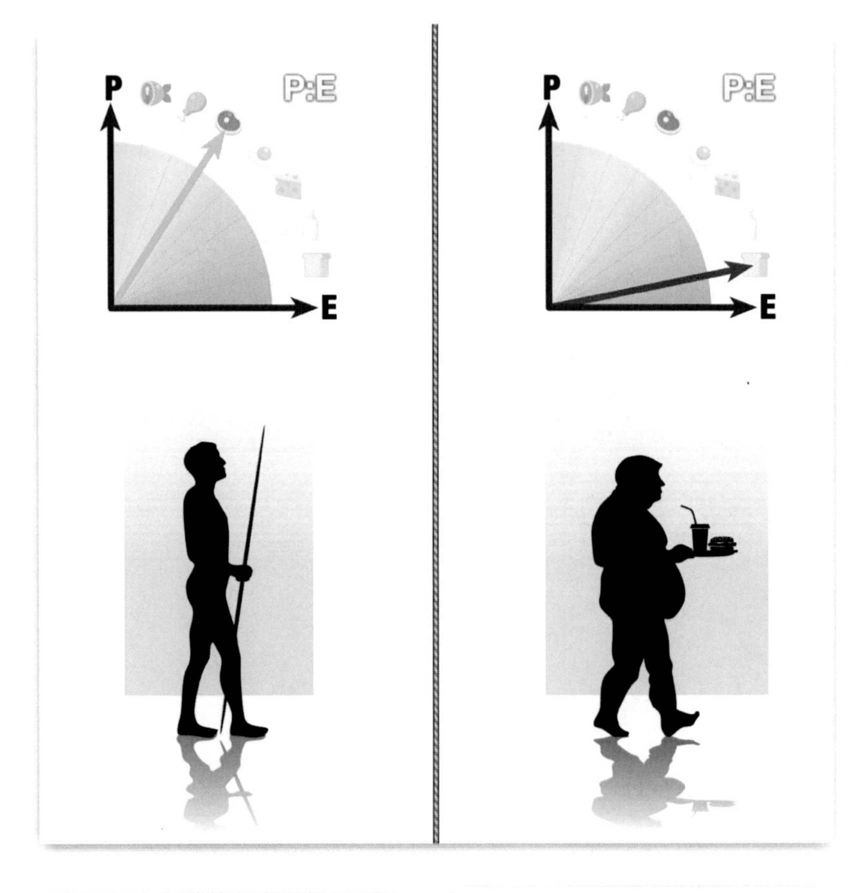

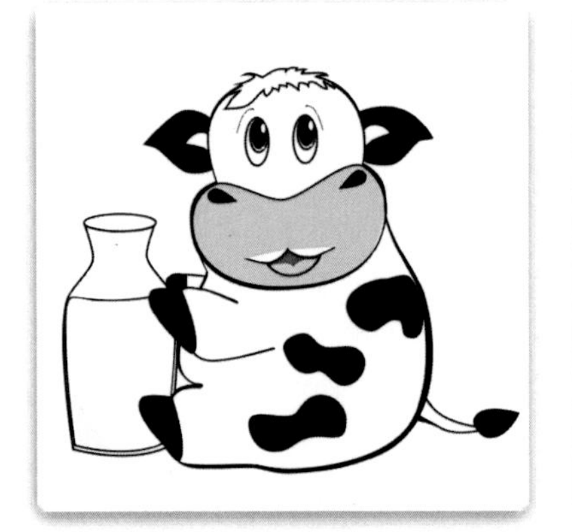

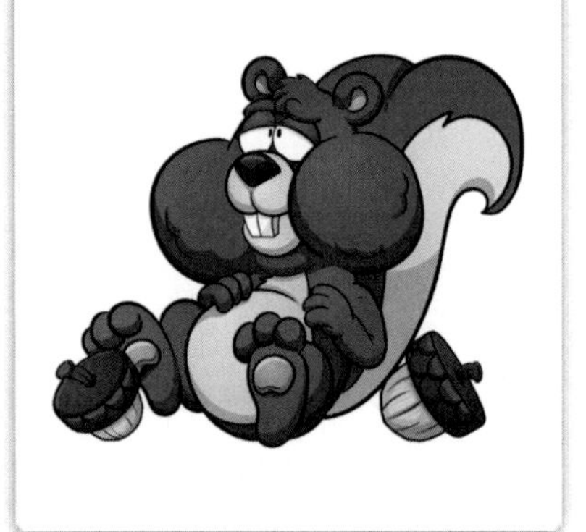

are at their fattest. So herbivores get the highest amount of carbohydrate energy from plants, and carnivores also get the highest amount of energy (animal fat from fatter animals). Omnivores get the best of both worlds, and your bear who is eating berries and acorns and fattier fish et cetera is going to gain plenty of extra fat energy on its body to help it survive the winter. In the winter, plant carbohydrates are scarce to non-existent. Similarly, animals are much leaner because they too are trying to find enough dietary energy to survive. As a result, the energy content of all plants and animals falls considerably. It is this wintertime diet—high in protein percentage but lower in carbs and fats—that we are trying to emulate with the Protein:Energy concept when our goal is fat loss.

So now we know that obesity is contributed to by carbs and

Fat and glucose are oxidized reciprocally in your cells.

The intracellular availability of GLUCOSE, not fat, controls the substrate that is oxidized for energy.

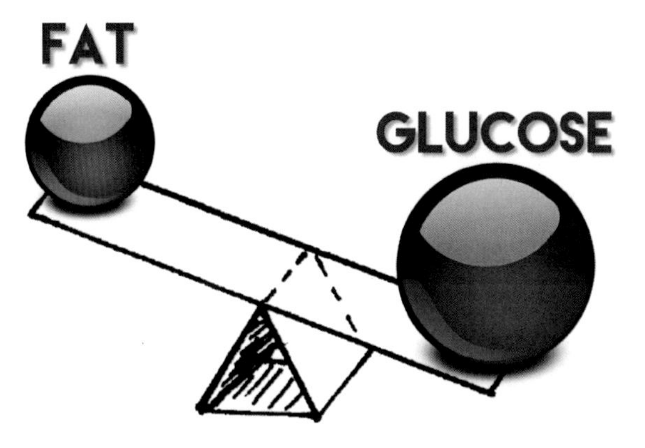

This system worked brilliantly for allowing maximum fat storage in times of high energy, back when increased carbohydrates and fats were only seasonally available.

But eating this way long-term breaks the system.

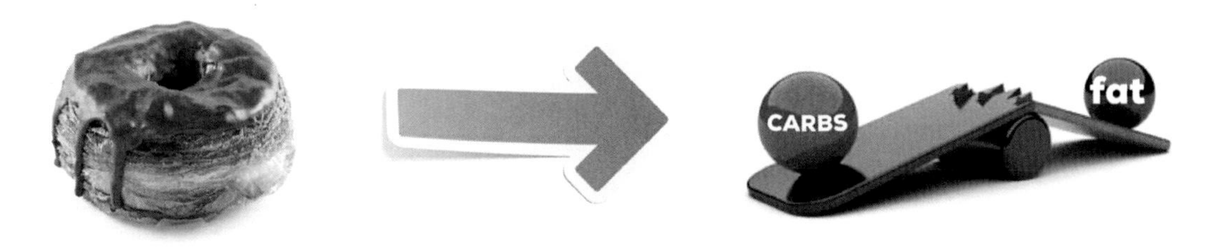

fats in two ways. First of all, this non-protein energy dilutes the protein and minerals in our diet to the point that we have to eat more energy just to satisfy our NUTRIENT HUNGER, or need for protein and minerals. Secondly, the rarely-found-in-nature-but-found-in-all-junk-food combination of carbs and fats together is uniquely rewarding and addictive and drives overeating in a way that was helpful during most of our human evolution—but has now turned against us in the modern food environment.

How do we fight back? Target protein and minerals, and simultaneously try to be either low fat or low

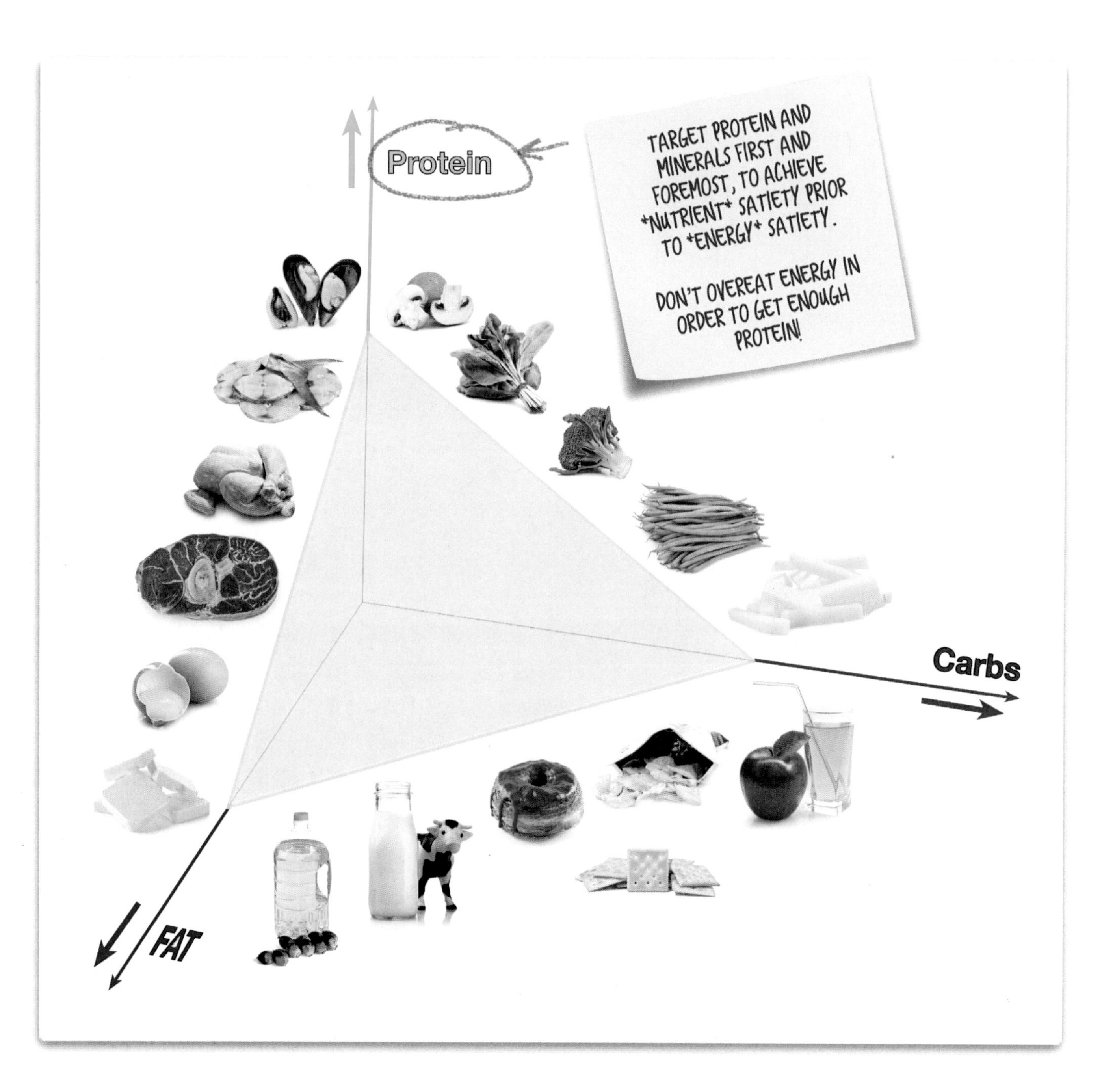

carb at all times. The Protein:Energy approach just so happens to check both of these boxes, which is why it is so darn effective. Eating whole foods is a pretty easy way to avoid the carbs+fat combo, as long as you avoid nuts and dairy (or at least MILK—fermented dairy seems to be better as the carbohydrates are mostly gone). Learn to recognize the fake man-made foods that surround us that use the deadly combination of carbs plus fat, as well as low protein and minerals.

Obesity is simultaneously pushed forward by the dilution of protein and minerals, and pulled forward by the frequent co-ingestion of carbohydrates and fat.

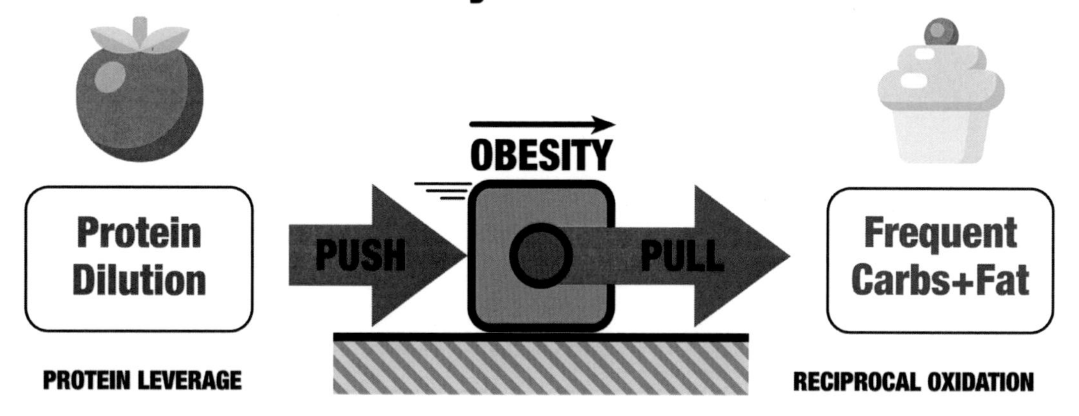

Dilution of protein and minerals with carbohydrates and/or fats requires overingestion of this non-protein energy to achieve the same protein satiety.

Carbs displace fat oxidation and fat passively accumulates. Subsequent glucose dependence and inadequate fat adaptation drives hunger.

Potential Solutions:

1. Low carbohydrate diet.
2. Low fat diet.
3. High protein diet.
4. Avoid refined carbohydrates and fats with any whole foods diet.

Potential Solutions:

1. Low carbohydrate diet.
2. Low fat diet.
3. High protein diet.
4. Any whole foods diet.
5. Eat less frequently (intermittent).

Nutrient hunger from protein dilution and the addictive nature of carbs and fats together both drive obesity.

AVOID THE TRIFECTA

Foods that are simultaneously high in carbs, fat, and energy density are the very worst. Avoid. Try not to eat high density carbs (sugar, etc). Try not to eat high density fats (oils, etc). And especially try not to eat these two together! Almost all successful diet strategies use this same technique, and avoiding this triple combination is one of the cornerstones of The P:E Diet.

What do we mean by 'energy density'? This is typically a refined carb or fat that has a high amount of energy per weight of food. For example, a steak and a potato would be carbs and fats together. But the energy density is low, thanks to protein in the steak and water in the potato. Ice cream, on the other hand, is just fat plus sugar with very little protein or fiber or water—thus very high energy density.

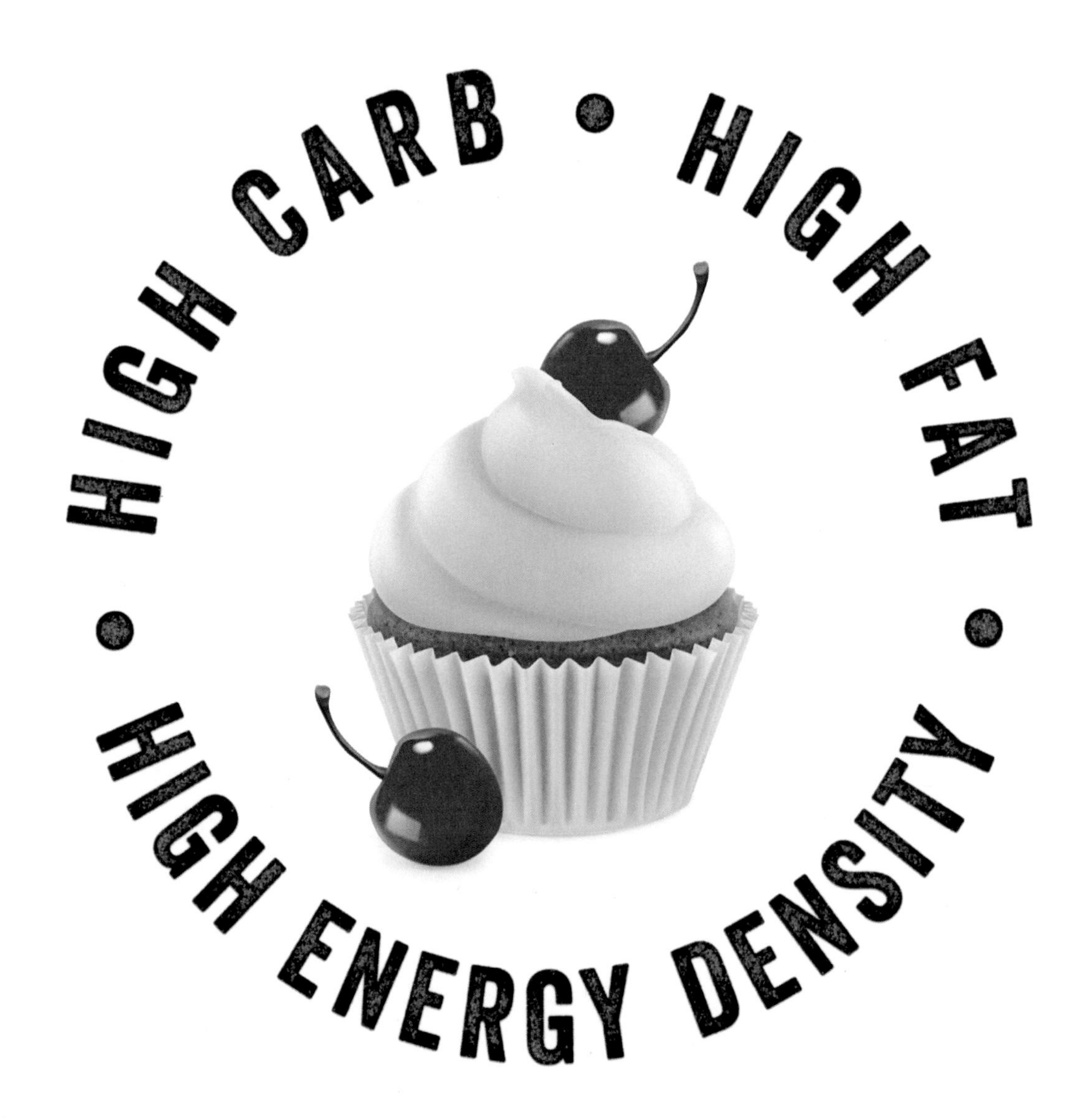

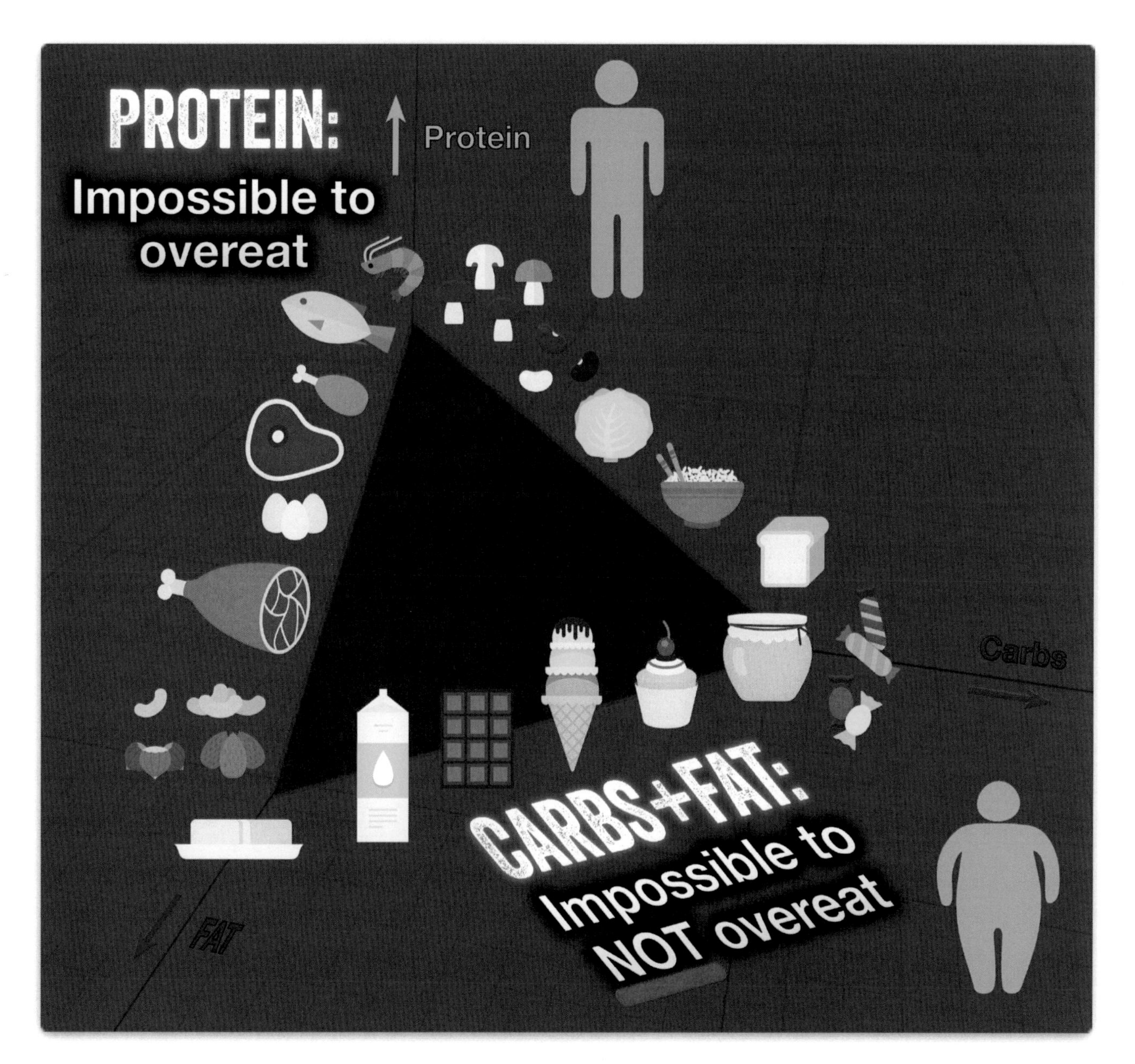

This is pretty much exactly how it works.

THE CAUSE OF OBESITY: OVEREATING EXPERIMENT

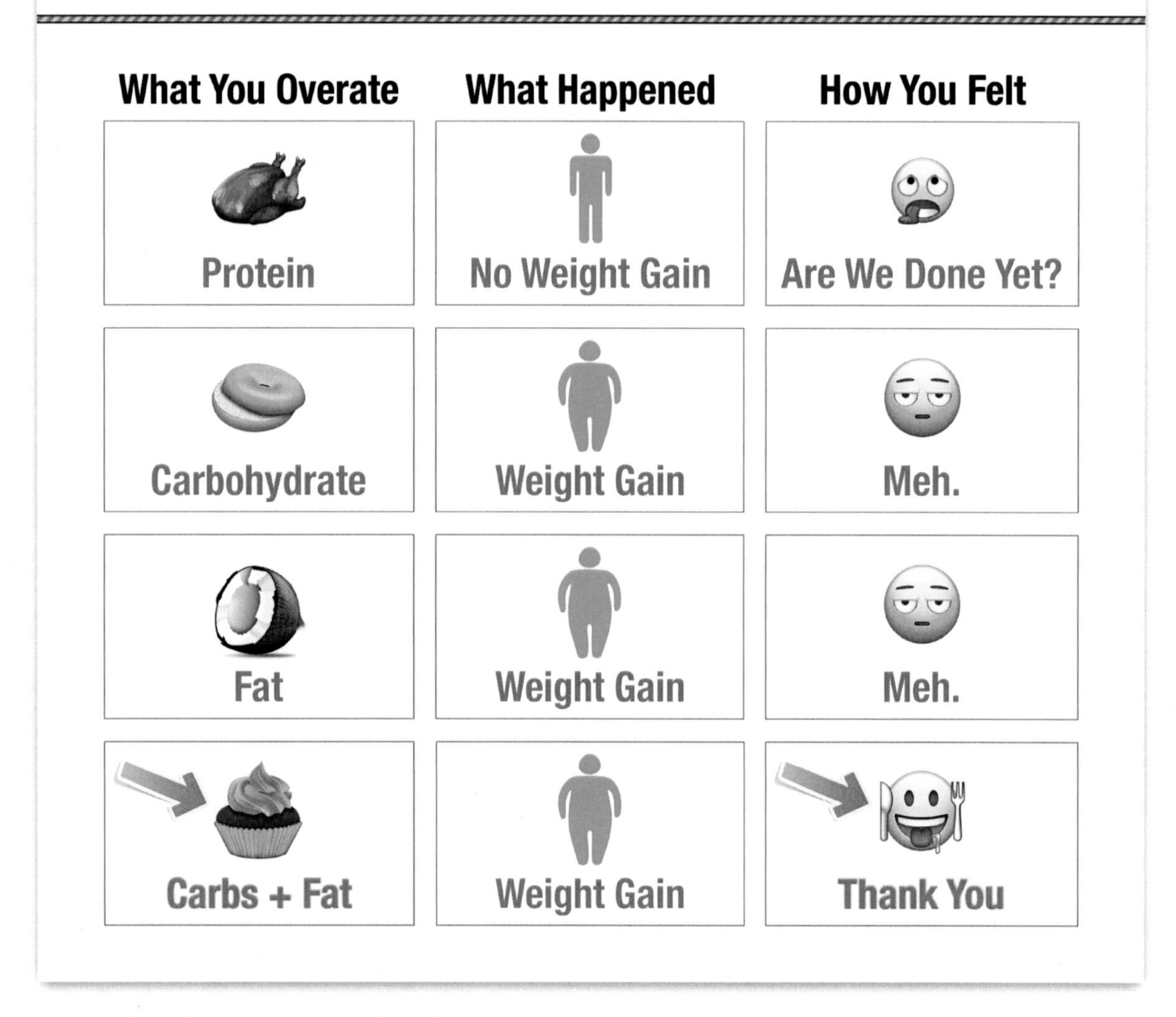

It is hard to overeat protein. But it is easy to overeat carbs + fat because these foods are so rewarding!

YOU ARE WHAT YOU EAT

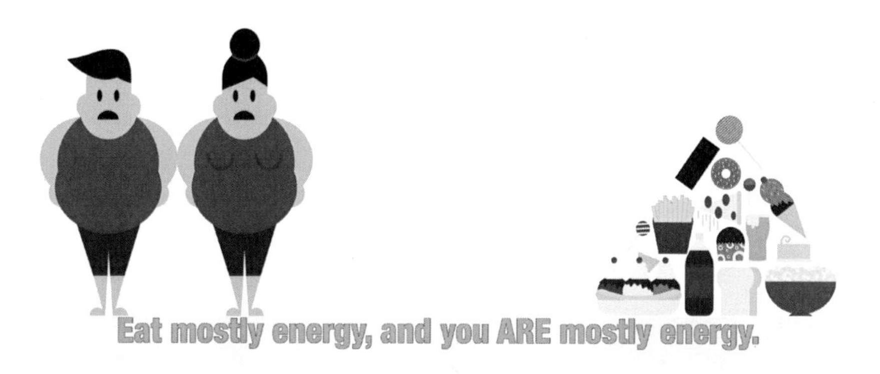

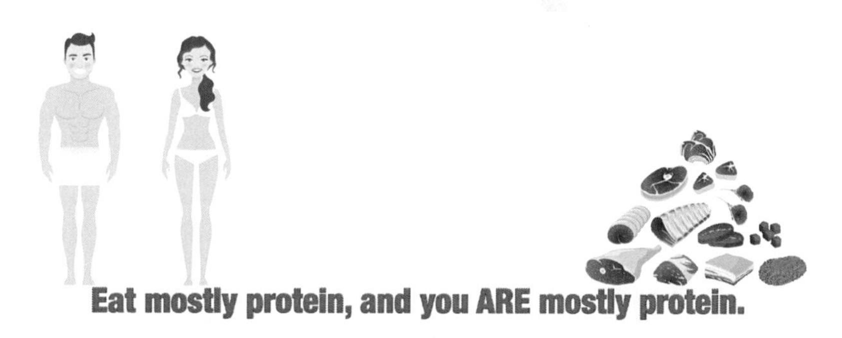

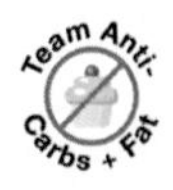

Sounds basic, but this is reality.

THE SECRET TO EVERY DIET

Every diet that offers long-term success will somehow allow for increased satiety when eating intuitively. This always involves a higher nutrient density, and always involves a higher protein to energy ratio.

However, while every diet can be properly formulated to yield success, it is also possible to formulate a diet POORLY and fail to get results. Paying attention to protein to energy ratio allows success with almost every approach.

All successful diets either reduce carbohydrate quantity, reduce fat quantity, increase protein percentage, or some combination of all three. In other words, all successful diets are following the Protein:Energy approach, even if they are unaware of it. Most successful diets are also somehow reducing the combination of carbs and fat together.

EVERY DIET WITH LONG-TERM SUCCESS IS DOING ONE OF TWO THINGS (OR BOTH):

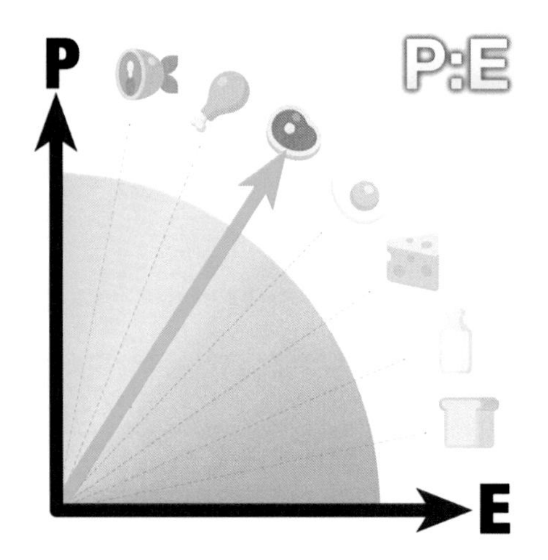

1. INCREASE P:E

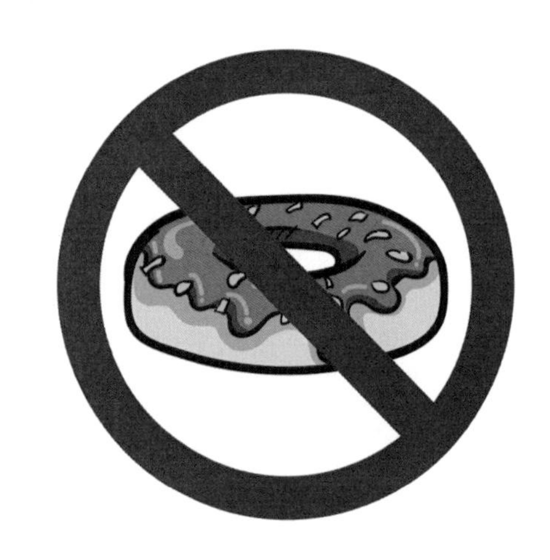

2. AVOID CARBS+FAT

LOW FAT

CORRECT: Fat is calorically dense and reducing fat will generally increase the protein to energy ratio.

INCORRECT: In natural foods, fat tends to 'come along' with protein. If your quest for reduction in fat leads to a lower protein diet, the result could be increased hunger and decreased satiety. Example: breakfast cereal and low-fat milk.

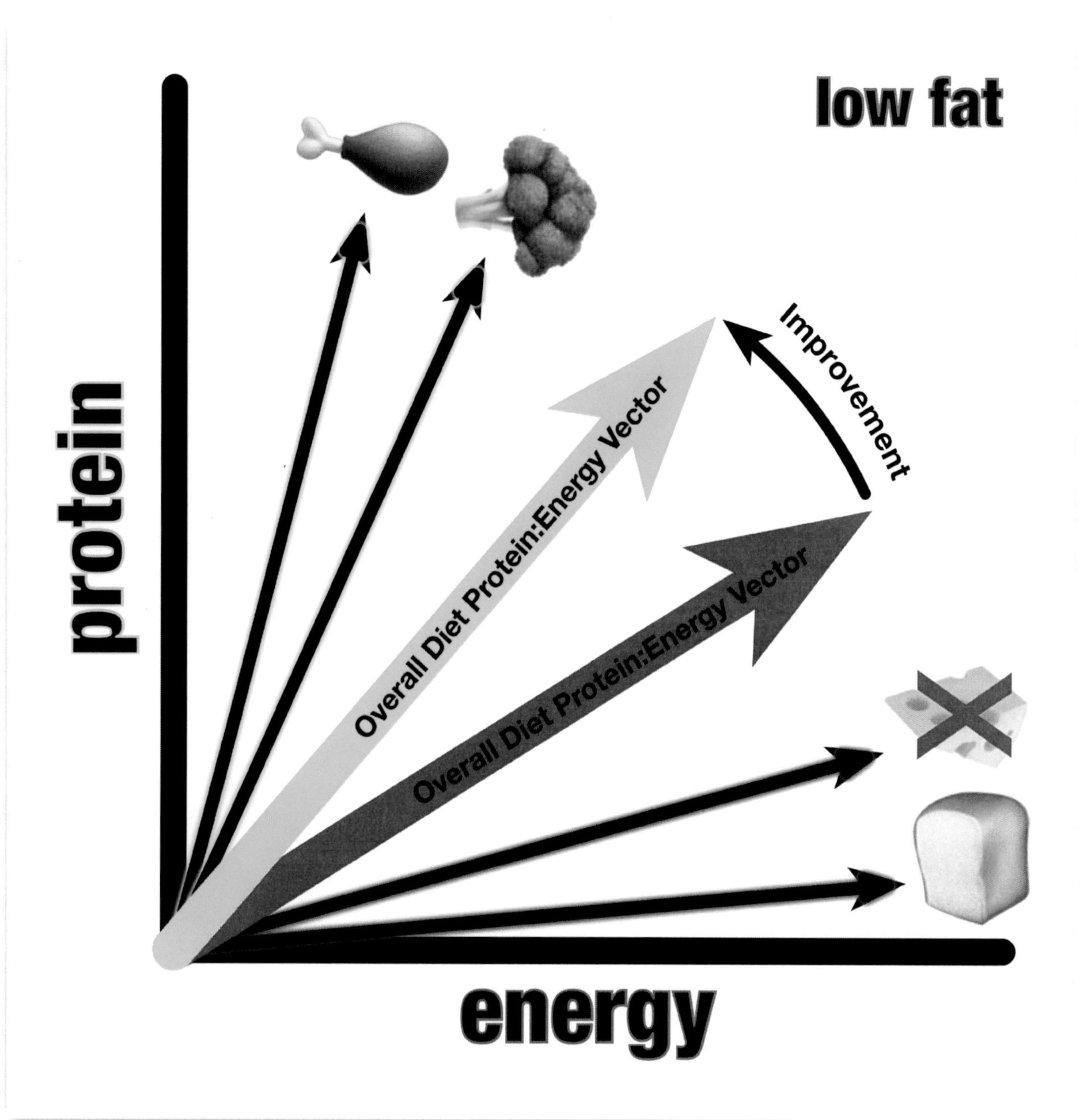

LOW CARB

CORRECT: Carbs are massively overeaten in our society and lead to a ton of protein dilution. Reducing carbs will almost always increase protein to energy ratio.

INCORRECT: Going out of your way to eat fat instead could fail to increase protein percentage. Example: 'butter-chugging' keto dieters.

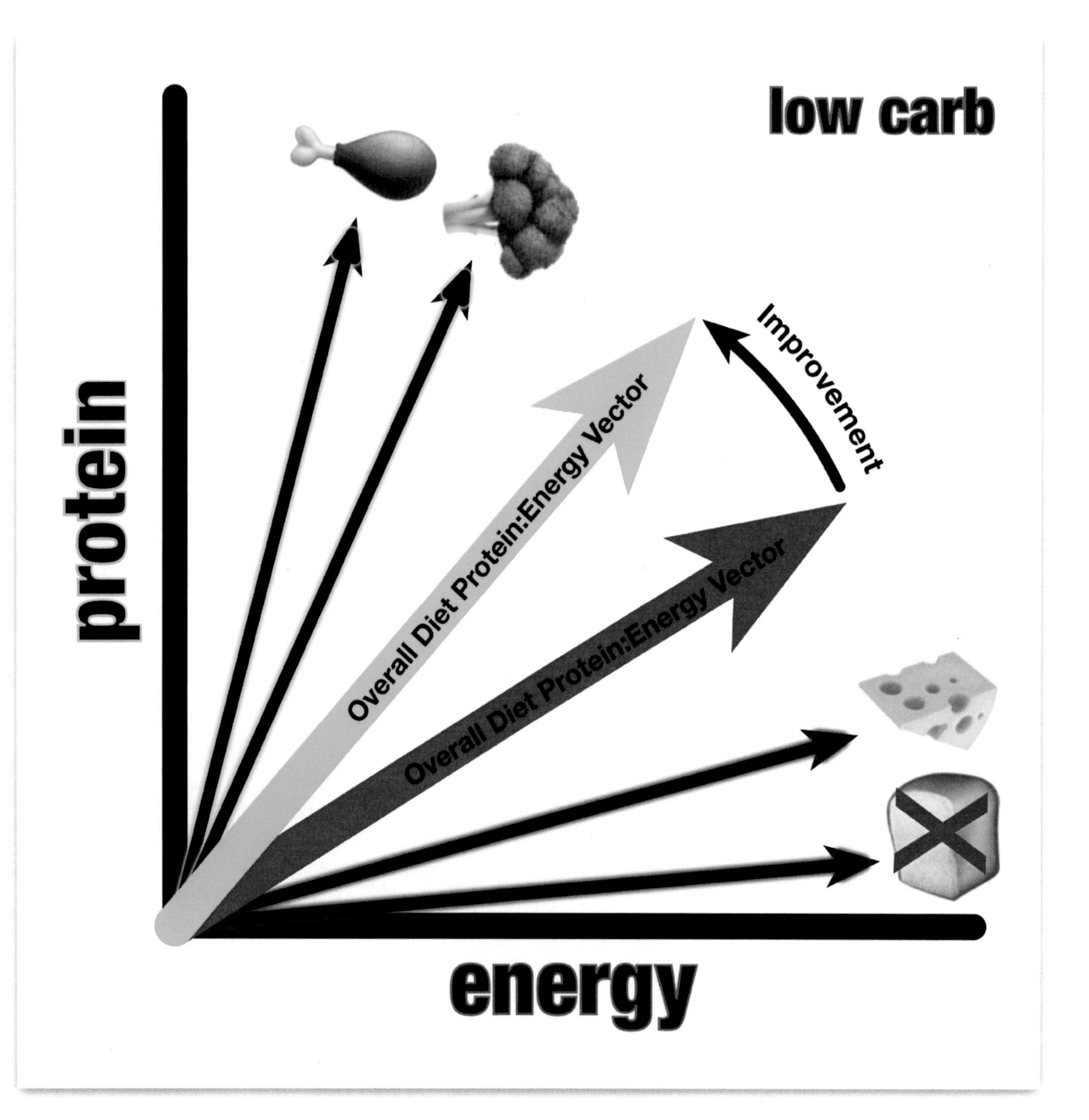

LOW CALORIE

CORRECT: Reducing calories almost always involves a reduction in both carbs and fats. If well-formulated, the result is a higher protein to energy ratio and successful weight loss.

INCORRECT: If you mistakenly restrict protein and increase carbohydrate, the result could be increased hunger and diet failure. Example: rice cakes and other 'diet' foods

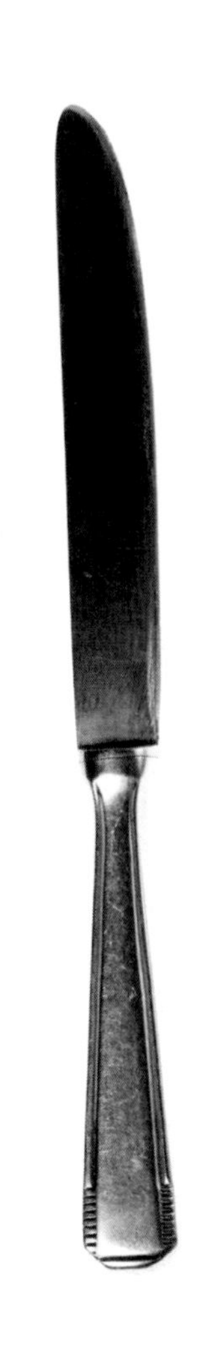

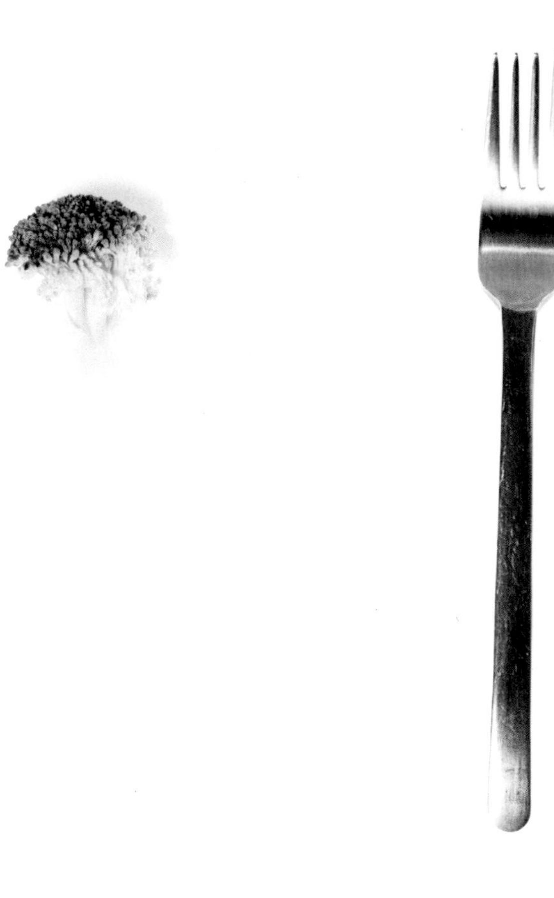

PALEO

CORRECT: Paleolithic eating skips a lot of the refined and added carbs and fats that came along with both agriculture and the industrial revolution. Typically just skipping the sugar and flour in the modern diet yields a huge upgrade in protein:energy ratio.

INCORRECT: A smoothie with dates and honey and bananas would be 'paleo' and would also contain about 100 grams of straight sugar with almost no protein.

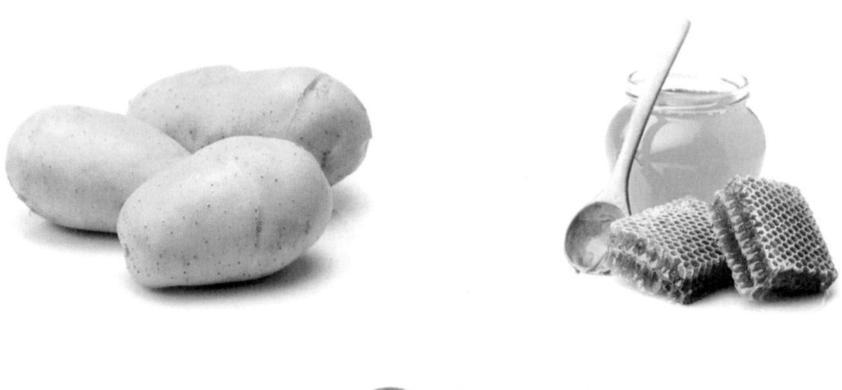

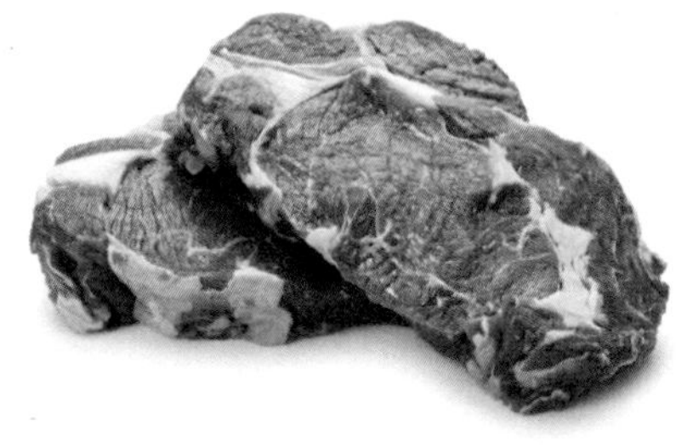

Exclude:

Bread

Pasta

Sugar

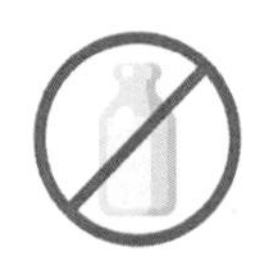

Milk

Corn

Beans

Rice

PLANT-BASED

CORRECT: Eating more legumes such as lentils and soy, plus more green vegetables, is a massive upgrade in terms of protein to energy ratio. Tofu, textured vegetable protein, gluten, and all of the plant protein fake meats that vegans eat, while far from optimal, actually have an extremely high protein to energy ratio, especially compared to the Standard American Diet. If you ditch the refined carbs in a 'junk food vegan' diet, you will get some pretty amazing results with this highly restrictive plan.

INCORRECT: See the phrase 'junk food vegan diet' above. Highly processed fake vegan foods can be some of the worst protein:energy foods on the planet.

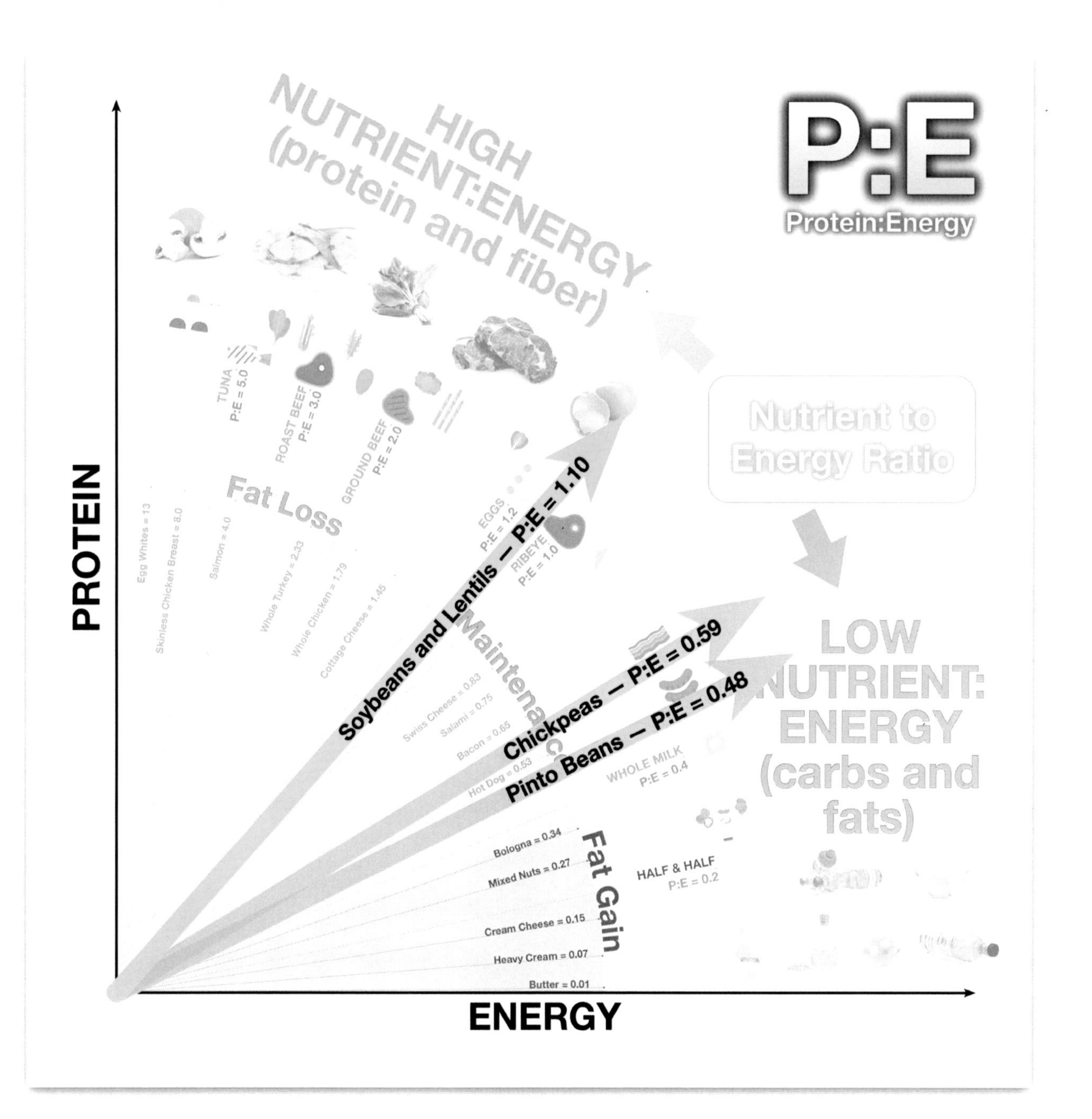

CARNIVORE

CORRECT: Because animal foods are, in general, always higher in protein:energy ratio compared to plant foods, this is pretty much an instant win for the average person.

INCORRECT: Processed meat such as bacon and hot dogs and sausage can have much higher fat grams than protein grams, and it is possible to actually gain weight on such a diet. If you go so far as to use high-fat dairy (butter and heavy cream) as 'carnivore' foods, you're probably going nowhere.

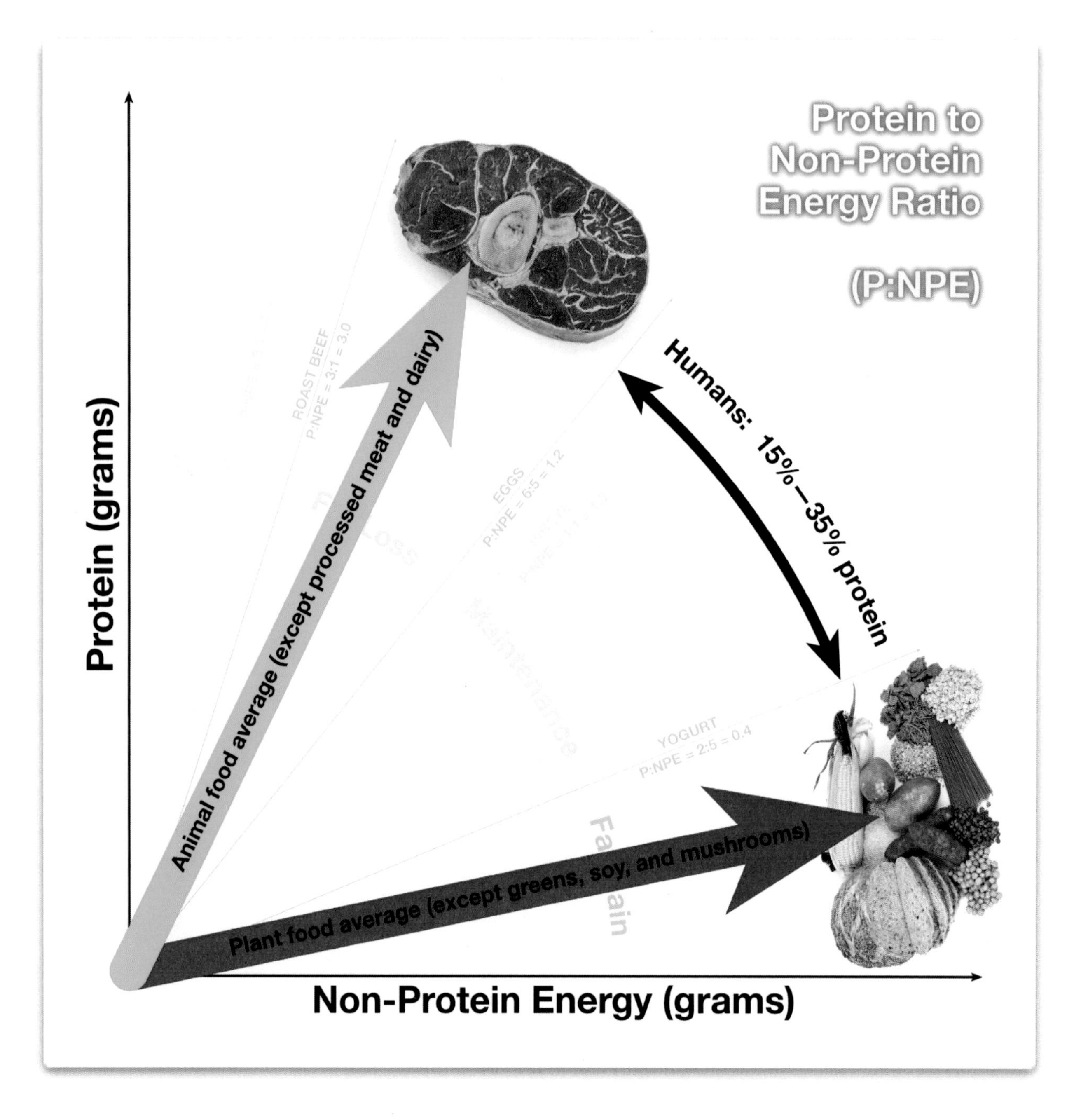

BODYBUILDING

CORRECT: All bodybuilders are really combining low carb AND low fat AND high protein, typically to the very highest level of success.

INCORRECT: If you ignore diet quality and nutrient density and simply use IIFYM ('If It Fits Your Macros') and basically eat toaster pastries but force yourself to greatly limit quantity, you will be STARVING and your body will fight back HARD.

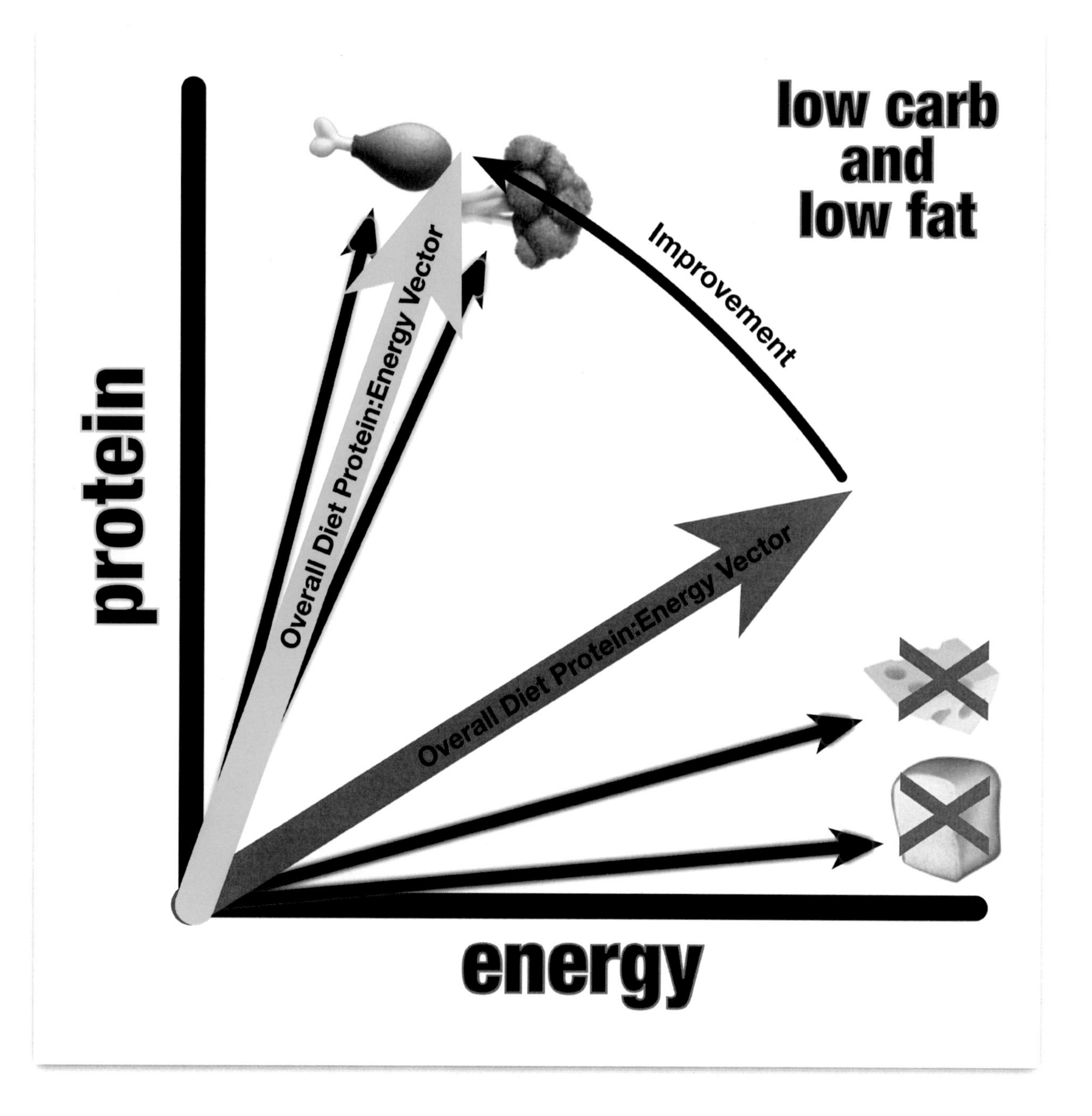

THE ENDLESS LOW CARB VERSUS LOW FAT WAR

Low fat! Low carb! These two camps have been fighting for as long as anyone can remember. What is going on here? Obviously someone here is right and someone is wrong, so who should we listen to?

If you really dive into the low fat rabbit hole, you will find all kinds of success stories. There are countless persons who have lost a ton of weight, reversed their type 2 diabetes, and transformed their health with very low fat diets. The majority of bodybuilders are following low fat diets, and have some extremely impressive results to show for it. Sometimes these low fat fans naturally gravitate towards plant-based diets, as plants tend to store their non-protein energy as carbohydrates—in stark contrast to animal-based diets, as animals tend to store their non-protein energy as fat. Therefore it is quite natural that LOW FAT diets go hand in hand with PLANT-BASED diets, as they have a lot of overlap. So you will find countless amazing stories of positive health transformations from those who have adopted low fat diets (plant-based or not).

BUT WAIT. Over on the low carb side, you will also find literally countless stories of amazing effortless weight loss and

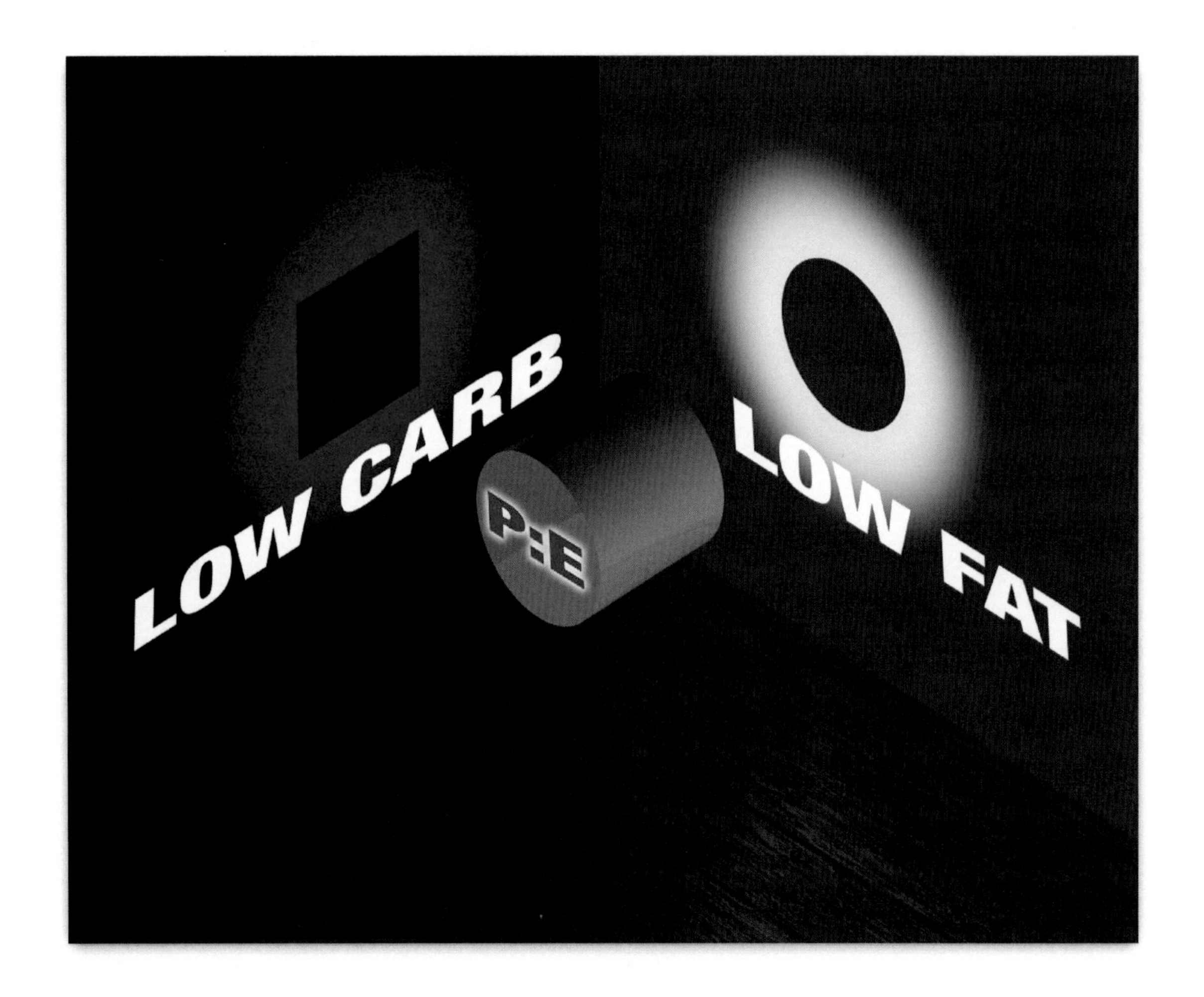

jaw-dropping body and health transformations. These diets tend, for reasons mentioned above, to be predominately animal-based, but this is only because stored carbohydrates mostly exist in the plant world. The low carb fans absolutely swear by low carb diets, and they have the results to back it up. Most of them are low carb converts for life.

All of this has left us with an enormous problem: NOBODY HAS ANY CLUE WHAT THE HELL THEY ARE SUPPOSED TO EAT.

You already know the answer. It is hidden deep inside your unconsciousness, you just haven't accepted it yet. You instinctively know that there is only one way on earth that you could have these two diametrically opposed camps of people who are rabidly devoted to either very low carb diets or very low fat diets. And the answer is:

THEY ARE BOTH RIGHT.

At first, it is a painful revelation. We humans want to belong to some sort of group, because this provides a lot of safety. In our evolutionary past, belonging to a group was literally quite often the difference between life or death. So we very much want to sign up for either the low fat or the low carb camp—how else can we be safe from dietary danger? So we naturally want to pick sides.

But slowly and gradually, your new-found knowledge turns into POWER. You realize that as long as protein percentage is high and you are well fat-adapted, you can frequently trade some of your fat energy calories in for carb calories, or vice versa. You realize that both low carb and low fat are accomplishing the same two primary goals:

1. **Higher protein percentage.**

2. **Avoidance of carbs+fat together.**

So by increasing your protein prioritization and eating meals centered around protein, and keeping meals either higher in carbs but not fat (or fat but not carbs), you have a lot more freedom.

Eating a fattier protein? No problem — keep the carbs lower at that meal.

Eating a 'carbier' [may not actually be a word] protein? Also no problem — keep the fats lower at that meal.

So now you can have a meal of fatty ribeye and eggs cooked in butter, as long as the carbs are low. And then later, you could have a meal of chicken breast and potatoes, as long as the fat is kept low. Protein is dominant at both meals, and you are avoiding carbs and fats together, so mission accomplished!

At this point, you are pretty much like Neo in 'The Matrix', because you can see the big picture. And this allows you to appreciate the benefits of being low fat and also the benefits of being low carb. And of course, you could always be somewhat low fat AND low carb at the same time, as this will give you the fastest and most powerful results. Congratulations, you have unlocked both diets.

WHAT TO EAT VERSUS *HOW MUCH* TO EAT

There are two basic approaches to dieting: WHAT to eat, and HOW MUCH to eat.

The 'how much' approach has dominated most of popular culture your entire life. Counting calories. Energy balance. Calories in, calories out. But this approach is inherently flawed. Why? Because we are surrounded by food-like GARBAGE that masquerades as real food. And if you choose that crap, not only will you be constantly hungry—you will probably gain weight, and, if taken to extremes, literally destroy your health.

The reality is that every mammal on earth has a specific diet that it is adapted to eat. A lion eats meat and a giraffe eats acacia leaves, and if you try to swap diets, both of them are doomed. Humans are a bit different. One of our superpowers is our adaptability. We can live in almost any environment, eating almost any diet. This is why you will find people who eat nothing but plants, nothing but animals, and everything in between. In a way this has led to some confusion: we have no clue what we are really supposed to eat. But, just like all mammals, humans DO have a diet that we are adapted to eat.

Humans are hunter-gatherers. If we dumped you out in the wilderness with nothing but a spear, believe us when we say that you would never have to worry about 'calorie balance' in order to avoid obesity. When humans eat wild, uncultivated plants and animals, we are typically eating a diet that is about three times higher in protein than the standard American diet—and HOW MUCH to eat ceases to be a factor entirely. You hunt animals, kill an animal, and eat until you are full. Or you gather some plant foods and eat them. Your body tells you how much to eat. You eat when you are hungry, and you stop when you are full. Everything works the way it is supposed

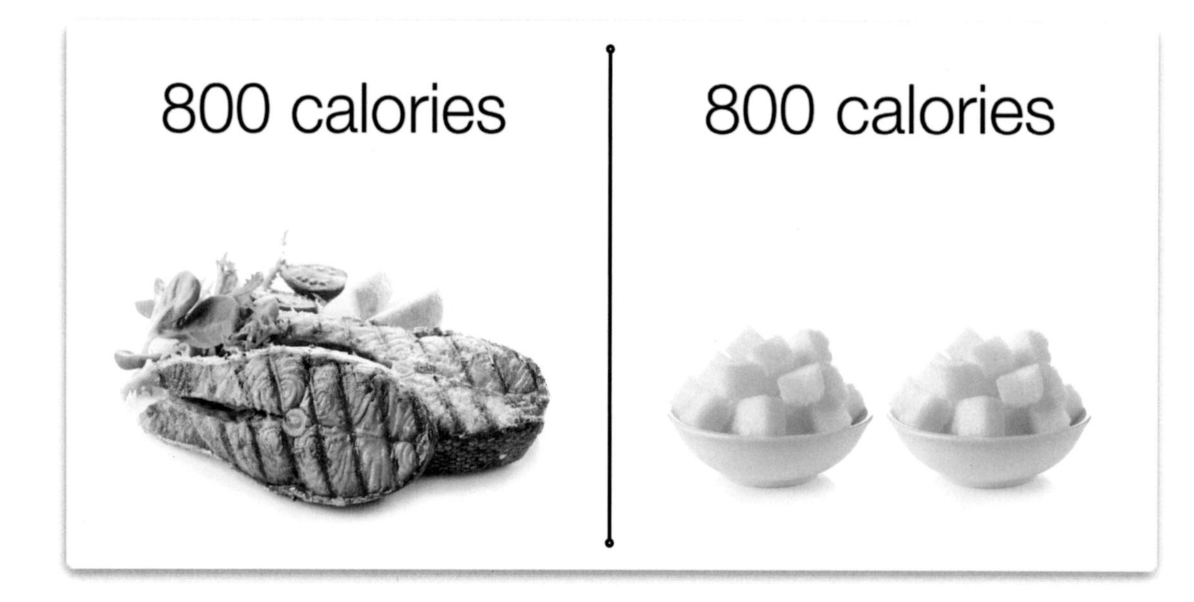

to. There are no addictive foods that are high in both carbs and fats. There are no empty calorie refined fats and carbs adding energy without protein or minerals. All food is in a CELLULAR form, so you automatically get a nice balance of cell wall membrane fats, proteins from cellular organelles, and minerals—in direct contrast to ACELLULAR foods like sugar and oil. This is why no wild animal on earth, eating the foods it is SUPPOSED to eat, has to worry about HOW MUCH to eat.

The entire diet section of this book is centered around the fact that for both body composition and overall health, it makes far more sense to focus on WHAT you eat rather than HOW MUCH. Why are domesticated animals, fed by humans, often just as fat as their human owners? Because of WHAT we are feeding them. No wild dog or cat is going to overeat the foods they are SUPPOSED to eat. But when humans get involved, everything goes to hell. We try to profit on dog and cat food by replacing expensive high-quality animal protein with cheap plant carbs and fats, like grain flour and seed oil.

Much of the obesity epidemic is purely economic. If you graph out the price of all of the foods in the grocery store versus macronutrients, you will find that it is all about the protein. The more protein in a food, the more expensive it is. In fact, if you are trying to get pure protein with less carbs and fats, this is most expensive of all. Adding carbs and fats to a food is never more expensive, and frequently foods are even LESS expensive with more carbs and fats. This

Choosing Low Protein "Food"?

Well then your body has a choice to make:

PROTEIN MALNOURISHMENT

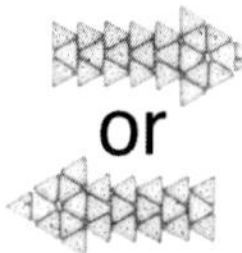

or

ENERGY EXCESS TOXICITY

Avoid energy toxicity, try to survive protein deficiency.

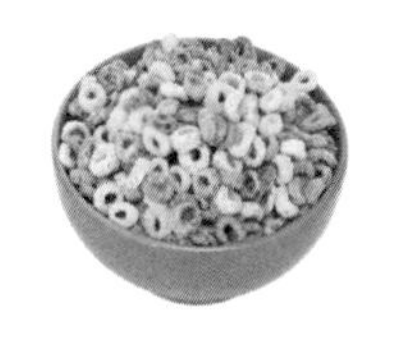

Avoid protein deficiency, try to survive energy toxicity.

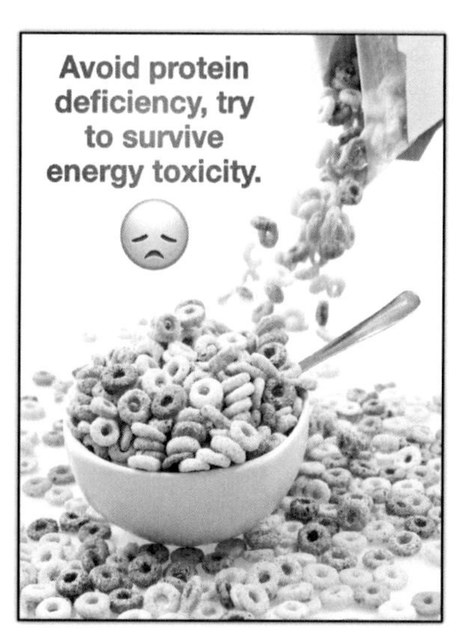

is why you can go almost anywhere on earth and draw a map of poverty and a map of obesity and they will typically overlap completely. Cheap plant carbs and fats are everywhere. In America, the farmers who produce these are often subsidized by the government. The shelf life of these empty calories is astronomically higher than protein. The profit margin is dramatically higher than protein. It costs more money to make a cereal BOX than it does to make the cereal IN the box. Protein is more expensive because it suffers from more logistical challenges. Protein requires more refrigeration. Transport is more difficult. Cooking is more of a factor. Shelf life is radically shorter compared to cereal grains and seed oils. All of these economic factors are driving obesity forward, and it is important to recognize this and understand the forces at work here.

REMEMBER: your obesity is so complicated that it will never be understood by even the brightest obesity researchers.

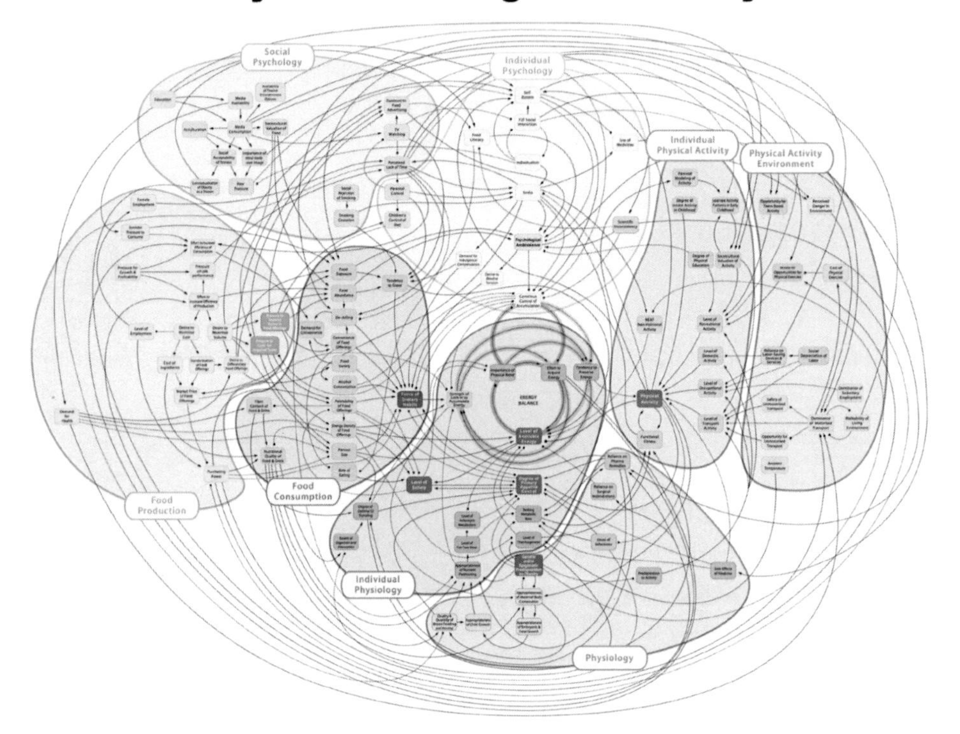

Unrelated, your pets are obese because someone tried to make more money by replacing their dietary animal protein with cheap plant carbohydrates. 😑

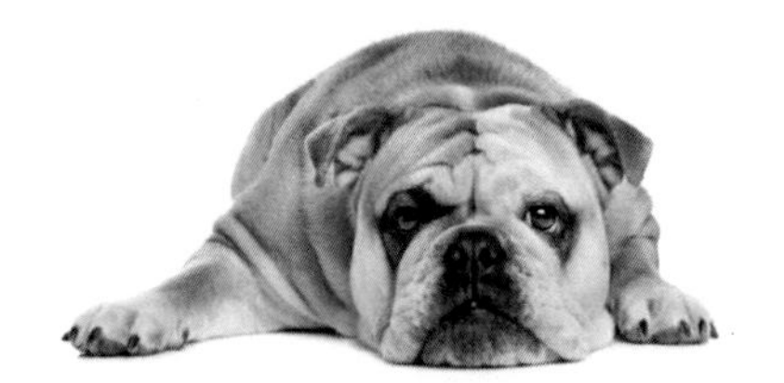

INGREDIENTS

Ground yellow corn, chicken by-product meal, corn gluten meal, whole wheat flour, animal fat preserved with mixed-tocopherols, chicken, soy flour, rice flour, propylene glycol, sugar, tricalcium phosphate, salt, phosphoric acid, potassium chloride, animal digest, mono and dicalcium phosphate, dried carrots, sorbic acid (a preservative), dried tomatoes, avocado, calcium propionate (a preservative), L-Lysine monohydrochloride, choline chloride, Vitamin E supplement, zinc sulfate, ferrous sulfate, Yellow 5, manganese sulfate, niacin, Red 40, Vitamin A supplement, Blue 2, copper sulfate, Vitamin B-12 supplement, calcium pantothenate, thiamine mononitrate, garlic oil, Yellow 6, pyridoxine hydrochloride, riboflavin supplement, Vitamin D-3 supplement, menadione sodium bisulfite complex (source of Vitamin K activity), calcium iodate, folic acid, biotin, sodium selenite.

Manufactured by: Nestlé Purina PetCare Company, St. Louis, MO 63164 USA

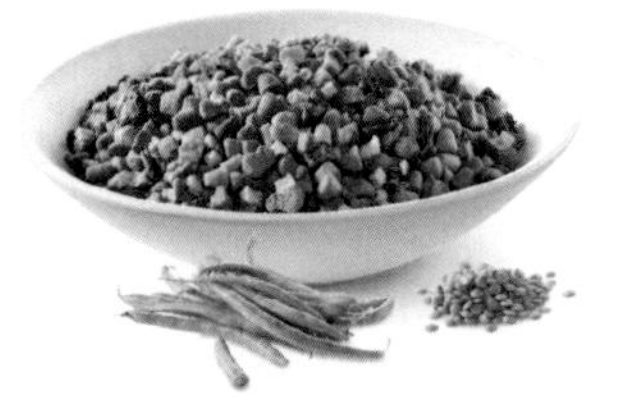

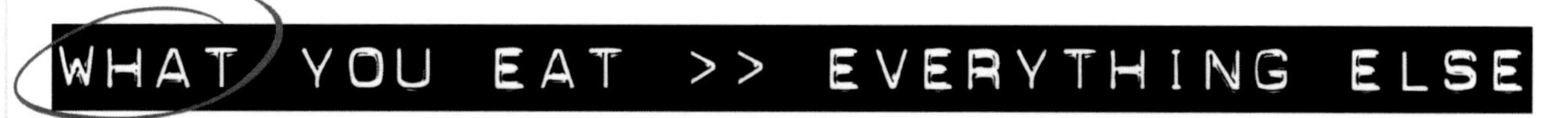

FOOD SELECTION

IS THE ONLY FACTOR IN OBESITY.

Don't believe us?

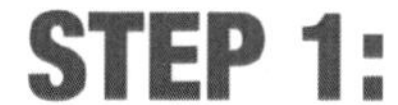

Perform a thought experiment where the foods pictured here are the only foods a person has access to.

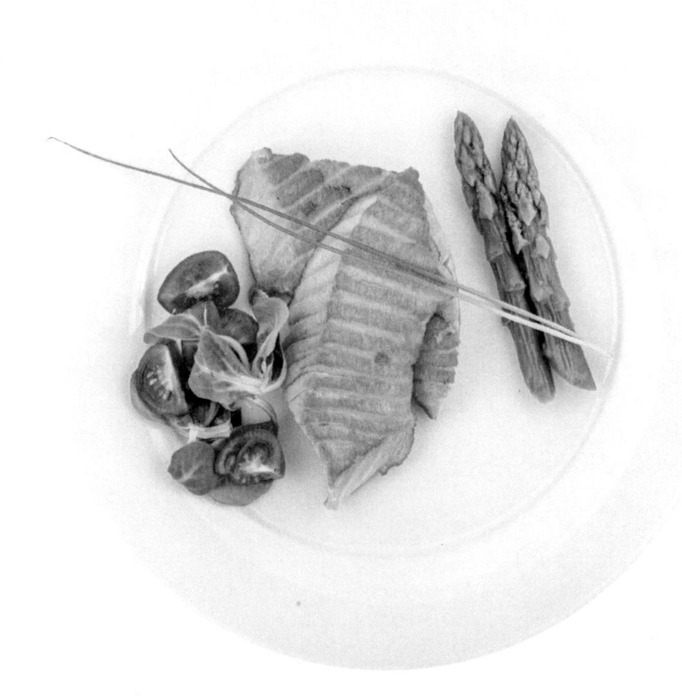

STEP 2:

Watch factors such as when you eat, how much you eat, and portion control fade away into insignificance.

**"Whenever you find yourself on the side of the majority,
It's time to pause and reflect."**

— Mark Twain

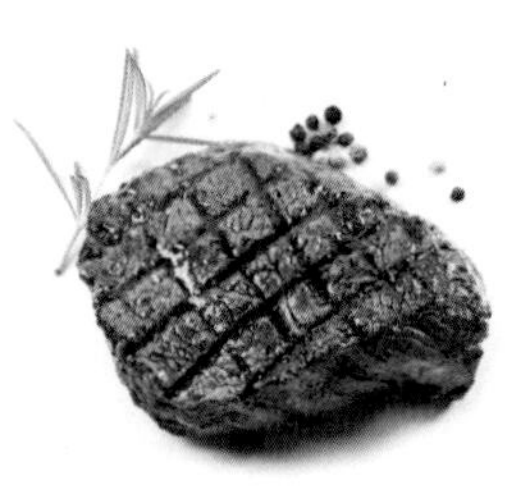

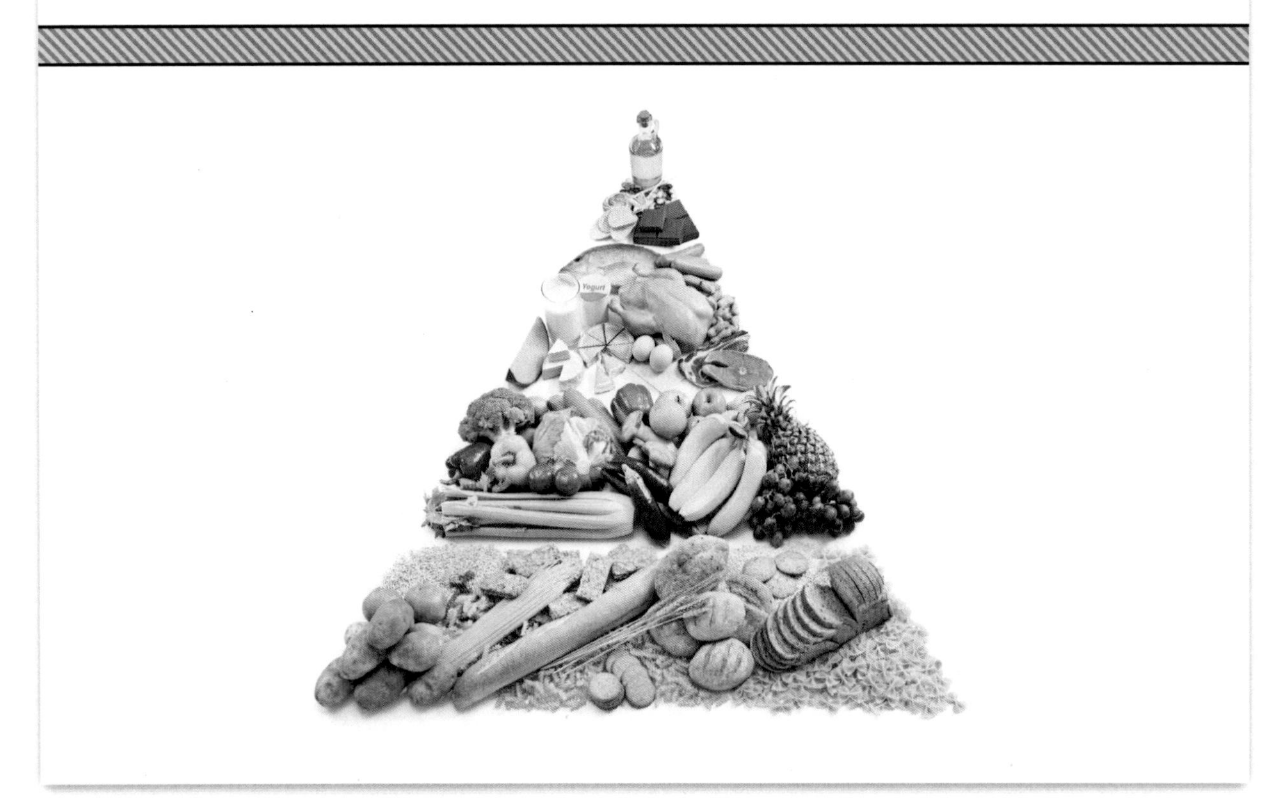

CARBS AND GLYCOGEN

As we discussed previously, GLYCEMIC carbs—non-fiber digestible carbs that break down to monosaccharides like glucose—exert a very powerful leverage on your entire metabolism. In this chapter, we are going to explore the powerful nature of dietary glucose.

Your body requires a continuous supply of glucose. You have cells in your body, such as red blood cells, that have no mitochondria—and without mitochondria, these cells cannot burn fat for energy. So these cells rely on glucose. Luckily, your liver is completely responsible for managing glucose, and your liver produces all the glucose you ever need through a process known as 'gluconeogenesis'. The liver primarily uses either amino acids (protein) or the glycerol backbones of triglycerides (fat) to create new glucose. This process is always occurring, and as a result, you really never have to eat any carbohydrates at all.

Your bloodstream can only hold about four grams—one teaspoon—of glucose. High blood glucose can be toxic, as evidenced by the diabetic complications seen in uncontrolled diabetics. Working muscles can immediately absorb and store some dietary glucose as glycogen (starch-like chains of glucose in storage form). But if your muscles are already full of glycogen—and this is their default state when you are not exercising—your liver is designed to absorb and store all of the extra glucose coming in from your diet.

Or at least your liver TRIES to do this. Most people can only hold about 100 grams of glucose in their liver at any given time. As your liver approaches capacity, you start converting some of this glucose into fat. Your body HAS to do this, because you have a pretty rigid ceiling on how much glucose you can store, while most of us have plenty of room for additional fat storage.

YOUR LIVER MAKES ALL THE GLUCOSE YOU NEED VIA GLUCONEOGENESIS

DIETARY GLUCOSE

GLUCOSE CREATED VIA HEPATIC GLUCONEOGENESIS

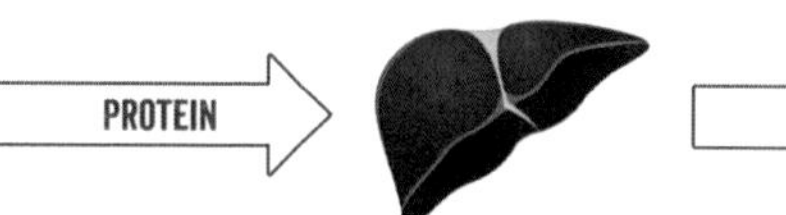

Liver glycogen and muscle glycogen have some very different properties. Muscle glycogen is there for emergency use. Because you can convert glucose from muscle glycogen into energy six times faster compared to fat, you always need this glycogen on board in case of emergency. Anytime you are running or fighting for your life, or performing any exercise at the highest intensity, your muscles are burning 100% glucose from glycogen. The glycogen in your muscles also STAYS in your muscles—the cells keep this glycogen for themselves and it cannot be shared with other parts of your body. So really the entire point of muscle glycogen is to STAY FULL and your body will do whatever it has to do in order to keep your muscles supplied with glycogen. This is a basic safety system for your body.

Liver glycogen is different. The job of the liver is to buffer any potentially toxic glucose load out of the bloodstream, in order to keep blood glucose in a narrow and tightly controlled range. When you eat dietary glucose, your liver sucks this glucose out of your bloodstream and stores it as glycogen. Your liver then immediately starts slowly releasing this glucose gradually over a period of hours, to be used by the rest of the entire body. Liver glycogen empties significantly (although never 100%) and, unlike muscles, the default state of the liver is to maintain a LOW level of glycogen so there is plenty of headroom to absorb more dietary glucose in the future.

As liver glycogen falls back down to baseline, your entire metabolism slowly transitions from the carbohydrate fed state to the fasted state. Blood glucose and insulin levels gradually go down, while at the same time the fasted state hormone glucagon rises, as well as free fatty acids. As liver glycogen dwindles and your body relies more and more on fat to run its metabolism, the liver starts generating ketones, which are really just water-soluble bits of fat that the brain can use instead of glucose for fuel.

By now, pretty much everyone has heard about ketogenic diets. Ketosis is really just the metabolic state that results when hepatic glycogen is low and your body is running on fat instead of glucose for fuel. This really is as simple as not eating carbs for 12 to 24 hours, depending on how packed with glycogen your liver and muscles were before you stopped eating glucose. You can speed up ketosis with high-intensity exercise, which burns glucose (from both muscle and liver)

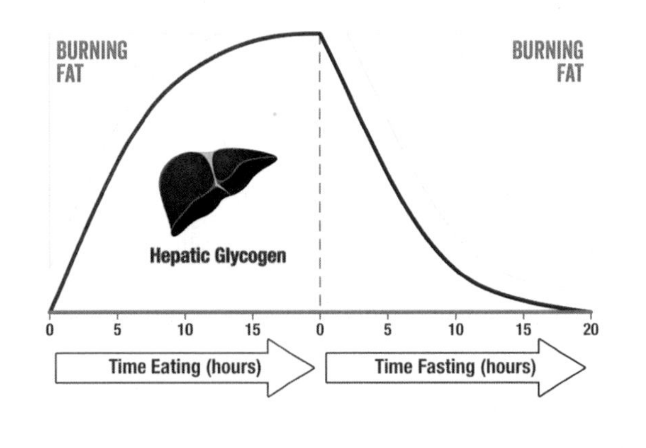

The liver is like a shock absorber for dietary glucose, sucking it out of your bloodstream and then slowly buffering it out over the next 12-24 hours.

FALLING LIVER GLYCOGEN IS THE TRANSITION FROM THE FED STATE TO THE FASTED STATE

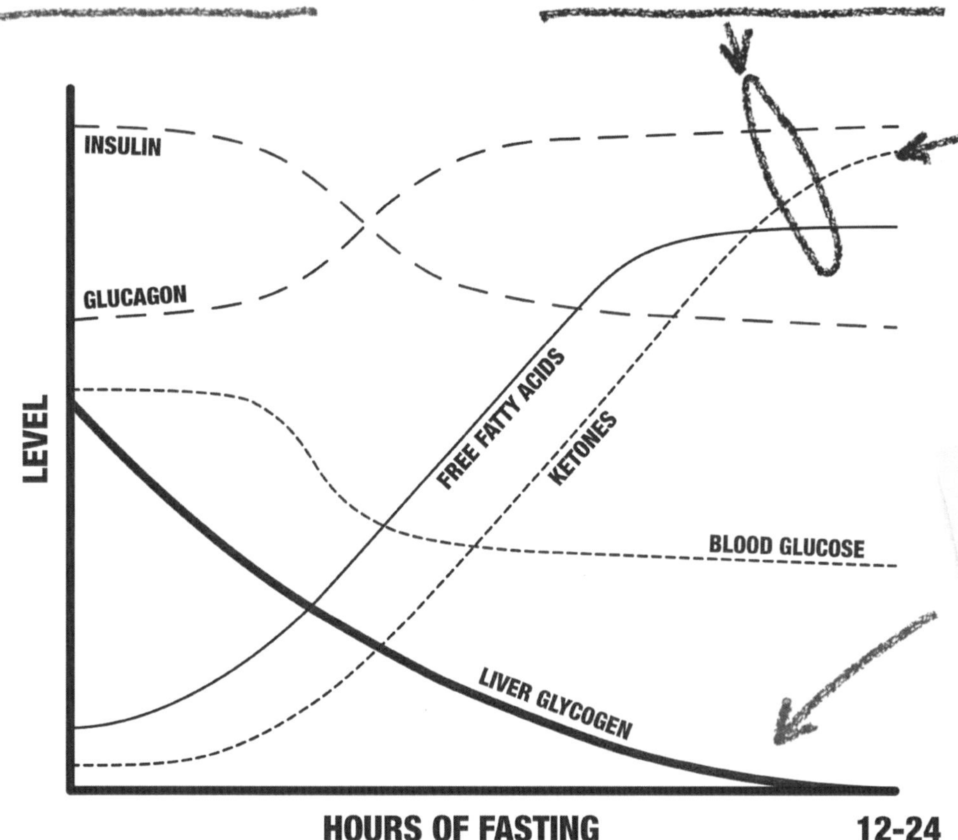

KETOSIS IS SIMPLY A STATE OF LOW LIVER GLYCOGEN.

LIVER GLYCOGEN IS ALWAYS SLOWLY DRIFTING DOWN TOWARDS ITS NADIR, AT WHICH POINT YOUR BODY IS FULLY IN THE 'FASTED' STATE AND RUNNING ON STORED BODY FAT FOR ENERGY.

quite rapidly. Contrary to the belief of many a butter-chugging keto dieter, you do not have to eat any fat at all to be 'in ketosis'. Ketosis is naturally occurring in anyone who isn't eating enough dietary glucose to fill liver glycogen.

The average American is eating EIGHT times a day, pretty much every two hours for sixteen hours out of every twenty-four hour day. During this time, we manage to consume about 300 grams of carbs, on average. As a result, we are in the 'fed' state more often than not, and the average person almost never allows liver glycogen to get low enough to allow for significant ketosis. Because elevated glucose displaces fat oxidation, we are all burning mostly glucose at the expense of fat oxidation for a good portion of our lives. This is not without several major consequences.

DIETARY CARBOHYDRATES TRANSIENTLY RAISE GLUCOSE, DISPLACING FAT OXIDATION...

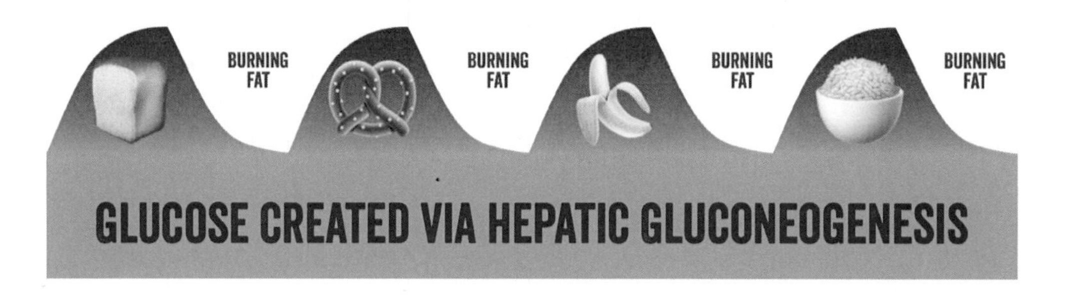

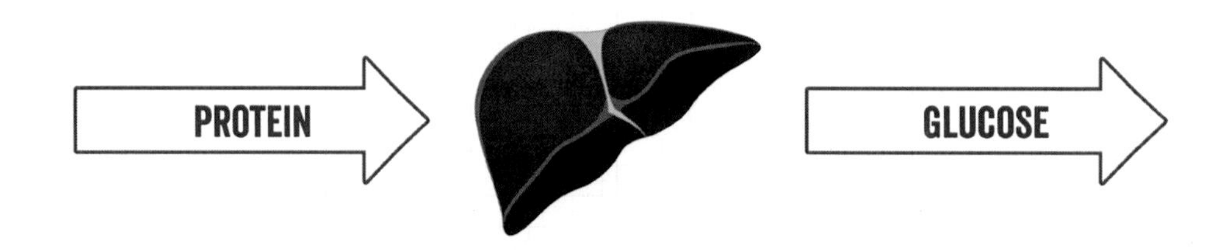

...BUT YOUR LIVER ALREADY MAKES ALL OF THE GLUCOSE YOU NEED VIA GLUCONEOGENESIS.

First of all, our metabolism will gradually up-regulate the machinery it takes to burn a particular fuel, and down-regulate the machinery we aren't using. This makes a ton of sense, and we would fully expect our bodies to adapt to the environment. So if you are eating a lot of carbs then you will be up-regulating the pathways for dealing with carbohydrate, at the expense of fat oxidation. And similarly, if you are NOT eating carbs, your body has to up-regulate the ability to run everything off of fat. There seems to be a sort of inertia to your metabolism, and what we have learned from studies where participants were switched from high carb to low carb diets, there seems to be a 1-2 week adaptation period. A lot of keto dieters refer to this as the process of 'fat adaptation', and it is a very real thing.

Becoming 'fat adapted' is a bit vague, and the exact biochemistry of this phenomenon has not been fully elucidated. However, pretty much everyone who has gone on an extended low carbohydrate diet can describe this to you. On a high carb diet, you are more tied to food. Because your liver glycogen, your main source of energy, is constantly falling, you have to eat much more frequently and you experience hunger quite a bit more frequently. Fat adaptation—the ability to live comfortably off stored body fat—allows for much less frequent meals, and a lower sense of urgency to eat when mealtime finally arrives.

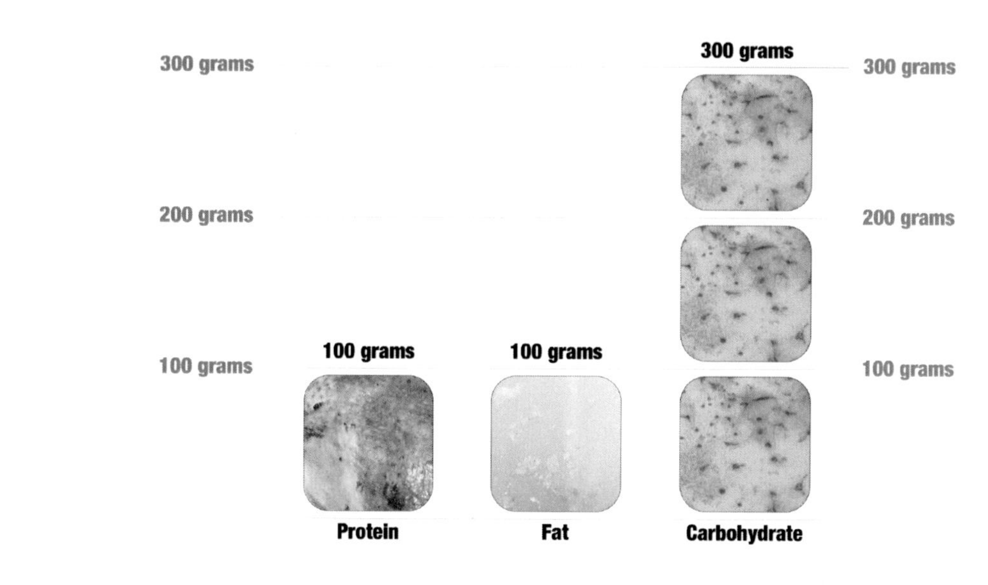

The average American is eating carbs 8 times a day — roughly every 2 hours of a 16 hour eating window, for a total of 300 grams of carbs daily. Most of us are trying to avoid the minor discomfort of low hepatic glycogen, and we are in a carb-fed state ALL DAY LONG.

FALLING GLUCOSE → HUNGER

In addition to the simple displacement of fat oxidation by dietary glucose, and the up-regulation of carb oxidation plus down-regulation of fat oxidation seen with chronically high carbohydrate diets, there is one other major factor at play here:

• Falling glucose makes you hungry. •

About 3-4 hours after eating a large amount of glycemic carbohydrates, we see a significant drop in glucose, and a significant rise in the hunger hormone ghrelin. What does this mean on a practical level? You get hungry. And specifically, you get hungry for more carbohydrates. In studies, participants who eat a high carbohydrate breakfast have significantly higher hunger scores a few hours later than those eating fewer carbohydrates. Many of us can relate to this on a personal level. You remember the time you only had juice and toast for breakfast, and three hours later you felt like you had to eat something or you were going to die of starvation.

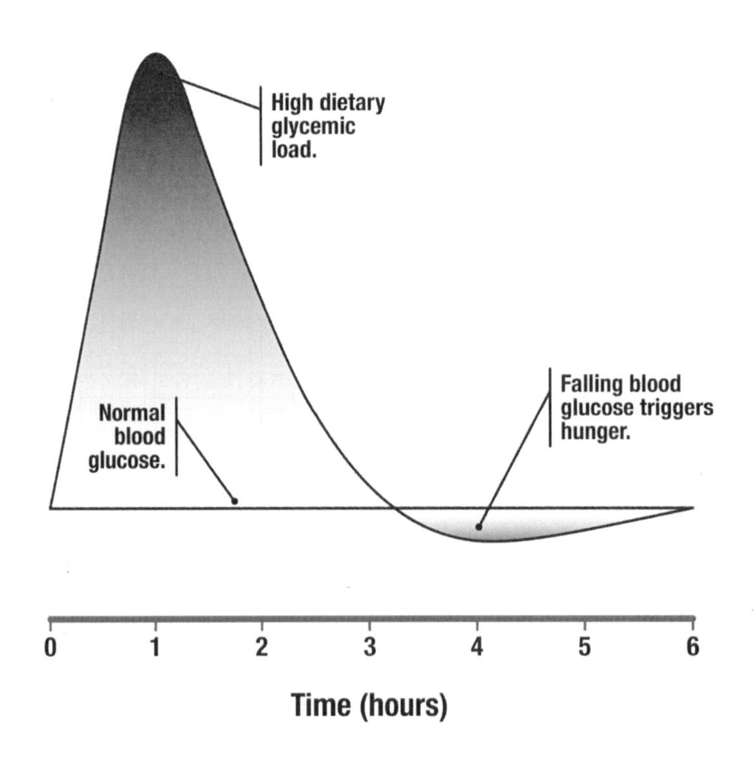

Carbs offer a lot of satiety acutely, for a couple of hours, but unlike protein and fat, that satiety wears off with a vengeance, followed by an increase in hunger that is often worse than if you had never eaten in the first place. You can see how we gradually got to the point where we eat the quantity and frequency of carbs that we do in modern society. As the direct result of our carbohydrate intakes, we have developed a state of relative dependence on dietary glucose, to the point that we have snack breaks at work and school that are perfectly timed to raise blood sugar just when the glycogen from our ridiculously high-carb breakfast cereal has worn off.

Time to reach for the S.A.I.D. (Specific Adaptation to Imposed Demand) principle again. If we decrease our carbohydrate intake, we force our bodies to adapt. We automatically up-regulate our fat oxidation pathways and slowly and gradually become less dependent on dietary glucose. This is almost like a form of metabolic exercise, and the reward is quite amazing. Those who endure the discomfort of eating less glucose will tell you that becoming 'fat adapted' eventually starts to feel like a superpower.

You are much less 'tied' to food and eating. Missing a meal goes from being a full-scale 'hangry' disaster to pretty much a non-event. Exercise no longer requires carb-loading before, during, and after.

Because they are buffered by the liver and then slowly released until they are metabolized, eating dietary carbohydrate is a time-based event. For this reason, it makes sense to pay attention not only to the QUANTITY of carbohydrate we are eating, but also to the FREQUENCY with which we eat them.

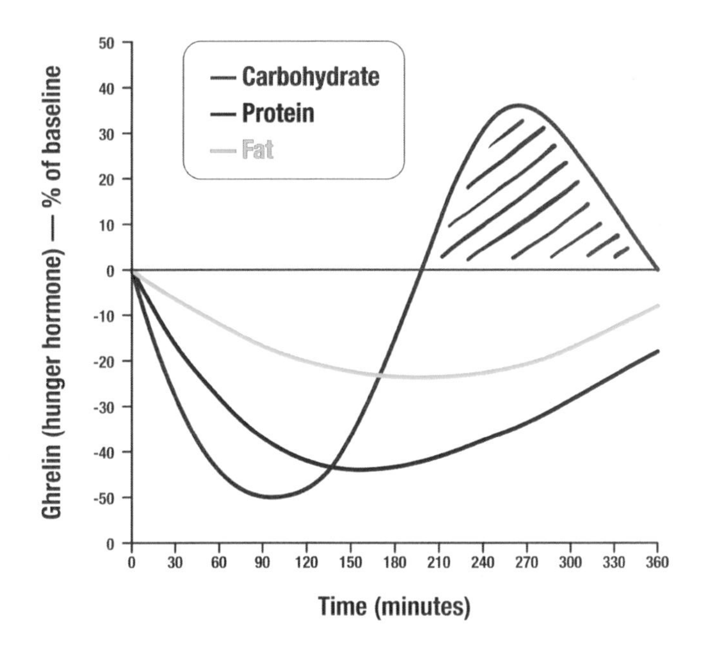

CARBOHYDRATE QUANTITY

Muscle glycogen is only depleted with high-intensity exercise. So if you haven't exercised with a high intensity recently, you are going to have to rely on your liver to dispose of your dietary glucose—either stored as glycogen, or in the case of overflowing glycogen stores, converted to fat—a liver process called 'lipogenesis'. Obviously if you are trying to lose fat you probably don't want a whole lot of this lipogenesis going on. Nor do you want the fat displacement, or 'fat-sparing', effect of a lot of carbohydrates. As the average person has room for about 100 grams of glycogen in their liver, it makes a lot of sense to recommend that a sedentary person, especially one who is trying to lose fat, might want to stay under 100 grams of carbohydrates a day. In fact, staying under 100 grams of carbs a day is probably one of the simplest fat loss plans on earth, and we highly recommend this for almost anyone who is trying to lose fat.

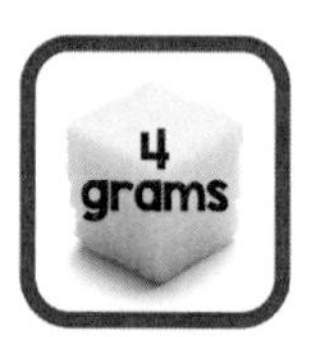

Your bloodstream can only hold 4 grams of glucose.

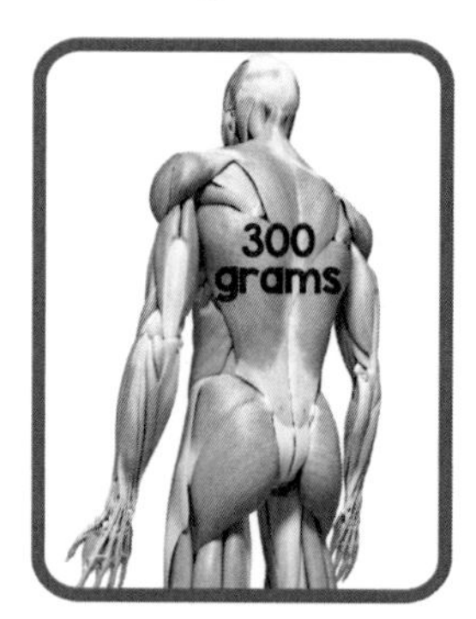

Your muscles can hold about 300 grams, but this is only used in very high intensity exercise.*

*About 90 minutes at high intensity to deplete.

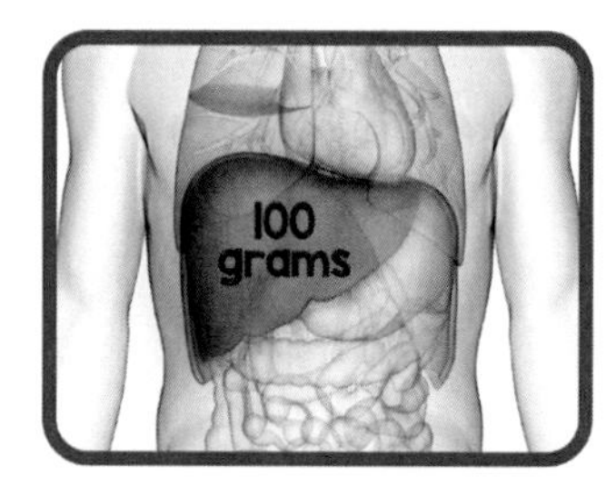

Your liver can hold around 100 grams of glucose, but it takes about 24 hours of fasting to deplete this.

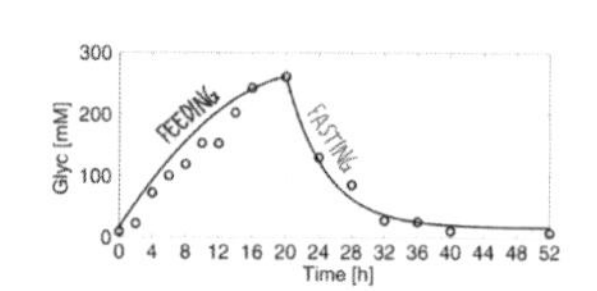

So unless you are engaging in high intensity exercise, you might want to limit yourself to 100 grams of net carbohydrates per day.

Which is roughly equivalent to four apples.

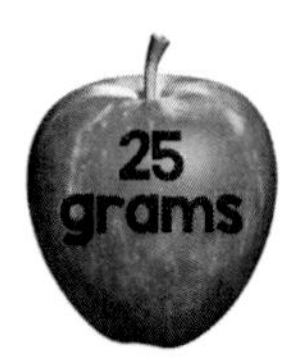

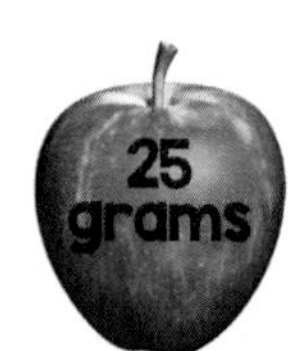

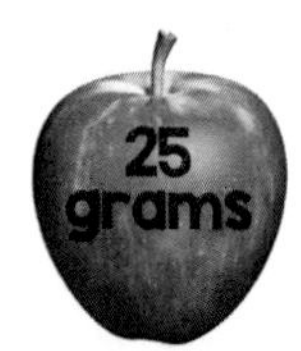

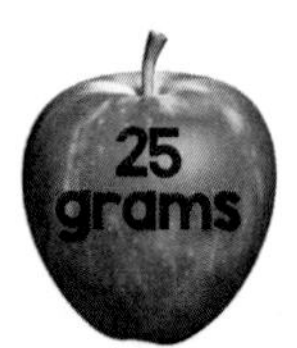

CARBOHYDRATE FREQUENCY

Because it takes 12 to 24 hours to fully deplete liver glycogen and enter the full-blown fat-burning state of ketosis, it makes a ton of sense to shrink down your carbohydrate frequency as much as possible. If you only ate carbs once a day, you will trigger the fasted state of ketosis daily even if you eat a fairly large quantity of carbohydrates at your single carbohydrate event. Therefore you can have almost as much fat-adaptation by limiting carbohydrate FREQUENCY as you will by limiting carbohydrate quantity. Of course, you can always combine the two—our personal favorite—and eat a limited amount of glycemic carbs once a day. It is quite likely that most of the benefits of intermittent fasting are due to the reduced frequency of eating carbohydrates and the expanded period of the day during which your body is forced to oxidize fat instead.

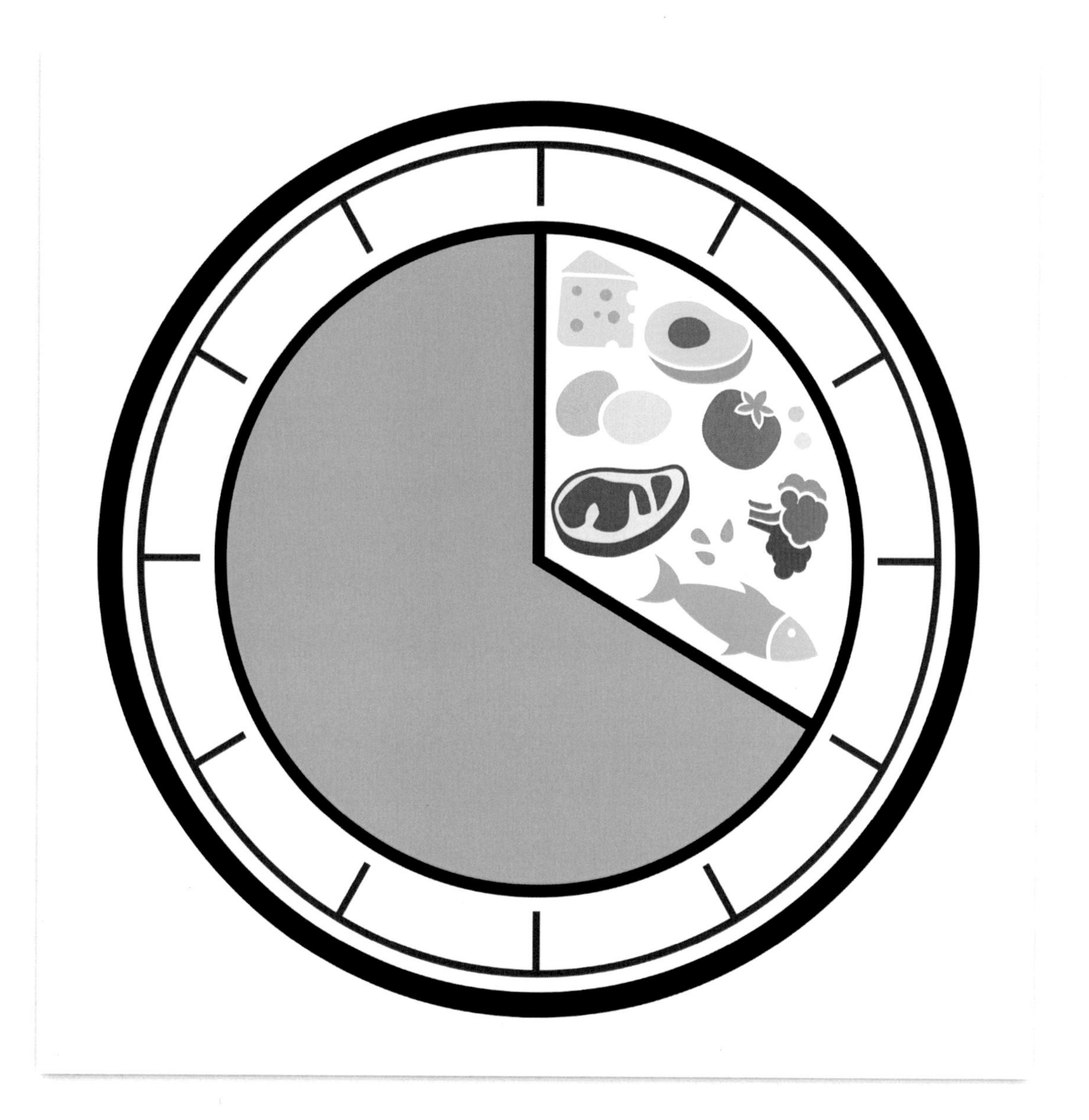

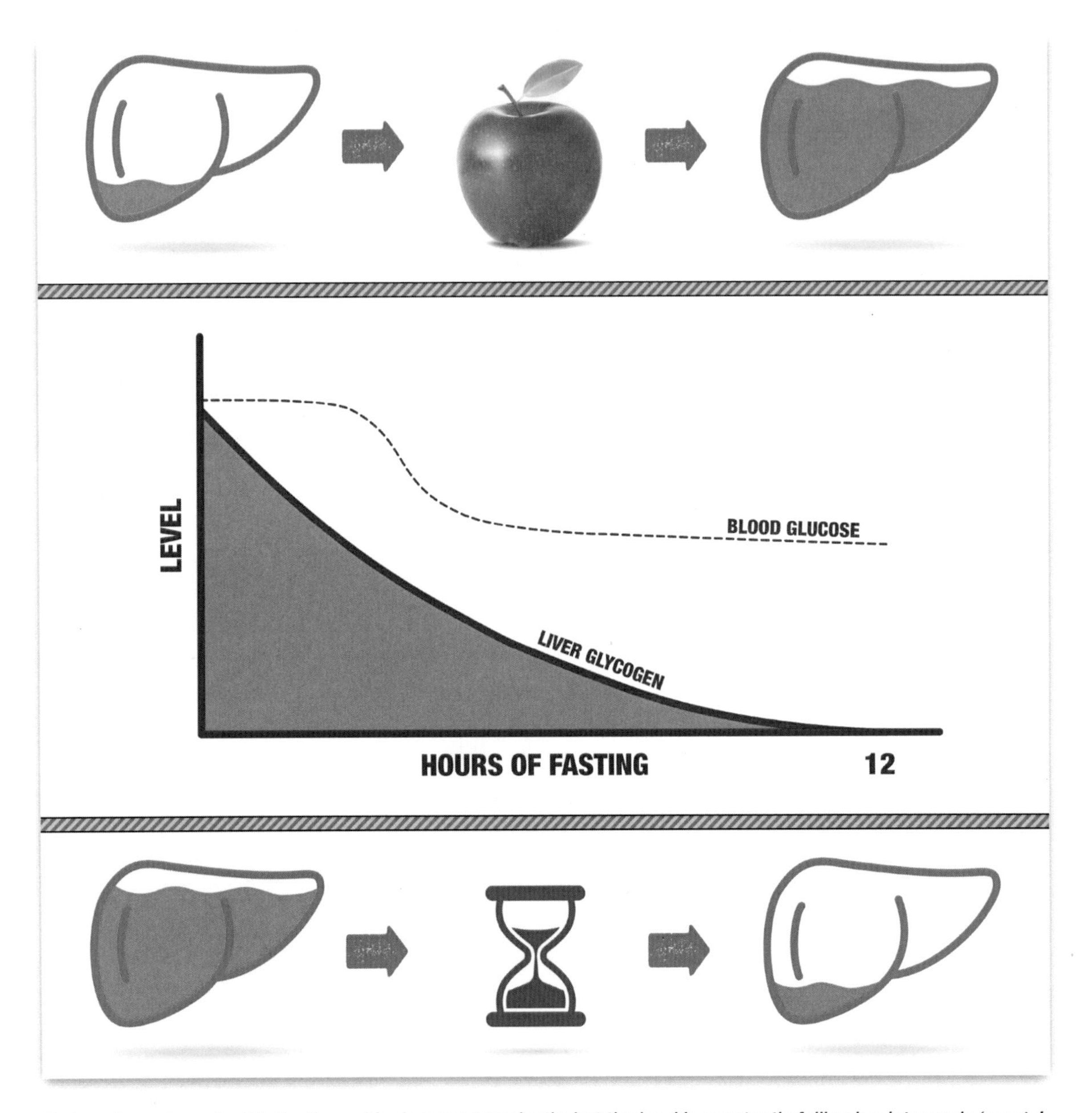

Eating glycemic carbs fills the liver with glycogen transiently, but the level is constantly falling back towards 'empty'.

METABOLIC FLEXIBILITY

The holy grail of metabolism is metabolic flexibility. What is metabolic flexibility? The ability to easily dispose of dietary fuels and easily switch from one fuel to the other without difficulty. For optimum metabolic flexibility, you need several things in place. First of all, you need some room in your adipocytes so you can easily store incoming dietary fat. If your fat cells are full and overflowing and there is increased fat energy in your circulation, you are not going to be metabolically flexible. Second, it helps to have plenty of disposal room for carbohydrates as well in your liver and your muscles. Regularly depleting liver glycogen with a decreased carbohydrate eating frequency is fantastic. Having more muscle tissue, and regularly depleting muscle glycogen, is also fantastic for glucose disposal headroom. Both of these, of course, require high-intensity exercise—resistance exercise to add muscle, and cardio to deplete glycogen (more on these later). So metabolic flexibility improves with leanness, high-intensity exercise (both resistance and cardio), and the fat-adaptation of periods of time without carbohydrate.

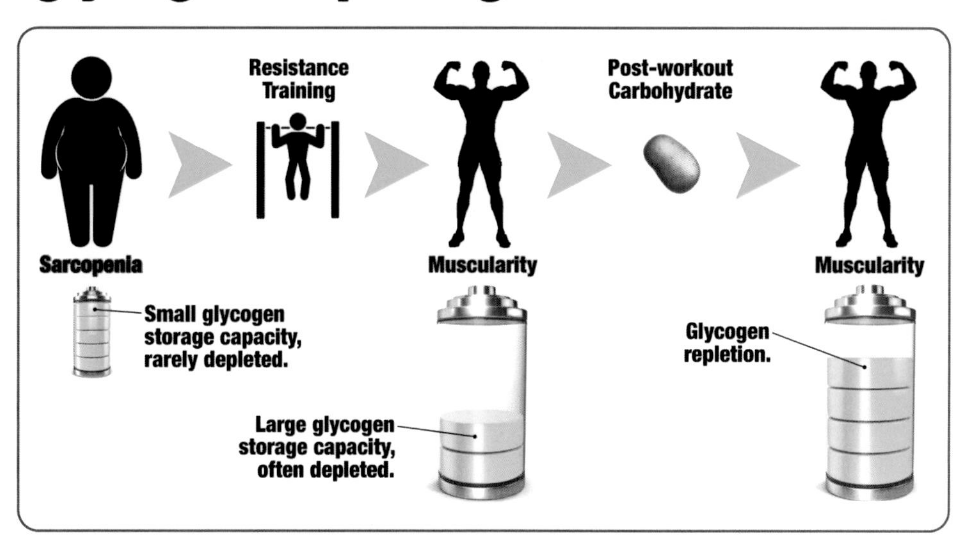

More muscle equals more metabolic flexibility — the ability to easily deal with dietary carbs OR fats.

THE CASE FOR CARBS

The ultimate strategy for maximally up-regulating fat oxidation? Never eat any carbs to begin with. This is certainly the strategy of those who go on a pure carnivore diet—and to be honest, this works pretty damn well for a growing number of people. But there are some reasons why you might want to include some carbs in your diet.

When your liver glycogen is completely empty, your sympathetic nervous system is more active. This is sort of your 'fight or flight' mode. People are usually more alert and more focused when they are low on liver glycogen. This is where some of the mental benefits of ketosis come from. It makes sense from an evolutionary perspective to be more alert and active when you have the highest need to look for food.

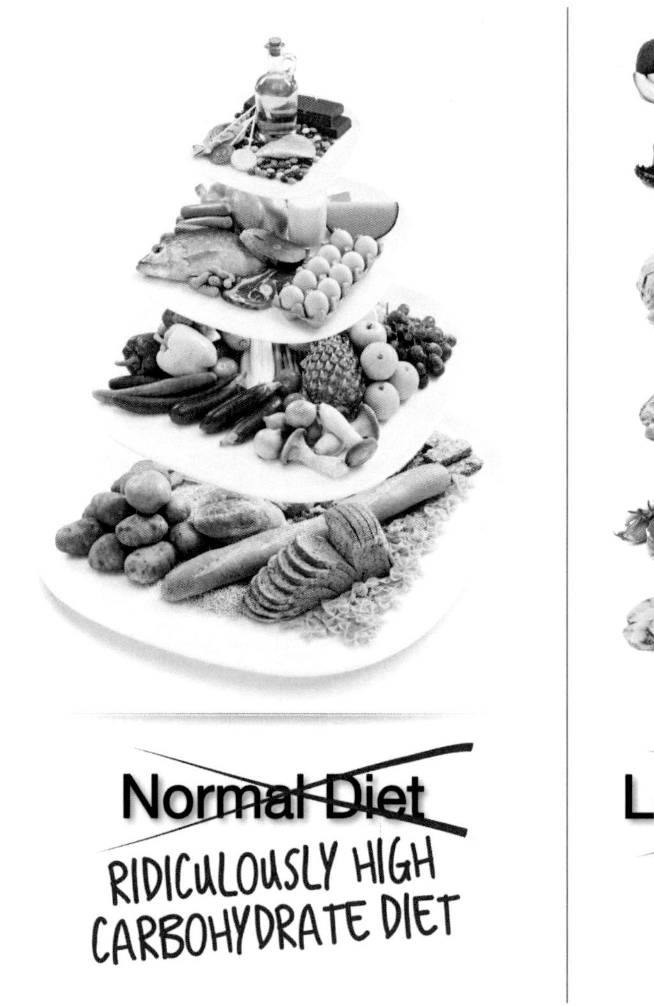

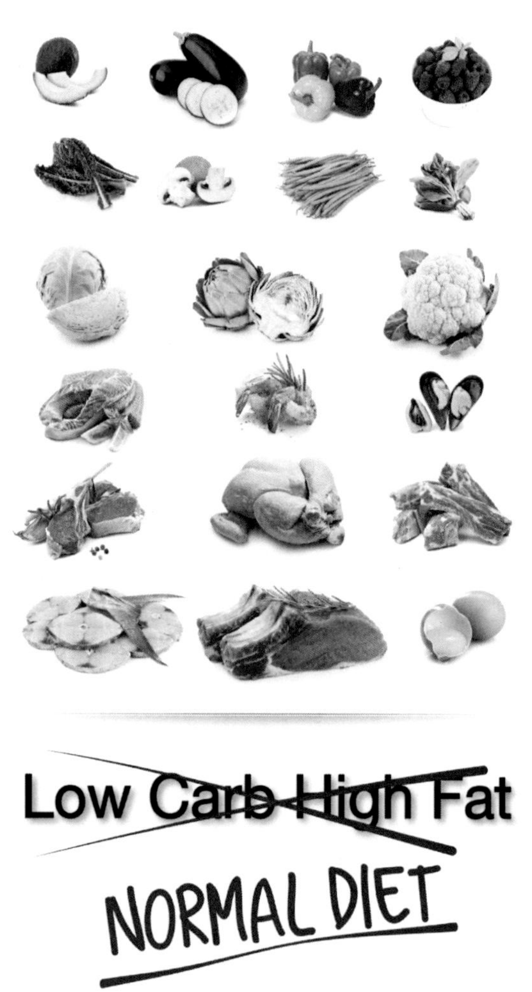

After a large carbohydrate meal, however, with lots of liver glycogen storage, our parasympathetic nervous system is activated—this is 'rest and digest' time. This is why we feel so tired and sluggish after a giant lunch of pasta or some other carbohydrate bomb. Once you understand how these two states operate, you can manipulate them at will. For example, if you have difficulty sleeping on a very low carbohydrate diet, you could eat carbs once a day (maybe 100 grams or so) and time this in the evening. Timing carbs in the evening has a few benefits. First of all, your sleep might benefit from the parasympathetic dominance of the carb fed state. And of course you will be more alert during the day, when your glycogen is low after your overnight fast. Secondly, by eating carbs in the evening, you are possibly less likely to be affected by the downstream hunger that can

Easiest Fat Loss Heuristic:

Eat foods to satiety as long as PROTEIN or FIBER is the dominant macronutrient.

PROTEIN:

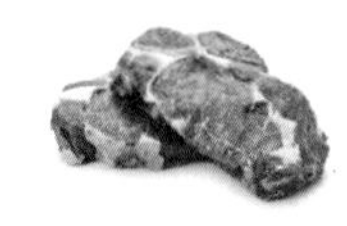
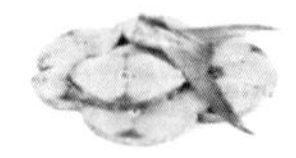
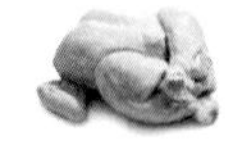
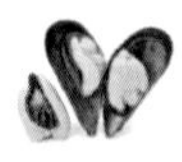
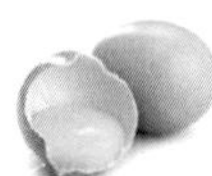

- beef
- fish
- pork
- chicken
- turkey
- veal
- lamb
- crustaceans
- shellfish
- cottage cheese
- eggs
- game
- whey

FIBER:

- arugula
- endive
- broccoli
- spinach
- kale
- turnip greens
- Chinese cabbage
- mushrooms
- artichoke
- cauliflower
- watercress
- collard greens
- celery

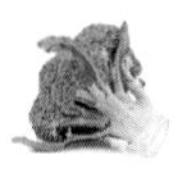
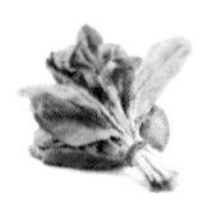
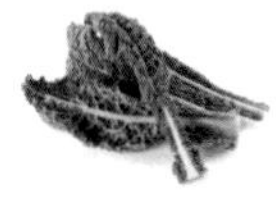
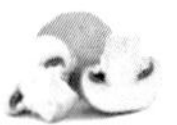
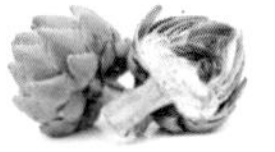

occur 3-4 hours after eating carbohydrate (although this can backfire on some who wake up hungry in the middle of the night so your milage may vary).

High-intensity exercise of extended duration will definitely require carbohydrates during the event. Even the most fat-adapted elite athletes can only participate in maximum intensity exercise for 2 hours at the very most before completely running out of muscle and liver glycogen and 'hitting the wall'—a state of hypoglycemia where your body pretty much stops doing what you have been asking it to do. Typically anyone who is engaging in very high intensity exercise for anything over an hour will benefit from some carbohydrate during the event.

Carbs may offer a significant satiety benefit for some people. For example, if you are hungry and you are in a low glycogen state, it might take hundreds of calories of fat and/ or protein for you to feel even slightly less hungry. But at that moment, some people might feel far more

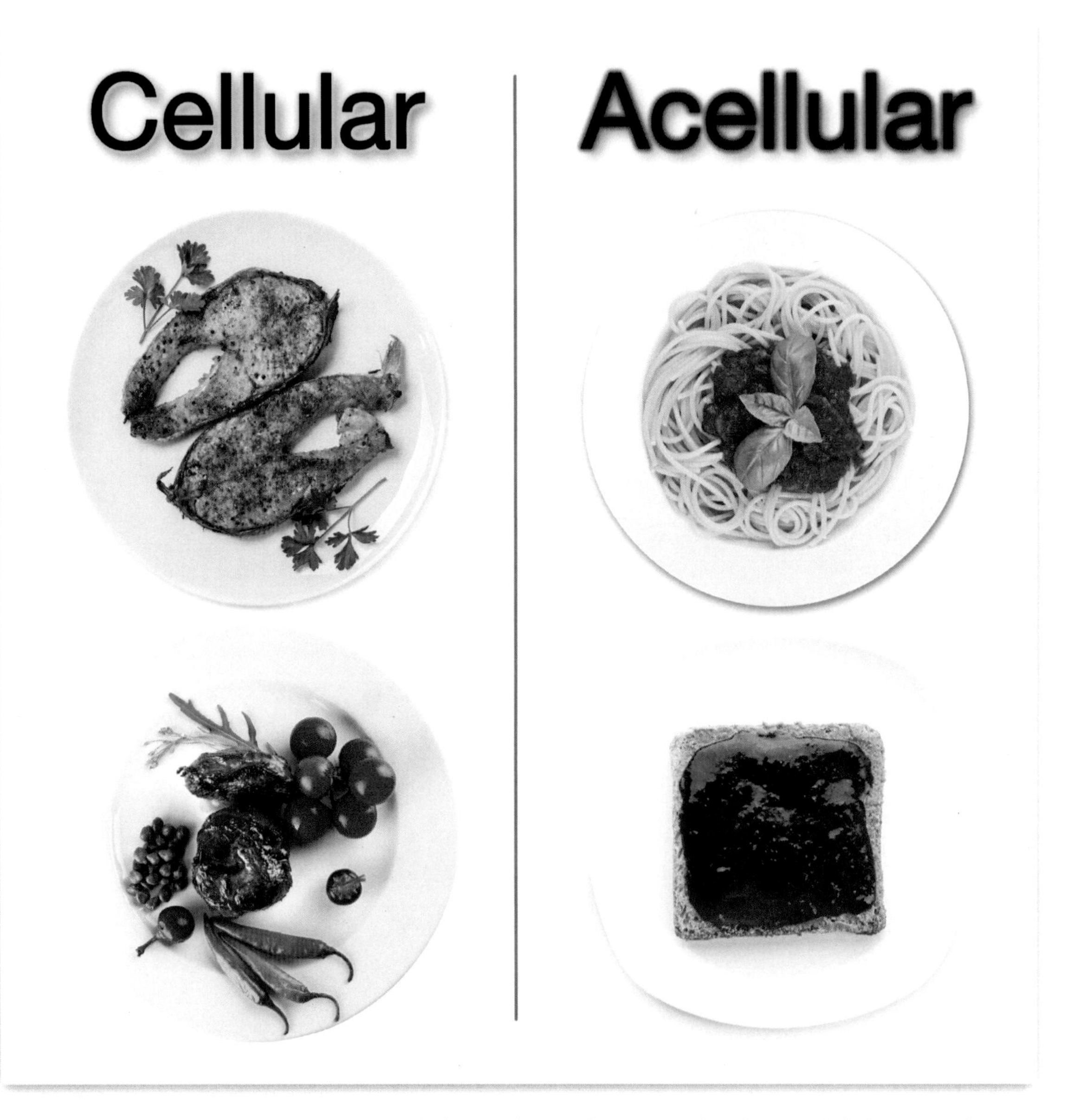

'Cellular' carbs, from unprocessed whole foods, always offer more satiety than 'acellular' processed carbs, such as sugar and flour.

satiety from just a small quantity of carbohydrate, as it is really that liver glycogen they are looking for rather than more fat and protein calories. When using carbohydrates for satiety, you really want to choose foods with the very lowest energy density. In other words, pick foods with as much water, fiber, and protein as possible. These foods will provide the highest satiety for the lowest actual carbohydrate content. If eating zero carbohydrates ever was the ultimate secret to leanness, every single bodybuilder would be on a zero carbohydrate pure carnivore diet. But that is not the case. Instead, physique athletes choose the foods that provide the highest satiety for the lowest amount of energy. In practice, these foods are usually very high in protein, fiber, water, and micronutrients—with very judicious and strategic use of carbohydrates and fats.

If you want to maintain maximal metabolic flexibility, it really doesn't make much sense to never eat any carbohydrates ever. But it DOES make sense to have very clear periods of time when you are in a carb-depleted state of maximal fat oxidation (read: ketosis), as well as times when you do have incoming dietary carbohydrate to deal with (instead of fat). Probably the easiest way to implement this is intermittent fasting, and limiting glycemic carbohydrate frequency. Our favorite way of accomplishing this in real life? Stay very low carb during the day and then have one higher carb meal at the end of the day—keeping protein percentage as high as possible, of course.

Finally, remember that in order to be successful long-term, your dietary strategy has to be sustainable indefinitely. You really want to be on the least

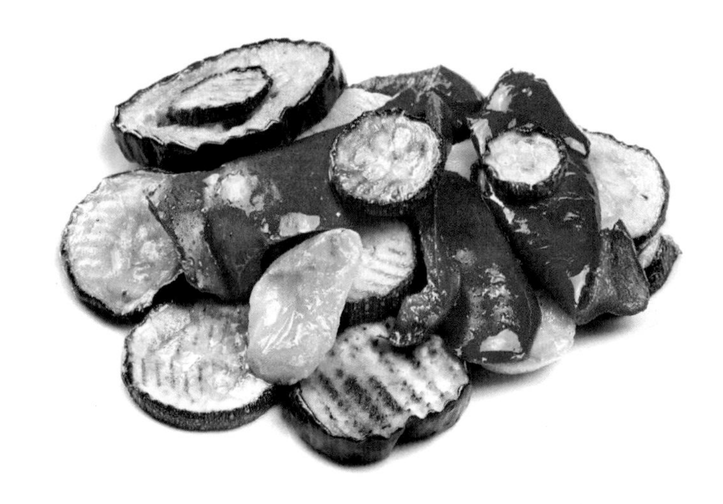

SAME AMOUNT OF NET CARBS

restrictive diet possible, to help out with long-term adherence. Being low carb most of the time with occasional carb-ups sounds a lot less restrictive versus swearing off all carbs forever—an unlikely scenario to begin with. Focus on the things you can realistically achieve. Can you permanently increase the overall protein percentage of your diet? Probably yes—and this will help you succeed at your body composition goals. Can you reduce your carbohydrate frequency on a long-term basis? I'm sure you could, and this is going to improve your metabolic flexibility.

WHAT SHOULD YOU ACTUALLY DO?

Consider a lower carbohydrate eating frequency, such as eating carbs once a day. This probably works best in the evening, at the end of your eating window, and after eating protein and fibrous veggies. Try to keep net carbs under 100 grams a day if you are not regularly engaging in high-intensity exercise. Choose carbs with maximal protein, fiber, and water content for satiety. 100 grams would be roughly equivalent to two potatoes, two cups of rice, or four apples.

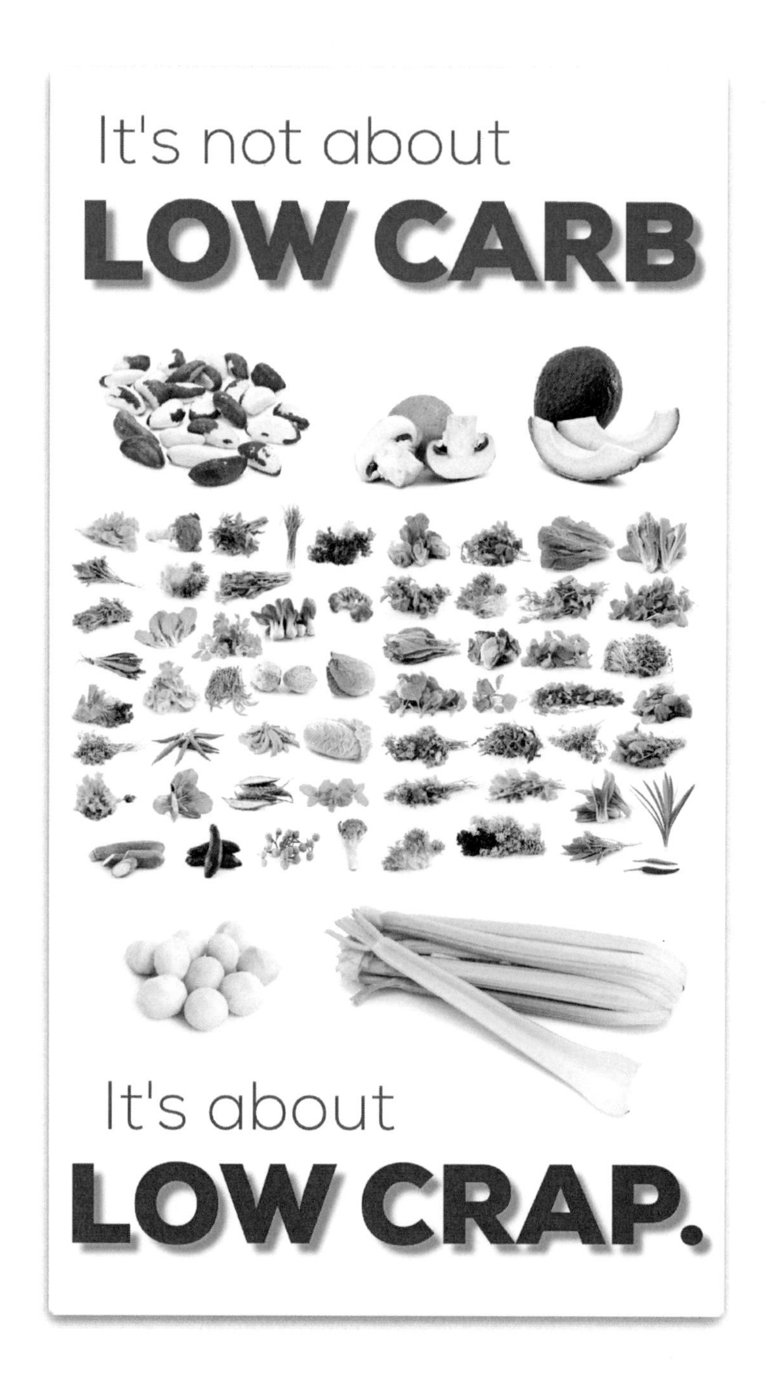

PROTEIN:ENERGY RATIO

Humans eat until they have reached an adequate quantity of protein and minerals. Minerals track very well with protein (which makes sense, as plants absorb nitrogen from topsoil along with other minerals). Therefore, in The P:E Diet, we target protein and foods with a high protein percentage, in order to increase the protein percentage of our diet. Protein offers both short-term and long-term satiety. Fat offers lower satiety. Carbs are unique in that they offer an initial satiety for a few hours, followed by a literal increase in hunger as blood sugar falls. More on this later! But for now, the goal is targeting protein first and foremost. That is the primary goal of the Protein:Energy approach.

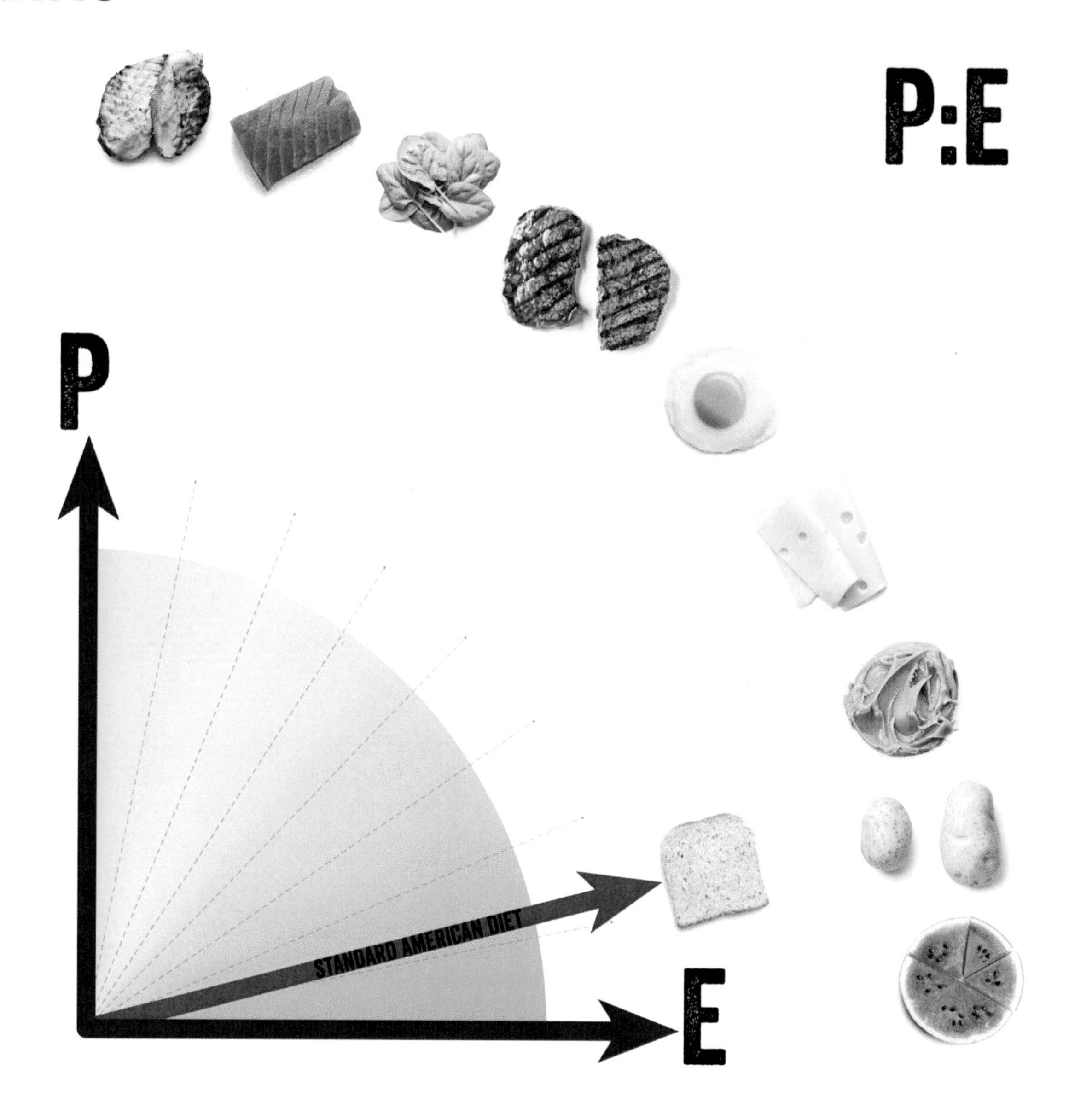

NUTRITIONAL INFORMATION

In order to calculate the Protein to Energy Ratio, we need to know the four basic mass quantities (in grams) printed on all nutritional labels for:

1. **Protein**
2. **Fat**
3. **Carbohydrate**
4. **Fiber**

Because fiber is indigestible and does not contribute directly to energy calories, we subtract fiber grams from total carbohydrate grams to yield 'net carbs' (carbs minus fiber). This gives us the total amount of carbohydrate energy.

So the equation is PROTEIN divided by FAT and CARBS minus FIBER. This could also be written as PROTEIN divided by FAT plus NET CARBS.

If you are eating a food without a label—and let's face it, this is always the healthiest choice—you can usually just 'google' the food and the word 'nutrition' and you will be given the USDA nutrition facts for the chosen food. You can also go directly to the USDA website here:

fdc.nal.usda.gov

Several other apps and web services are very helpful for providing nutritional information. Our favorites are:

cronometer.com

and

myfitnesspal.com

Once you have the nutritional information, you can use it to calculate your P:E ratio. Feel free to try our free P:E calculator at:

PtoER.com

$$\frac{\text{PROTEIN}}{(\text{FAT} + \text{CARBS} - \text{FIBER})}$$

$$\frac{\text{PROTEIN}}{(\text{FAT} + \text{NET CARBS})}$$

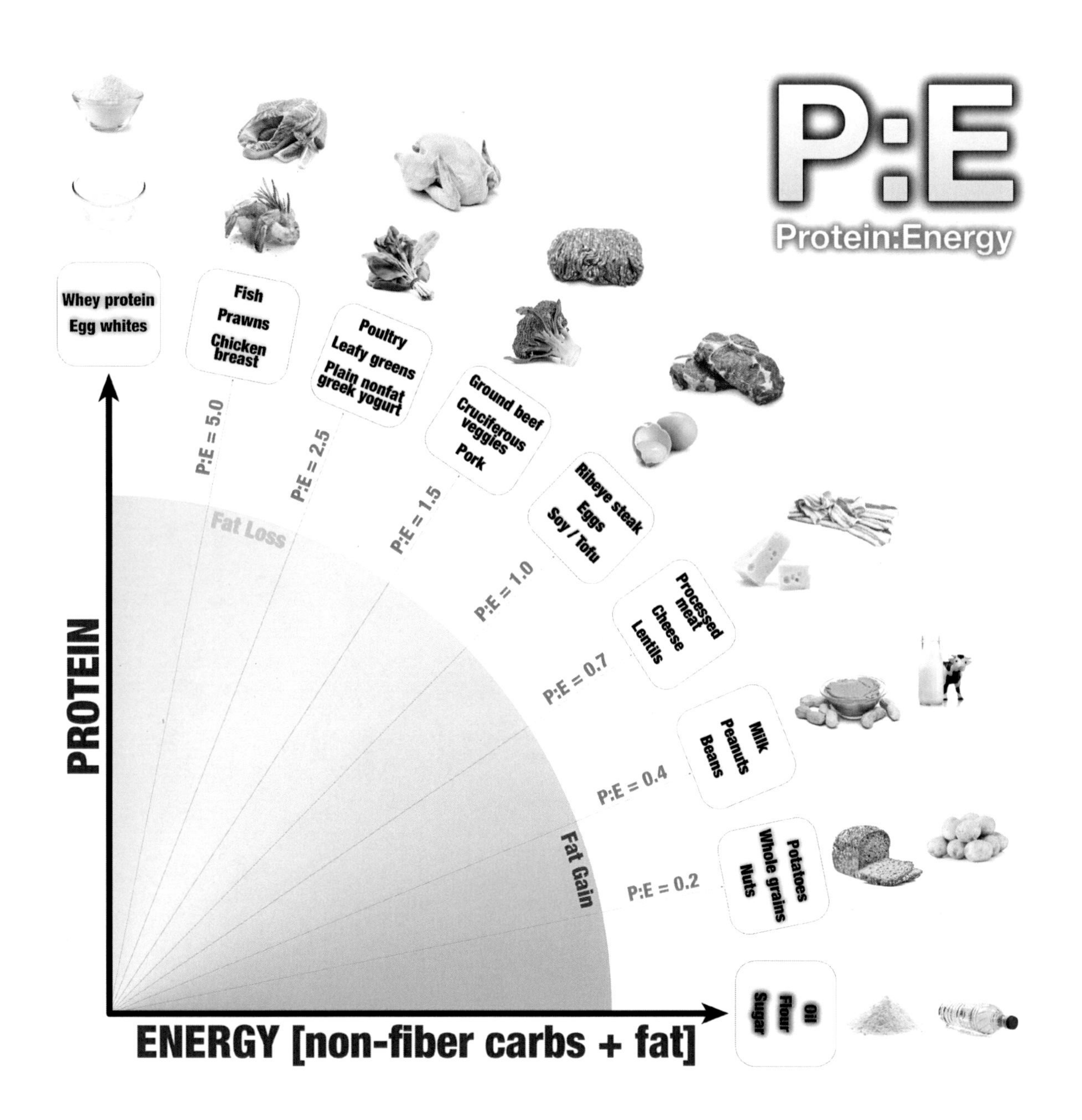
P:E
Protein:Energy
Whey protein
Egg whites
Fish
Prawns
Chicken breast
Poultry
Leafy greens
Plain nonfat greek yogurt
Ground beef
Cruciferous veggies
Pork
Ribeye steak
Eggs
Soy / Tofu
Processed meat
Cheese
Lentils
Milk
Peanuts
Beans
Potatoes
Whole grains
Nuts
Oil
Flour
Sugar
P:E = 5.0
P:E = 2.5
P:E = 1.5
P:E = 1.0
P:E = 0.7
P:E = 0.4
P:E = 0.2
Fat Loss
Fat Gain
PROTEIN
ENERGY [non-fiber carbs + fat]

PRACTICAL IMPLEMENTATION

Below we will provide some examples of using the P:E calculation for actual foods. When you use the Protein to Energy system, protein and fiber are essentially 'good', and carbs and fats are 'bad'. Of course you have to eat SOME energy and you can't live on nothing but whey powder and egg whites (100% protein). The idea here is not to get the highest score and eat pure protein—instead you want to INCREASE your current protein to energy ratio in order to increase the protein to energy ratio of your body. A good target might be 1.0, which is roughly equal grams of protein and non-protein energy. As this is near the average for worldwide hunter-gatherers, this is probably a good place to start. You will need MORE energy if you are highly active and LESS energy if you are sedentary; ideally if you eat the RIGHT foods your body should let you know HOW MUCH to eat.

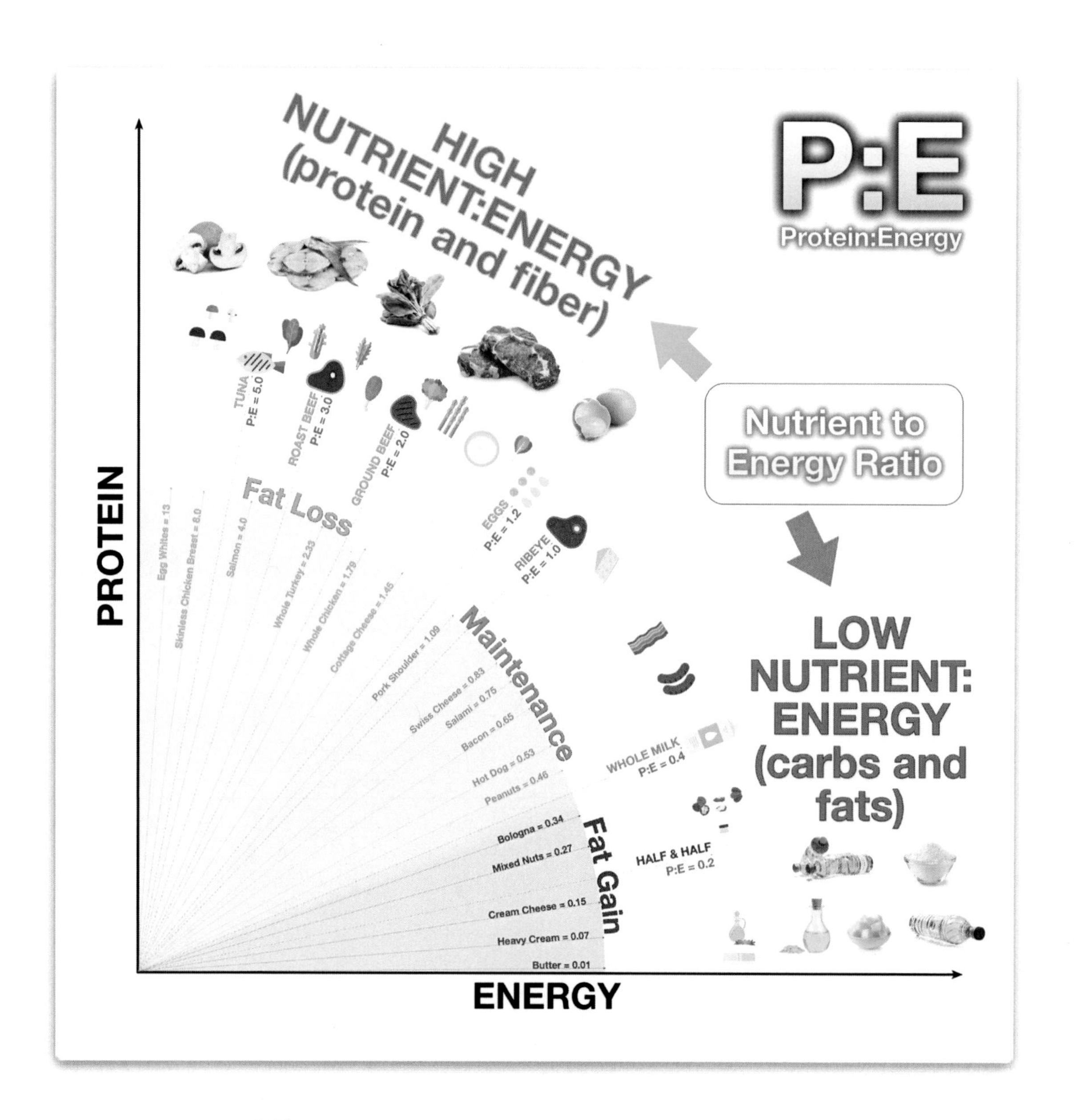

When you start to evaluate foods this way, you quickly come to a few realizations. First of all, meat is awesome. For example, shown below is

GROUND BEEF at various fat percentages. Leaner ground beef is a slightly higher score than higher fat percentages, but all of them are EXCELLENT. And guess what: ground beef is in fact an amazing food.

Grains, however, are an entirely different story. Here are all of your grains shown below. Oats seem to be the 'best', but are still pretty much terrible. Rice, unsurprisingly, scores terribly here.

Your average ANIMAL food is scoring higher than your average PLANT food. And let's remember that 84% of all human calories on earth are currently coming from PLANTS—a statistic made far more terrible because 60% of all plant calories come from wheat, rice, and corn—some rather suboptimal grains.

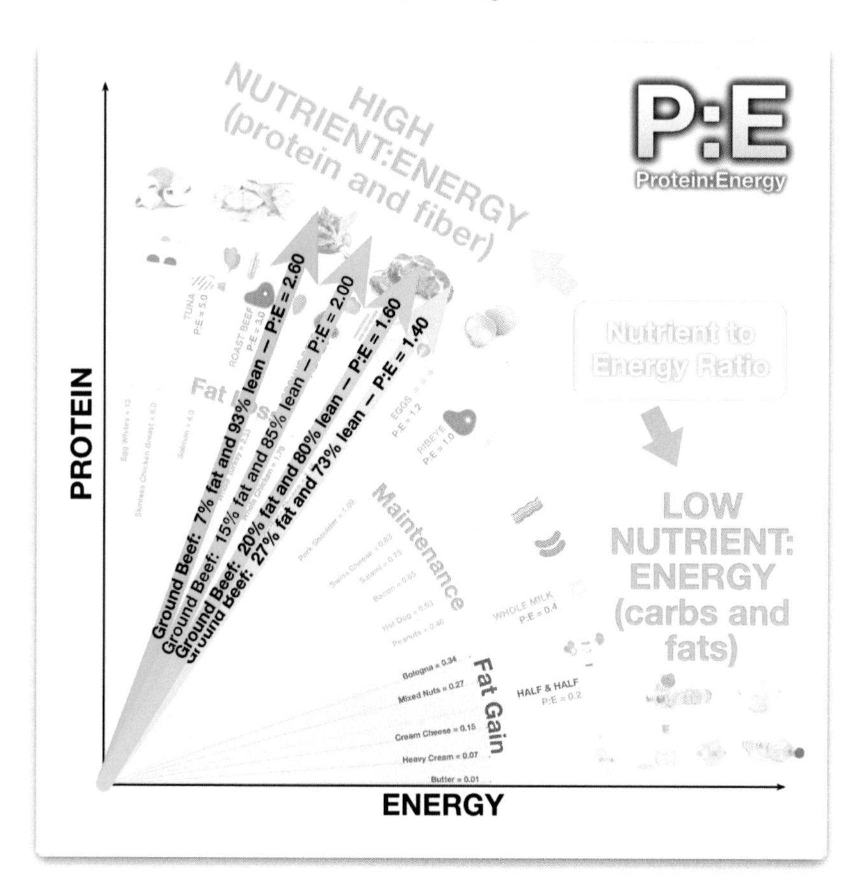

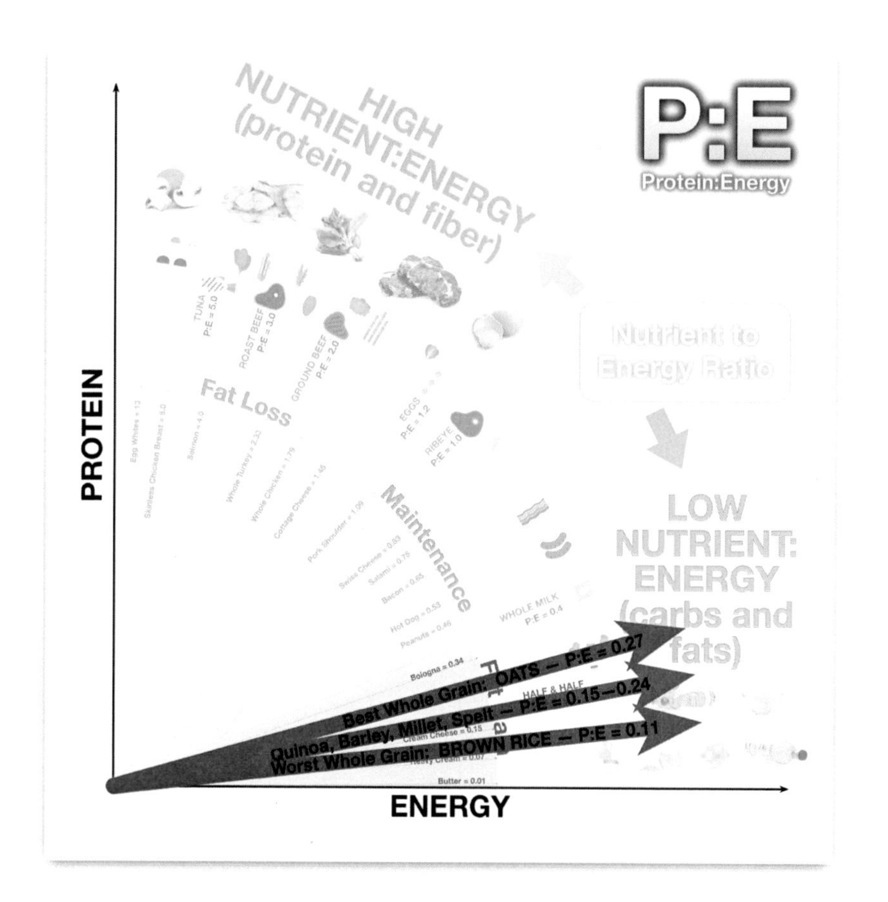

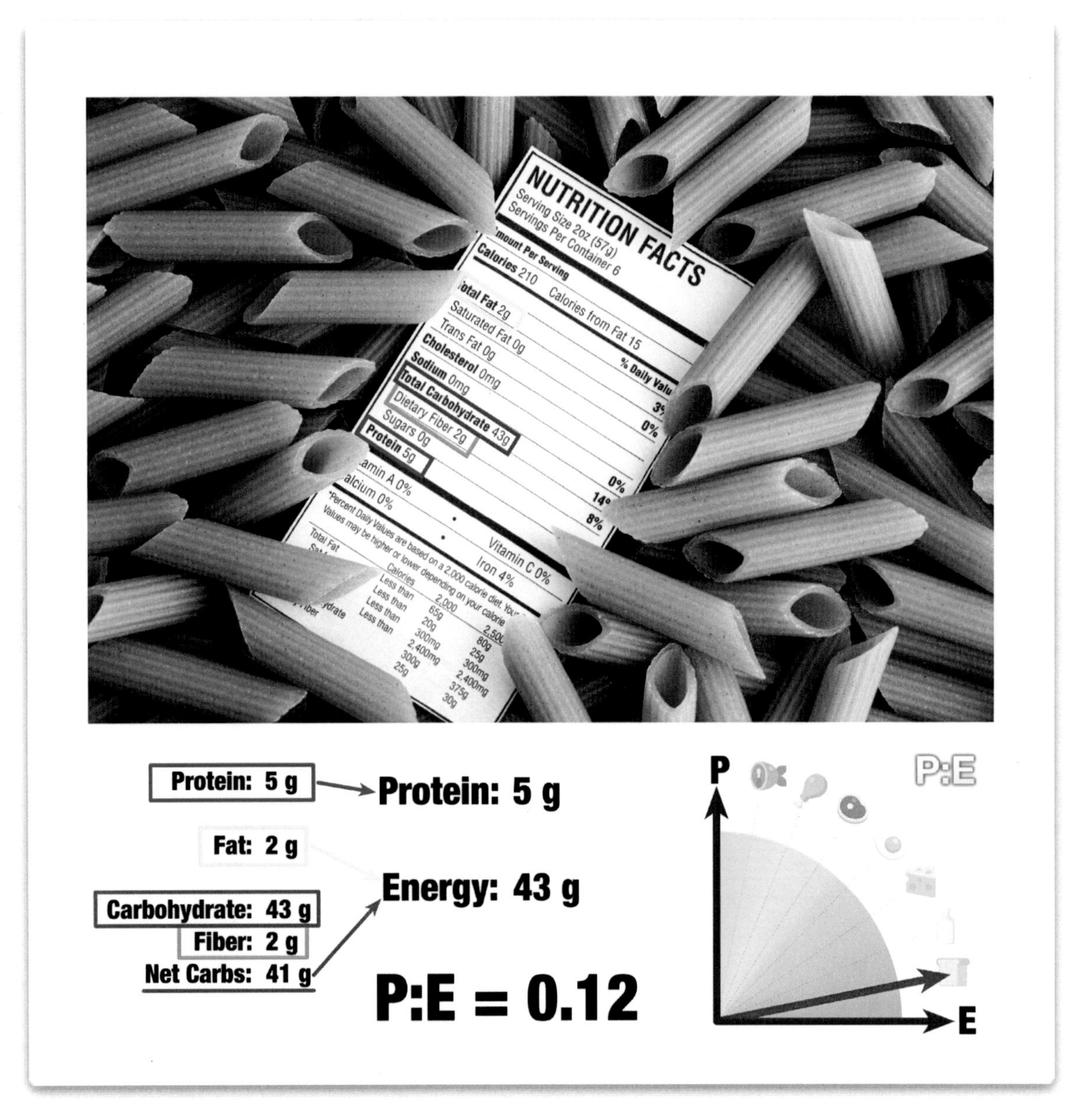

Pasta, like anything else made from grain flour, is pretty low on the P:E scale. Better than sugar or oil, but not by much!

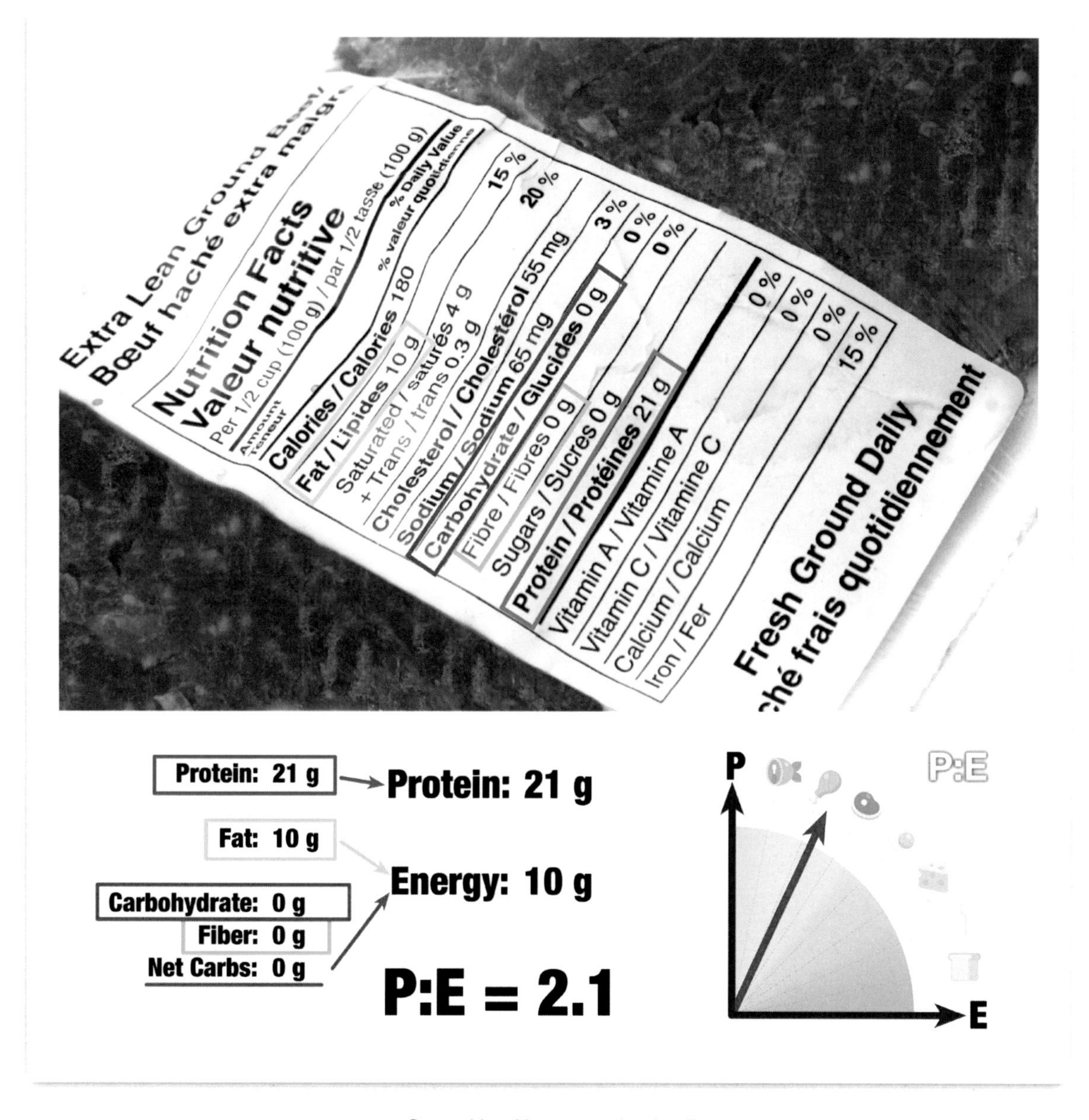

Ground beef is an amazing food!

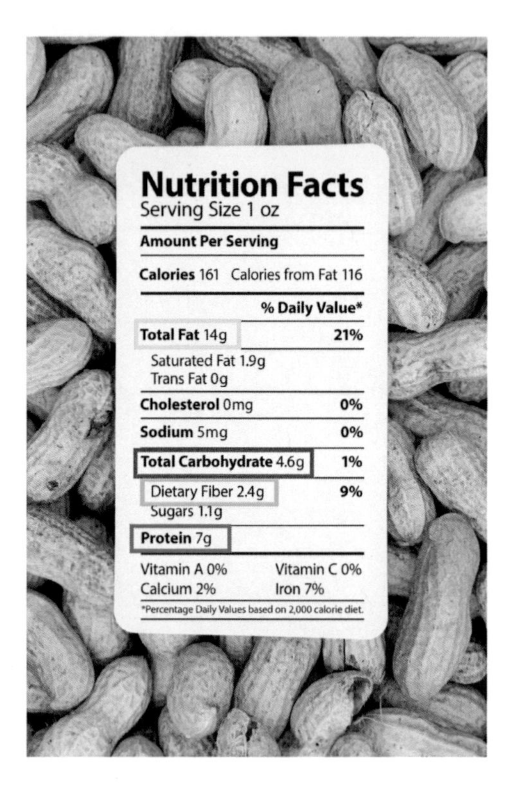

Nutrition Facts
Serving Size 1 oz

Amount Per Serving	
Calories 161	Calories from Fat 116
	% Daily Value*
Total Fat 14g	**21%**
Saturated Fat 1.9g	
Trans Fat 0g	
Cholesterol 0mg	**0%**
Sodium 5mg	**0%**
Total Carbohydrate 4.6g	**1%**
Dietary Fiber 2.4g	**9%**
Sugars 1.1g	
Protein 7g	
Vitamin A 0%	Vitamin C 0%
Calcium 2%	Iron 7%

*Percentage Daily Values based on 2,000 calorie diet.

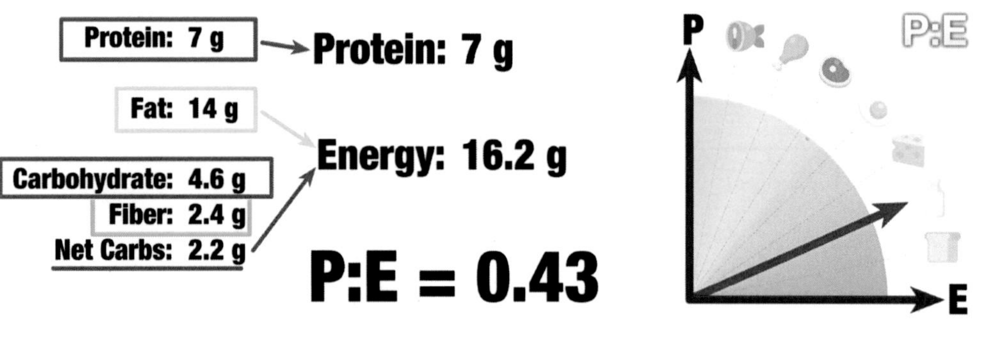

Peanuts are higher than other tree nuts, but they still aren't a good fat loss food by any stretch.

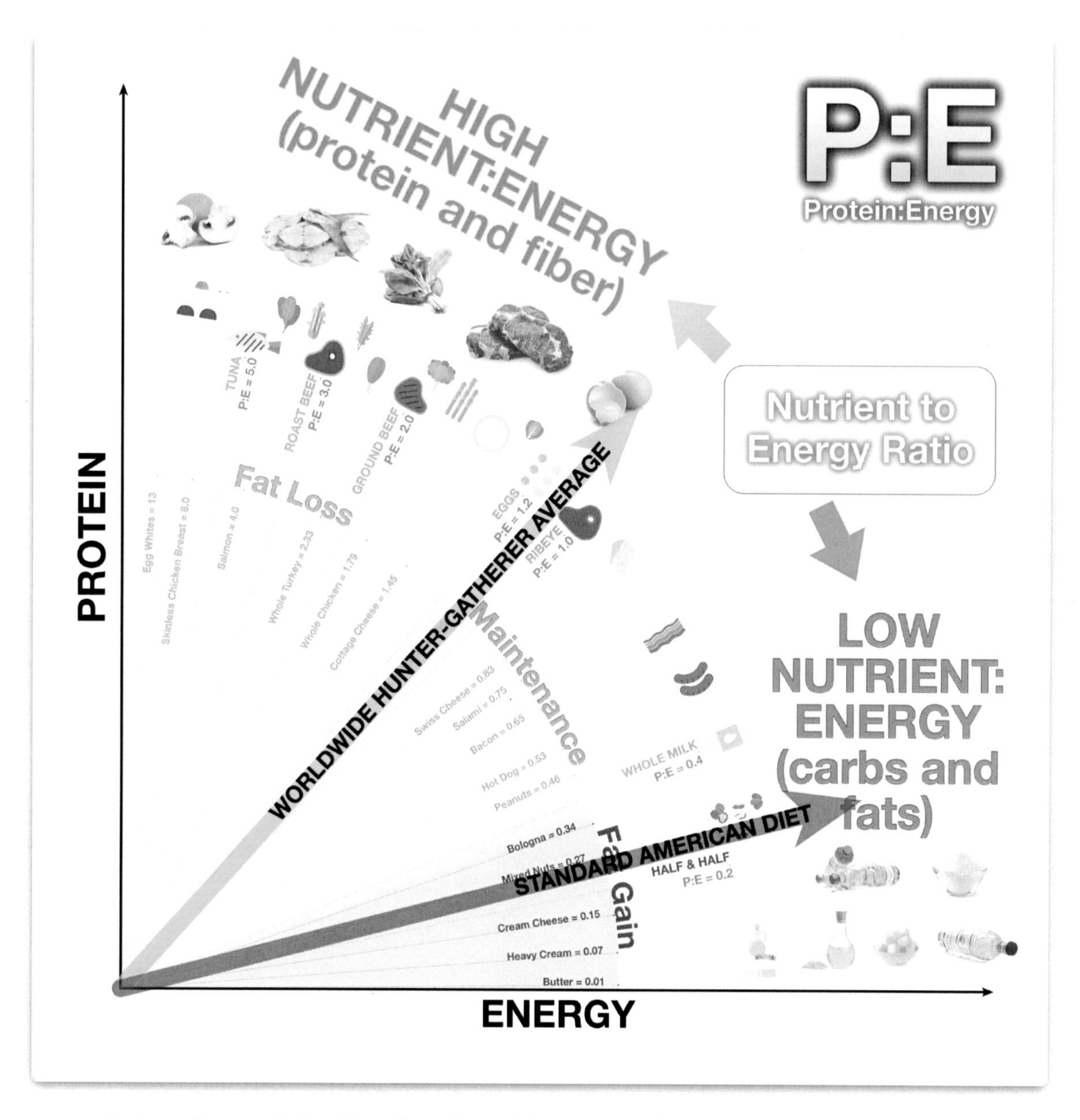

Hunter-gatherers eat about three times the protein percentage that we do. This explains their results.

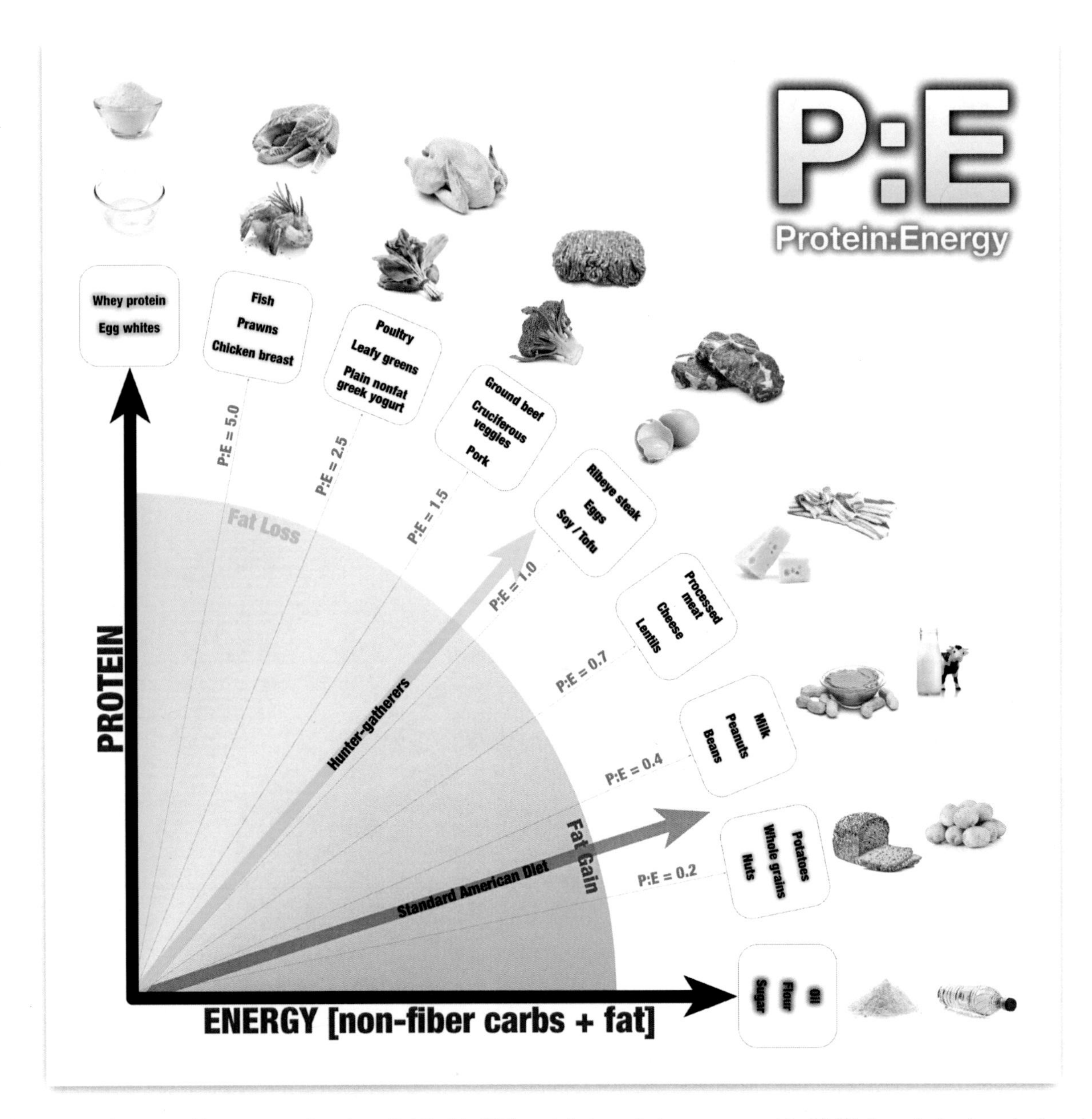

The average hunter-gatherer on earth eats a diet that is 33% protein by calories, compared to 12.5% by calories here in America.

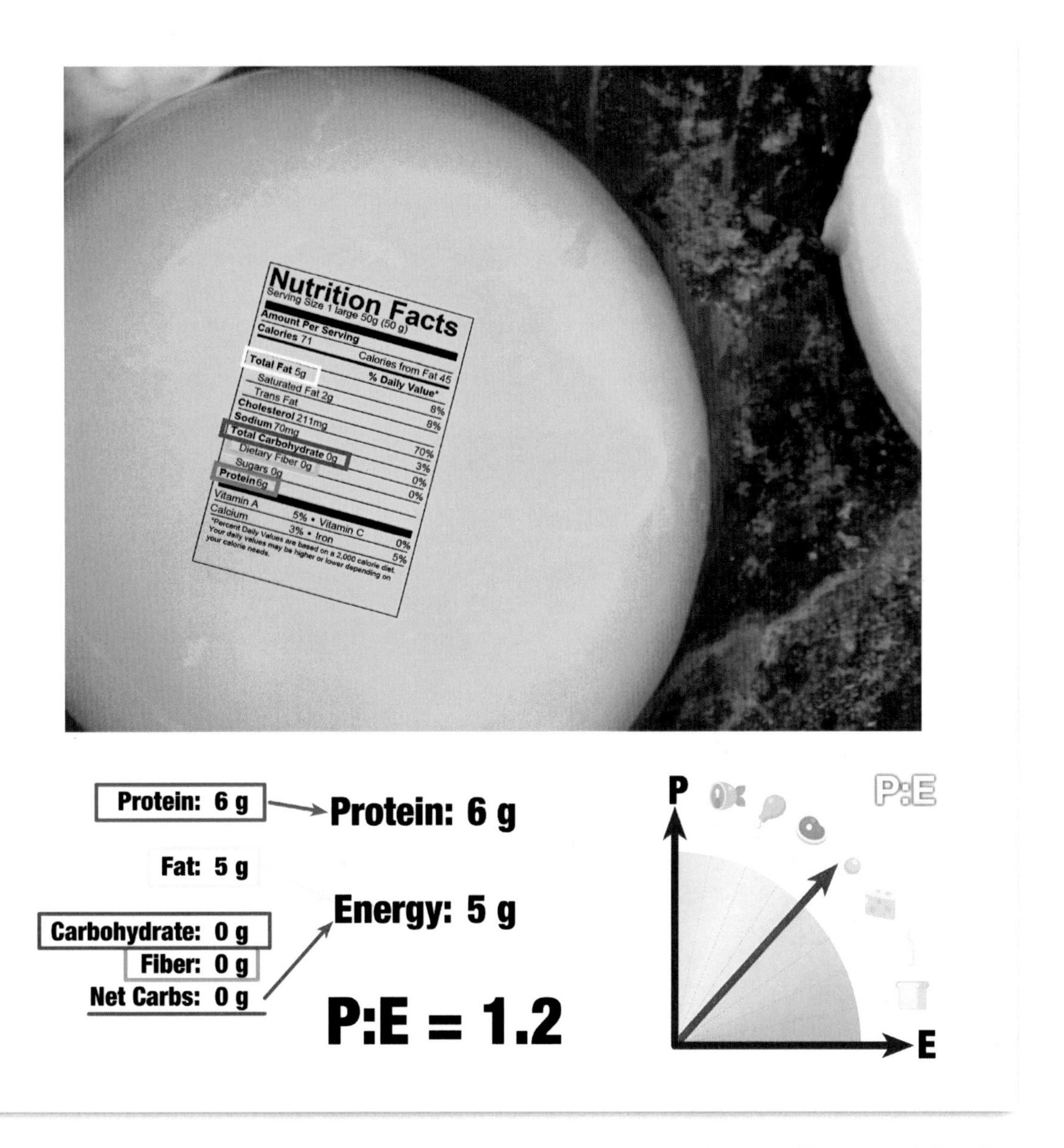

Eggs have a great P:E ratio, and are one of the most nutritious foods you could ever eat. These contain literally everything it takes to create and sustain life. Plus they taste amazing.

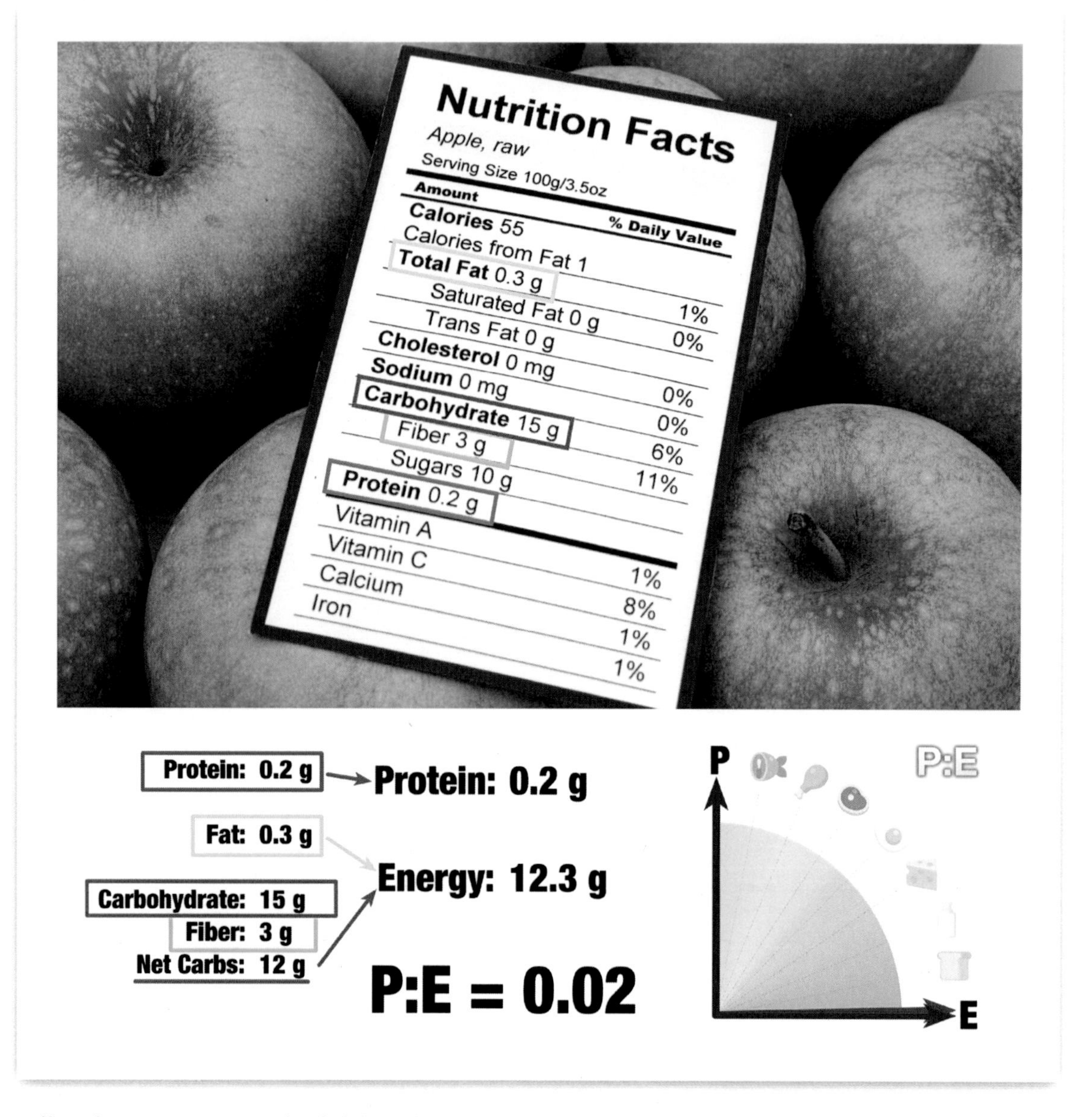

If you have to eat some carbs, fruit has a low energy density and is therefore much more satiating than refined carbs like sugar and flour. Not a great source of protein however, so be strategic with these carbohydrates.

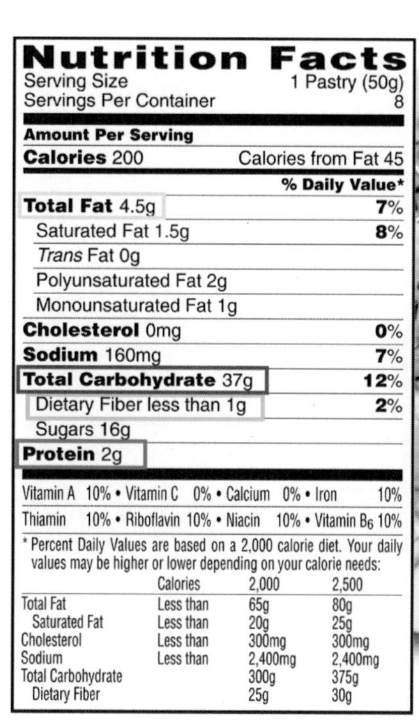

Nutrition Facts

Serving Size	1 Pastry (50g)
Servings Per Container	8

Amount Per Serving

Calories 200	Calories from Fat 45
	% Daily Value*
Total Fat 4.5g	**7%**
Saturated Fat 1.5g	**8%**
Trans Fat 0g	
Polyunsaturated Fat 2g	
Monounsaturated Fat 1g	
Cholesterol 0mg	**0%**
Sodium 160mg	**7%**
Total Carbohydrate 37g	**12%**
Dietary Fiber less than 1g	**2%**
Sugars 16g	
Protein 2g	

Vitamin A 10% • Vitamin C 0% • Calcium 0% • Iron 10%

Thiamin 10% • Riboflavin 10% • Niacin 10% • Vitamin B6 10%

* Percent Daily Values are based on a 2,000 calorie diet. Your daily values may be higher or lower depending on your calorie needs:

	Calories	2,000	2,500
Total Fat	Less than	65g	80g
Saturated Fat	Less than	20g	25g
Cholesterol	Less than	300mg	300mg
Sodium	Less than	2,400mg	2,400mg
Total Carbohydrate		300g	375g
Dietary Fiber		25g	30g

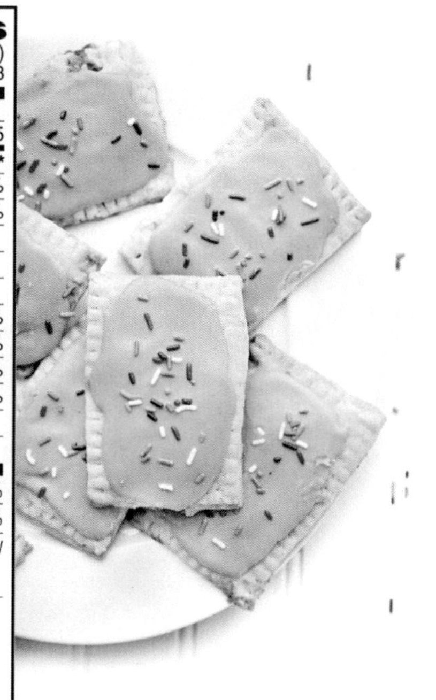

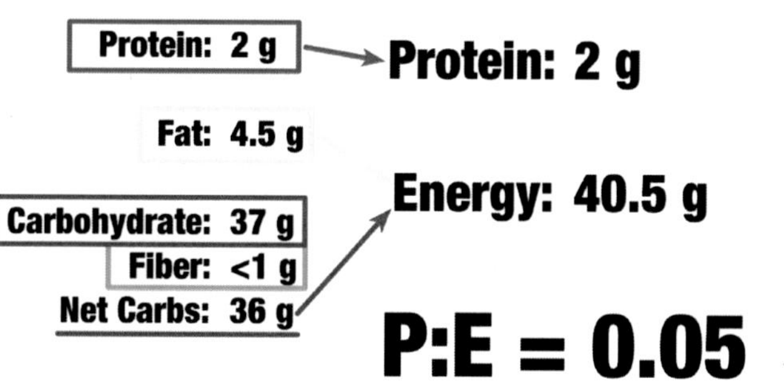

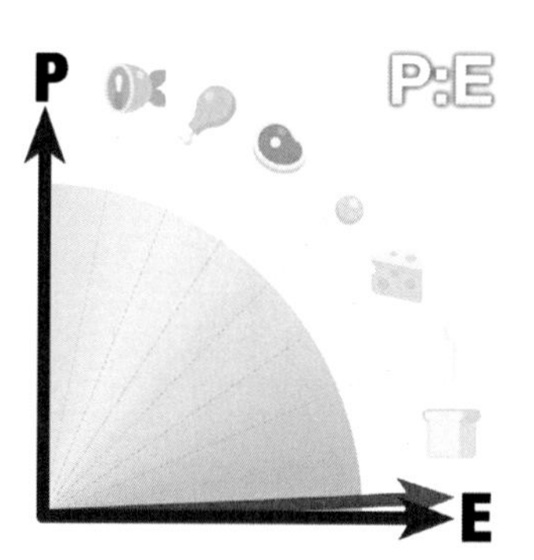

Yeah, pretty much awful. Just like you would expect.

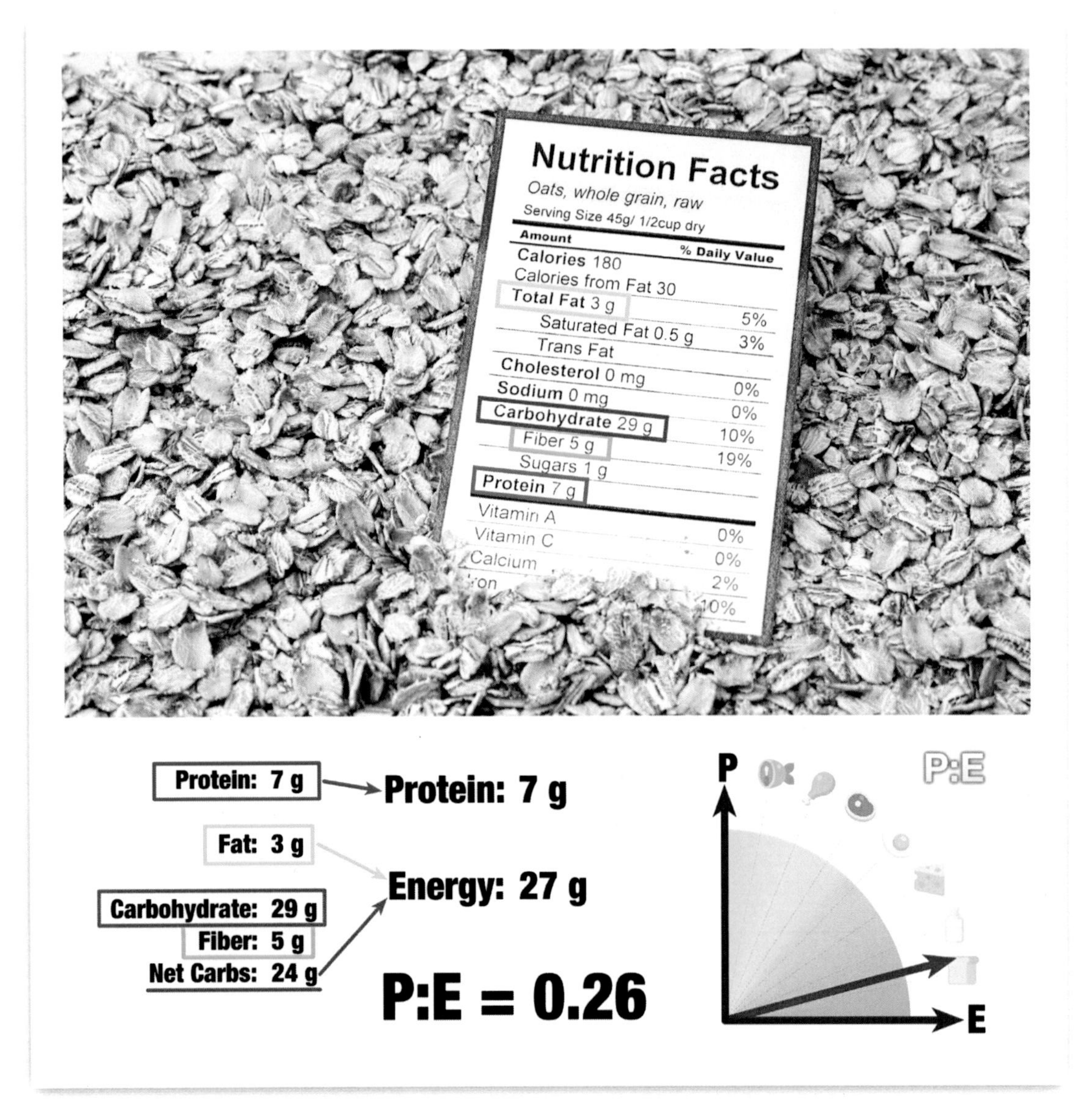

Oats offer more protein and fiber and satiety than pretty much any other grain, so if you have to eat some carbs they are one of your better options. Still not great from a P:E standpoint, so you are better off eating animal protein first and foremost and using this strategically as a reasonably high satiety carbohydrate choice.

HOW TO USE THE P:E RATIO

Ok, so you have done some rough P:E calculations on a few different foods, and now you are starting to get the point. Meat, eggs, and green vegetables are good; grains are bad. Fish is the greatest thing ever, and sugar and oil are the worst things ever. But now how do you incorporate this into everyday life?

The P:E Diet is all about *FOOD CHOICE*. You are specifically CHOOSING one food, over other possible food options, because it is going to provide you with a higher level of nutrient satiety—allowing you to eat less energy overall. So what you want to do is make small and sustainable substitutions, in a gradual and progressive fashion, to slowly and surely improve your diet quality in a way that will lead you to naturally eat less energy.

In the example pictured here, we have eggs at a P:E of about 1.0 (equal grams of protein and fat), bacon at about 0.7 (higher fat grams than protein grams), and buttered toast way down near 0.1

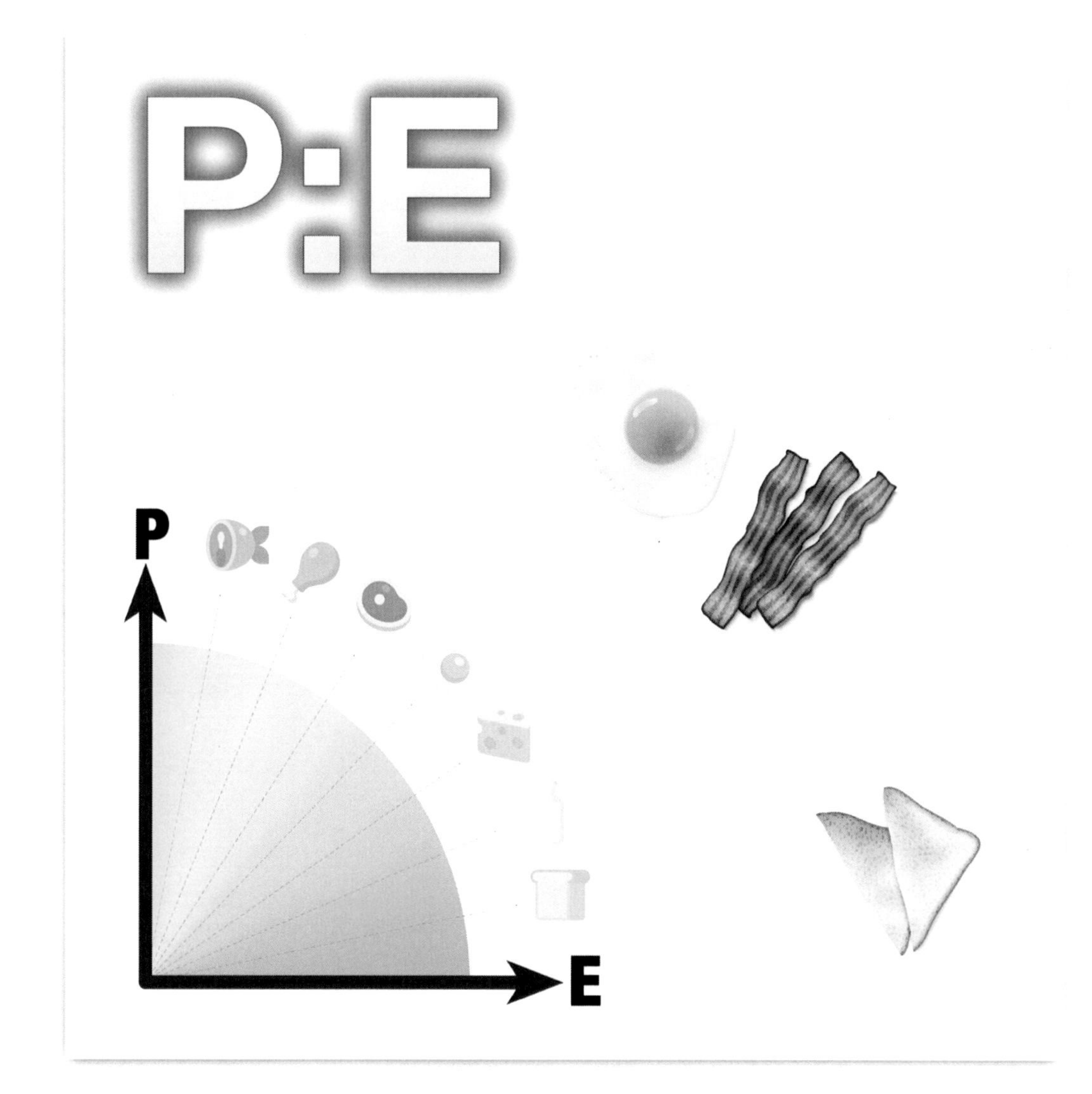

Eggs, bacon, and buttered toast. With The P:E Diet, you would prioritize these foods in this order: eggs > bacon > toast.

(way more grams of carbs and fat than grams of protein). So your general approach would be choosing eggs over bacon and toast if possible. Now if your breakfast was always toast, you would actually be progressing your diet if you switched entirely to bacon for breakfast. But eggs would be an upgrade from bacon as well!

The goal is NOT to eat 100% protein at all times. In fact, a P:E of 1.0 (pretty much steak and eggs) would be an excellent maintenance ratio for most people—and if you are highly active and need a ton of energy calories, you might even be very lean and healthy at a P:E of 0.5. But since the Standard American Diet is way down around a 0.25, we know that most people have a lot of room for improvement.

And that is the goal—slow, steady, gradual improvement of your diet, one food substitution at a time. Switching from a doughnut for breakfast to oatmeal would significantly raise the P:E of that meal. And then switching to bacon would be another improvement. And then steak and eggs would be even higher. You could even go for a much leaner meat—our favorites for breakfast are Canadian bacon and turkey bacon, both of which are quite lean and have a P:E way up around 5.0 or so!

We don't expect anyone to use this system to track every single food, or their entire day, or their entire lives—that is the exact opposite of what we are suggesting. Instead, we recommend familiarizing yourself with the general P:E ratio of the foods you eat most often. Then, armed with this knowledge, you can look for ways of substituting out certain foods for other choices that are a little bit higher on the P:E scale. Maybe there is a version of the food you are eating that has higher fiber? Or lower fat. Or fewer carbs. Or more protein. Or maybe you decide to skip that food entirely, based on its low P:E score, and replace it with an entirely different food.

You don't have to walk around the grocery store with a slide rule or a calculator. But get into the habit of looking at labels and doing a quick mental calculation. Look for grams of protein. Then look for grams of fat as well as net carbs (total carbs minus fiber). If the energy grams (fat plus net carbs) are dramatically higher than the protein grams, you might want to keep looking. But if protein grams are equal to energy grams, or even higher? Perfect!

Focus on small, steady, gradual, and most importantly SUSTAINABLE changes. You want a diet that you enjoy, and than you can stick to for life. So maybe in the example above, you choose to eat a few more eggs and a few less pieces of toast? Or you trade in your bacon for turkey bacon? Or you make toast out of some low carb bread? Any of these small swaps would be pretty easy and likely sustainable—and would help you get closer to your goals.

Every food you eat is either moving you closer to your goals, or farther away—keep this in mind. Luckily, you have the power to make these choices every single day! Choose wisely!

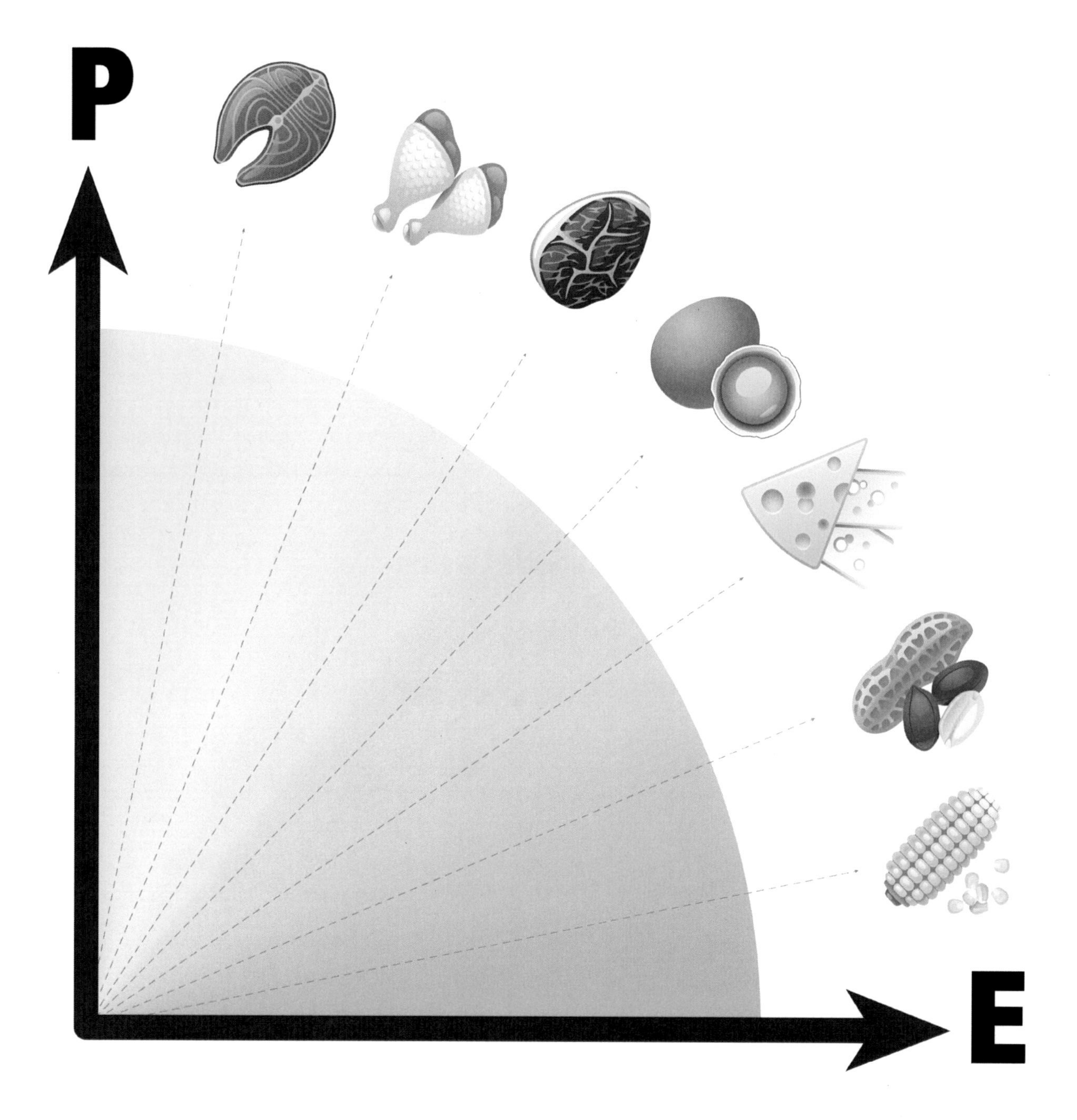
P
E

40 grams of protein.

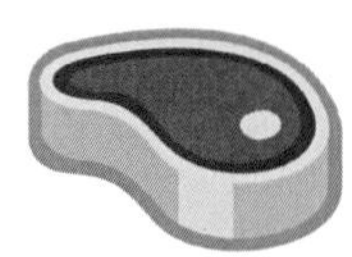

Also 40 grams of protein.

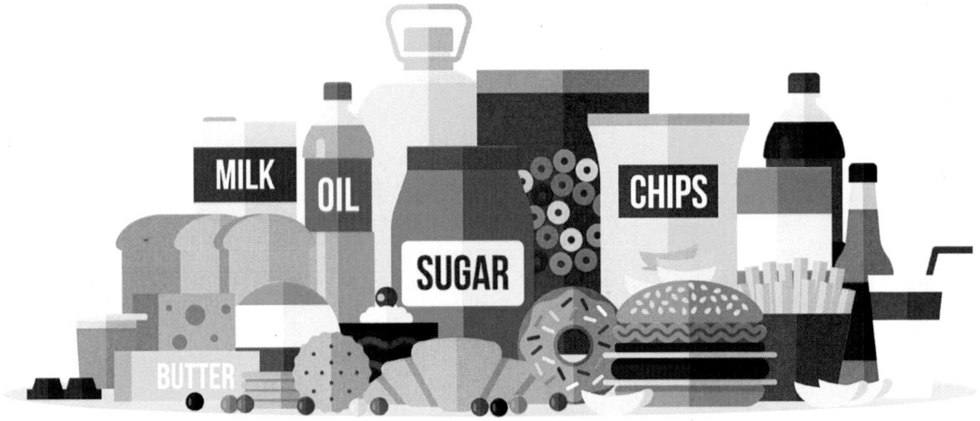

This is what protein dilution looks like. It is all around us.

WHAT TO EAT

You are only going to MAINTAIN your results if you enjoyed the process that got you there in the first place.

— Ted Naiman

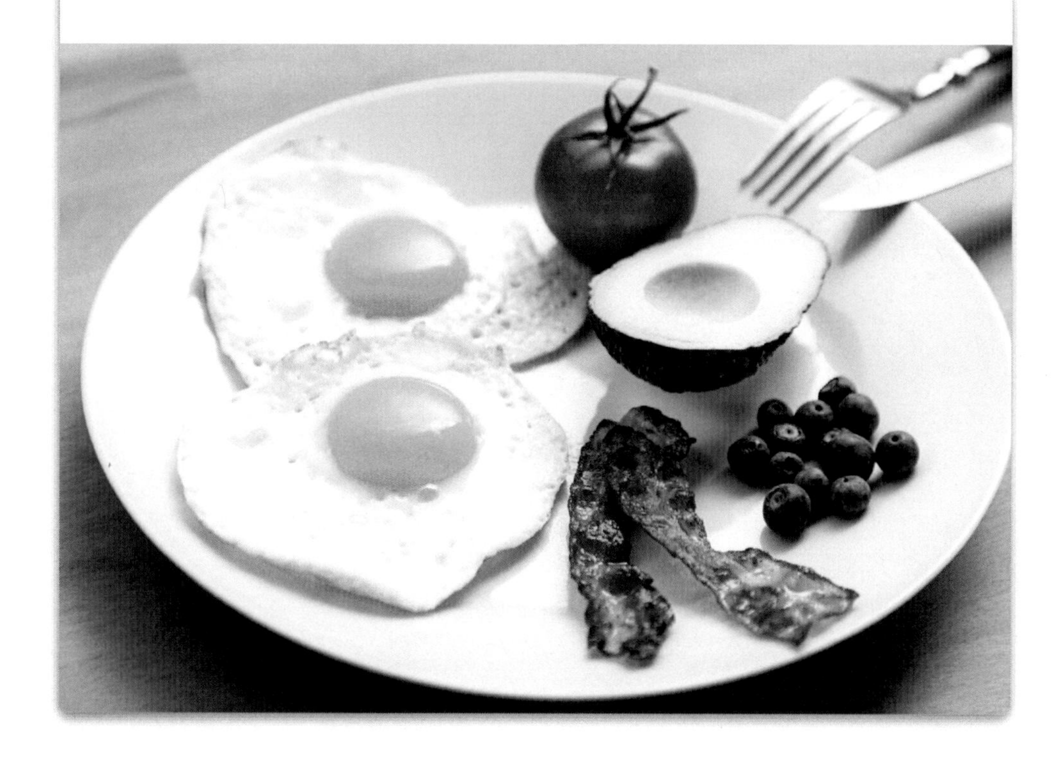

SPECIES-APPROPRIATE DIET

Humans are hunter-gatherers, and we do have a SPECIES-APPROPRIATE diet. We prefer to start with a basic Paleo-ish template as a starting point, although there are tons of modern processed foods that are just fine on the P:E scale (plain Greek yogurt, cottage cheese, and whey protein would be excellent examples).

You'll want to base your meal around protein. Any high quality protein is fine—including beef, lamb, pork, poultry, fish, seafood, and fermented dairy like greek yogurt or cottage cheese.

Aim to consume grass-fed beef, wild caught fish, and pastured chickens and eggs when possible for the optimal nutrition.

Properly raised animals eating their species appropriate diet (like cows eating grass) means more omega 3s in your protein! This will help reduce inflammation in the body.

Start with one or two protein sources in your meal (e.g. beef and eggs) and then include some veggies. Simple as that!

Animal foods are inherently higher in protein and minerals compared to vegetarian options, as they are at a higher trophic level. However if one chose to be a vegetarian for ethical reasons, good choices would include eggs and fermented dairy (cottage cheese and yogurt). An ethical vegan could also make this work using legumes (with soy and lentils at the top of the list) and plant proteins (tofu, textured vegetable protein, wheat gluten, and plant protein concentrates).

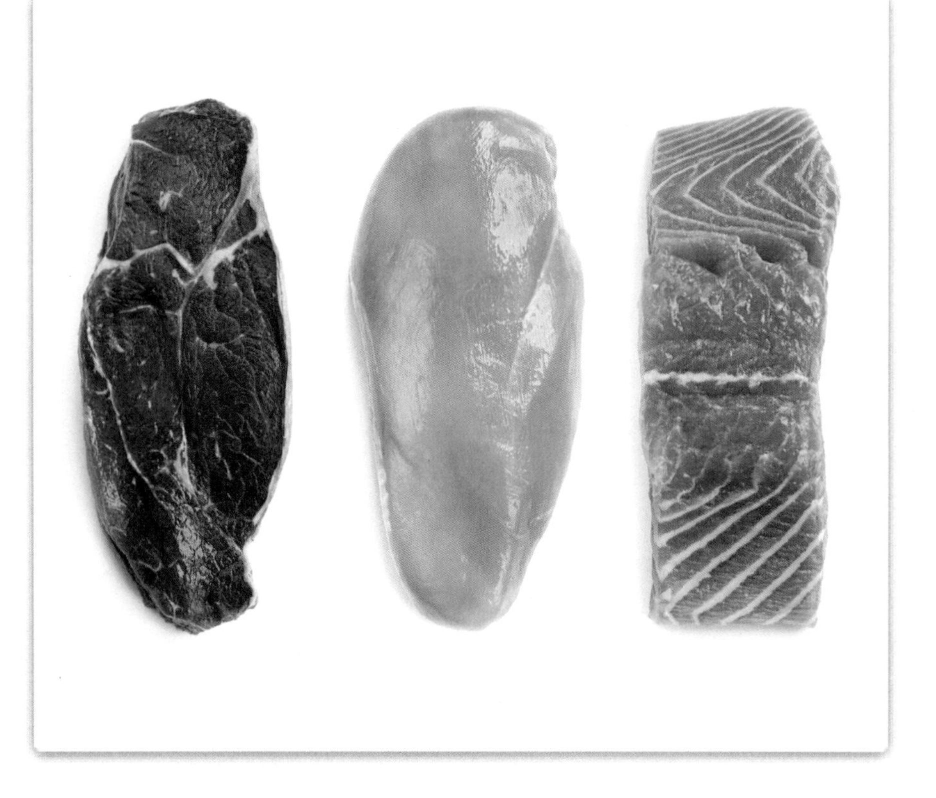

MEAT

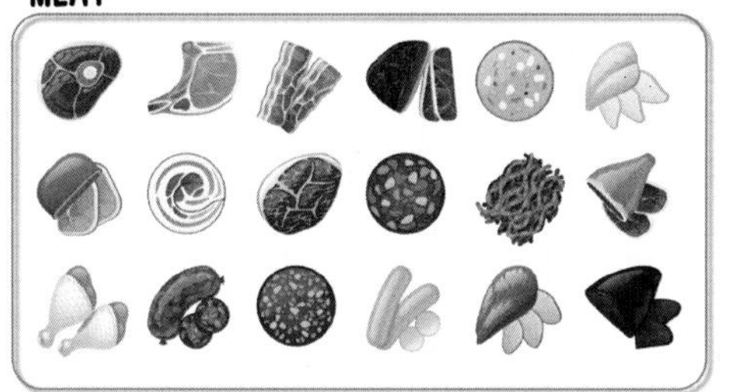

EGGS

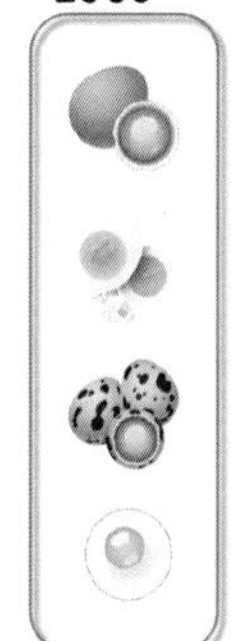

SEAFOOD

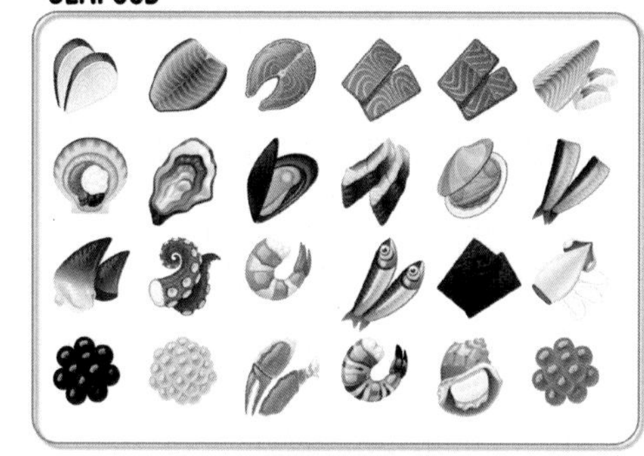

HERBS AND SPICES

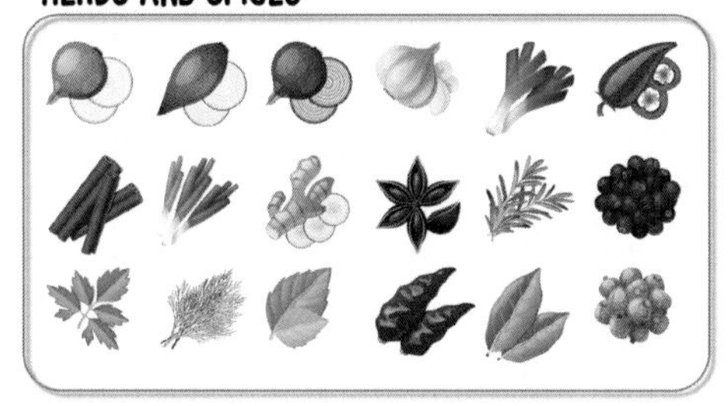

The P:E Diet

High Protein to Energy Ratio (P:E)

thePEdiet.com

FERMENTED DAIRY

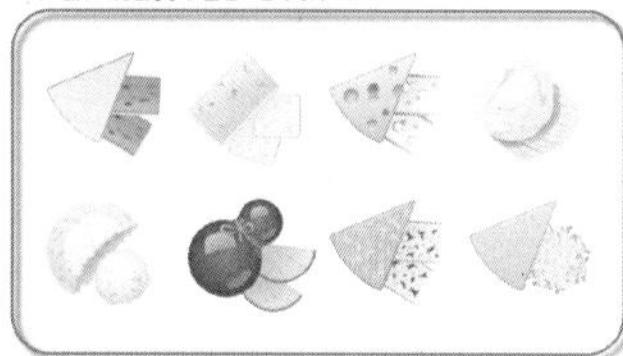

VEGETABLES

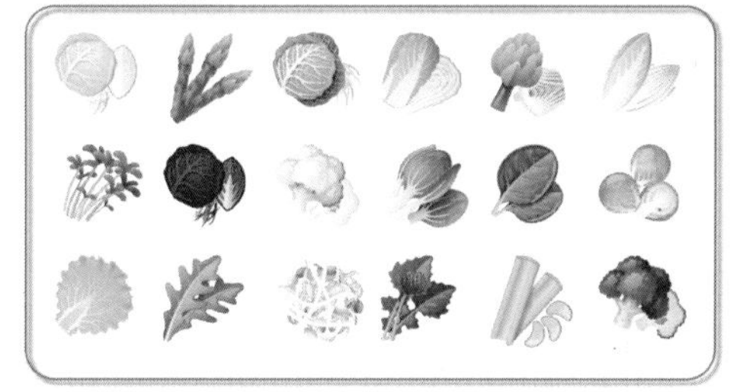

MUSHROOMS

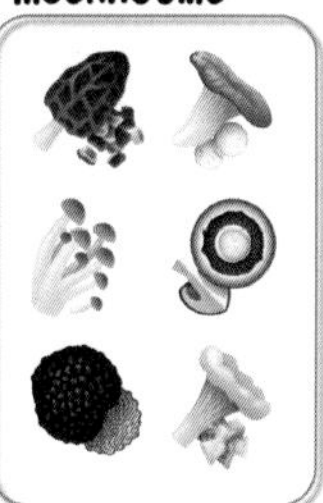

LOW SUGAR FRUIT

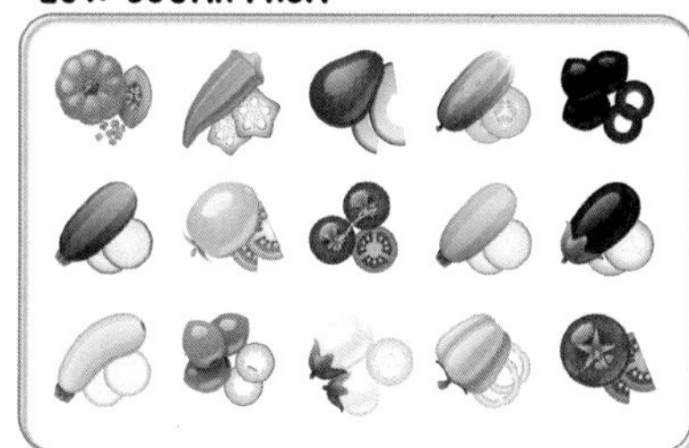

NUTS AND SEEDS

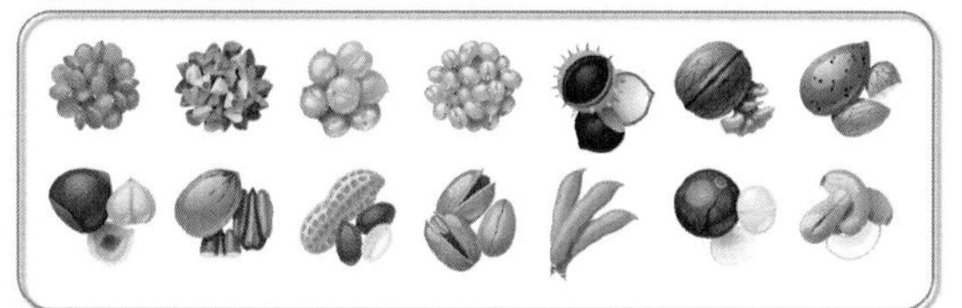

TUBERS

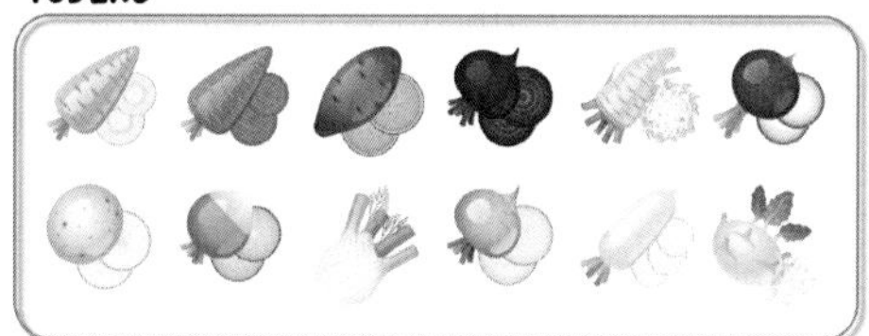

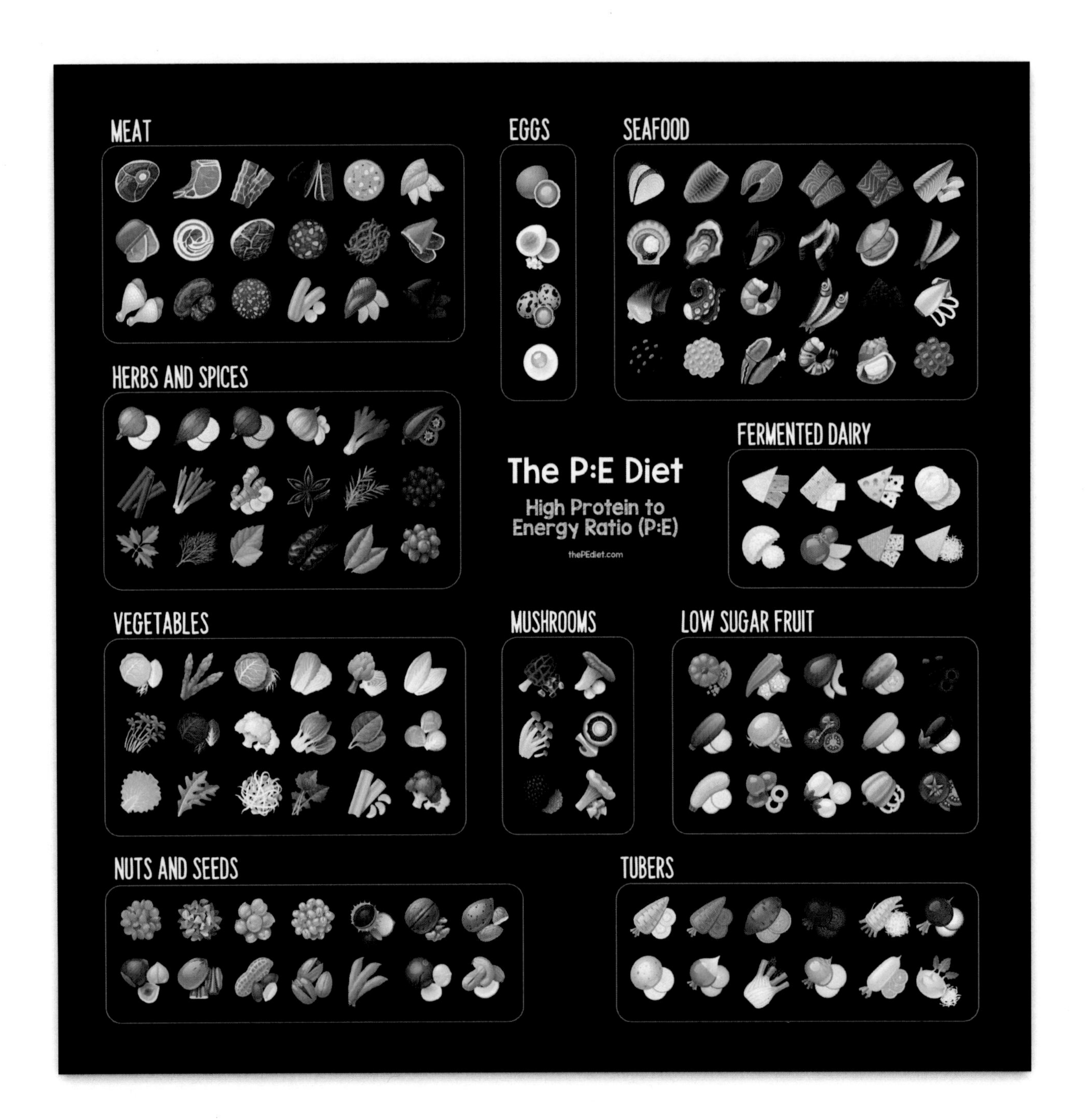
MEAT
EGGS
SEAFOOD
HERBS AND SPICES
The P:E Diet
High Protein to
Energy Ratio (P:E)
thePEdiet.com
FERMENTED DAIRY
VEGETABLES
MUSHROOMS
LOW SUGAR FRUIT
NUTS AND SEEDS
TUBERS

PROTEINS

Best options include:

- **Ruminants (beef, lamb, bison)**
- **Poultry**
- **Fish**
- **Seafood**
- **Eggs**
- **Wild game**
- **Pork**
- **Legumes**
- **Fermented dairy (plain greek yogurt and cottage cheese)**

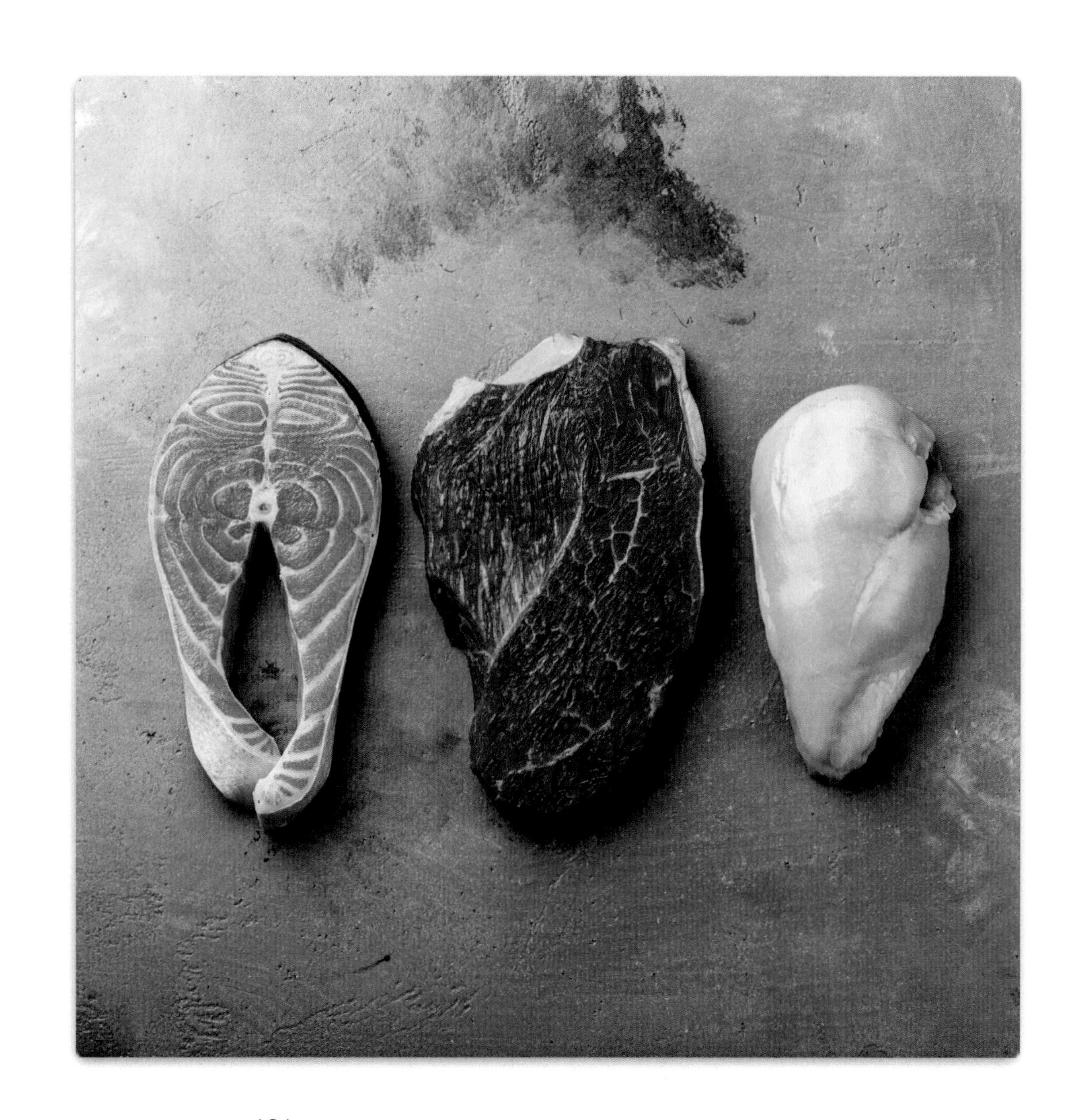

Always choose animals that are eating what THEY are supposed to be eating.

Opt for grass-fed meats, free range organic chicken, and pastured pork when possible. Opt for pasture-raised, organic eggs when possible. Opt for wild-caught fish and seafood when possible.

Always buy the highest quality that you can afford.

FATS

Remember, you want to keep dietary fat moderate. This isn't popular Keto where you're dousing everything in butter and MCT oil. It's best to simply consume whole food fats—meaning the fats you're already getting from your meat, eggs, and seafood sources.

We recommend minimizing nuts, cheeses, butter, dark chocolate, avocados, and other high fat foods—these extra fat calories can add up fast! Rather, prioritize protein-dense foods like beef and eggs while incorporating fibrous leafy greens and other high protein and mineral foods.

For cooking, use just enough fat to grease the pan or whatever surface you're working with.

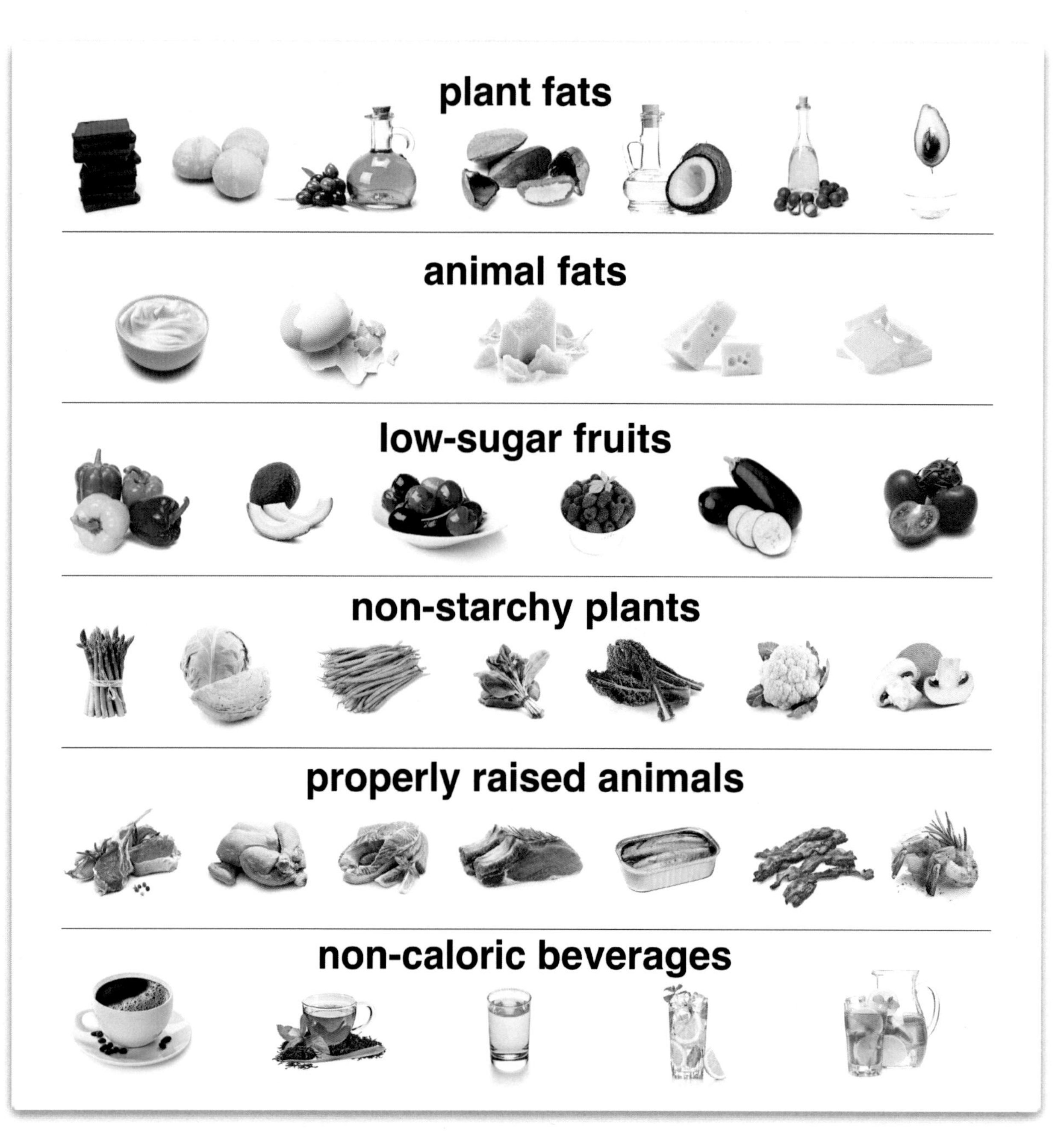

Best Cooking Fats:

- **Avocado oil**
- **Ghee**
- **Grass-fed butter**
- **Beef tallow**
- **Lard**
- **Coconut oil**
- **Olive oil**

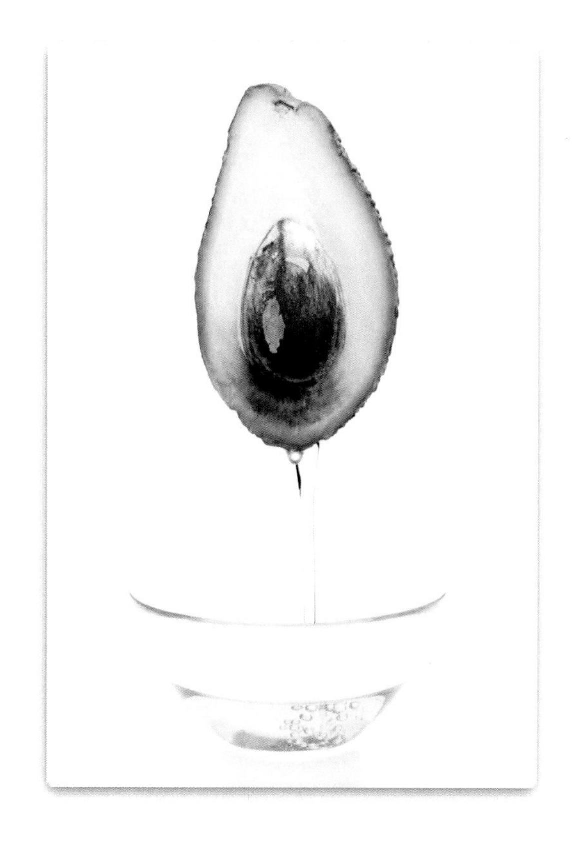

High Fat Snacks to be consumed sparingly:

- **Avocados**
- **Low sugar dark chocolate**
- **Hard cheeses**
- **Salami**
- **Nut butters**
- **Any nuts or seeds (macadamia, pumpkin seeds, almonds, etc.)**

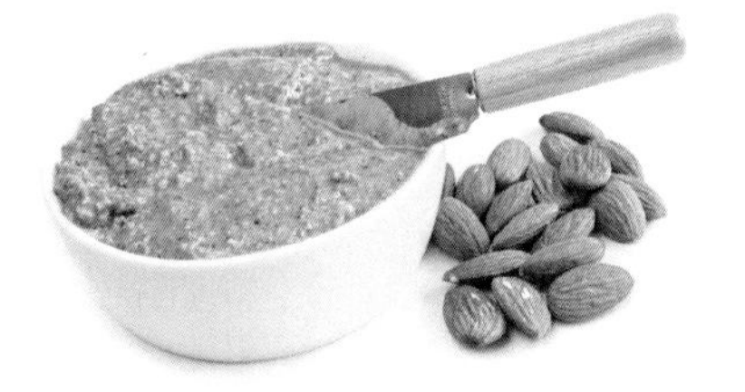

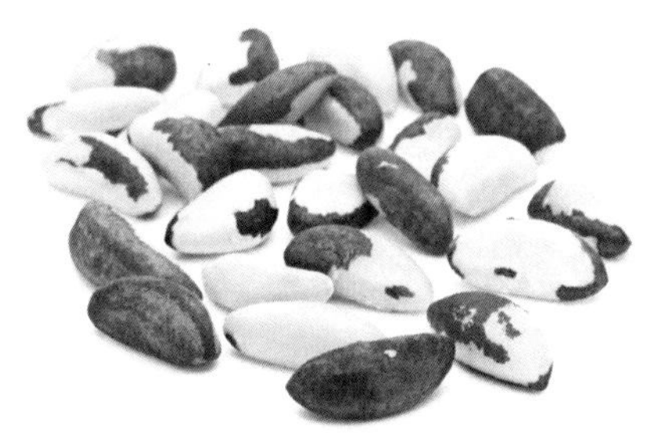

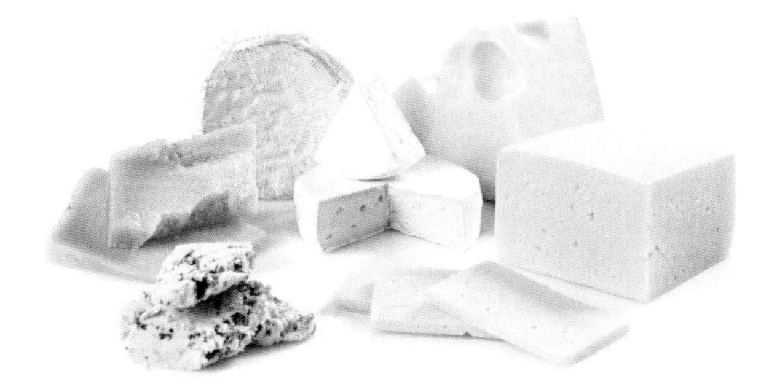

CARBS

Keep carbs as low as possible if you haven't reached your goal weight yet! If you're still in a weight loss or fat burning stage, limit your carbs to non-starchy vegetables like spinach, broccoli, kale, and asparagus. Also include some low sugar fruit, such as tomatoes, avocados, berries, etc.

If you are at your goal weight and/or perform lots of high intensity, glycolytic exercise like CrossFit, sprinting, mountain biking, soccer or football—you can probably get away with small amounts of fruit and starchy tubers. The best time to consume these is often around exercise (before or after intense exercise).

You can trade in some of your fat calories for carbs if that's the case. If consuming some occasional carbs, try to avoid eating fat at the same meals. Fruit and tubers are excellent choices.

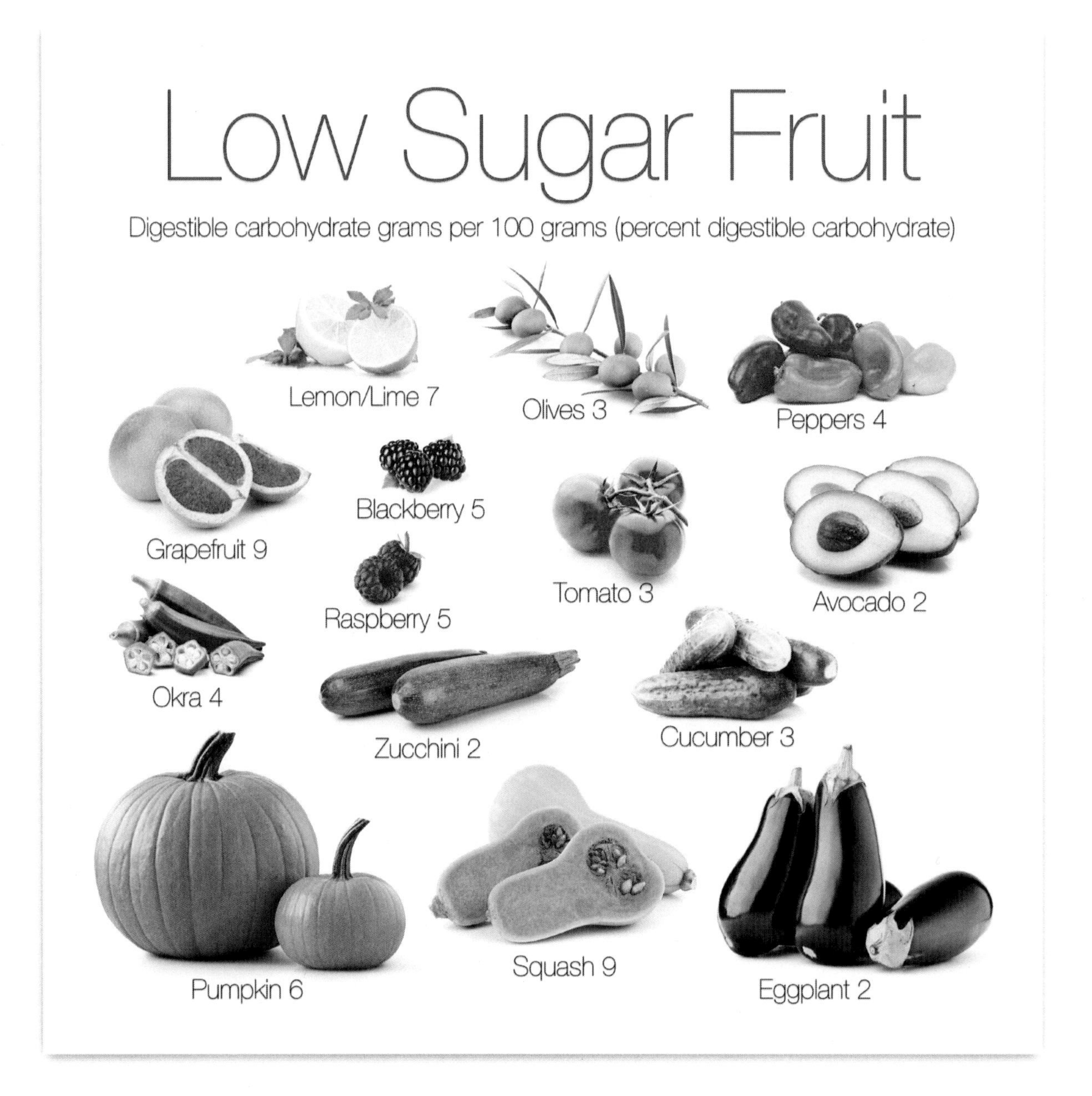

DESSERTS

Since we're focused on nutrient dense whole foods—there aren't too many dessert options! If your goal is fat loss, limit these and just eat more protein-rich food and veggies at your meals!

<u>Some good dessert options:</u>

- **Berries.**
- **Dark chocolate (70% or higher).**
- **Greek yogurt mixed with stevia and cocoa powder.**

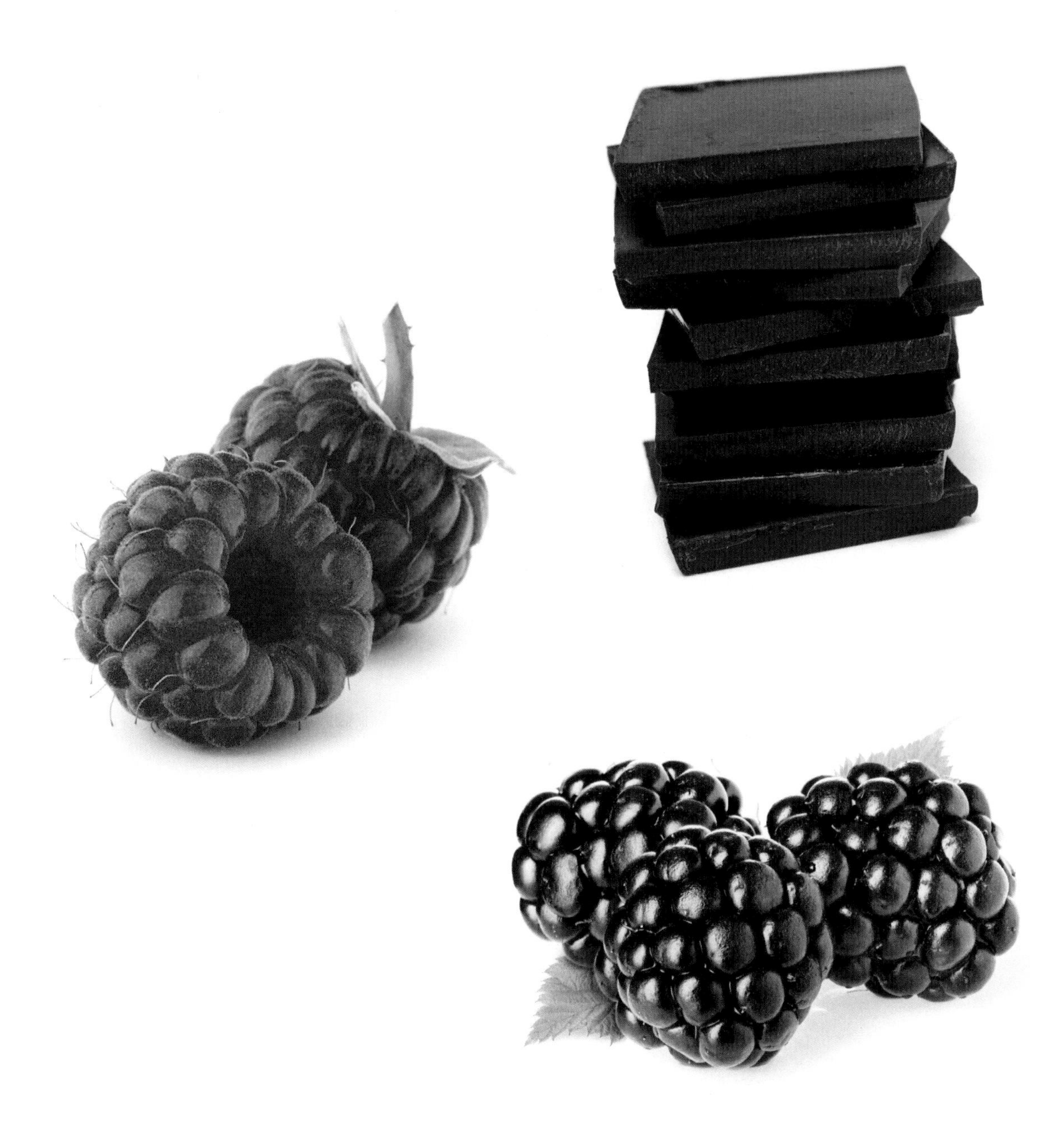

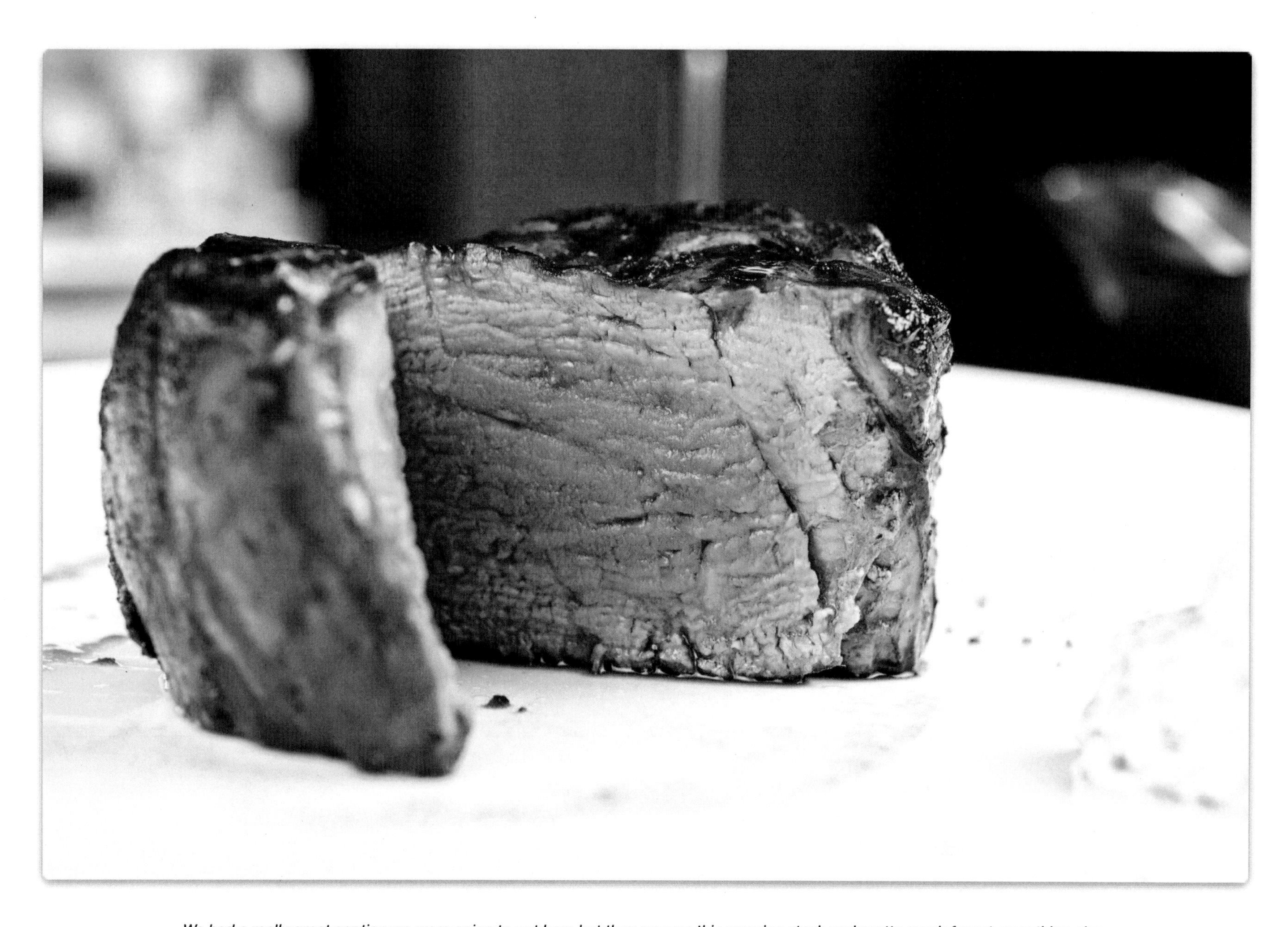

We had a really great caption we were going to put here but then we saw this amazing steak and pretty much forgot everything else.

KNOW YOUR BIOLOGY

We are specifically hard-wired to seek out foods with the very highest energy density, while using the very least energy expenditure in the process. This kept us alive for millions of years. Unfortunately we now have to intentionally head in the opposite direction. Knowing exactly how this works and what to do is half the battle, and that's where this book comes in. Be sure to set yourself up for success with an environment that offers plenty of tasty high protein whole foods that are low in either carbs or fats (or both), and try to avoid subjecting yourself to a lot of junk food. Willpower is a finite resource, and if you have junk food in your pantry you are GOING to eat it at some point.

Exercise is similar. We are actually hard-wired to AVOID exercise completely, in an attempt to conserve as much energy as possible. Prior to the industrial era, we all had to do tons of manual labor just to stay alive, so lack of exercise was unheard of. Now however, it is a constant threat to the majority of persons in first-world society. Again, understanding what your natural inclinations are towards exercise is very helpful when it comes to a strategy for dealing with these inclinations. This is one of the main reasons that the exercise VOLUME we will recommend in upcoming chapters is, by most standards, quite tiny! Read on for more.

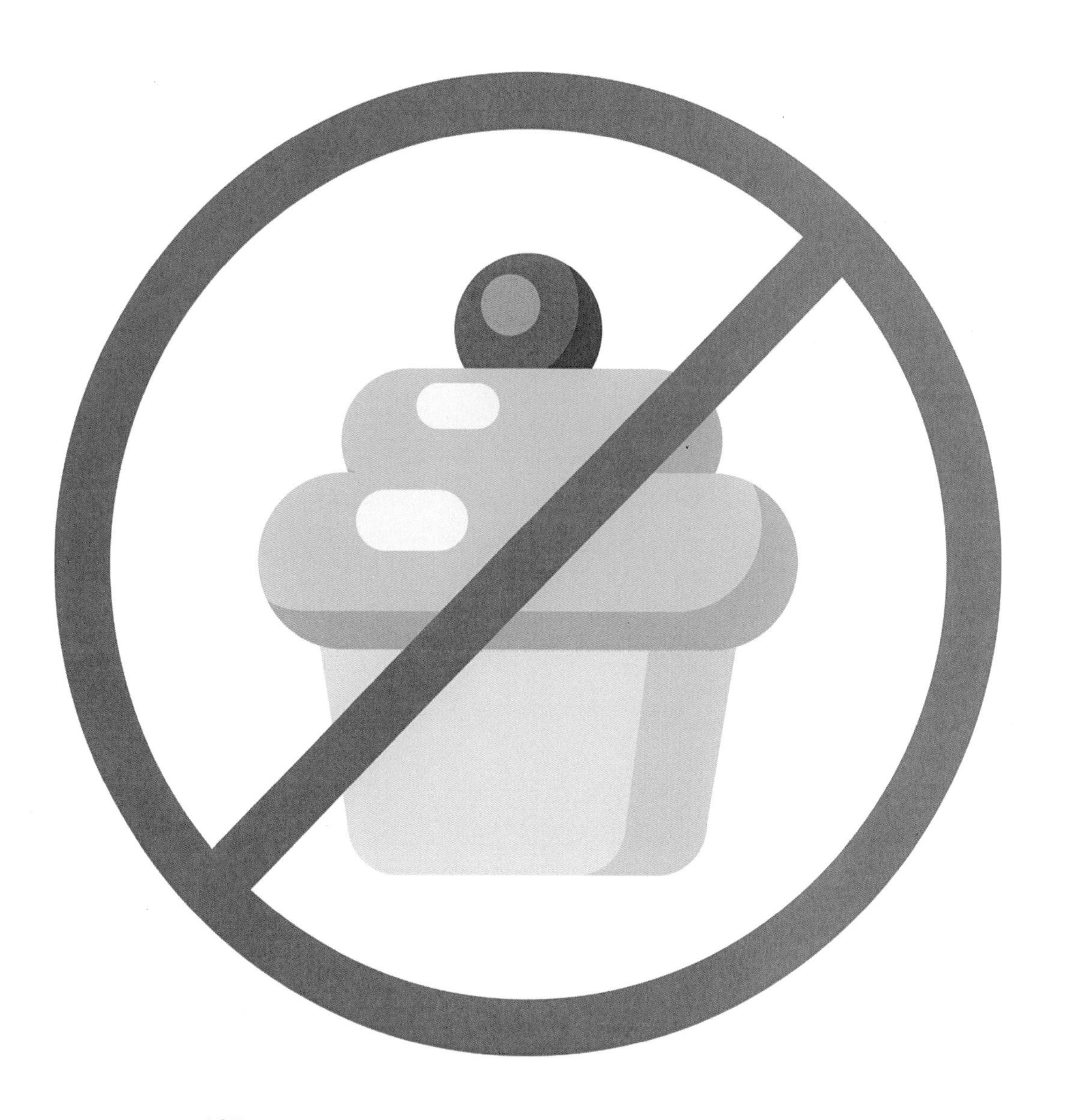

FED VS FASTED

Your body is designed to smoothly transition between two different and opposing states: 'Fed', and 'Fasted'.

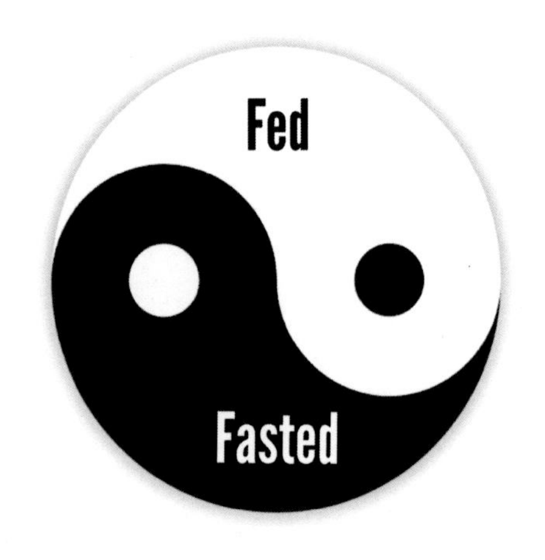

In the fed state, insulin is elevated, and this signals your body to store excess calories in your fat cells. In the presence of insulin, the burning of fat is reduced, while the body burns glucose (from your last meal) instead.

As we mentioned before, the primary signal of the 'fed' state is glucose entering the body from the diet and being stored in the liver as glycogen. In the 'fasted' state, liver glycogen has gradually drifted down to baseline, and with it declines blood glucose and insulin. In the fed state, insulin and glucose and glucose oxidation (burning) are all increased, while in the fasted state, insulin is low—while glucagon and fat oxidation are elevated. When you are in the fasted state, the body ramps up its mobilization of stored body fat from your fat cells and is actively burning this fat for energy (instead of glucose).

The practical importance of all this? You are more likely to burn stored body fat while in the fasted state, and you are more likely to store body fat while in the fed state.

Unfortunately, over time we seem to be spending less and less of our time in the fasted state and more and more time in the fed state. As a result, our bodies and our cells spend less and less time mobilizing and burning stored body fat

FALLING LIVER GLYCOGEN IS THE TRANSITION FROM THE FED STATE TO THE FASTED STATE

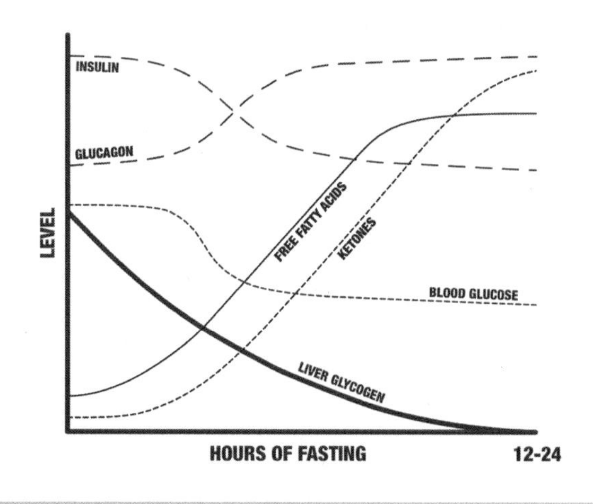

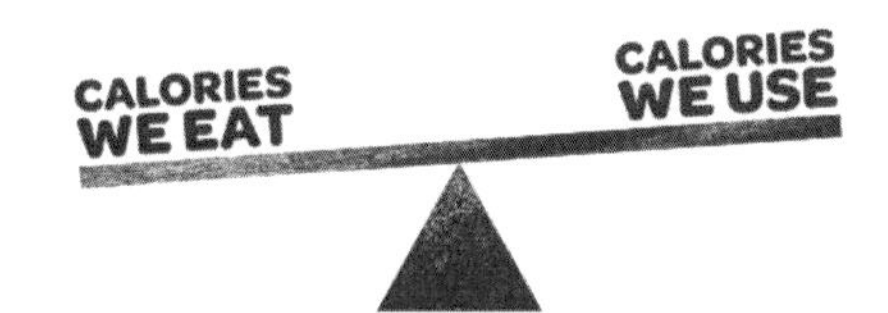

Fed State

- insulin high
- glucose high
- burning glucose
- storing fat

Fasted State

- insulin low
- glucose low
- liberating fat
- burning fat

for energy, and the glucose-burning pathways are overused.

Right now, the average American is eating something with carbohydrate in it an average of EIGHT times a day, spread out over a SIXTEEN hour eating window, for a total of about 300 grams of carbs per day. If we never ate any fat we could probably get away with this, like some sort of crazy "30 bananas a day" vegan YouTuber. Sadly however, we tend to overeat carbs and fats together, and of course now you know why—this combo is irresistibly tasty and addictive. Over time, this overeating leads to excessive fat gain and the subsequent energy toxicity of insulin resistance, or 'metabolic syndrome': abdominal fat storage, high triglycerides, low HDL or "good" cholesterol, and elevated glucose with eventual type 2 diabetes (1 in 12 humans on earth currently have full blown type 2 diabetes, while 35% of adults and 50% of older adults have Metabolic Syndrome, or pre-diabetes).

Most people with insulin resistance are disproportionately burning glucose on the cellular level, and they often displace burning body fat due to the amount of dietary glucose coming in from carbohydrates. When these people run out of glucose from their last meal, instead of easily transitioning over to the fasted state to burn fat, they become hungry for more glucose (from carbohydrates) as their bodies and cells have decreased capacity for mobilizing and burning fat for energy.

Let's put it this way. Why would a highly obese person EVER be hungry? They have enough fat stores to last a very long time. The world record for fasting went to

Some Proven Benefits Of Intermittent Fasting

- Promotes fat loss
- Improves insulin sensitivity
- Improves metabolism
- Starves "bad" bacteria in the colon
- Promotes longevity
- Improves hunger
- Improves mindful eating
- Improves appreciation of real whole foods
- Improves eating patterns
- Improves brain function
- Improves immune system
- Fights cancer cells (glucose-dependent)
- Reverses diabetes
- Improves fatty liver
- Improves neurodegenerative disorders
- Reduces inflammation
- Improves cellular regeneration and repair
- Improves lipid parameters
- Normalizes blood pressure
- Improves allergies
- Rest for digestive organs

a 456 pound man who fasted for 382 days, consuming only water and vitamins and losing 276 pounds with no ill effects. But the average overweight person is used to being in the fed state, has very little practice in the fasted state, and is continually burning glucose rather than fat at the cellular level. They have changes in their cellular metabolism. The cells can burn either glucose (sugar) or fat for fuel, and over time they will have a preference for one over the other; "sugar burners" have increased the cellular pathways that burn glucose and decreased, or down-regulated, the underused pathways for burning fat. So what happens to the overweight "sugar burner" who stops eating for a few hours? As they run out of glucose from their last meal, instead of seamlessly transitioning to the fasted state and mobilizing and burning stored body fat, they become HUNGRY for MORE GLUCOSE, from carbohydrates! They will spend most of the day trapped in a cycle of eating every few hours, spiking glucose, and then becoming hungry when blood sugar drops. A good analogy is that of a tanker truck on the freeway filled with oil. If the tanker truck runs out of gas it stops moving, despite the fact that it has 10,000 gallons of potential fuel on board. Why? Because it prefers to run on refined gas and is incapable of burning oil for fuel.

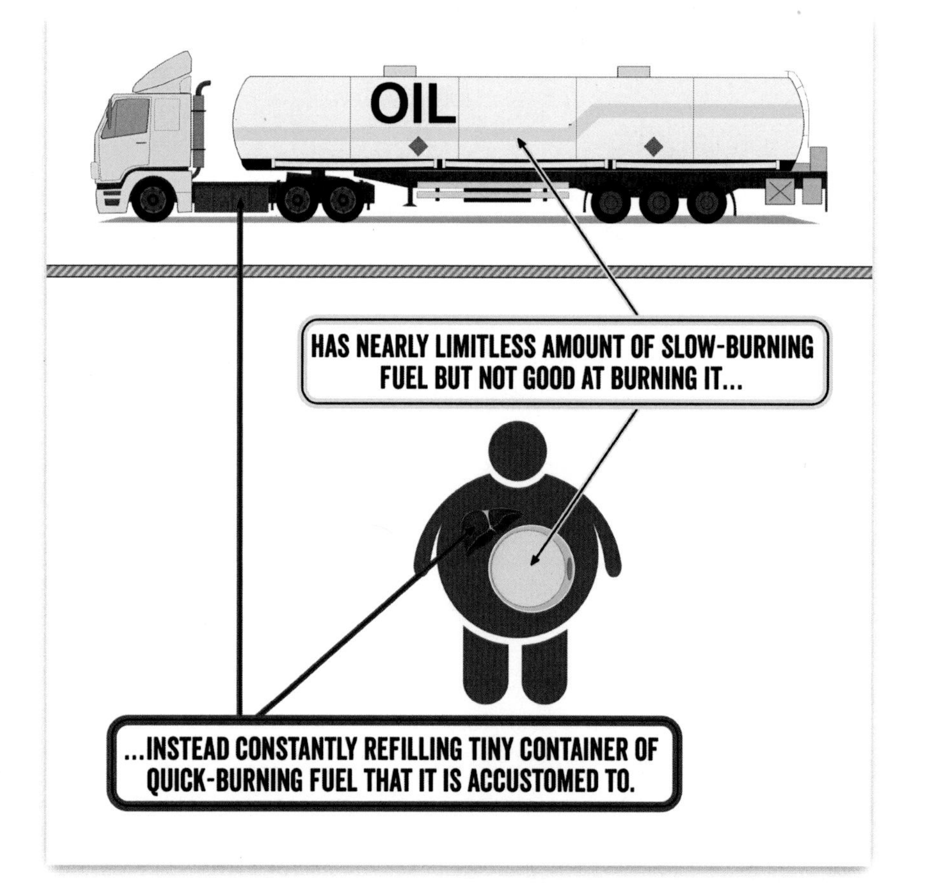

FAT ADAPTATION

Humans have the ability to become 'fat-adapted' and improve their ability to fuel themselves with stored body fat instead of glucose. However, this takes time and practice, and your body has to do a number of things to slowly up-regulate (or increase) your fat-burning pathways. This includes improving insulin sensitivity to lower insulin and promote fat mobilization into free fatty acids from the adipocytes (fat cells) as well as up-regulating the fat-burning pathways at the cellular level.

There are several ways to improve 'fat adaptation' or

the ability to successfully burn stored body fat for energy, and these include the following:

- Low carbohydrate diets. Eating a low carb diet improves the body's ability to utilize fat for energy rather than glucose.

- Exercise. High-intensity exercise depletes glucose and glycogen rapidly, forcing the body to switch over and utilize more fat for fuel. Exercise also improves insulin sensitivity.

- Caloric restriction. Eating fewer calories also equals less glucose available for fuel, so the body is more frequently forced to rely on stored body fat for fuel. You will always naturally eat the lowest calories when you are maximizing nutrient density by eating whole, natural, unprocessed, real foods found in nature (avoid processed foods). Once again, we see that satiety is CRUCIAL, and that means targeting a high nutrient density diet.

- Intermittent fasting, and spending more time in the fasted state, which gives the body more 'practice' at burning fat.

METABOLIC EXERCISE

The purpose of this section of our book is to highlight INTERMITTENT FASTING as a strategy for exercising and strengthening the body's ability to exist in the fasted state, burning fat instead of continually burning sugar (glucose) from the fed state.

Just like anything else, this ability can be strengthened over time with practice. But this ability also atrophies or shrinks over time with lack of use, just like your muscles atrophy when you break your arm and have to wear a cast for a few weeks.

Spending time in the fasted state is actually a form of exercise—a METABOLIC WORKOUT.

In fact, there are a lot of parallels between exercise and fasting.

Exercise does all of the following great things:

- Decreases blood glucose.

- Decreases insulin level.

- Increases insulin sensitivity.

- Increases lipolysis and free fatty acid mobilization.

- Increases cellular fat oxidation.

- Increases glucagon (the opposite of insulin).

- Increases growth hormone (the opposite of insulin).

BUT did you know you can also accomplish all of the above by doing ABSOLUTELY NOTHING?

The secret is *FASTING*. Extending the amount of time that you spend during your day in the FASTED state (as opposed to the FED state) accomplishes all of these, very similar to exercise. Extending your time in the fasted state is actually a form of metabolic 'exercise', in which you train your body to rapidly and efficiently mobilize free fatty acids from your adipose stores (fat tissue), something you absolutely can get better and better at with the metabolic 'practice' of fasting. Just as overweight and out of shape people struggle to jog or lift weights or participate in other forms of physical exercise, they are also generally out of practice when it comes to rapidly and efficiently mobilizing and burning and living off of stored fat for fuel. Intermittent fasting and spending more of your day in the 'fasted' state (and less time in the 'fed' state) is a great form of metabolic 'exercise' which has many health benefits, including fat loss!

LESS FEEDING, MORE FASTING

One of the best ways to achieve effortless and long-lasting fat loss? Train yourself to eat two meals a day (and eliminate snacking). The easiest and best way to accomplish this? Leverage your natural overnight fast by skipping breakfast (drinking coffee makes this easier and more enjoyable, plus coffee has numerous health benefits). No breakfast, lighter lunch, and larger dinner also maximizes the body's natural shifts between sympathetic ("fight or flight") and parasympathetic ("rest and digest") nervous system tone, with higher alertness and activation from sympathetic tone during the day while under-eating, and higher parasympathetic resting tone in the evening during the fed state.

Typically, the fed state starts when you begin eating and for the next three to five hours your body digests and absorbs the food you just ate. Insulin rises significantly, to some degree shutting off fat-burning and also triggering excess calories to be stored as fat. After the first few hours mentioned above, your body goes into what is known as the post–absorptive state, during which the components of the last meal are still in the circulation. The post–absorptive state lasts until 8 to 12 hours after your last meal, which is when you enter the fasted state. It typically takes 12 hours after your last meal to fully enter the fasted state.

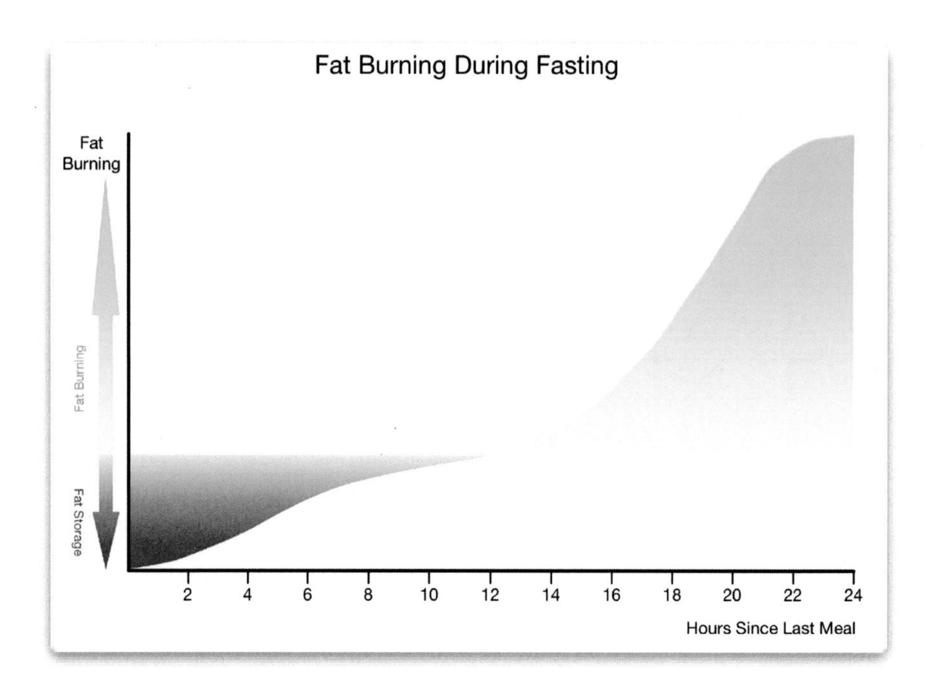

When you're in the fasted state your body can burn fat that has been inaccessible during the fed state. Because we don't completely enter the fasted state until around 12 hours after our last meal, it's rare that our bodies are in this fat burning state in the modern food environment. This is one of the reasons why many people who start intermittent fasting will lose fat without changing what they eat, how much they eat, or how often they exercise. Fasting puts your body in a fat burning state that you rarely get to enter during a normal eating schedule.

MINIMIZE CARB FREQUENCY

Eating carbohydrates, especially refined carbohydrates with no fiber, overdrives the 'fed' state, as carbohydrates raise both glucose and insulin higher than other macronutrients. In general, when you eat a meal, your body spends a few hours processing that food and burning what it can from what you just consumed. Because it has all of this readily available, easy to burn energy in its blood stream (thanks to the food you ate), your body will choose to use that as energy rather than the fat you have stored. This is ESPECIALLY true if you just consumed carbohydrates, because these are rapidly converted to glucose and your body has to burn sugar as energy before any other source (you have limited glucose storage, and high glucose is toxic; your body burns extra glucose preferentially to get rid of it, much in the same way that the body burns alcohol consumed for energy prior to other energy calories--alcohol therefore also sabotages fat loss).

EXERCISE HELPS

Exercise helps greatly with fat adaptation. Your glycogen (the storage form of glucose in your muscles and liver that your body can burn as fuel when necessary) is depleted during sleep and fasting, and will be depleted even further during training, which can further increase insulin sensitivity. This means that a meal immediately following your workout will be stored most efficiently—mostly as glycogen for muscle stores or burned as energy immediately to help with the recovery process, with minimal amounts stored as fat. Compare this to a regular day (no intermittent fasting): the overeaten carbs from foods consumed will see full glycogen stores, and thus be more likely to be stored as fat.

FASTING MYTHS

There are many myths about fasting:

"Breakfast is the most important meal of the day!"

We have all been told to eat breakfast. Unfortunately this is terrible advice. When you first wake up in the morning, your insulin level is quite low and most people are just starting to enter the fasted state, 12 hours after eating the last meal of the previous day. The worst thing you could do is to eat a ton of food, spiking insulin and glucose and immediately shutting off fat-burning. A much better choice would be to push the first meal of your day out at least a few hours, during which you can fully enter the fasted state and burn stored body fat. The VERY WORST would be to eat a high carbohydrate breakfast, spiking insulin and glucose as high as possible; in addition to reducing fat-burning for as many as 12 hours, this will drive as many calories as possible into fat stores as well as providing further reinforcement of the burning of glucose rather than fat. Also, high spikes of insulin and glucose always lead to large drops in glucose a few hours later, which triggers HUNGER (if you want to have hypoglycemia or low blood sugar and ravenous hunger, just eat a breakfast of pure carbohydrates and then wait 2-3 hours to see how you feel). Interestingly, many properly fat-adapted people aren't very hungry in the morning and have no problem skipping breakfast. This is appropriate, as throughout our evolution humans have always been hunter-gatherers and rather than eating a large breakfast first thing in the morning we would hunt and gather throughout the day, having a larger meal later in the day. We highly recommend mimicking this pattern by skipping breakfast and eating most of your calories later in the day (referred to as a 'reverse taper' of calories, with none in the morning and most in the evening). Some individualization is present here, however. Some people do find that they have higher satiety and they function better by eating breakfast and eating earlier in the day—this is of course fine if it works for you! But for many, skipping breakfast is both the easiest and most convenient way to intermittently fast.

"Eat small frequent meals."

There has been plenty of worthless advice here. We have been told to eat frequently to "keep your metabolism going" and "don't let your body enter starvation mode". This is all the exact opposite of the truth: in order to burn fat, you want to spend more time in the fasted state and get very very efficient at living on stored body fat rather than caloric intake from constant eating.

"Fasting leads to burning muscle instead of fat."

Many people are concerned that if they start fasting they will either stop making muscle or maybe even burn muscle. While this is certainly true of starvation (days without food), it is definitely not true of intermittent fasting (hours, rather than days, without food). If this were true, humans would not be here today. In fact, growth hormone is increased during fasted states (both during sleep and after a period of fasting). Growth hormone might as well be called "fasting hormone", as it rises by as much as 2,000% after 24 hours of fasting. Growth hormone prevents muscle breakdown, and is used in combination with testosterone by bodybuilders who want to simultaneously build as much muscle and burn as much fat as possible. Growth hormone elevates in fasting to help preserve muscle in times of fasting, and this makes sense. In our hunter-gatherer ancestors, if fasting for short periods of time and going for a few hours or even a few days without food made you weaker and slower you would never catch or find any food and you would die and humans would become extinct. In fact the opposite is true; while fasting for short periods (less than 24 hours), muscle is preserved or can even grow if you are doing resistance training (highly recommended). Also, people experience an increased level of focus and alertness during intermittent fasting thanks to the release of epinephrine and norepinephrine (earlier in our evolution, this increased energy and alertness helped us catch prey when necessary).

"Your metabolism slows down when you are fasting."

While this is true of starvation (days or weeks without food), in the short term this is completely false. A number of studies have proven that in fasting up to 72 hours, metabolism does not slow down at all and in fact might speed up slightly thanks to the release of catecholamines (epinephrine or adrenaline, norepinephrine, and dopamine) and activation of the sympathetic nervous system (sympathetic nervous system is often considered the "fight or flight" system, while the opposite is the parasympathetic nervous system or the "rest and digest" system). It makes sense that this fight or flight sympathetic nervous system would be activated during the daytime, when hunter-gatherer humans are most active and in the fasted state (looking for food), followed by parasympathetic "rest and digest" mode in the evening after eating a large meal.

"If I don't eat I will get low blood sugar [hypoglycemia]."

Studies have shown that healthy persons who have no underlying medical conditions, who are not taking any diabetes medications, can fast for extremely long periods of time without suffering from any hypoglycemia. In fact, almost all sensations of hypoglycemia or low blood sugar (in non-diabetics) results from eating a very high glycemic index carbohydrate food a few hours prior (blood sugar spikes, then insulin spikes, then blood sugar drops rapidly). However if you are a diabetic, especially if you are on any diabetes medications, you definitely need to check with your doctor before starting a fasting protocol. Some diabetes medications can lead to severe hypoglycemia when fasting (mostly insulin and sulfonylurea drugs like glipizide, glimepiride, and glyburide). [Be sure to check with your doctor prior to starting a fasting protocol if you have any medical problems, diabetes or otherwise.]

HOW TO FAST INTERMITTENTLY

There are a number of ways to actually perform intermittent fasting, but the easiest and most popular varieties involve taking advantage of your natural overnight fast by skipping breakfast and pushing the first meal of the day forward a number of hours. Once you have passed the 12 hour mark from dinner the night before, you are truly in a fasted state and you begin to rely on stored body fat for fuel. The longer you stay in the fasted state, the more metabolic practice you will get at burning stored body fat and the deeper your fat adaptation will get. In fact, if you can maintain this intermittent fast for 20 to 24 hours you will achieve a very high rate of lipolysis (breakdown of stored body fat into free fatty acids, available for burning in the cells) and fat oxidation (burning of fat in the mitochondria).

When you first start out with intermittent fasting, you can have quite a bit of hunger and low energy and other symptoms. In this case we recommend starting out with "baby steps", by just pushing breakfast out an hour or two at first, then slowly increasing the fasting interval. As time goes by and you become more "fat adapted", it is easier and easier to fast. This is identical to exercise in those who are sedentary: it is painful and extremely difficult at first, and then once you are adapted it gets easy and even enjoyable.

LOW CARBOHYDRATE DIET

It is much easier to fast if you are already on a low carb diet, as these diets naturally lead to quite a bit of fat adaptation and are naturally lower in the secretion of insulin as well as the utilization of glucose as a fuel. In fact, we HIGHLY recommend the combination of a very low carb diet with intermittent fasting. The closer you get to a ketogenic diet (extremely low in carbohydrates) the easier it is to go for hours and hours without eating, thanks to the fat adaptation that these diets lead to.

For those who do incorporate carbohydrates in the diet, we would recommend that these contain a lot of FIBER, which is indigestible and does not contribute to the elevation of glucose and insulin. If you do decide to eat digestible carbohydrates, we would recommend that you consider avoiding these early in the day, as this might sabotage the fat adaptation process, as well as setting you up for a blood sugar and hunger roller coaster for the rest of the day. Instead, we would recommend eating digestible (non-fiber) carbohydrates in the evening, and ideally only after either intermittent fasting to deplete liver glycogen and/or exercising with a high level of intensity to deplete muscle glycogen (eating digestible carbohydrates when your muscle and liver glycogen are already full is more likely to lead to fat storage and worsening insulin sensitivity, the exact opposite of what you are looking for).

INTERMITTENT FASTING PROTOCOLS

There are several popular ways to accomplish intermittent fasting and we will discuss the three most popular varieties next. All of these involve lengthening the overnight fast by skipping breakfast and postponing the first meal of the day. All of these also involve eating no calories at the beginning of the day and the majority of your calories very late in the day, a concept called a caloric 'reverse taper'.

Keep in mind that for the purpose of these discussions we will consider the baseline standard diet to involve 12 hours of fasting (overnight) plus 12 hours of an eating window during the day consisting of three meals, breakfast, lunch, and dinner.

The sad reality however is that most people are actually eating first thing in the morning until late at night, with lots of snacking, so the eating window for the average American is actually closer to 16 hours!

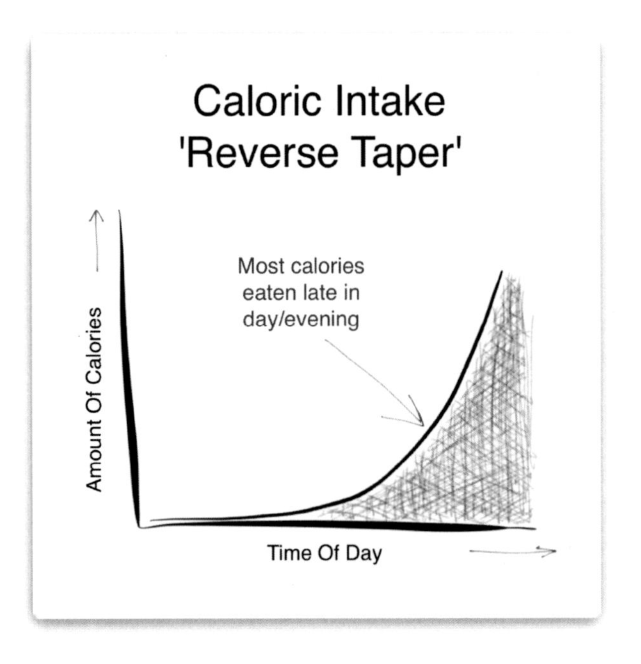

LEANGAINS

Leangains, as popularized by bodybuilder Martin Berkhan, is by far the most popular method of fasting intermittently. This form of fasting consists of skipping breakfast every morning and pushing the first meal of the day to lunch. Basically you skip breakfast and then eat a normal lunch and dinner in an eight hour window. The idea is to fast for 16 hours (overnight plus the first ~6 hours of your day), then eat all your calories in an 8 hour window. For example, let's say you get up at 6:00 a.m. You would skip breakfast and eat nothing for six hours, then lunch at noon and dinner at 8:00 p.m. Snacking inside your eating window is allowed (although we will say that generally speaking you want to try to consolidate calories into larger meals rather than snacking). This 16:8 split (16 hours fasting and 8 hours eating) is recommended every single day. If you had one day off from this protocol and followed this the other six days of the week, that would amount to an additional 4 hours of fasting per day compared to the standard 12:12 split that we are assuming to be baseline (12 hours fasting and 12 hours eating). Four hours per day times six days per week equals about 24 hours of total additional fasting per week. [4 hours fasting per day times 6 days per week = 24 hours]

WARRIOR DIET

The Warrior Diet, as popularized by Ori Hofmekler, consists of fasting during the majority of the day, then eating all of your calories in the evening. The goal is to skip breakfast and lunch, then eat a huge dinner in a four hour window at the end of the day. This is a 20:4 hour split (20 hours of fasting and then a 4 hour eating window at the end of the day). This method of fasting does allow you to eat very large very satisfying meals at the end of the day, and might be perfect for someone who was going out to dinner to

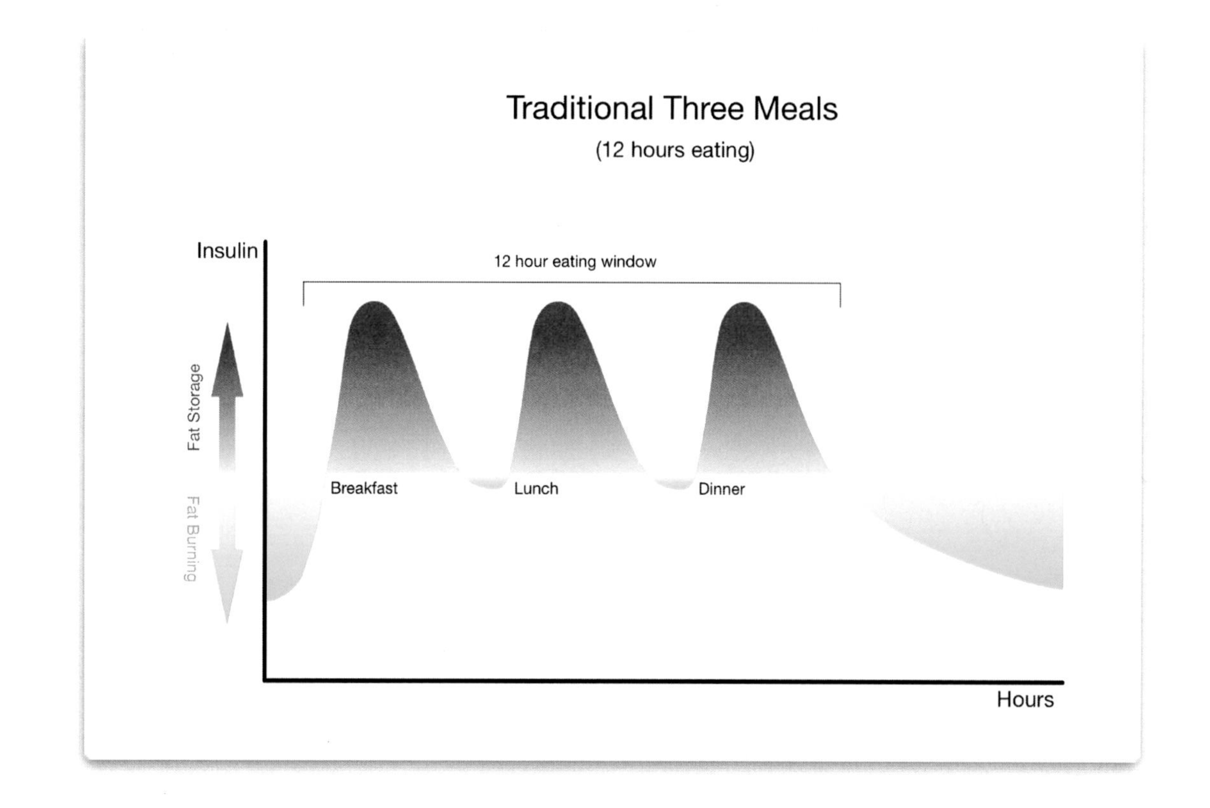

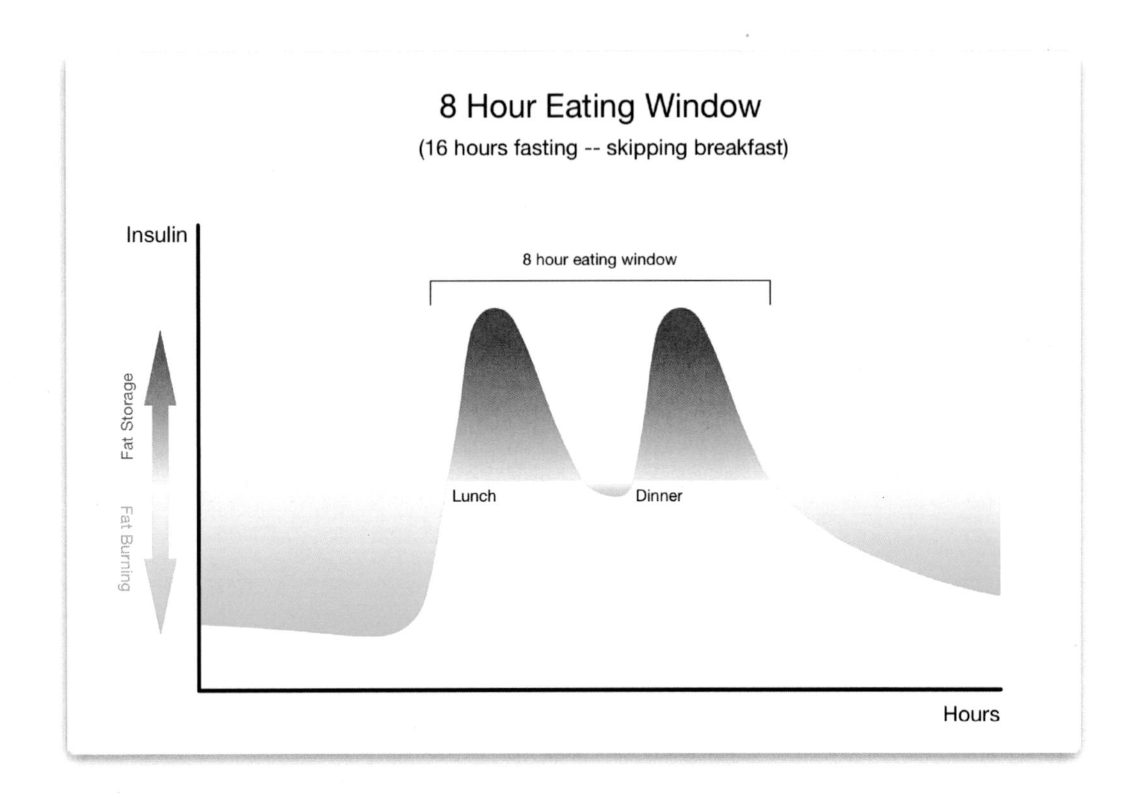

eat in a social setting, where a ton of calories and food might be involved. Fasting this long during the day is more difficult but does lead to a deeper level of fat adaptation and low insulin (which helps improve insulin sensitivity). If one followed this protocol roughly every other day (let's say three days a week), that would equate to eight hours of fasting compared to the 12:12 baseline standard diet, times three days per week would also equal about 24 hours of total additional fasting per week. [8 hours fasting per day times 3 days per week = 24 hours]

EAT STOP EAT

Eat Stop Eat, as popularized by bodybuilder Brad Pilon, involves fasting for an entire 24 hours, two days per week. Let's say you eat your last meal of the day at 8:00 p.m. the day before. You fast overnight and then all the following day, skipping breakfast and lunch, and then pushing dinner out to 8:00 p.m. (for a full 24 hours with no calories). This is quite difficult and is only recommended two days per week (nonconsecutive). While this is quite difficult, by the end of the 24 hours you do reach a very deep level of lipolysis and fat oxidation, with very low insulin levels, and this is quite desirable. Many people think that the following day they will binge on so much food that the benefits of the fasting on the previous day will be negated, but this is not true. Studies have repeatedly shown that persons will overeat by hundreds of calories the next day, but still not come anywhere close to eating as much as they would have by eating normally both days (in other words, you are still left with a large net caloric deficit even after eating more food the day after your fast). Each day that you fast in this fashion adds 12 hours of fasting compared to the standard 12:12 split we are calling baseline, and two days per week of this again equals about 24 hours of total additional fasting per week. [12 hours fasting per day times 2 days per week = 24 hours]

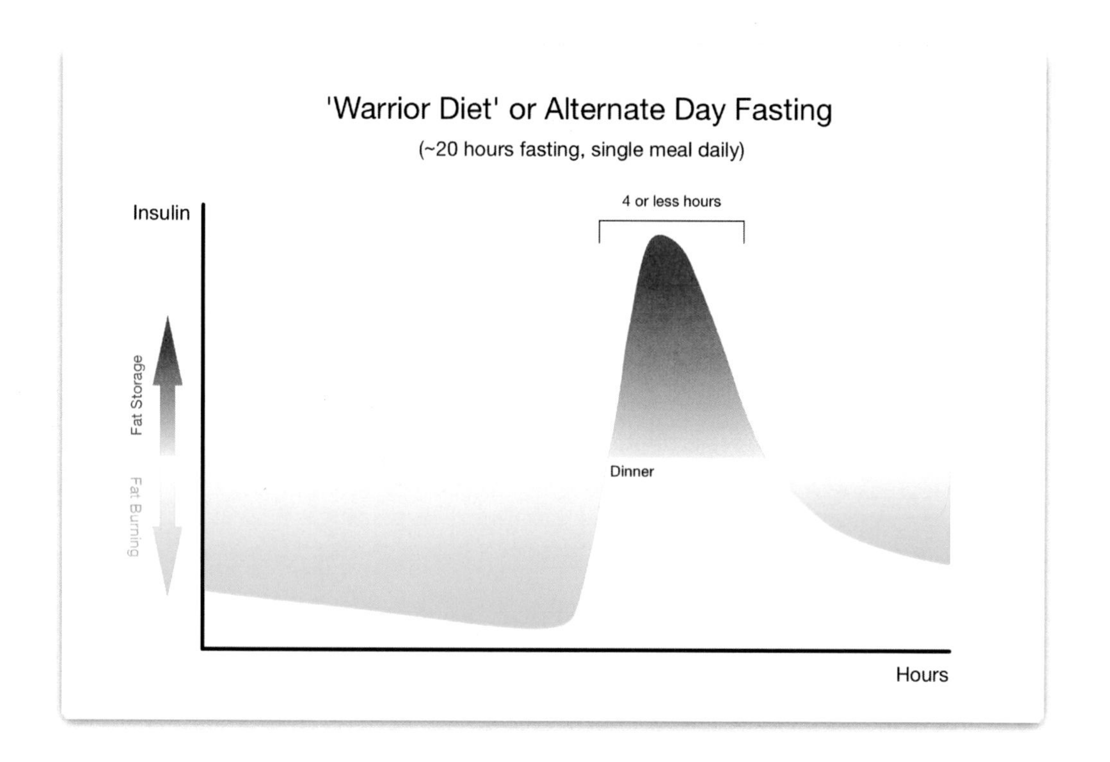

IT'S ALL GOOD

With all of these fasting methods, the goal is to skip breakfast, avoid snacking, and consolidate calories near the end of the day. All of these methods are quite effective, and you can in fact mix and match these as much as you would like. We would highly recommend keeping it flexible. Fast for as long as is convenient on any given day, and break your fast whenever you need to or want to. Anything beyond a 12 hour window is going to be at least somewhat beneficial towards anyone's goals. If you planned on fasting 16 hours but only make it 13, that's ok and you are still much better off than if you had eaten all day long with early and late calories plus lots of snacking.

We think a good goal would be 24 hours per week of additional fasting (additional to the standard 12:12 baseline). This could be 2 days of 12 extra hours (Eat Stop Eat), 3 days of 8 extra hours (Warrior Diet), or 6 days of 4 extra hours (Leangains). You could also mix and match as desired. Keep it flexible and go with whatever best suits your schedule and your lifestyle and your current level of fat adaptation.

COFFEE = AWESOME

During the fasts feel free to drink ANY noncaloric beverage you want, including but not limited to: water, coffee (with or without noncaloric sweetener such as stevia), tea (hot or iced, sweetened with stevia if desired), diet soda with no calories, or any other beverage with no calories. However you really don't want anything with lots of calories here. Fat is the macronutrient that spikes insulin the very least, which is why so many people are using Bulletproof coffee or some other method of adding fat (butter, coconut oil, etc) to coffee in the morning. However, we would NOT recommend this or any other source of calories while fasting, as this will be detrimental to what you are trying to accomplish with fasting.

If you will absolutely die without at least a tiny splash of cream in your coffee well then do it, you will be better off with it than if this prohibition against cream in your coffee keeps you from trying to fast intermittently at all (95% fasting much better than 0% fasting)! However we would try to keep the cream in your coffee to an absolute MINIMUM quantity, and you should also use this opportunity to learn to drink coffee black (this is something anyone can learn over time, believe it or not). We *HIGHLY* recommend the use of black coffee or tea in the morning to make your fast easier and more enjoyable. Both coffee and tea have numerous health benefits, and they both contain compounds that help with fat burning, energy, and alertness.

ENJOY YOUR NEWFOUND FREEDOM FROM FOOD

Once you are properly fat adapted, intermittent fasting is actually easy, fun, enjoyable, and liberating—while making you leaner and healthier in the process! Let's say you are following the Leangains protocol. Breakfast every day during the work week is now JUST BLACK COFFEE, how easy is that? No more worrying about what you are going to grab for breakfast as you rush around in the morning and struggle to get to work on time. This saves you a ton of time and work and effort and is literally a form of metabolic exercise in the meantime, improving your insulin sensitivity and strengthening your fat adaptation. This is a win in many ways. It also frees you to eat very large and satisfying meals in the evening, without feeling the deprivation of watching calories or restricting yourself. And on days where you skip breakfast and lunch, you will be amazed at how much extra time you will have when you don't have to worry about what to eat, where to get it, and when to find time to eat it. Your productivity will be higher as concentration and focus is higher in the fasted state (thanks to the sympathetic nervous system activation and catecholamines), and you will have more free time.

SOME POINTERS

Of course you are going to check with your doctor before you do ANYTHING in this book. But you REALLY want to check with your doctor before initiating intermittent fasting if you are diabetic and on diabetes medications.

You can generally take any vitamins or supplements you want while fasting as long as they don't have calories, but you don't need any supplements as you will be eating plenty of nutrient-dense foods every day.

You don't have to worry about losing muscle from lack of protein during your fast, as long as you eat adequate protein at the meals before and after fasting.

You will not lose muscle while fasting as long as you are exercising regularly, and we specifically recommend resistance training such as lifting weights or doing bodyweight calisthenics—more on this coming up!

Following a low carb diet pairs nicely with intermittent fasting, as both improve fat adaptation a great deal. However it is not at all necessary, and in fact the REAL power of intermittent fasting probably lies in the way it decreases

CARBOHYDRATE FREQUENCY. So even those on a high carbohydrate diet will see the 'fat adaptation' benefits of intermittent fasting. In fact, those on a high carbohydrate diet might have the highest benefit of all. It is certainly ok to eat more carbohydrates and utilize intermittent fasting!

It is perfectly fine to exercise while fasting, either cardio or lifting weights (lifting weights is better for fat loss and body composition and we highly recommend resistance exercise for everyone, as this will further your goals considerably).

Drink plenty of water and non-caloric beverages while fasting; coffee and tea in the morning make fasting considerably more enjoyable in addition to health and fat-burning benefits and are therefore highly recommended.

Don't use intermittent fasting as an excuse to eat tons of junk food when you are eating—continue to eat responsibly, sticking with whole natural foods with high nutrient density and avoiding processed foods as much as possible.

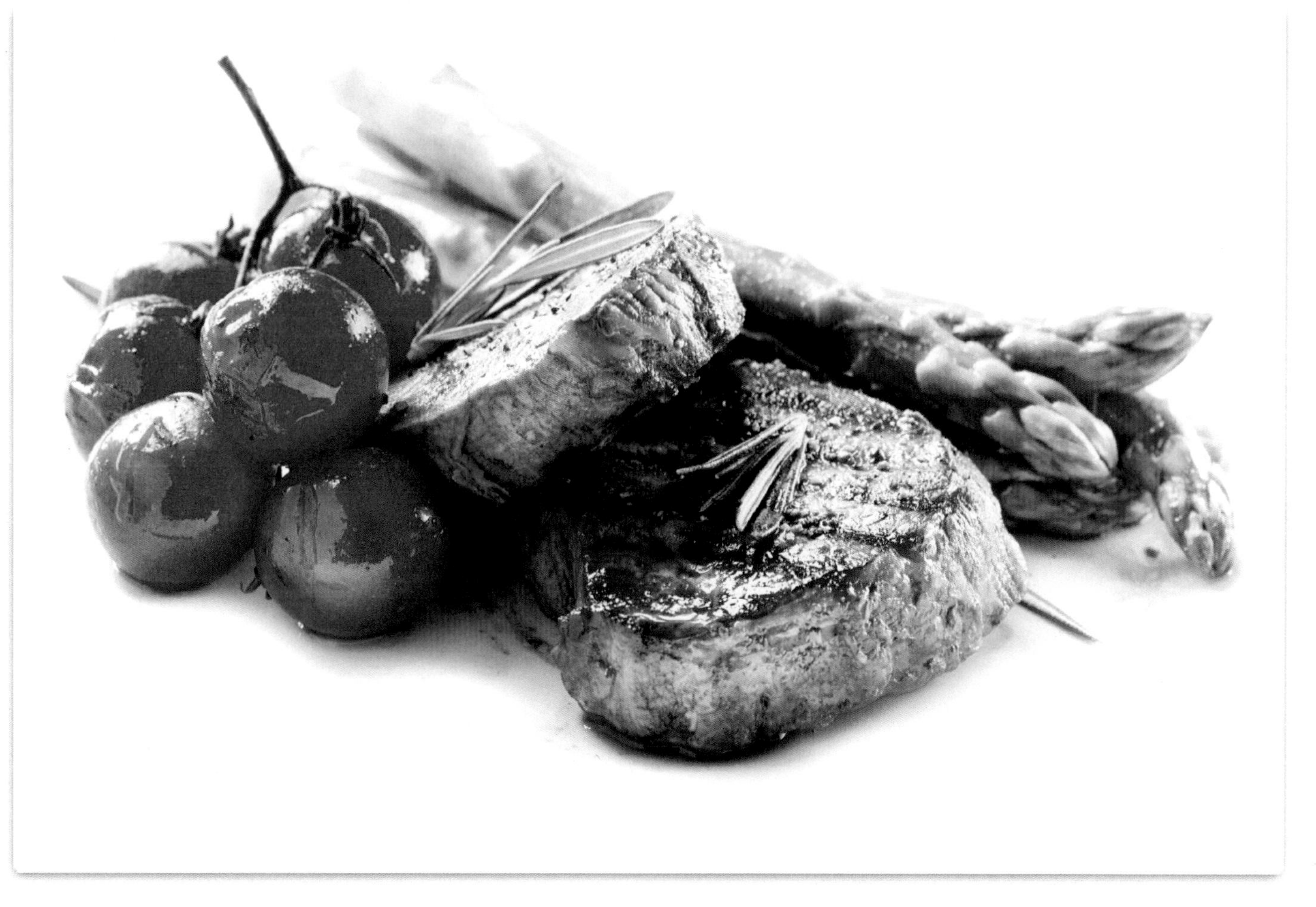

THE THREE HUNGERS

Hunger and satiety are extremely complicated. We typically eat for some combination of three reasons. First of all, we need nutrients. Secondly, we need energy. And finally, eating is enjoyable! Let's unpack each of these a little bit here, and explore how we can manipulate these for optimum success!

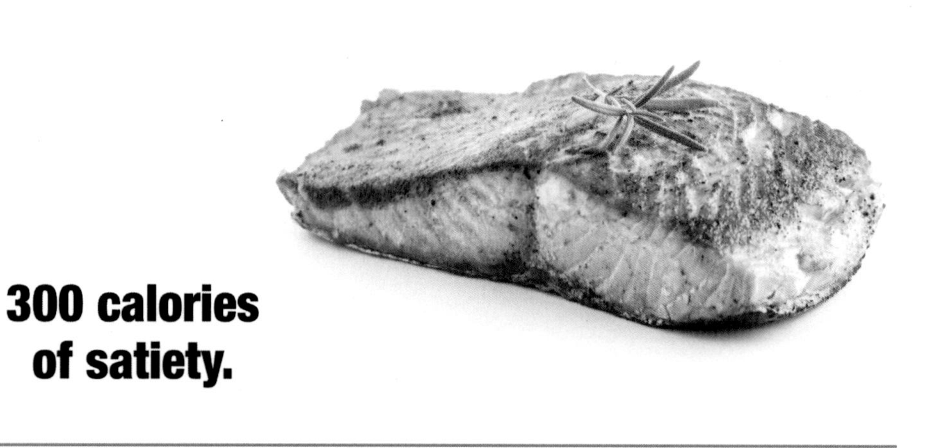

300 calories of hunger.

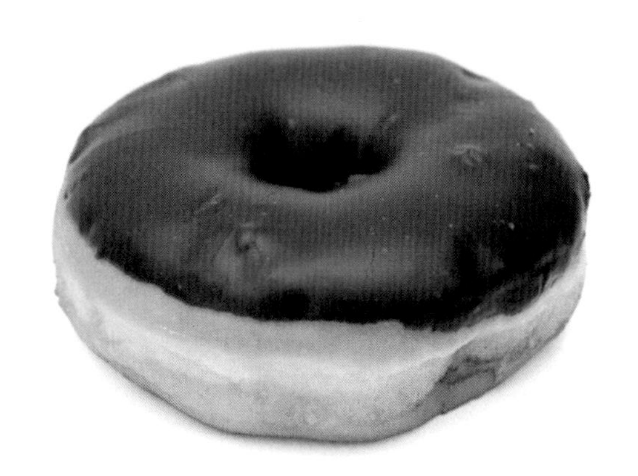

Think about how hungry you will be three or four hours from now.

1. **NUTRIENT HUNGER.**
2. **ENERGY HUNGER.**
3. **HEDONIC HUNGER.**

NUTRIENT HUNGER

Your body is the most complicated chemistry lab in the entire universe. Every second, there are trillions of chemical reactions taking place in your body. In order for all of this to function, you need a lot of STUFF. And except for air and water and sunlight, all of this 'stuff' comes directly from your diet. You need dozens of vitamins and minerals and essential amino acids and essential fats from your diet, and if you don't get these, things are going to stop working properly. Thankfully, your body gives you some hints when you are low on raw materials —but the main signal of hunger is a bit non-specific. We know from human and animal studies that if you have a specific dietary deficiency—protein or minerals, for example—you will be hungrier and more driven to eat. What your poor body doesn't know is that most of the food in your environment is food-like garbage. So you eat and eat, but you might not get what your body is looking for. Non-protein ENERGY is everywhere—but protein and minerals are few and far between. So we are getting fatter in our ill-fated attempts to supply our bodies with the things they really need.

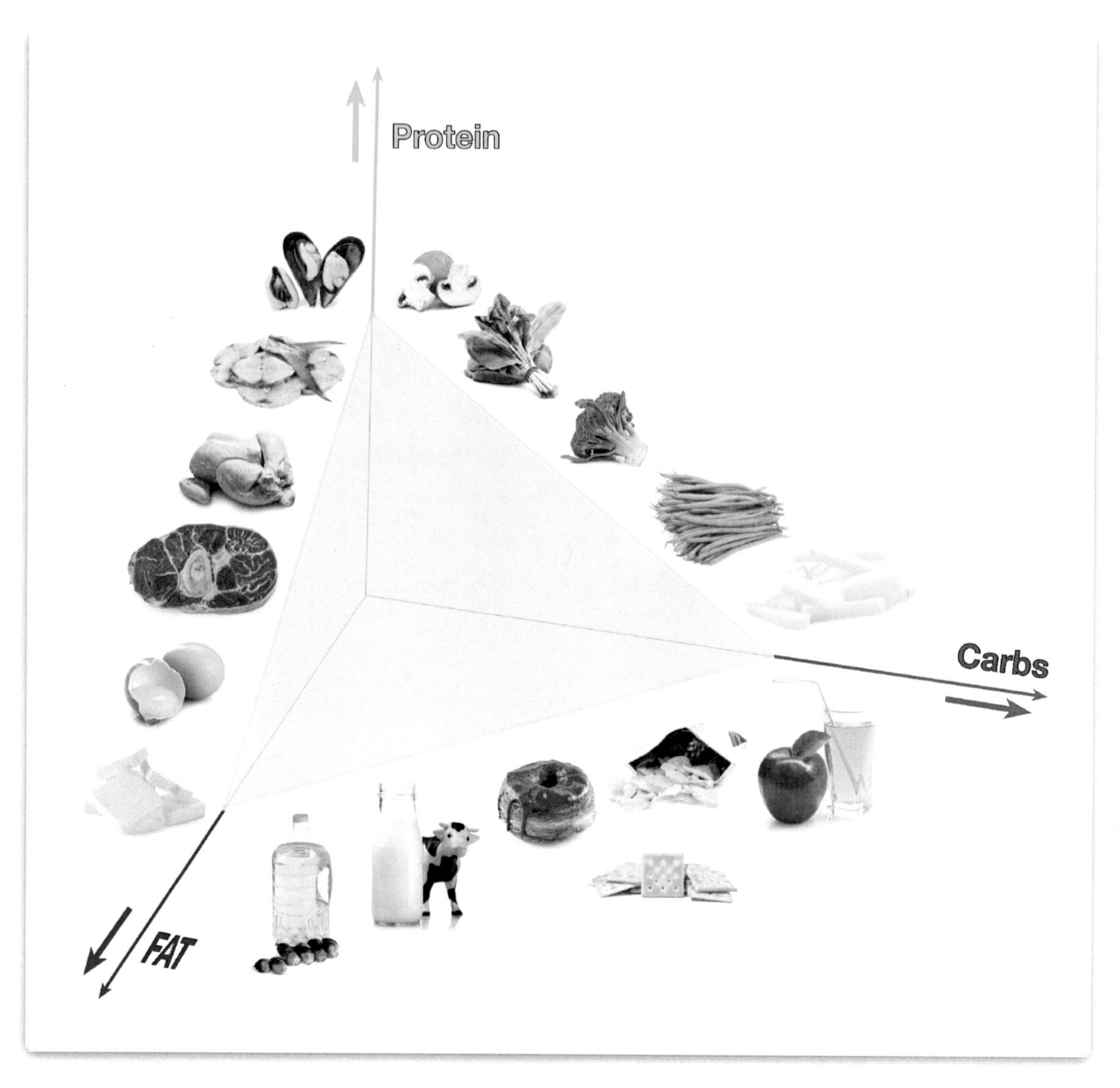

Protein tracks together with minerals and other micronutrients. Targeting protein — and aiming high on this pyramid — is the best way to maximize nutrient satiety.

ENERGY HUNGER

The primary goal of your body is to keep your DNA alive long enough to pass it on to the next generation. In order to do this, it is imperative that you have plenty of extra energy around, just in case. Not so much that you can't escape from a predator, but enough so you don't die during the wintertime when plant foods are nonexistent and all of the animals you hunt for food are low on energy themselves. So your body is constantly trying to conserve the energy it has, while also looking to acquire more. In today's food environment, we are drowning in energy. In fact, our biggest current threat is the energy overload and energy toxicity that leads to obesity and the entire spectrum of chronic degenerative diseases. Sometimes we have difficulty distinguishing nutrient hunger from energy hunger. For this reason, your very best strategy is targeting NUTRIENTS first, by eating protein and other nutrient-dense foods first and foremost. Once you can be sure that you have consumed adequate protein and minerals, and your nutrient hunger is satisfied, then you will be in a much better position to properly interpret energy hunger. Often times, if someone has plenty of extra fat to burn, they find that after eating protein and minerals they really don't have any energy hunger.

800 calories

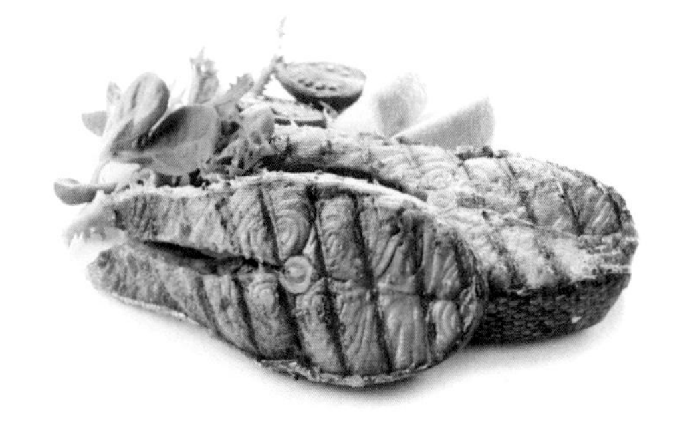

800 calories

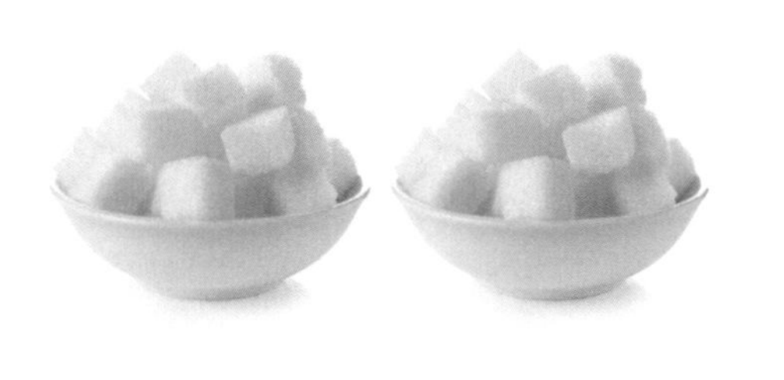

Sometimes we also struggle to differentiate LOW GLYCOGEN hunger (lack of 'fat adaptation') from a true global low energy hunger. This is yet another reason to reduce your carbohydrate frequency, to improve fat adaptation. If you are properly 'fat adapted', and you target protein and minerals first, you find that you can get by with the very smallest amounts of non-protein energy (carbs and fats).

In practical terms, every meal should start with lean protein and low carb vegetables if possible. Energy can be added in if you still have leftover 'energy hunger'.

Don't worry if you don't have a really good idea of how this actually looks or feels! Many people are unfamiliar with these concepts and it takes some time to get used to them. Intermittent fasting and reduced carbohydrate frequency can be very helpful when it comes to getting in touch with all of the forms of hunger and fullness.

HEDONIC HUNGER

As we established, eating high energy density carbs and fats together is extremely rewarding and, for many, extremely addictive. Your best strategy is understanding what is going on with your biology when it comes to these foods.

Lower energy carbs and fats together aren't nearly as problematic. For example, imagine eating a steak and a salad. The steak has some fat, and the salad has some carbs. But the energy density of the steak is low thanks to protein, and the energy density of the salad is low thanks to fiber. As long as protein and fiber are present, you are probably fine.

But mix together a high energy density carbohydrate, like a potato, with a high energy density fat, like oil? Now you have french fries or potato chips — these are extremely hyperpalatable and you can overeat the hell out of these!

Anything with high energy density carbs and fats together is going to be extremely tasty. You are definitely going to eat these foods, but treat them with the caution and respect they deserve.

How do you deal with these foods? Our favorite is eating these AFTER a nutritious meal of protein and veggies, so your nutrient hunger is taken care of and the danger factor is lower. Eat these foods with a lot of INTENTION and MINDFULNESS. Try not to buy these foods and have them in your house, but rather only eat these at social outings, and only buy one serving. Enjoy these cheats and don't deprive yourself of these foods on occasion — but try to make these the exceptions to an otherwise nutrient dense baseline diet. Most of all, be hyperaware of what these foods are doing to you and how they are affecting your behavior. Some highly addicted people find it best to avoid these completely, almost like an alcoholic who avoids alcohol 100% of the time. This is a legitimate strategy, and the only person who knows what works best for you is YOU.

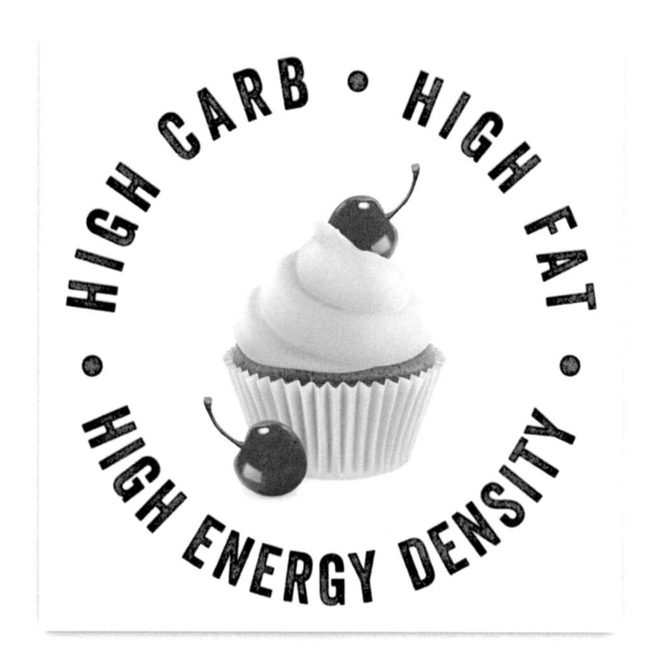

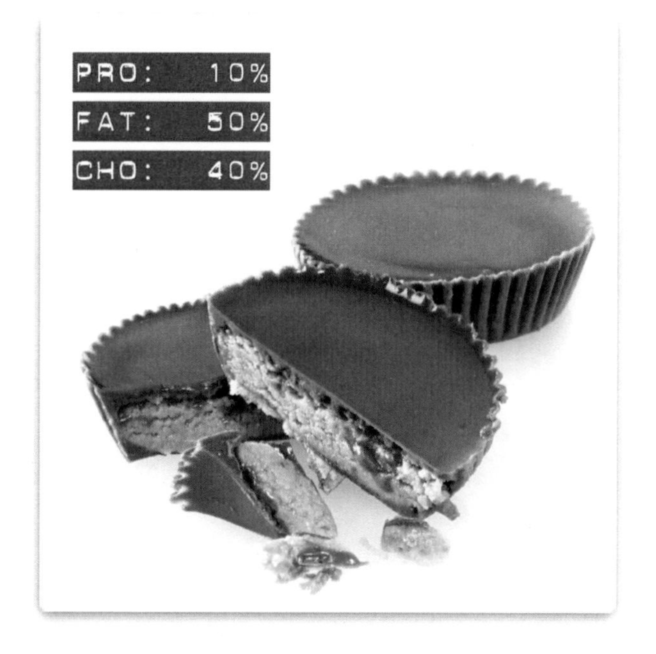

PRACTICAL APPLICATION:

Now that you know about the three hungers, you can strategize:

1. EAT LEAN PROTEIN AND VEGGIES FIRST.

Targeting protein and minerals allows you to achieve NUTRIENT satiety first. This allows you to be more in touch with ENERGY hunger and fullness.

2. MINIMIZE CARBOHYDRATE FREQUENCY TO ALLOW FOR FAT ADAPTATION.

Once you are 'fat adapted', or more comfortable living in a low carb/glycogen state, you are FAR better equipped to be in touch with your overall energy hunger and fullness.

3. EAT ADDED ENERGY (CARBS AND FATS) LAST AND ONLY IF NECESSARY.

If you have a lot of available energy already in your body, you might be surprised to find just how little additional energy (added carbs and fats) you need to eat.

4. BE EXTREMELY CAUTIOUS WITH HIGH ENERGY DENSITY CARBS AND FATS TOGETHER.

You probably don't have to deprive yourself of these foods forever, but they need to be treated with extreme respect and caution, as they can drive a lot of overeating!

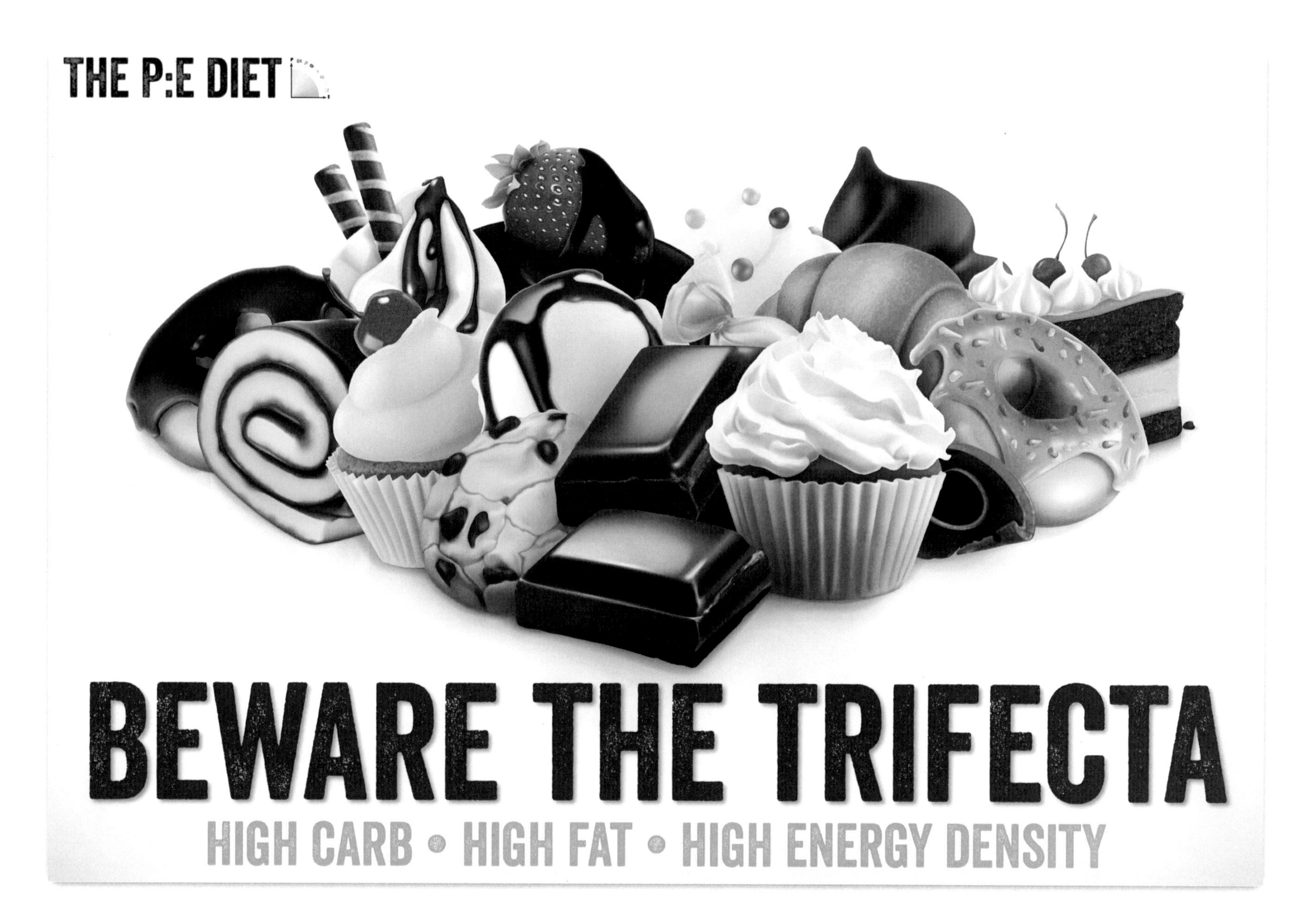

Treat these foods with a LOT of respect, because they are extremely powerful!

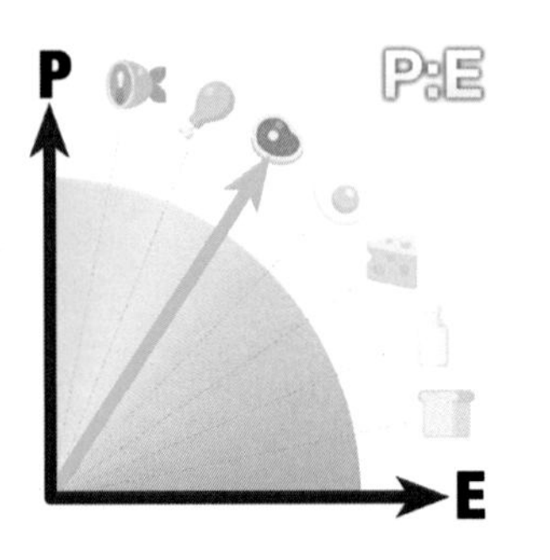

1. MAXIMIZE SATIETY.

TARGET PROTEIN AND MINERALS FOR HIGHEST NUTRIENT DENSITY.

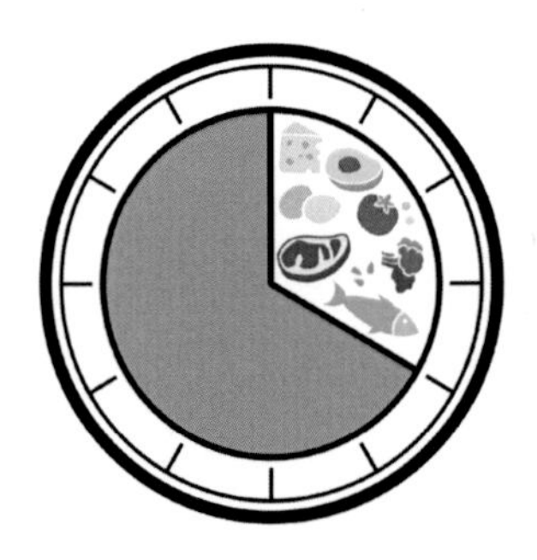

2. MAXIMIZE FAT ADAPTATION.

USE INTERMITTENT FASTING WITH LOW CARBOHYDRATE FREQUENCY.

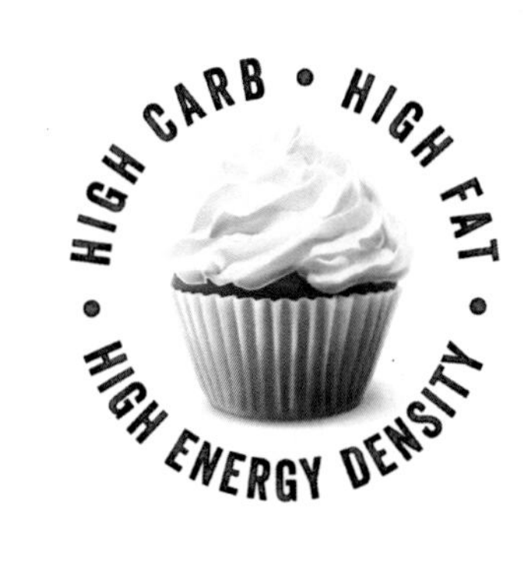

3. AVOID THE TRIFECTA.

HIGH CARB + HIGH FAT + HIGH ENERGY DENSITY = OVEREATING.

The three pillars of The P:E Diet.

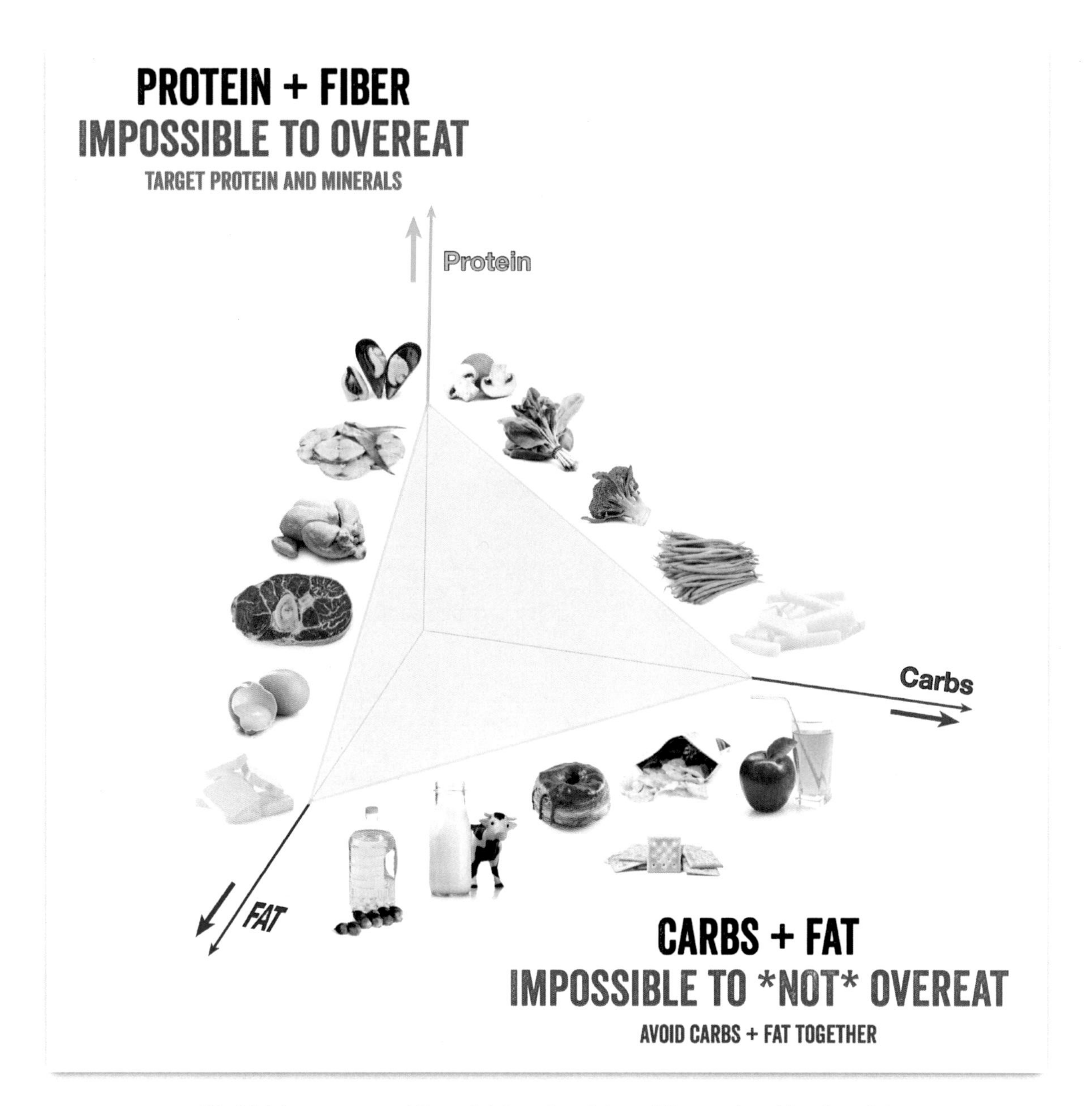

We think by now you get the point: target protein and fiber, and avoid carbs + fat.

OBESITY AND HYPERINSULINEMIA ARE SYMPTOMS OF ENERGY TOXICITY.

Which is caused by—you guessed it—overeating energy.

THERE ARE ONLY TWO REASONS ANYONE OVEREATS:

1. YOU NEED TO EAT MORE.

Cause #1: Nutrient Hunger.

Mechanism: Protein and mineral dilution due to excess refined carbs and fats.

Best Solution: Target protein [P:E ratio].

Possibly Helpful: Paleo Diet, Whole Foods Diet.

Cause #2: Energy Hunger.

Mechanism: Glucose dependence and lack of fat adaptation from frequent carbs.

Best Solution: Less frequent carbs via low carb diet and/or intermittent fasting.

Possibly Helpful: Low Carb Diet, Ketogenic Diet.

2. YOU WANT TO EAT MORE.

Cause: Addiction.

Mechanism: Dopamine reward of rare combination of carbs and fats together.

Best Solution: Stay low carb, low fat, or both most of the time [P:E ratio].

Possibly Helpful: Low Carb Diet, Low Fat Diet, Vegan, Carnivore, Whole Foods.

NOTE ZERO MENTION OF THE FOLLOWING TERMS:

Calories, energy output, energy balance.

Know the main reasons for overeating so you are better equipped to circumvent them.

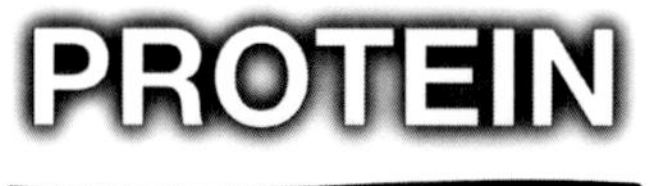

can do anything that carbs and fat can do.

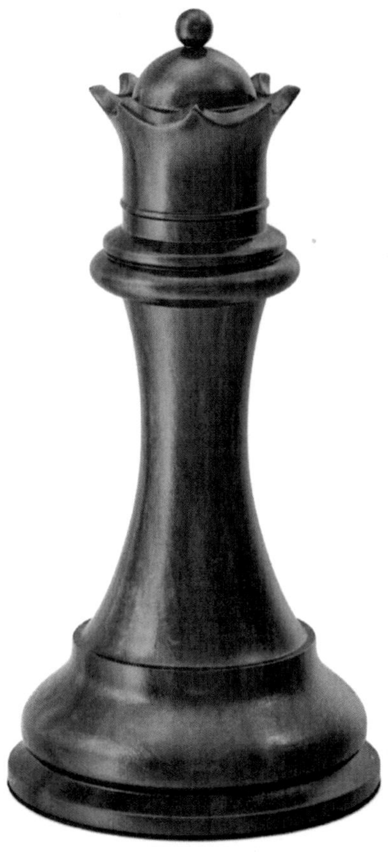

But carbs and fat can't do anything that protein does.

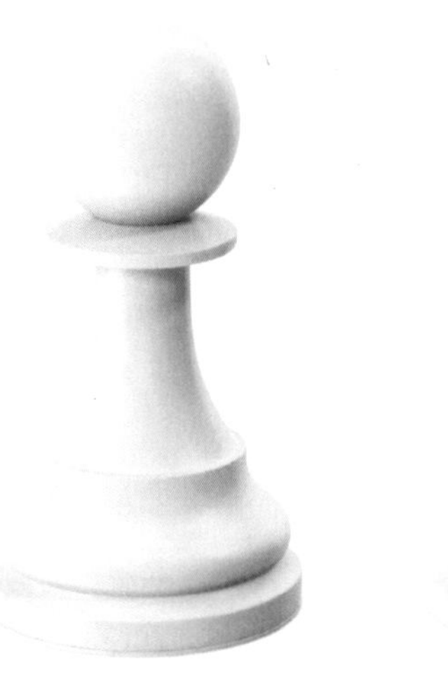

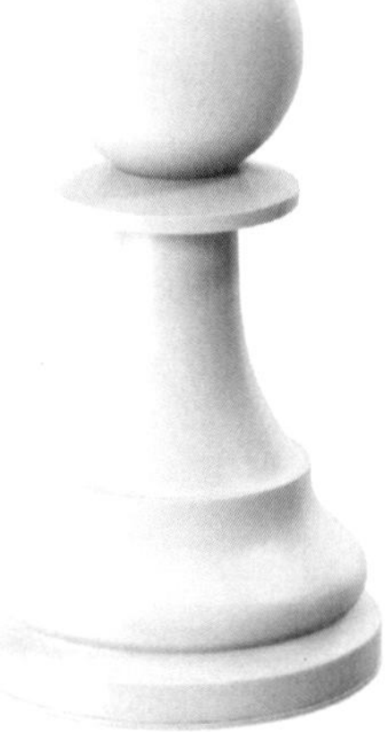

Which macro should you build your diet around?

Your body can convert protein into carbs or fat — but it CANNOT convert carbs or fat into protein!

PROGRESSING 'FAT ADAPTATION'

It is a scientific fact: there is ZERO requirement for carbohydrate in the human diet. But the reality is that you DO need glucose, at all times, just to stay alive. Your liver can make all the glucose you need out of protein, but this is a little more difficult than just eating all your glucose (especially eating glycemic carbs 8 times a day, for 16 hours out of every 24, like the average American).

In theory, shrinking down your carbohydrate frequency SOUNDS great —but it can be VERY difficult, especially to the uninitiated! Trying to meet all of your energy needs in a low glycogen state, running solely off of stored body fat and some glucose created by your liver out of protein, is the metabolic equivalent of jogging or any other type of exercise.

And just like exercise, it is a LOT OF WORK when you first start out. Neophytes often notice low energy levels, decreased exercise tolerance, and general fatigue and brain fog.

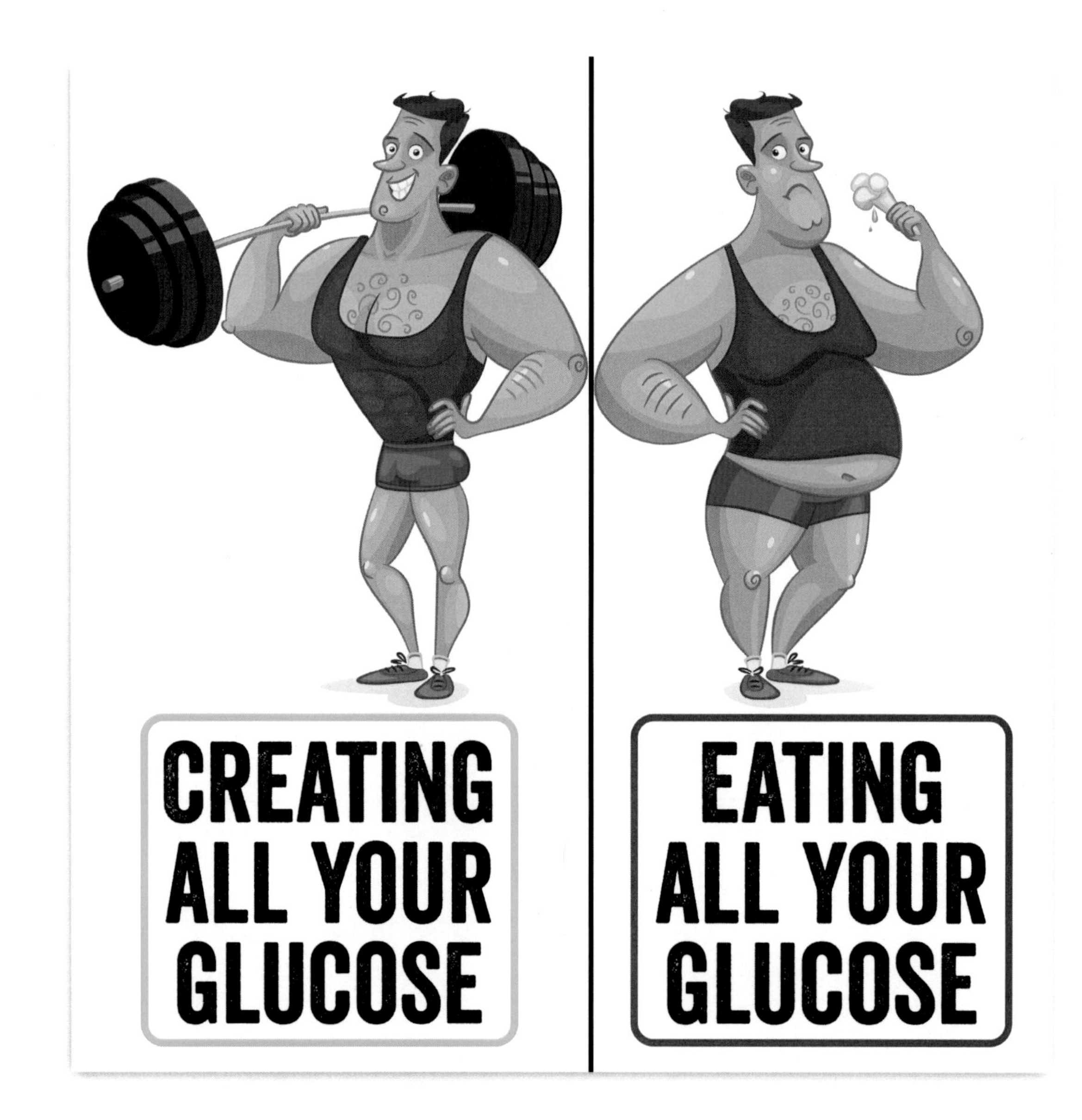

You have two options when you embark on a reduction in glycemic quantity and frequency. The first option is just diving in headfirst, embracing the suck, and powering through for the one or two weeks it takes to get through the majority of the discomfort—with the caveat that it could be MONTHS before you have the same athletic capacity that you had before in a carb-loaded state. The second option is to gradually progress your reduced carbohydrate frequency, little by little.

If you do choose to slowly progress this ability, we highly recommend you start with BREAKFAST. Try to see if you can eliminate carbohydrates from breakfast, by replacing them with protein-rich foods such as eggs, meat, or plain Greek yogurt. At this point, you would continue eating carbohydrates for lunch and dinner. Once you are comfortable with this, start whittling away at lunchtime carbs. Take the bread off your sandwich and wrap it in lettuce. Be sure to double your meat and cheese, increasing the protein, so you aren't hungry.

Last to go? Dinnertime carbs. And in fact, if you NEVER got rid of those, and only ate significant net carbohydrates once per day, you would probably be fine. Most people could reach adequate fat adaptation with this degree of carbohydrate restriction. In fact, many people struggle to achieve energy satiety every day unless they eat at least around 100 grams of net carbohydrates. Evening is usually the largest craving for these glycemic carbs, which makes sense, as they do trigger the parasympathetic state ("rest and digest"). If you are going to continue to eat these carbohydrates, please feel free to do so—but be sure to keep protein high at this meal, and in fact we recommend eating PROTEIN FIRST. There are a number of studies, mostly performed in Japan, looking at the timing of protein, vegetables, and carbohydrate (rice) with mealtimes. These studies show that eating protein and vegetables first, and rice last, at the same meal, leads to higher satiety and improved outcomes. The reasons for this are likely due to satiety hormones from the small intestine which are beyond the scope of this book, but let's just say that your grandparents, who told you to eat dessert AFTER dinner, were really on to something.

A few final notes about fat adaptation. Exercise is phenomenal for improving fat adaptation. If you are performing a ton of glycolytic exercise (exercise of a very high intensity that burns mostly glucose), you might not have to worry about reducing carbohydrate frequency. There are also genetic factors here, and some persons are perfectly well fat-adapted despite a high carbohydrate diet. We are happy for these people, and most of the advice here is for the REST of us.

As with everything else when it comes to diet, the only person who really knows what works best for you is YOU, so don't be afraid to try things and see what happens.

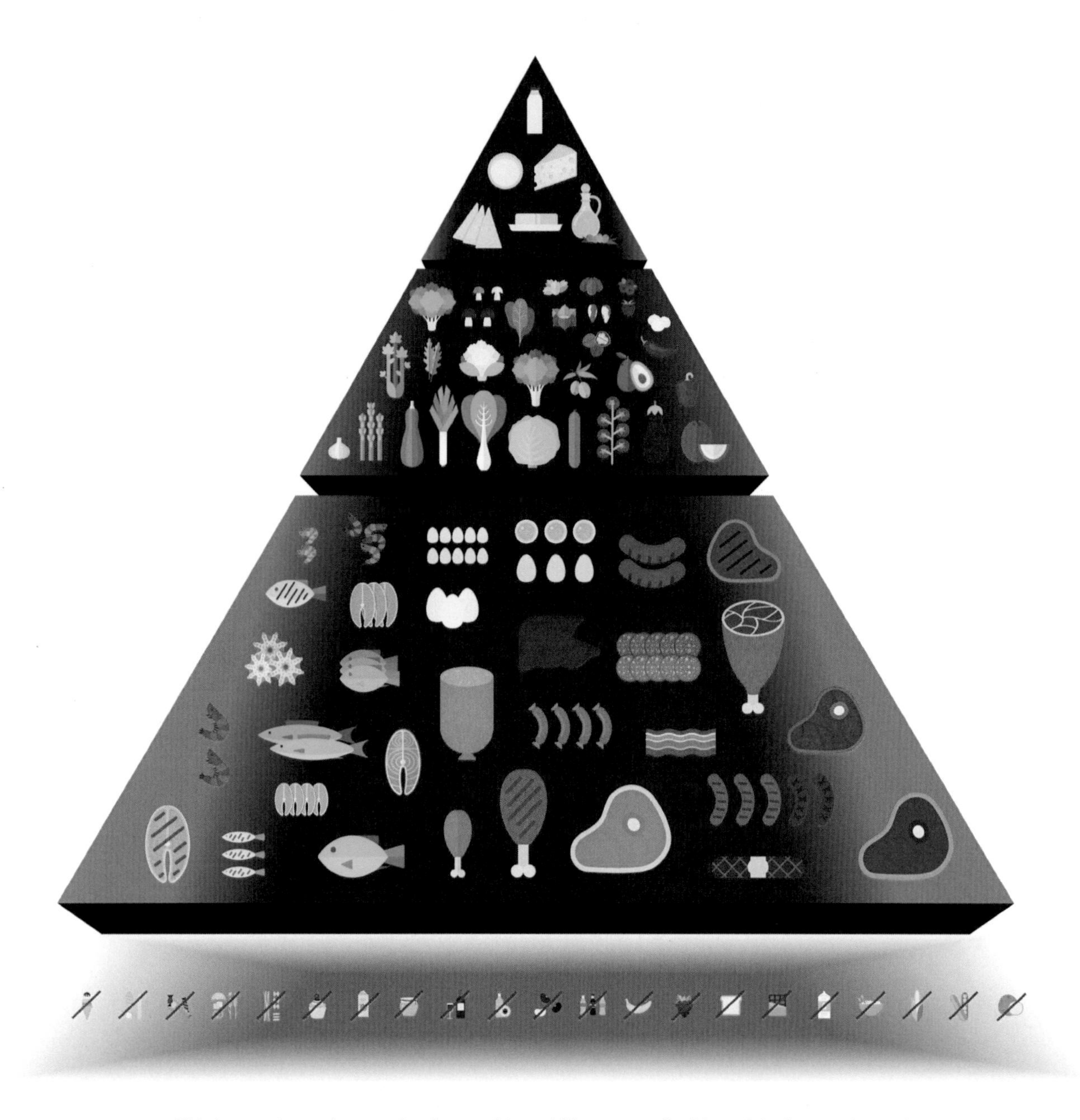

This low carb carnivorous food pyramid would be an excellent template for most people.

5 STEPS TO FAT LOSS

1. **REPLACE CARBS WITH PROTEIN.** →
2. (OH SORRY THERE WAS JUST ONLY THAT ONE STEP—YOU'RE DONE)
3.
4.
5.

If your average person replaced some of their carbohydrates with protein, they would improve body composition immediately.

PROTEIN : ENERGY

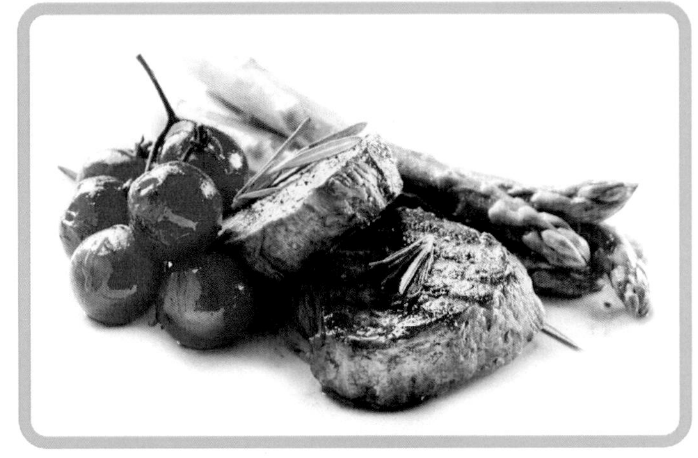

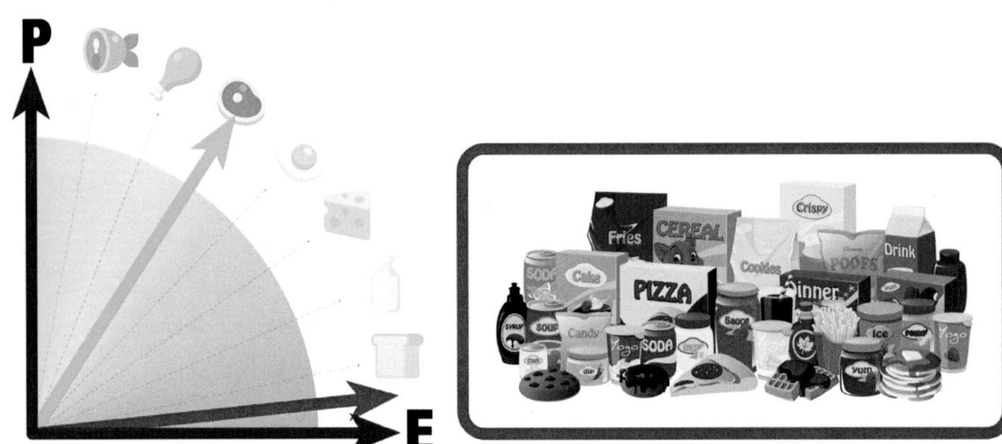

No surprise: real food usually has an excellent P:E ratio, and fake packaged food usually has a terrible one.

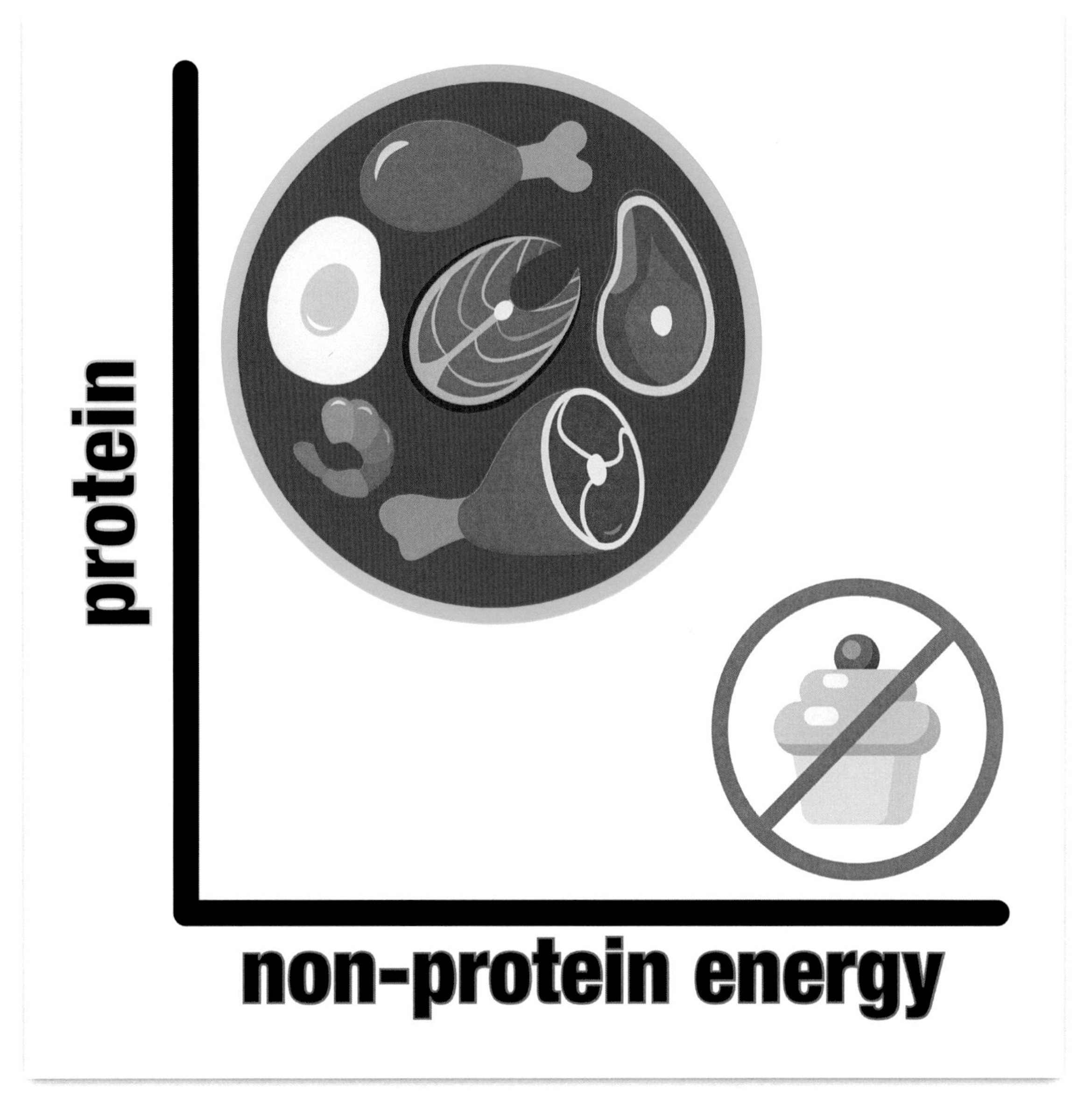

The primary strategy of The P:E Diet is targeting more protein and less non-protein energy (non-fiber, or glucose-producing carbs, plus fats).

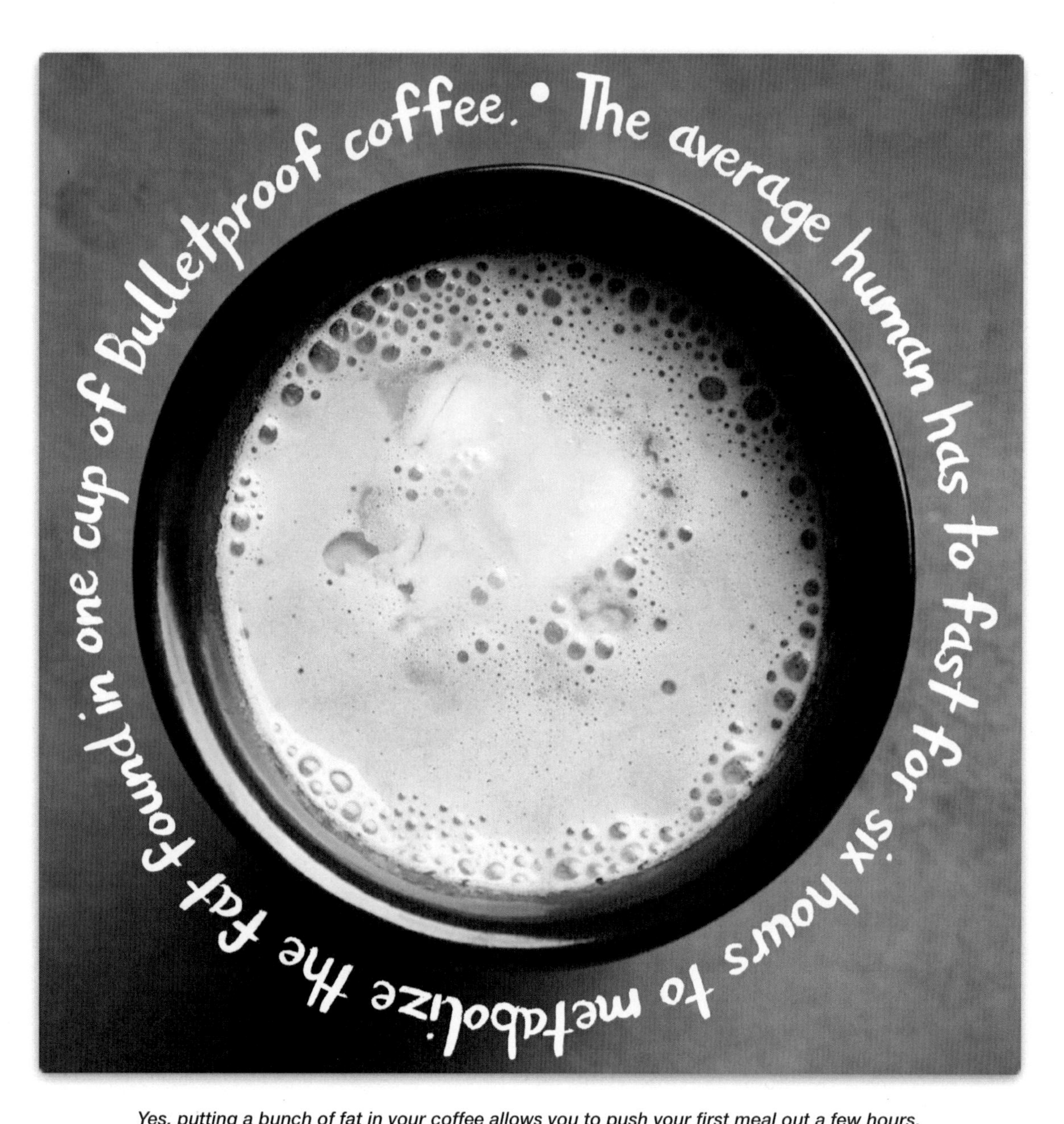

Yes, putting a bunch of fat in your coffee allows you to push your first meal out a few hours. But this fat is nutritionally empty and is just more fat you have to burn to reach your goals.

SUPERFOODS?

No, we're not going to go on a rant about some rare and all-powerful berry from the Amazon or something. But there are a few high nutrient density foods that are so amazing that they deserve a place in everyone's 'baseline' diet. Try to make these staples and you will up your chances for success!

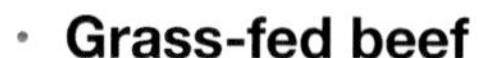

- **Grass-fed beef**
- **Pastured eggs**
- **Wild-caught salmon**
- **Plain Greek yogurt**
- **Low sugar fruit**
- **Shellfish**

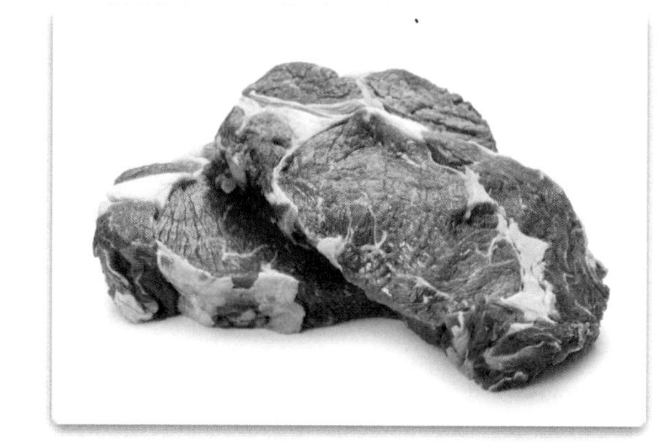

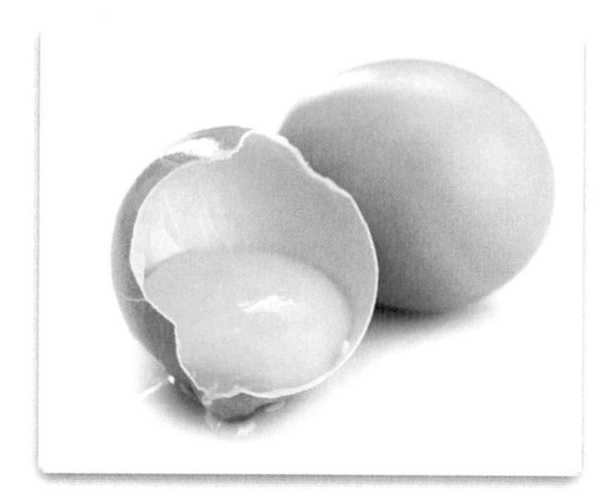

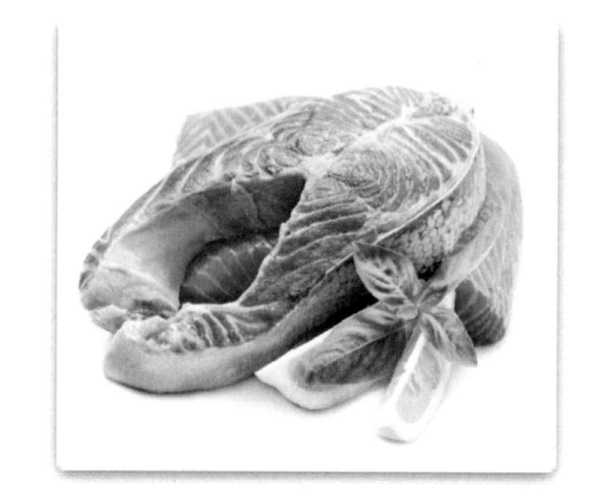

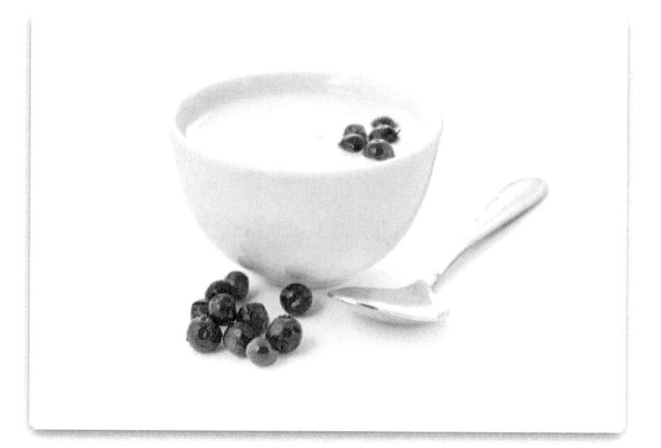

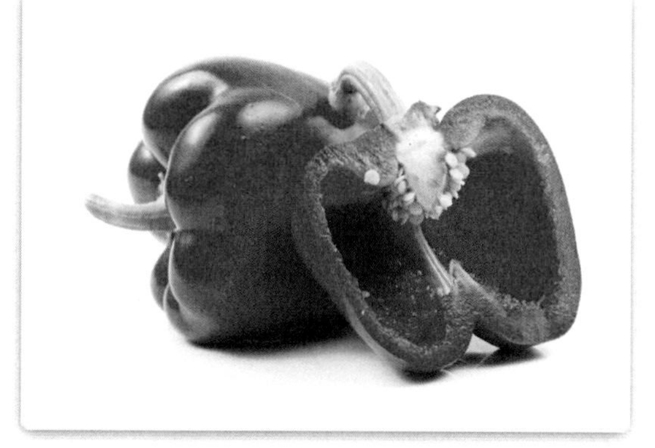

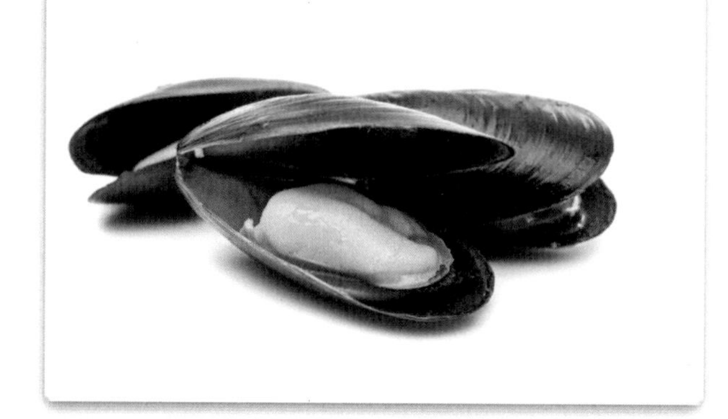

YOUR 'BASELINE' DIET

You should have a basic diet template that you follow on a regular basis. You should have a few staple protein sources that you are extremely familiar with. Maybe these are pastured eggs, wild-caught salmon, and grass-fed beef. You should know how to buy and cook these foods. You should at least be vaguely familiar with the macronutrients in these foods and their P:E ratios. You should have them on hand most of the time. You can deviate from this 'baseline' diet as much as you want, but this always gives you something to fall back on when you aren't sure what to eat. We have foods like ground beef, Greek yogurt, canned sardines, canned salmon, pastured eggs, and chicken breasts around almost all of the time. Set yourself up for success by having these foods available as often as possible. Keep emergency protein sources nearby—our favorites are hard-boiled eggs and individually packaged grass-fed beef sticks (without sugar). If you are eating carbohydrates, make sure you have some low energy density high satiety choices available, like apples, carrots, berries, and potatoes. If you need something super convenient, consider some whey powder and a shaker bottle for the times when you are starving but you have no time at all. Having all of this in place makes you far less likely to fall off the wagon and end up in the drive-through of your favorite fast food place.

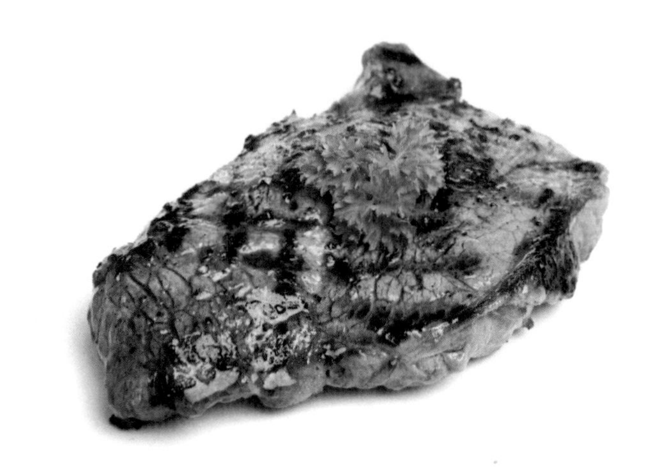

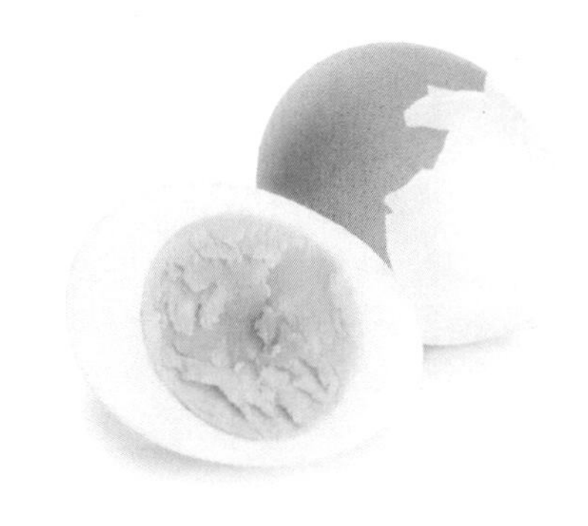

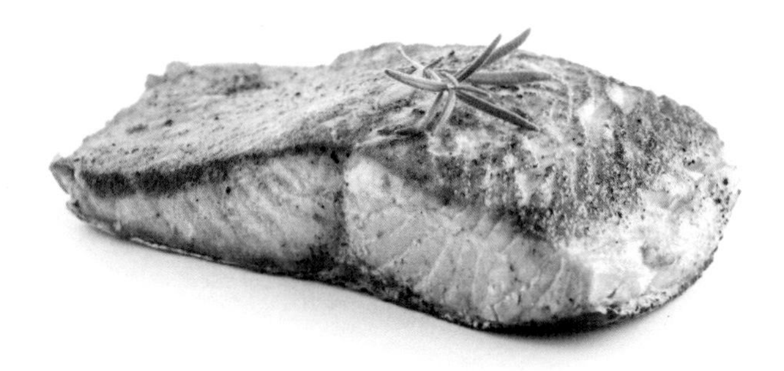

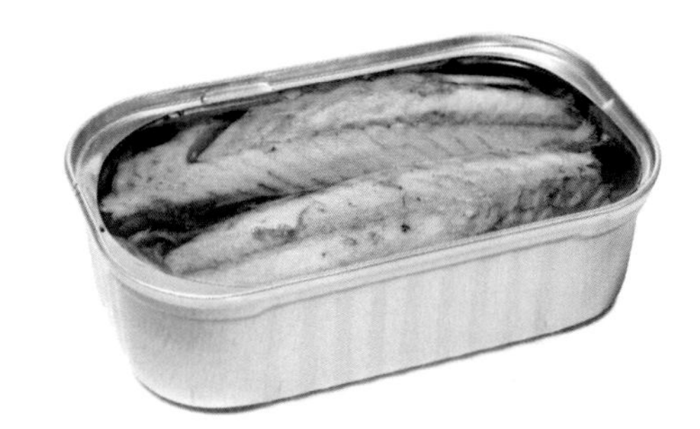

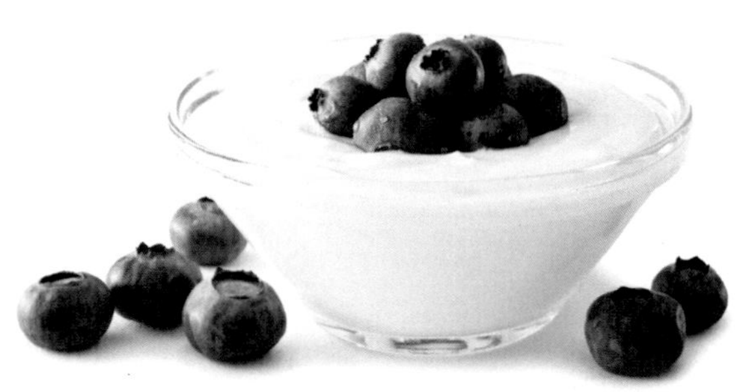

Easiest Fat Loss Heuristic:

Eat foods to satiety as long as PROTEIN or FIBER is the dominant macronutrient.

PROTEIN:

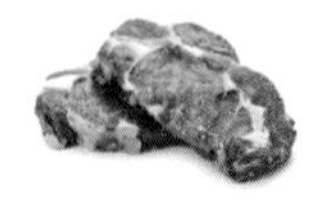
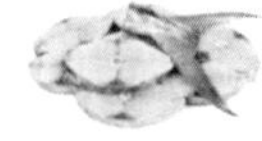
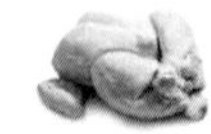
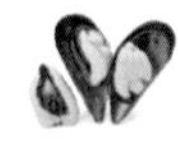
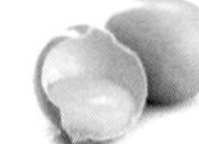

beef
fish
pork
chicken
turkey
veal
lamb
crustaceans
shellfish
cottage cheese
eggs
game
whey

FIBER:

arugula
endive
broccoli
spinach
kale
turnip greens
Chinese cabbage
mushrooms
artichoke
cauliflower
watercress
collard greens
celery

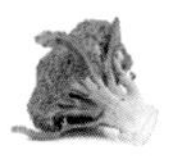
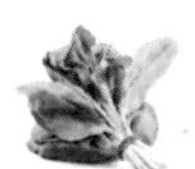
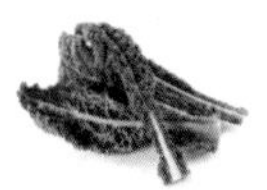
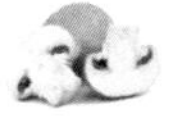
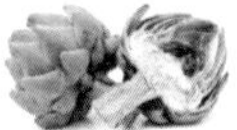

Target protein and fiber, while limiting added fats and non-fiber carbohydrates.

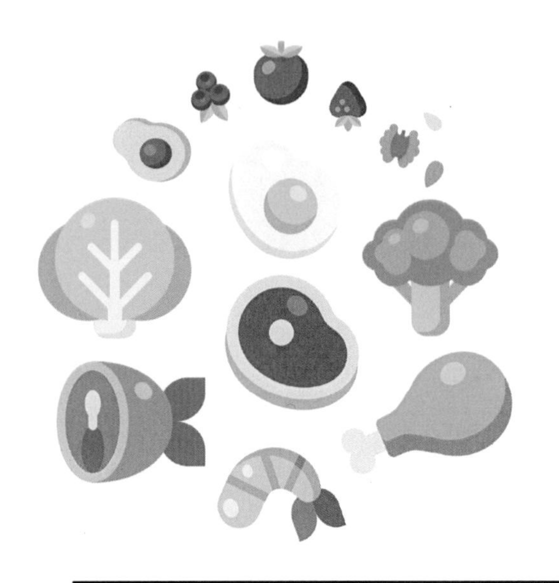

TARGET PROTEIN AND MICRONUTRIENTS

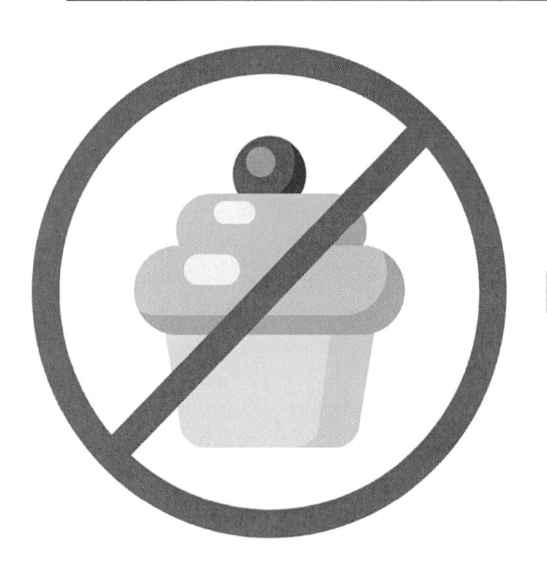

AVOID NUTRITIONALLY EMPTY CARBOHYDRATE AND FAT ENERGY

No caption necessary. 😁

THEN:

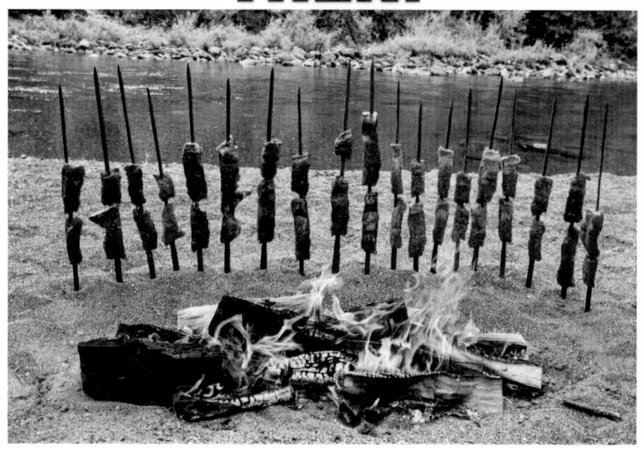

FOOD PROCESSING

INCREASES

nutrient density

NOW:

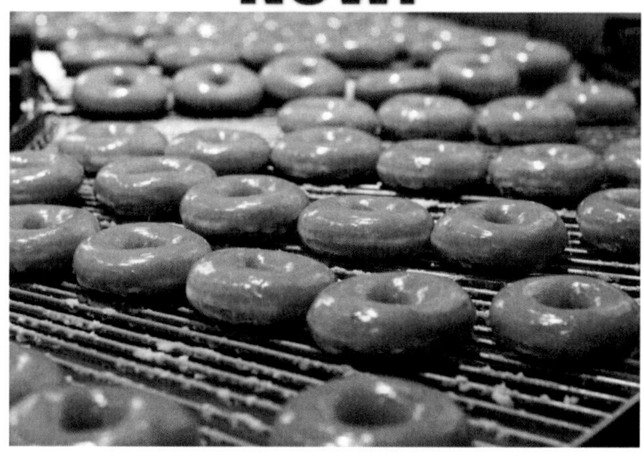

FOOD PROCESSING

DECREASES

nutrient density

Before you eliminate all 'processed' foods and go on a 'raw' diet, consider this. Humans are 'cucinivores', which means that we literally evolved eating cooked food. Cooking meat (and some plant foods) allows for higher digestibility and nutrient extraction, while destroying some parasites and anti-nutrients. Cooking and otherwise 'processing' food literally made us human.

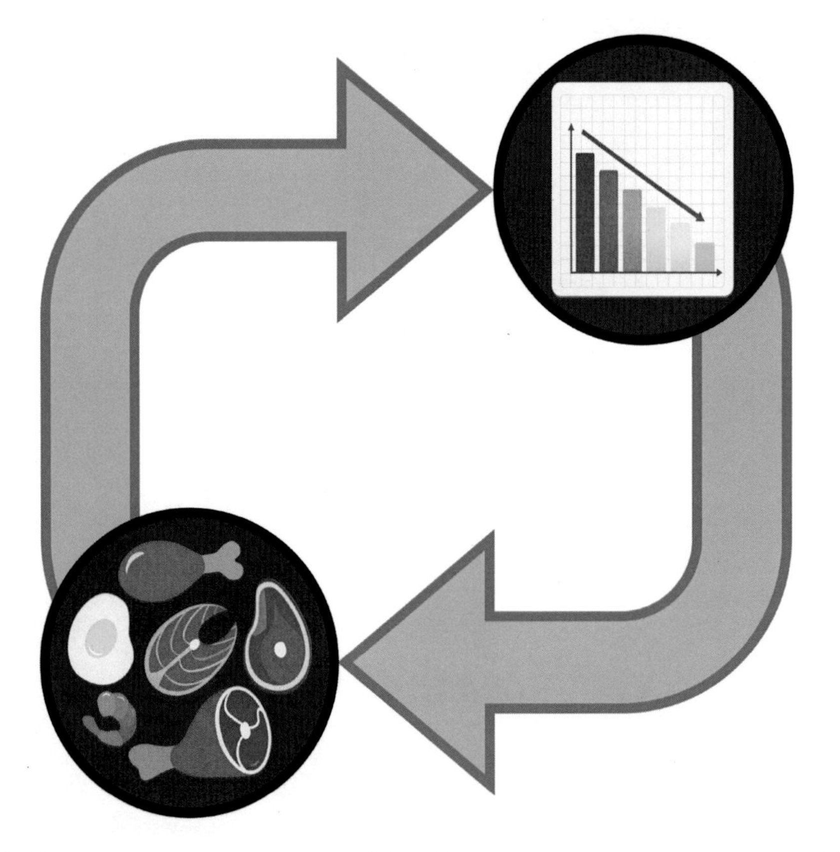

If you wanted to sum up this entire book into one graphic, this would be it.

true cause of obesity:

EMPTY CALORIES

sugar

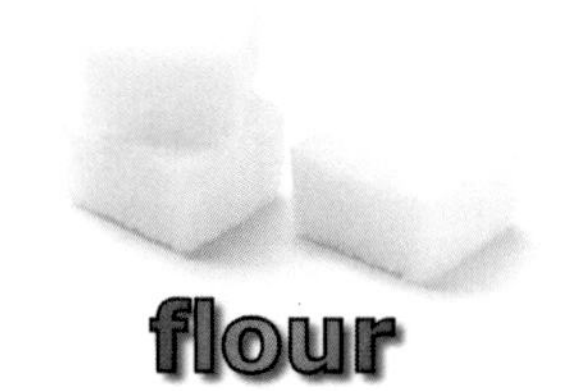

flour

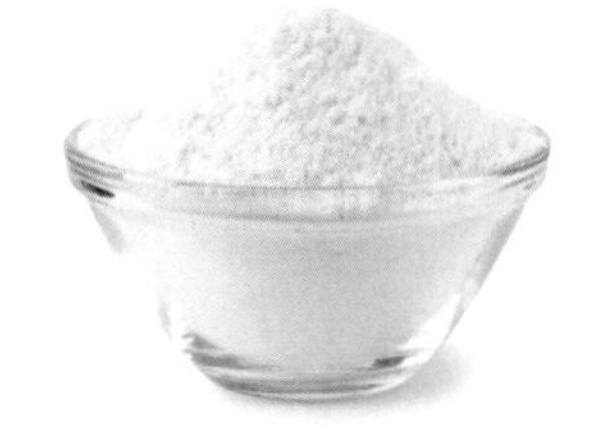

vegetable oil

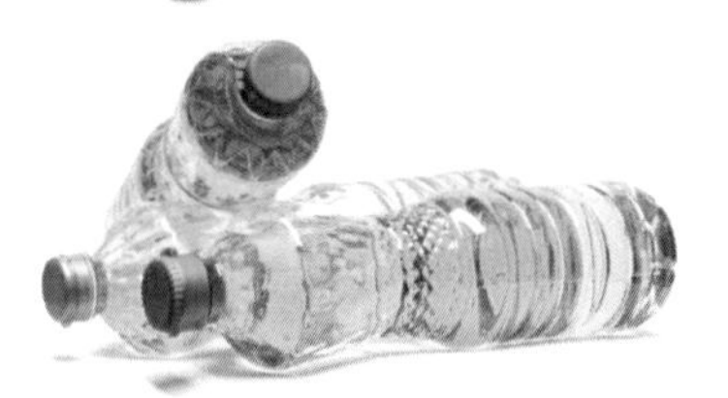

solution:

MAXIMUM NUTRIENT DENSITY

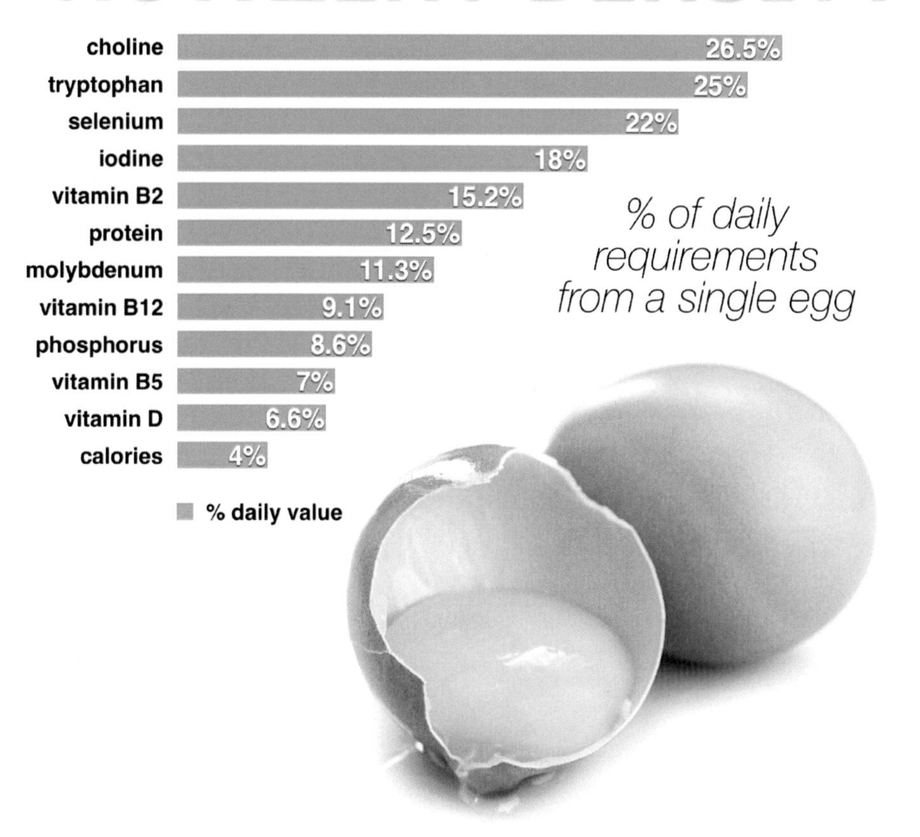

Eggs really are one of our most perfect foods.

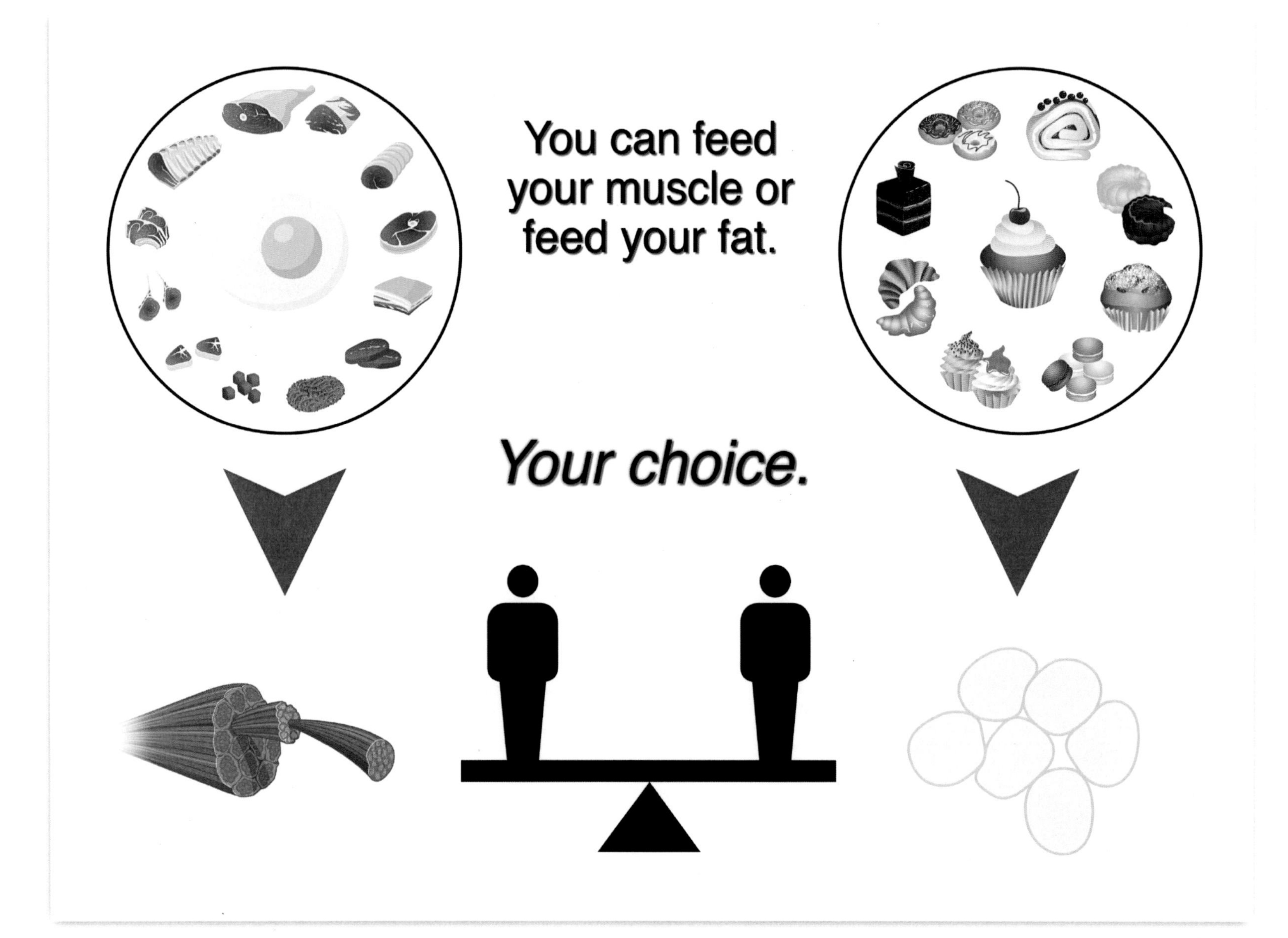

You get to choose — every single day, and even every single meal.

BY 8 YEARS OLD,
CHILDREN TODAY HAVE
EATEN MORE SUGAR
THAN AN ADULT ONE
CENTURY AGO ATE IN
THEIR ENTIRE LIFETIME.

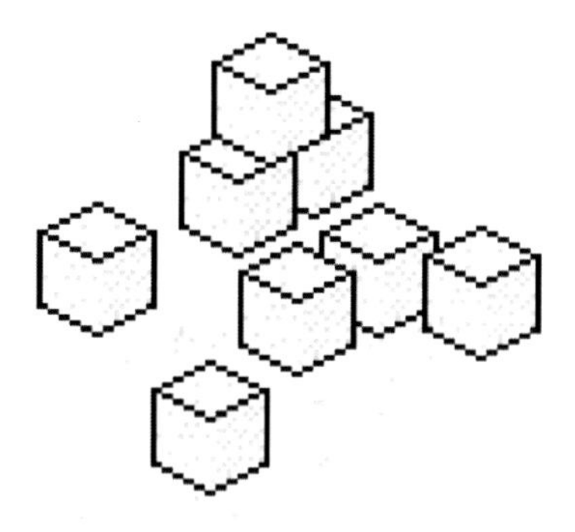

If you don't believe that sugar is addictive, you have never tried to take candy from a child.

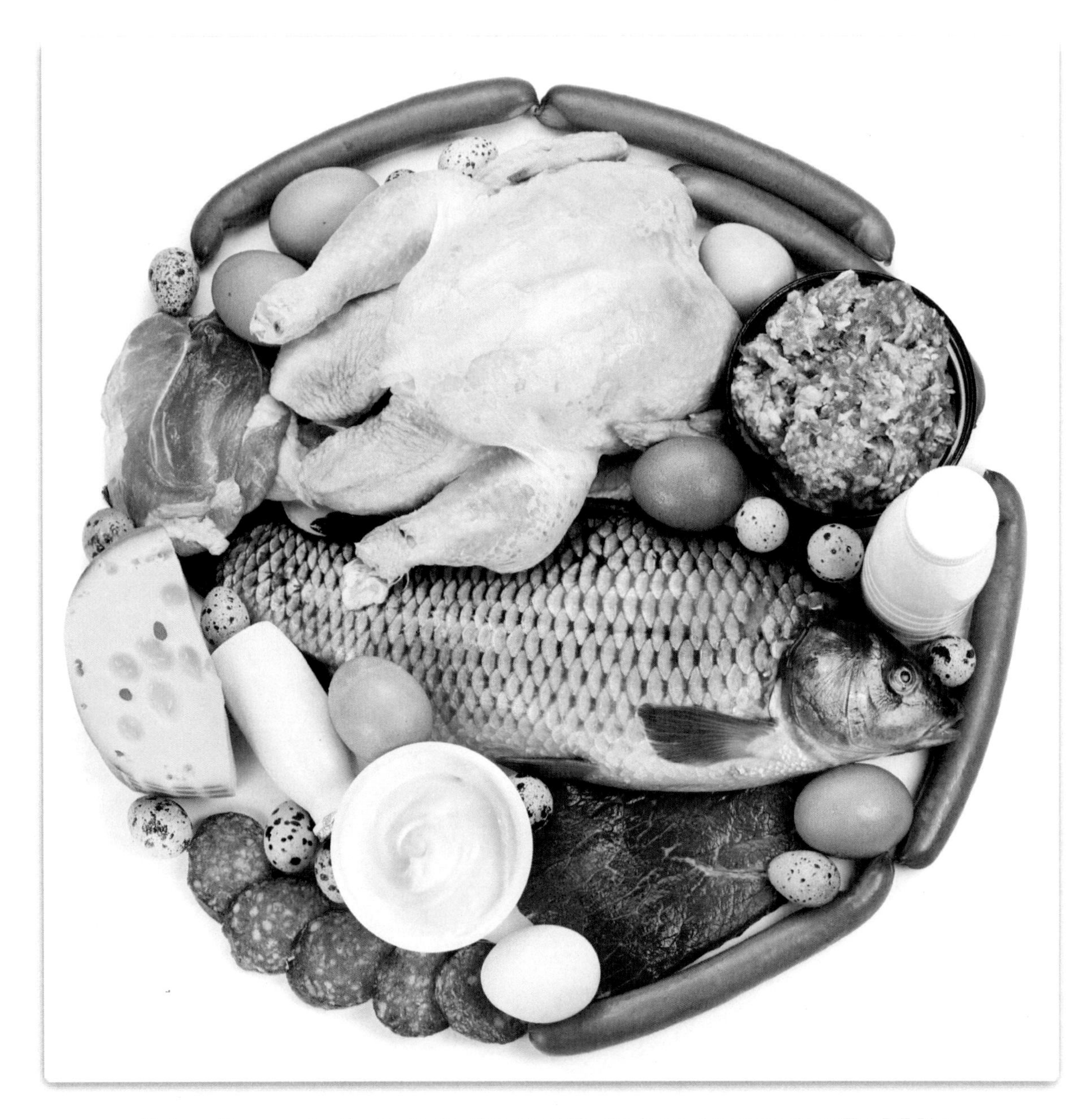

High-quality, properly raised animal protein should be the focus of most meals on The P:E Diet.

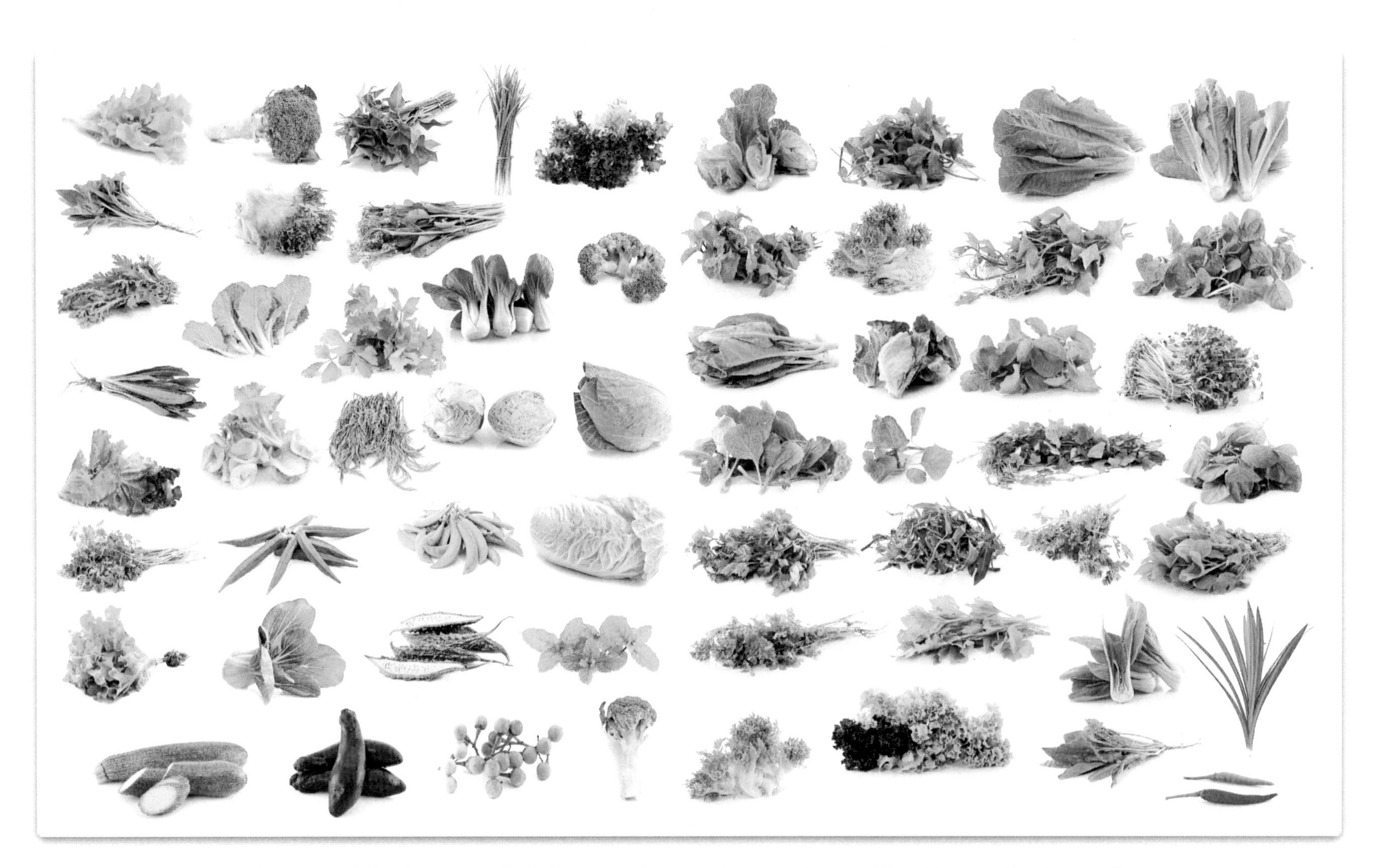

Anyone should be able to eat unlimited amounts of green and non-starchy vegetables without tracking these at all.

The Amoeba Diet™

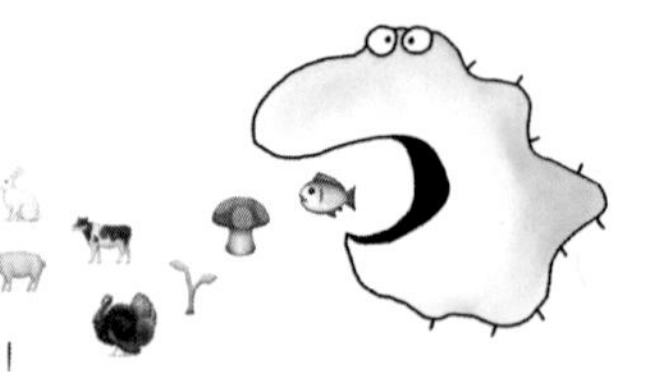

- The ultimate 'whole foods' diet!
- Try to eat animals and plants in their entirety!

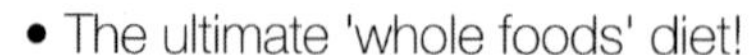

- Stop eating concentrated empty calorie sugars (and fats)!

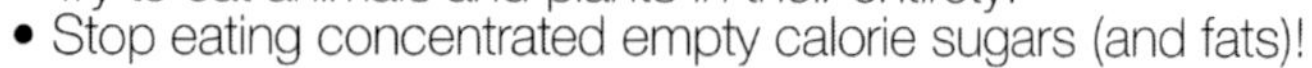

Best: as close to entire animals and plants as possible for maximum nutrient density.
bones • skin • connective tissue • organ meats • fiber • cellulose

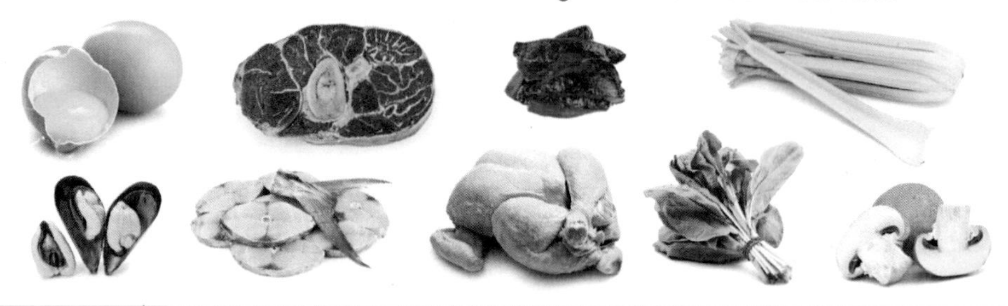

Not so good: individual components of animals and plants, chosen for sugar or fat content.
oils • concentrated plant sugars (fruit/juice, tubers, endosperm) • flour • processed dairy

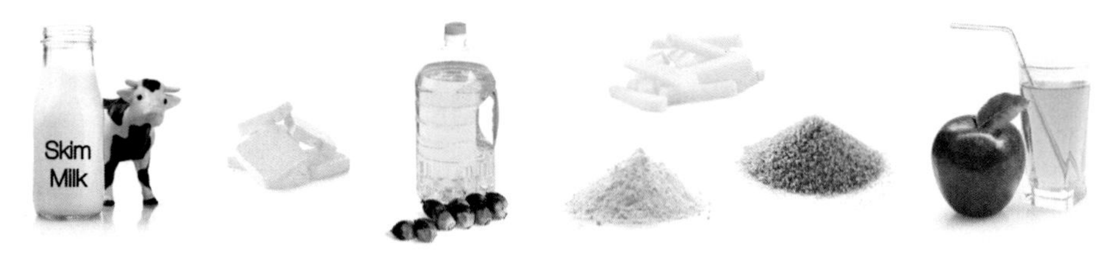

Horrible: nutrient-devoid processed combinations of empty-calorie carbs and fats.

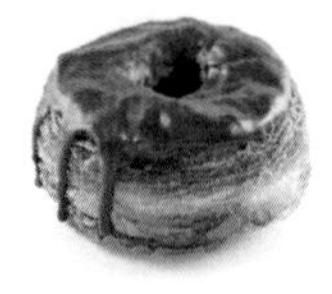

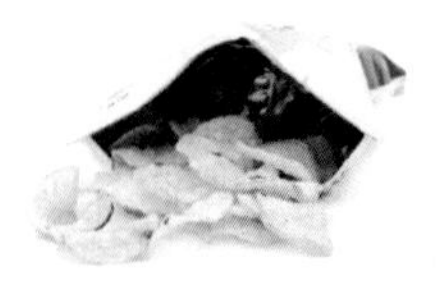

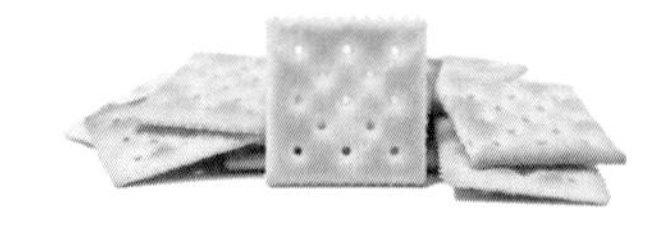

The name of 'The Amoeba Diet' is just a joke, but the general idea is pretty solid: if you focus on eating plants and animals in their entirety, rather than just taking the highest energy parts of plants and animals, you will be getting a fantastic P:E ratio as well as a full spectrum of micronutrients.

PLANT-BASED?

Let's start with the facts: 84% of all human calories on earth already come from plants. And we hate to say it, but at the moment, things aren't going so well. Of course, 60% of these plant-based calories come from three things: wheat, rice, and corn. Yup. These grains have a horrifically low P:E ratio, so we are not surprised that the health and body composition of the average person is suboptimal.

We are currently facing a deluge of plant-based propaganda, despite the fact that humans are clearly omnivores and eating meat is part of what made us human. The reality is, plants versus animals is a false dichotomy, and humans have clearly eaten both for our entire evolution. Some plant-based proponents argue that a plant-based diet is inherently healthier than an animal-based diet. Sadly this is the exact opposite of the truth. First of all, the greatest contributor to the global obesity epidemic is EMPTY CALORIES. Empty calories are, by definition, pure energy—with no protein or minerals. These are essentially SUGAR and OIL. And where do we get sugar and oil? That's right: FROM PLANTS. It is possible to eat a 'plant-based' diet that is comprised of abject food-like garbage. Secondly, animals are at a higher trophic level than plants. Because they are higher on the food chain, they automatically bioaccumulate more protein and minerals and micronutrients, and eating animals always provides higher quality protein and a higher density of nutrients.

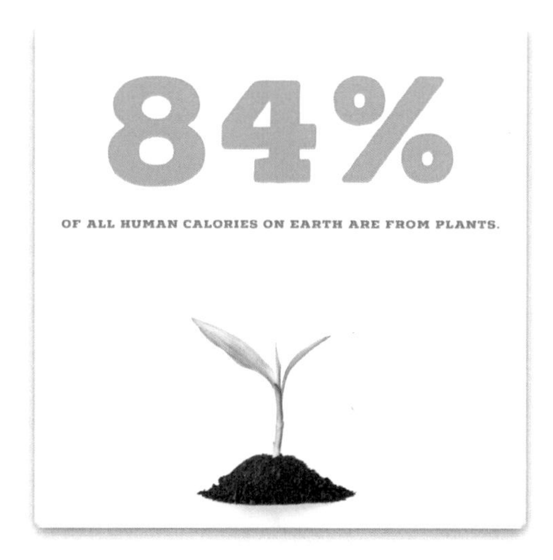

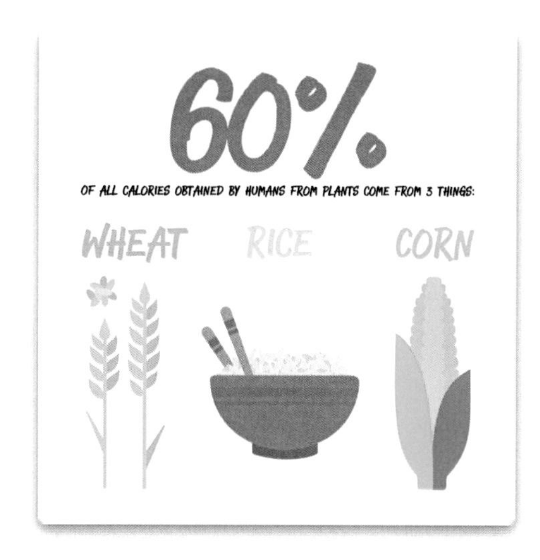

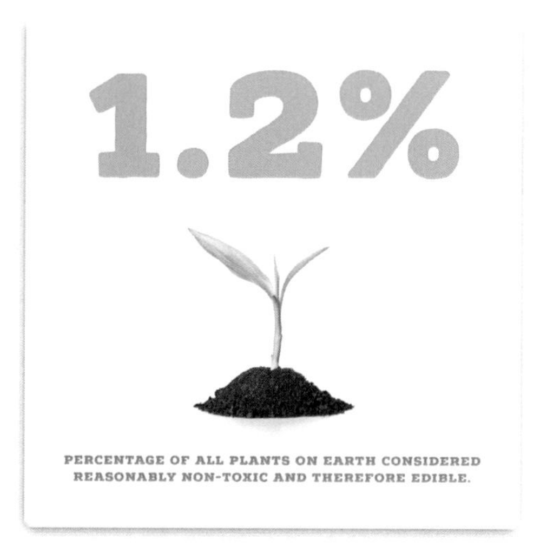

Now don't get us wrong: some plant foods are fantastic. If you are smart about it and take some supplements and prioritize protein, it is possible to be completely healthy on a plant-based diet. However, the reality is that a plant-based diet is merely POSSIBLE, rather than OPTIMAL.

If you do choose to be a vegan for ethical reasons, we have tons of respect for you and we wish you well. And we also encourage you to target the hell out of protein. Vegan foods high in protein include seitan (wheat gluten), soybeans (including tofu, tempeh, and edamame), lentils, chickpeas (garbanzo beans), nutritional yeast, spelt, teff, hempseed, green peas, spirulina, amaranth, quinoa, oats (oatmeal), wild rice, chia seeds, and nuts. Certain vegetables also have a ridiculously high protein to energy ratio, including broccoli, spinach, asparagus, artichokes, and Brussels sprouts. If you are eating only these high-protein vegan foods, and maybe also using plant protein supplements (powders based on soy, rice, pea, hemp, etc), you could actually have a reasonably healthy diet. Don't forget a B12 supplement and possibly a few other supplements to make up for the inherent deficiencies in a plant-based diet (iron, vitamin D, and the omega-3 fatty acids DHA and EPA are probably at the top of the list).

If you are vegetarian and you do eat eggs and dairy, then we would encourage you to eat the heck out of those animal foods that you DO eat, as these are typically the best way to maximize protein and nutrients.

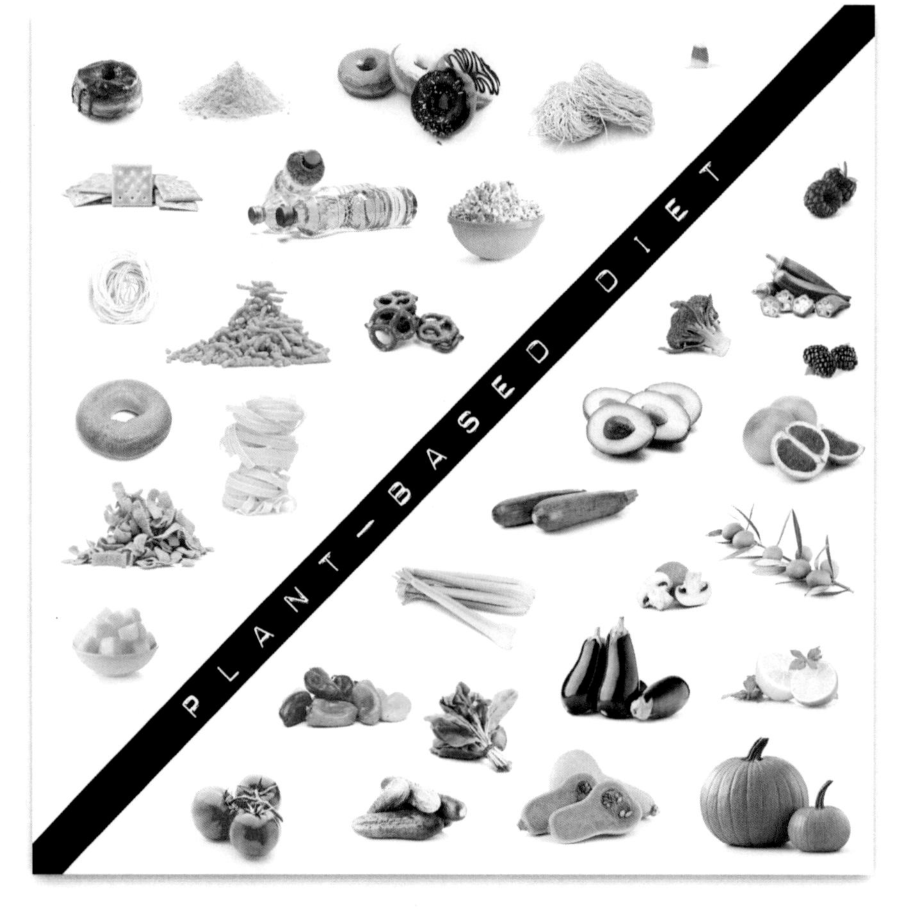

'Plant-based' does not automatically equal healthy. Some plant foods are amazing, but it is sadly also possible to eat a 'plant-based' diet that consists of pure food-like garbage.

Optimal Vegetarian

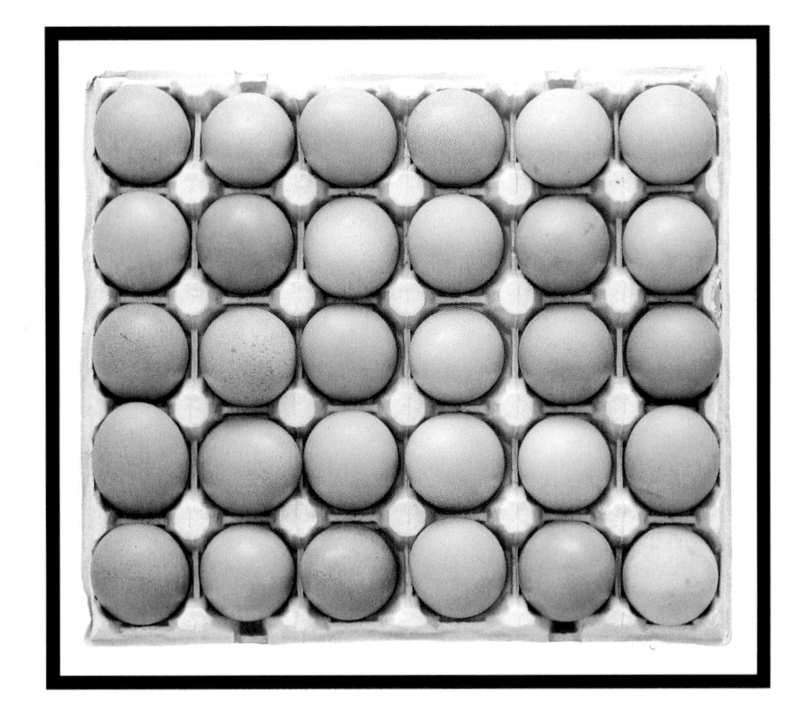

FOOD PYRAMID

This is a slight exaggeration...but if you don't eat a lot of meat (or ANY meat), choose the few high protein animal foods that you DO eat and eat a LOT of them!

Cave paintings by early hominids provide valuable clues about the diet that enabled their success.

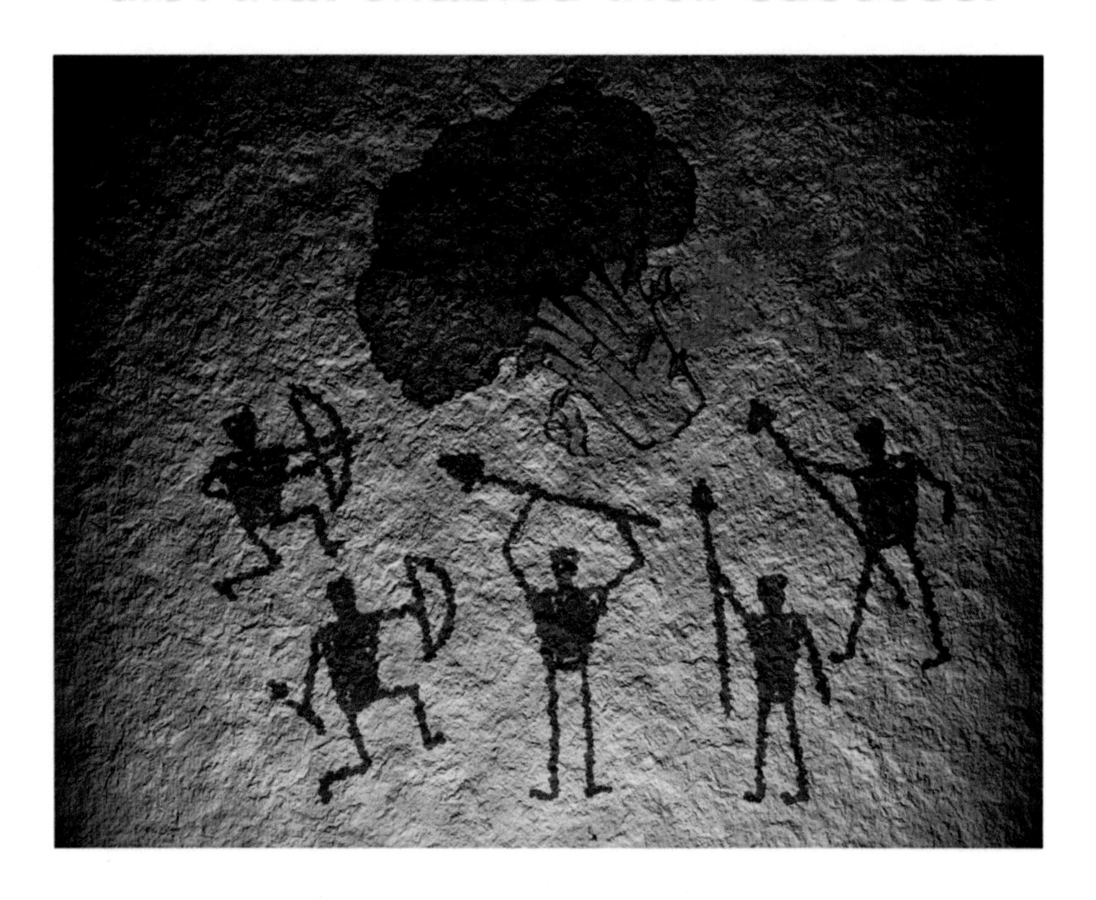

Um, no.

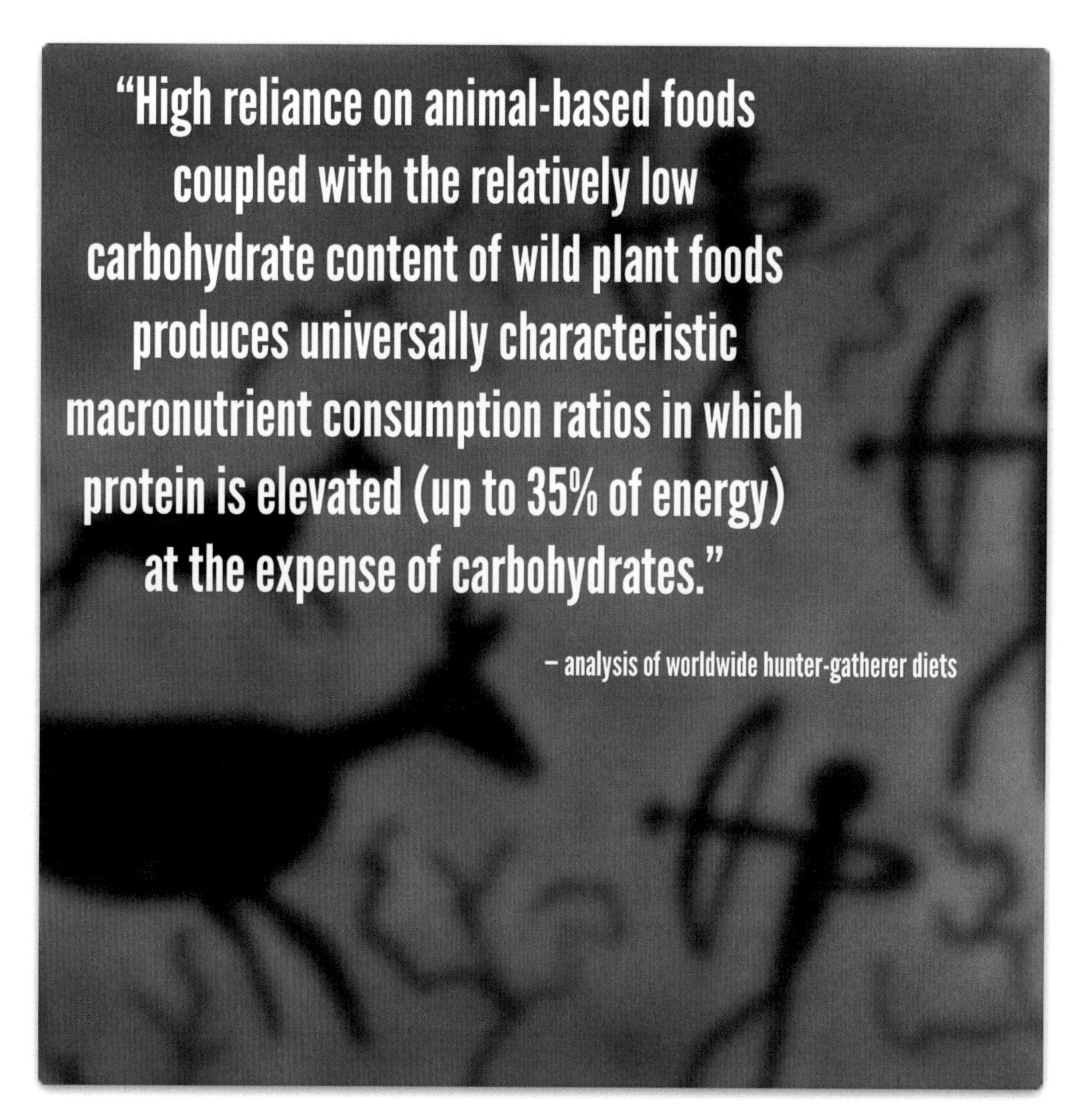

Last time we checked, hunter-gatherers had a rather low rate of obesity and type 2 diabetes.

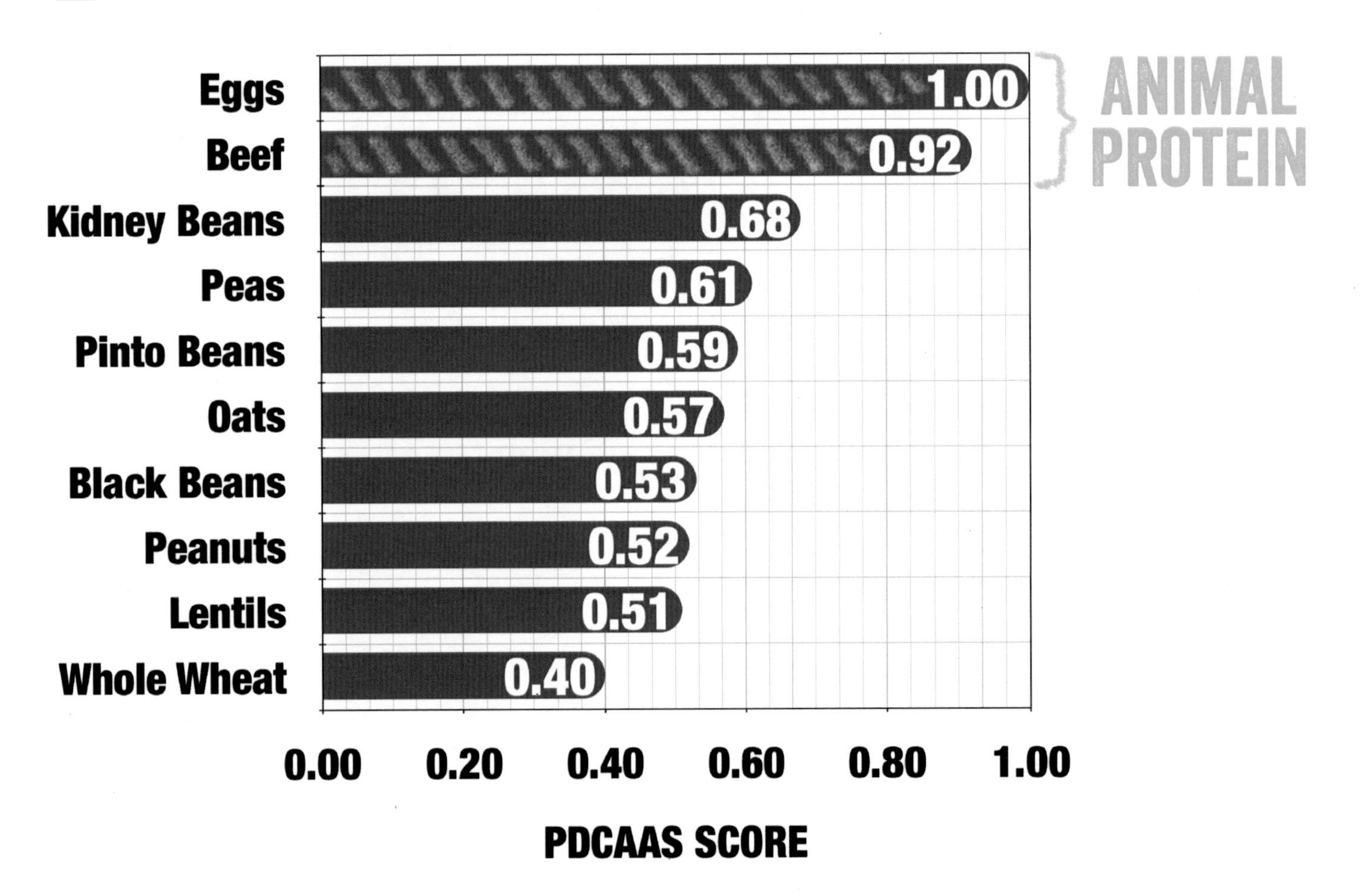

We're sorry, but it is a scientific fact that animal protein is of a higher quality than plant protein.

Grams Of Protein Per Serving In Plant And Animal Sources

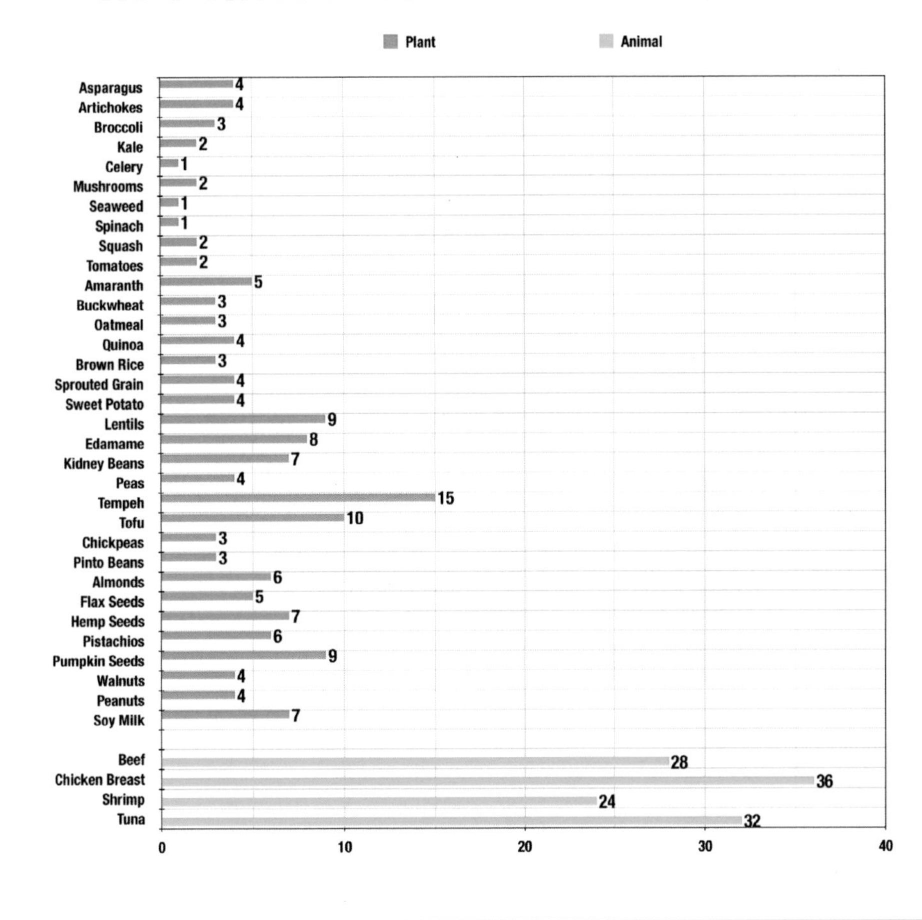

Plants are cool, but they really have trouble competing with animal foods when it comes to the P:E ratio.

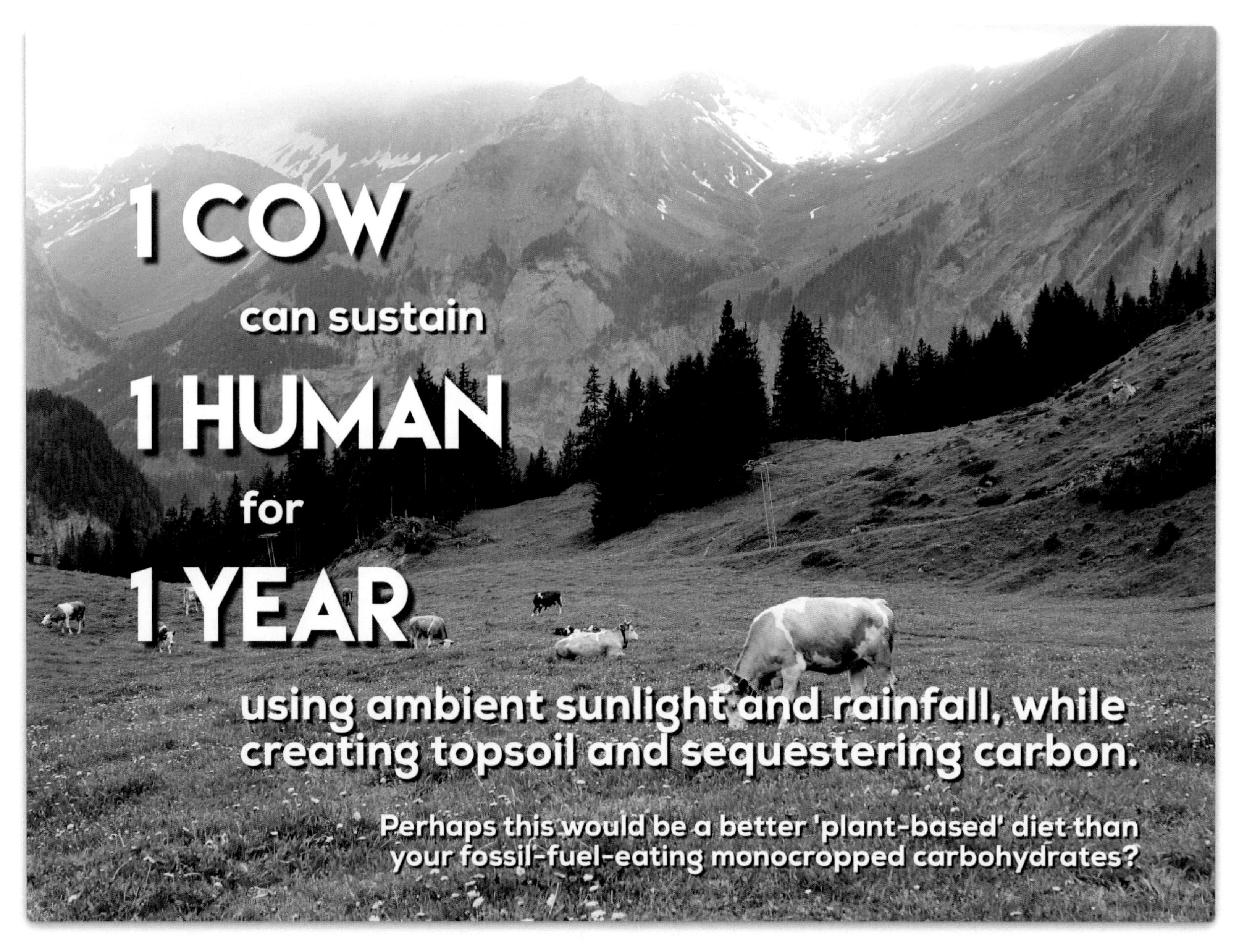

Properly raised grass-fed beef is not only one of the healthiest foods in the grocery store, but also one of the most environmentally friendly choices.

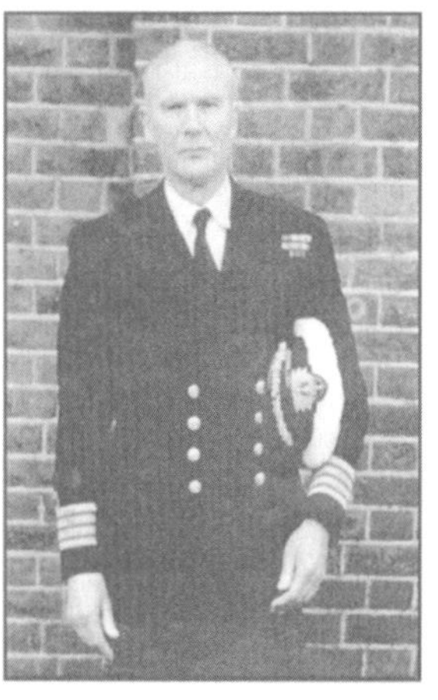

"For a modern disease to be related to an old-fashioned food is one of the most ludicrous things I ever heard in my life."

–Surgeon Captain T.L.Cleave, FRCP
(London, 1906-1983)

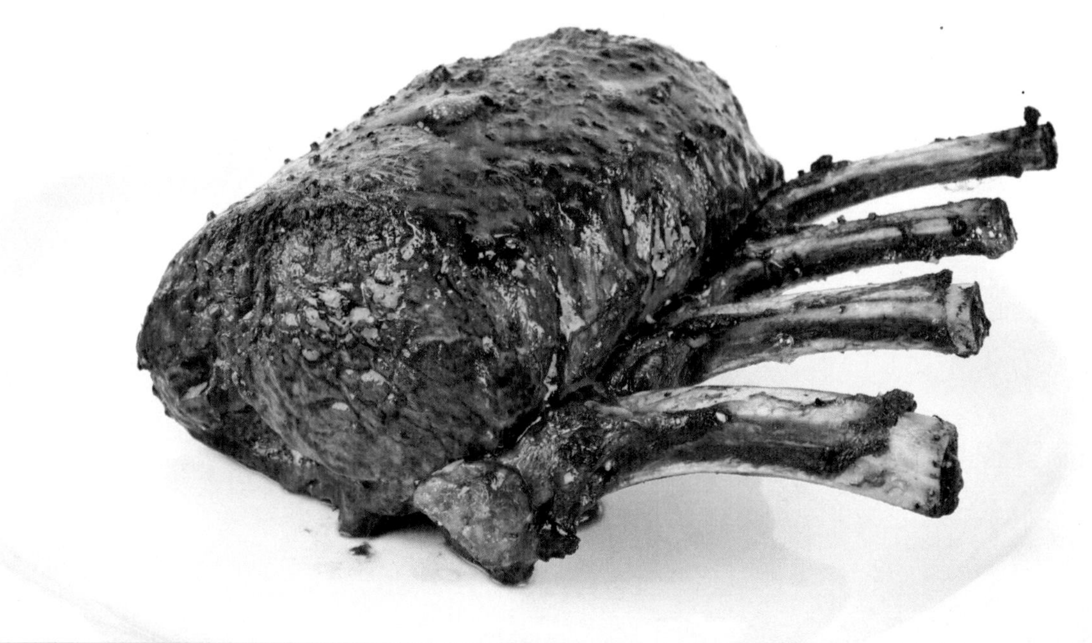

Sorry vegans—meat does not cause diabetes.

Naiman's Razor

To estimate the value of any particular food, perform the following thought experiment:

> **"How would I look and feel if I ate nothing but this food for an entire year?"**

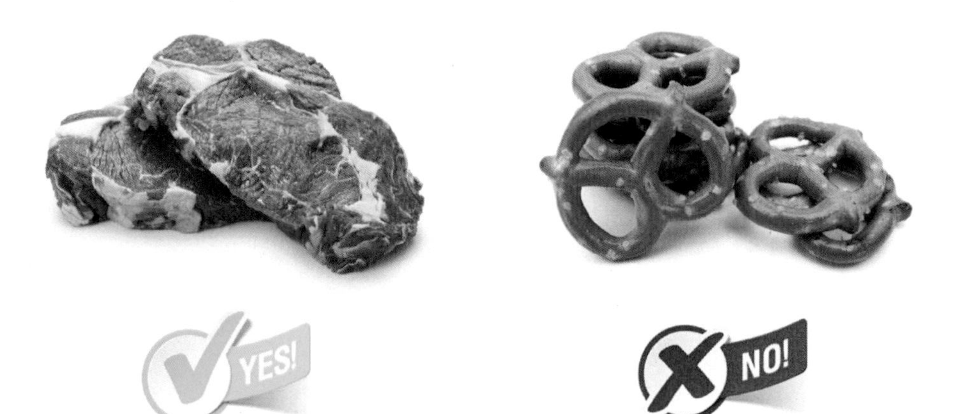

Yes you can absolutely live on nothing but red meat and water. Not sure you want to try that with any other food!

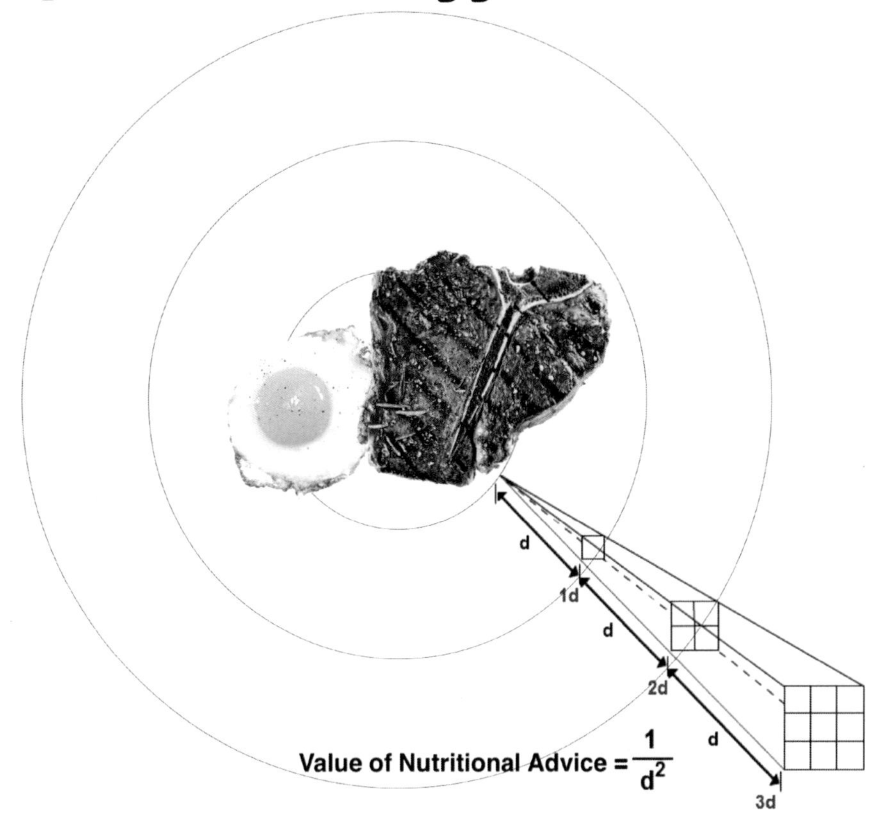

Dr. Naiman's favorite meal: steak and eggs.

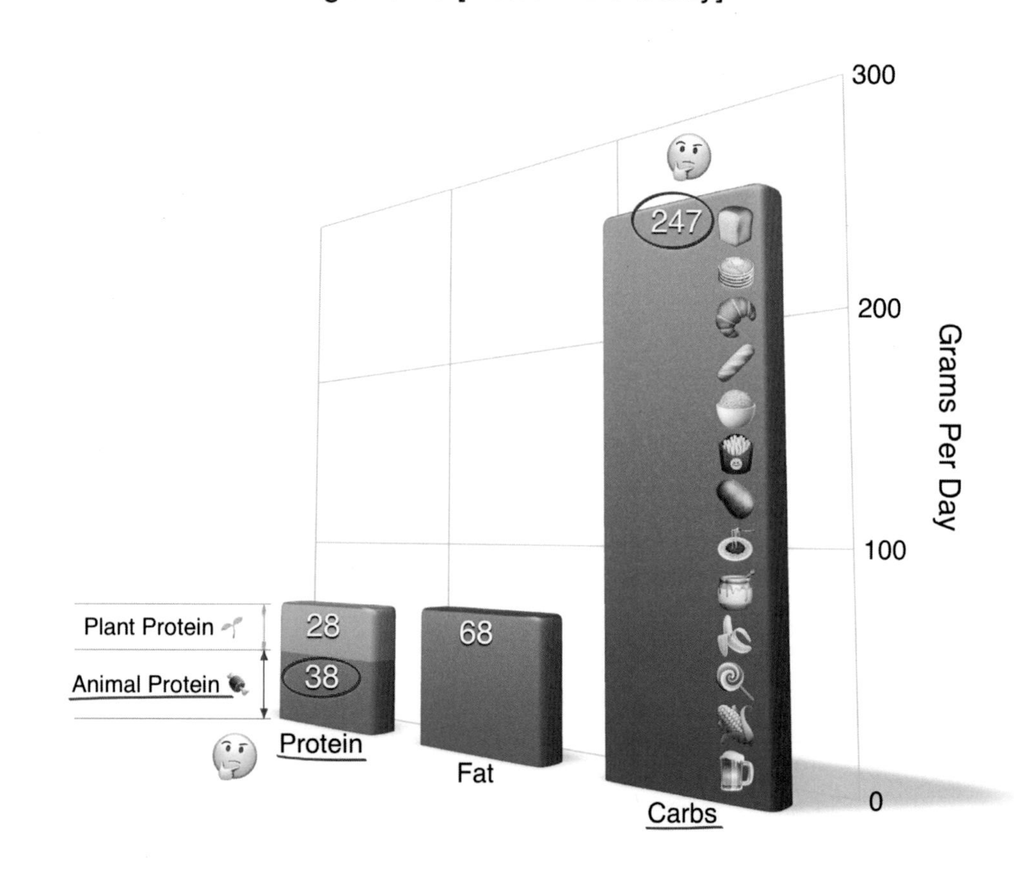

Your average older American is in horrible health due to a sedentary lifestyle and a low protein high carbohydrate diet!

MACROS

The whole point of The P:E Diet is choosing foods that have a higher P:E ratio so you can eat intuitively and have higher satiety at a lower energy intake, without really having to track anything. But if you find that your fat loss has stalled, or if you really want some extreme results, the next step would be tracking your macronutrients.

Start with a good app for your smartphone—our favorite is Cronometer [cronometer.com]; second favorite is MyFitnessPal [myfitnesspal.com]. Both of these allow you to enter everything you are eating and they will keep track of your grams of protein, carbohydrate, and fat.

Because your goal is the highest lean mass at the lowest fat mass, you want protein grams higher than energy grams. A good rule of thumb is targeting protein at about 1 gram per day per pound of IDEAL body weight (not what you actually weigh, but what you probably SHOULD weigh). A rough estimate of ideal body weight for women is 100 pounds for the first five feet of height and then 5 pounds for every additional inch over 5 feet. For men, the estimate would be 110 pounds for the first five feet and then also 5 pounds for every additional inch over 5 feet. For example, the average male in America is almost 5 feet 10 inches tall, so the ideal body weight would be around 160 pounds. Let's ignore for a moment the fact that the average male in America currently weighs 198 pounds! The average female in America is 5 feet 4 inches tall, so her ideal body weight would be 120 pounds—and again, we can stop for a moment and lament the fact that the average adult American female weighs 171 pounds.

IDEAL BODY WEIGHT ESTIMATION

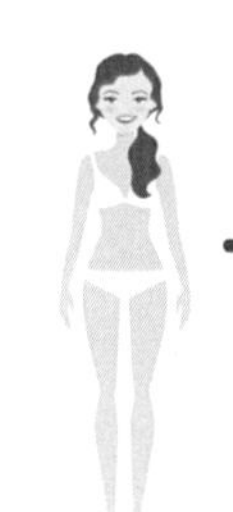

WOMEN:
100 POUNDS
FOR THE FIRST 5 FEET...

MEN:
110 POUNDS
FOR THE FIRST 5 FEET...

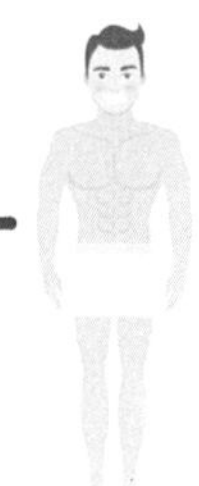

BOTH:

...THEN 5 POUNDS FOR EVERY ADDITIONAL INCH OVER 5 FEET.

So a male 5 feet 10 inches tall would want to target 160 grams of protein per day, and a female 5 feet 4 inches tall would want to target 120 grams of protein per day. Keep in mind that these are MINIMUM targets and it would be ok to EXCEED this number.

What about fat and carbs? Well, since the idea is to eat more protein and less energy, fat and carbohydrate goals are LIMITS to stay beneath, rather than a TARGET to meet or exceed (like protein). If you are looking for really aggressive fat loss, target fat grams at HALF of your protein target and carb grams also at HALF of your protein target (so 80 grams each for our 5'10" male and 60 grams each for our 5'4" female). You may have to liberalize the non-protein energy calories (fat and carbs) if you are highly active and very hungry on this plan, but this would be a good starting point.

Easy Fat Loss Macros—The Protein "Over / Under":

Keep protein grams OVER your desired body weight (in pounds), and keep non-protein energy (fat + NET carbs) UNDER same target

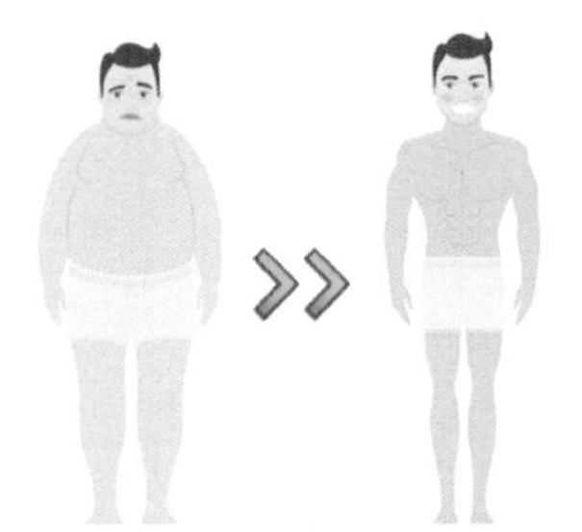

Desired body weight (in pounds): Example = 160 lbs

$$\frac{\text{Protein (grams)} \geq 160 \text{ g}}{\text{Fat (g)} + \text{Net Carbs (g)} \leq 160}$$

Protein ≥ 160 g
Energy ≤ 160 g

Prioritize foods with PROTEIN or FIBER

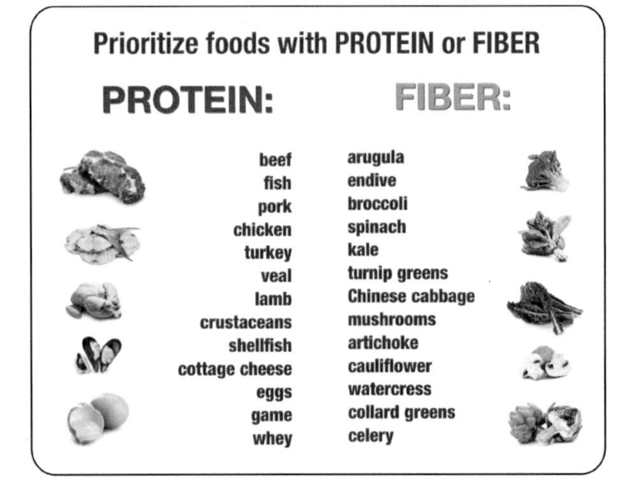

PROTEIN:	FIBER:
beef	arugula
fish	endive
pork	broccoli
chicken	spinach
turkey	kale
veal	turnip greens
lamb	Chinese cabbage
crustaceans	mushrooms
shellfish	artichoke
cottage cheese	cauliflower
eggs	watercress
game	collard greens
whey	celery

Maintain high Protein:Energy ratio

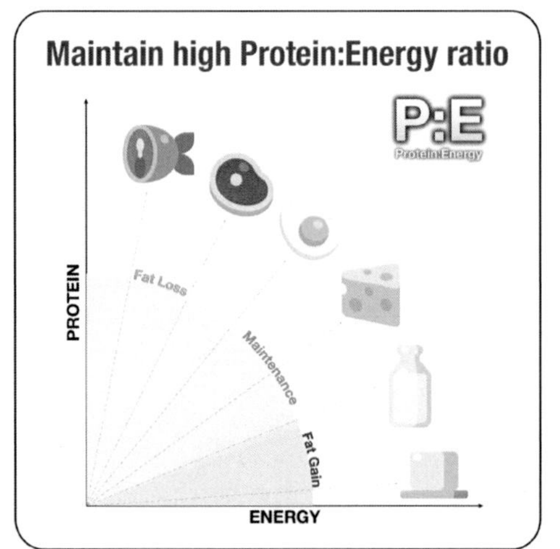

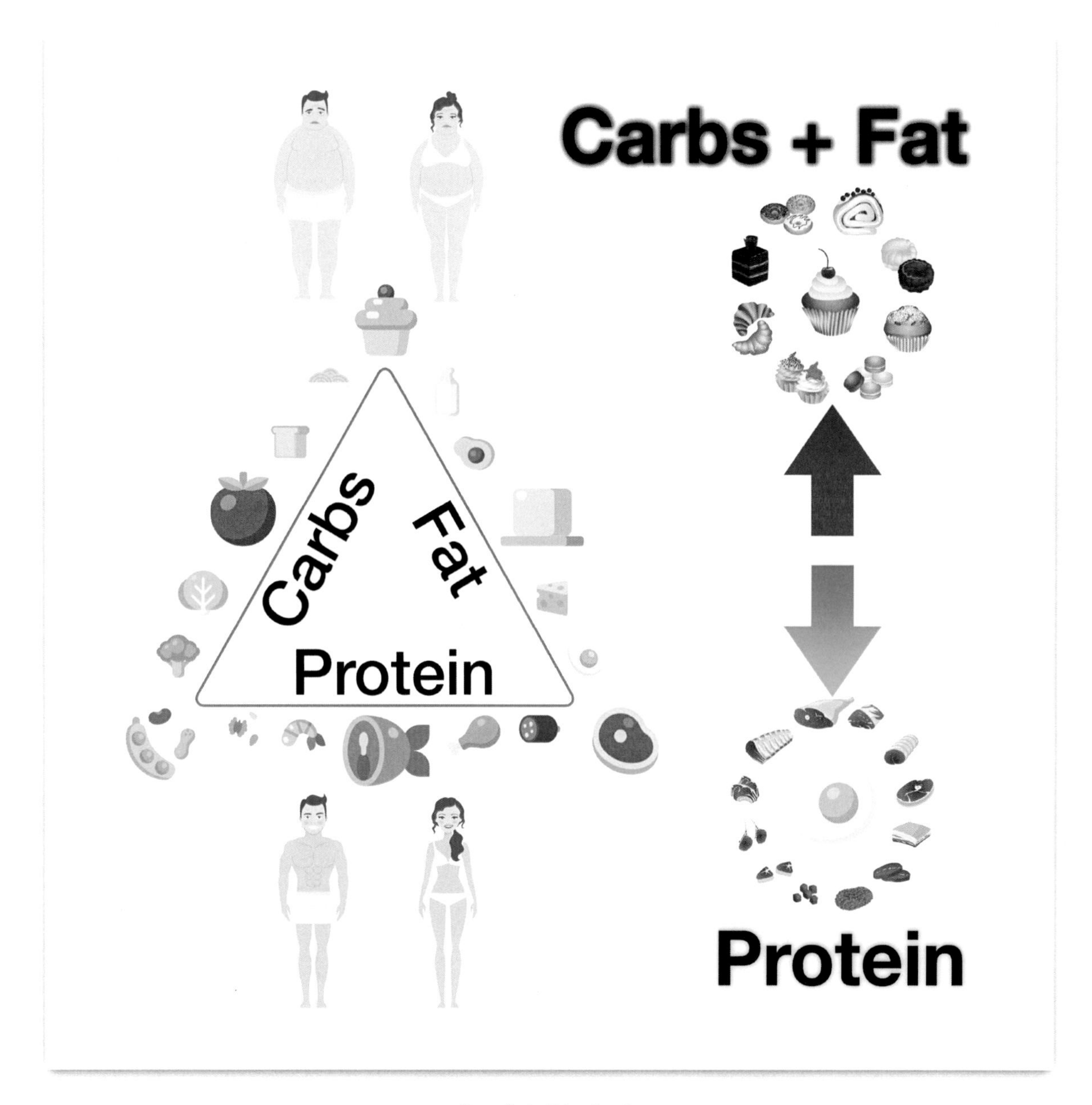

It really is this simple.

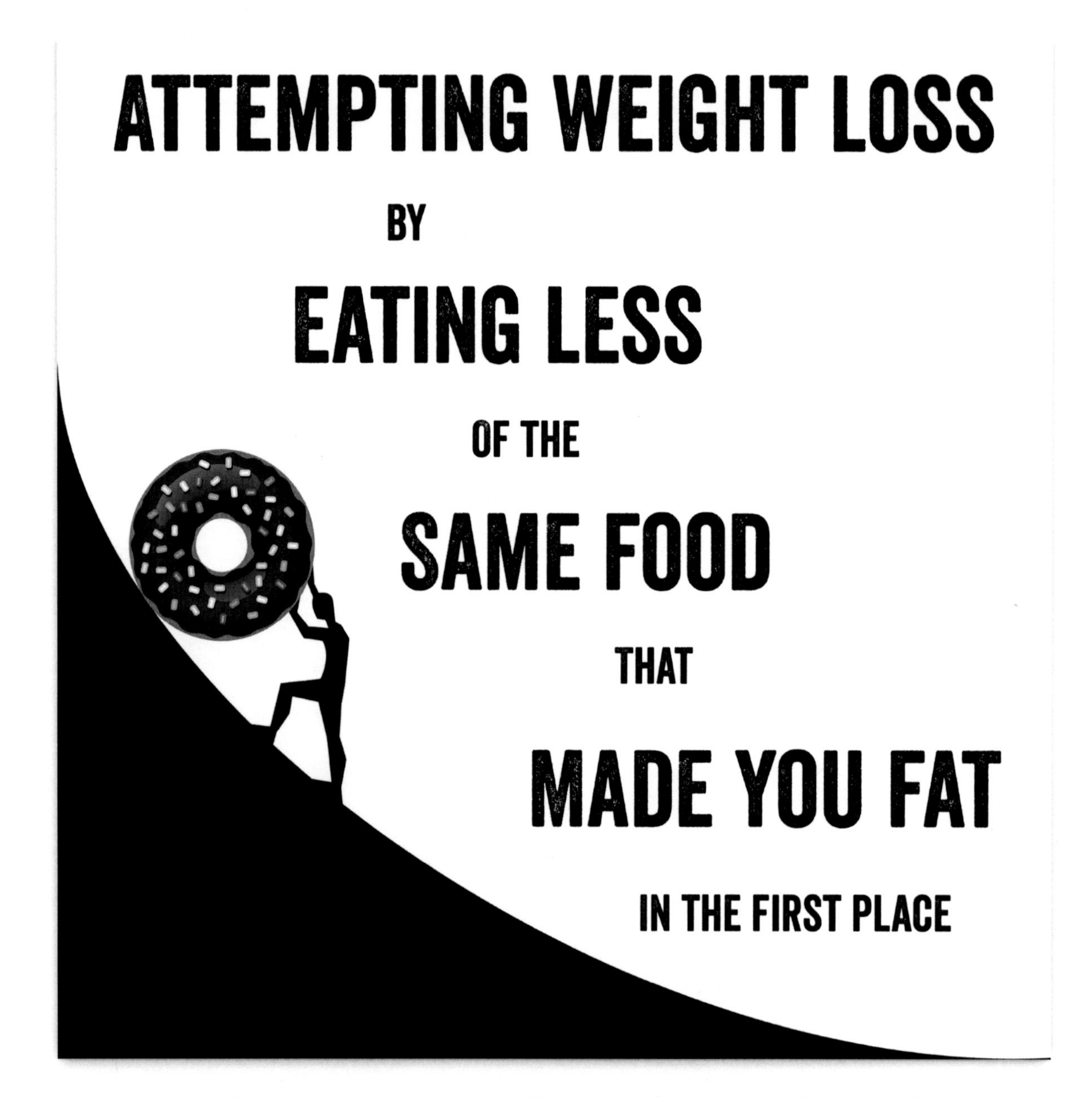

Trying to lose weight by simply eating less of the Standard American Diet is doomed to failure.

ENERGY DENSITY AND SATIETY

There is one more factor that we want to discuss, and it has to do with the energy density of food. By energy density, we are referring to the amount of energy calories per gram of food. Why would anybody care about this?

As it turns out, humans eat about 3-4 POUNDS of food every single day. And believe it or not, there are many studies that suggest that we eat this weight of food somewhat independent of how many calories are in the food. So if you are trying to lose weight, you want to eat food that weighs the most but contains the least amount of carbs and fat. When it comes to eating the highest weight of food at the lowest energy calories, you have three secret weapons:

1. **PROTEIN**
2. **FIBER**
3. **WATER**

ENERGY DENSITY AND SATIETY

HUMANS EAT, ON AVERAGE, FOUR POUNDS OF FOOD DAILY.

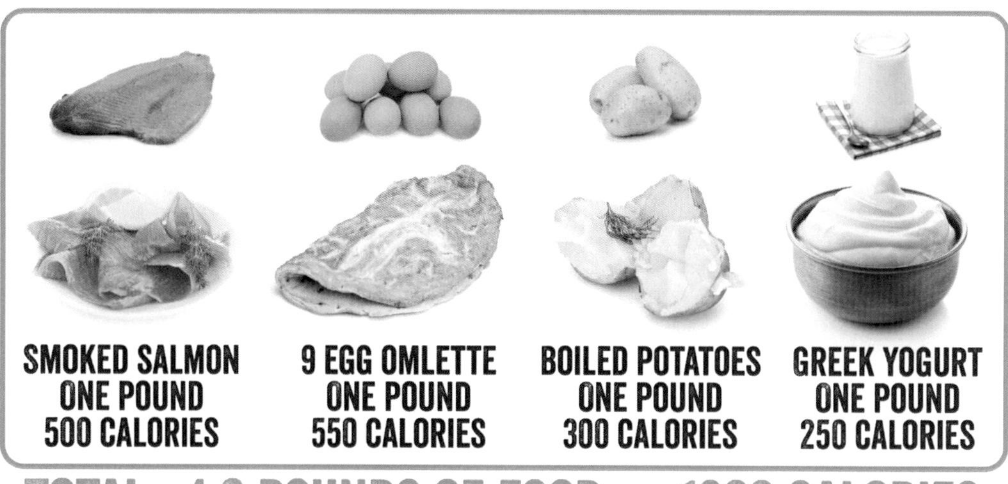

TOTAL: 4.0 POUNDS OF FOOD — 1600 CALORIES

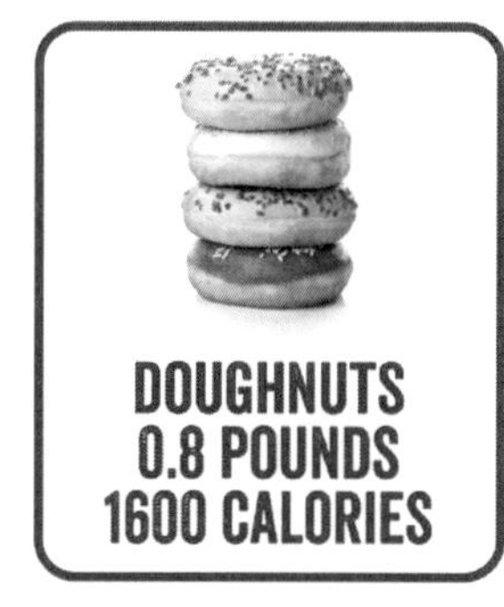

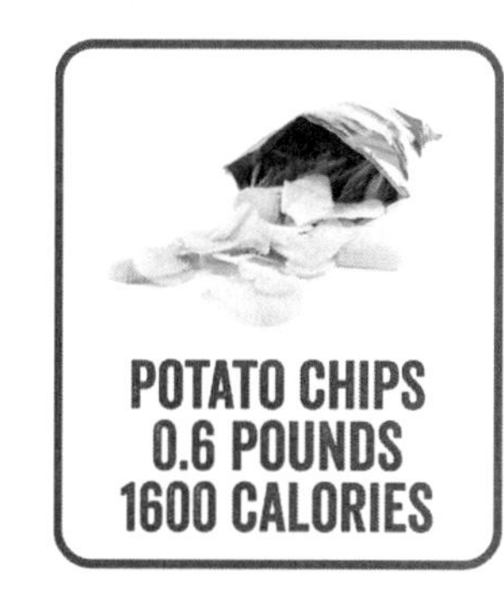

In the example pictured here, we demonstrate how someone could eat FOUR ENTIRE POUNDS OF FOOD and still only consume 1600 calories. Yes, you will be full FOR A VERY LONG TIME if you eat these four pounds of food—with 186 grams of protein—despite the fact that all this food only yields 1600 calories. Almost any reasonably active adult is going to lose weight on 1600 calories per day. If you choose to eat 1600 calories of potato chips, that is only a meager 10 ounces of chips (0.6 pounds), with only a paltry 15 total grams of protein. You are going to be STARVING in a few hours, despite the fact that you already ate your entire day's allotment of calories if your goal is weight loss. Oh, and don't forget the fact that if you are losing weight on a LOW PROTEIN diet, half the "weight" you lose will actually be LEAN MASS (muscle and bone)! Not good! In contrast, if you lose weight on a high protein diet, and you are reasonably active, a much higher percentage of your weight lost will be pure fat, instead of muscle.

Many bodybuilders eat a lot of carbs, and this is something that a lot of low carb fans can't really understand. But these high carb fitness competitors have two secret weapons. First of all, they keep fat intake quite low. As we discussed previously, you can get away with a lot more carbohydrates if you simultaneously reduce your fat intake. Secondly, they are usually very smart about WHICH carbohydrates they are eating. They will very frequently choose carbs that have the very highest weight for the lowest calories, by choosing foods with a ton of protein and fiber and water. This is why you might see a bodybuilder prioritizing oats, for example, over other grains. Or apples, over other fruit—apples have a fairly low energy density, thanks to fiber and water. Or carrots, or zucchini, or other low energy density fruit and grains and tubers. By choosing these foods, it is possible to engineer the very highest satiety at the very lowest energy intake. This will also keep protein and minerals as high as possible, and is basically just an extension of the P:E concept!

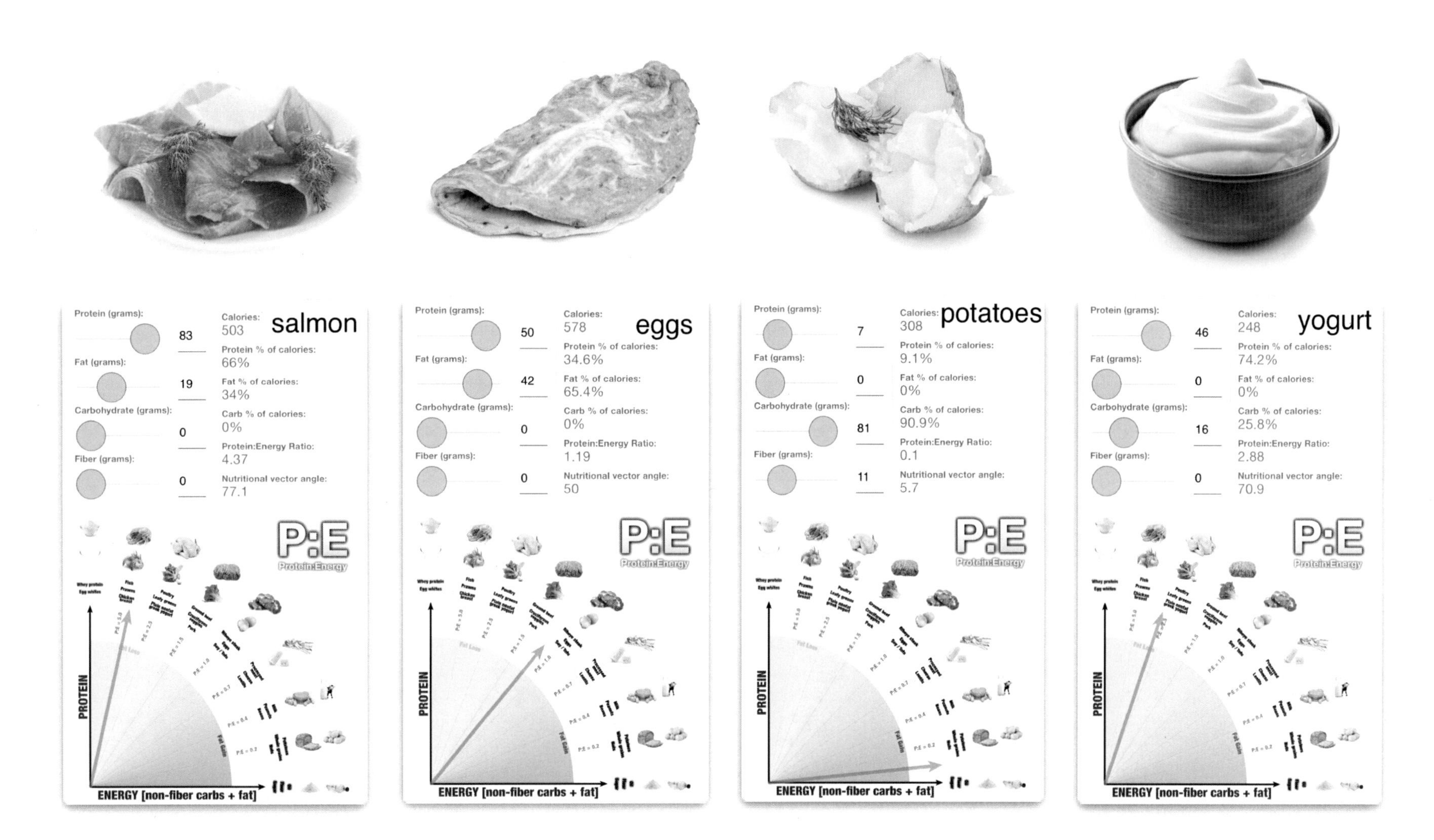

In our example, we use one pound of smoked salmon, one pound of eggs, one pound of plain boiled potatoes, and one pound of fat free Greek yogurt. Yes, that is a LOT of food!

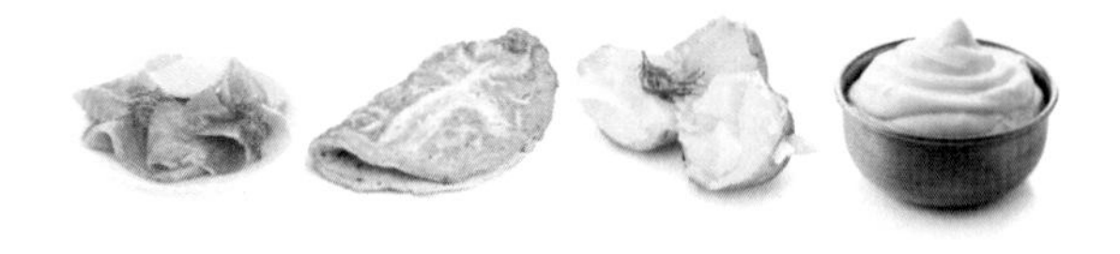

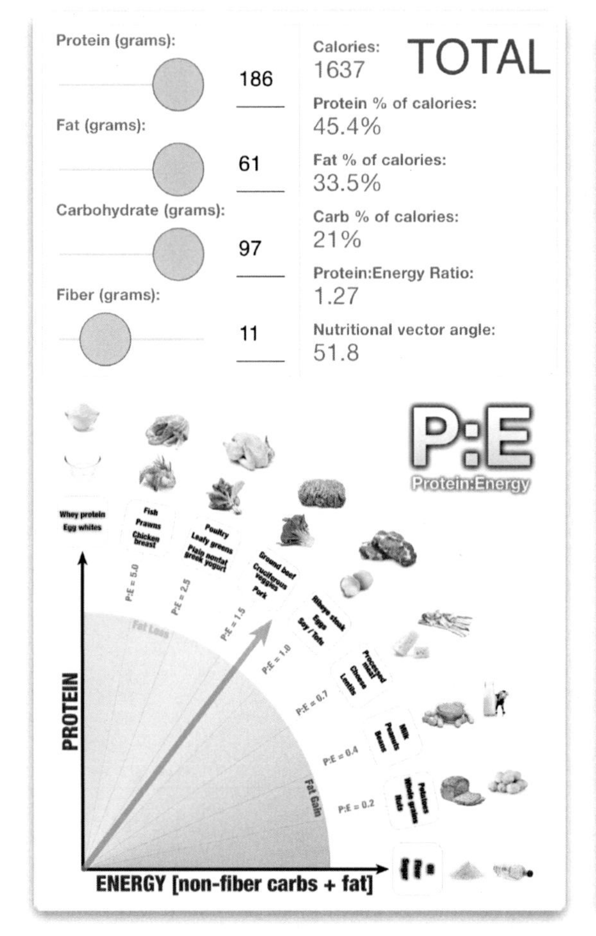

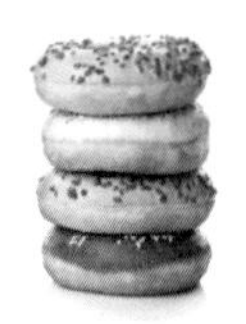

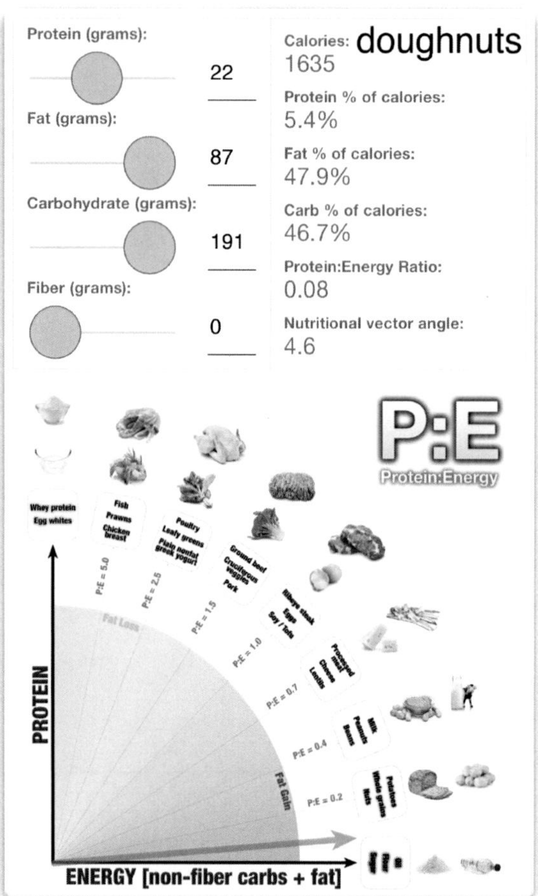

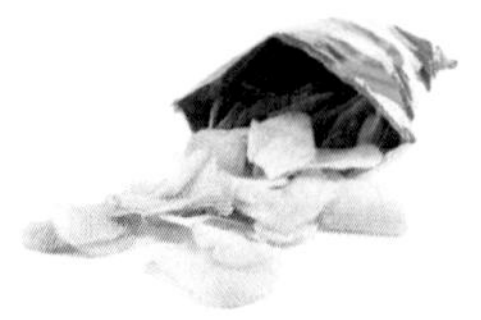

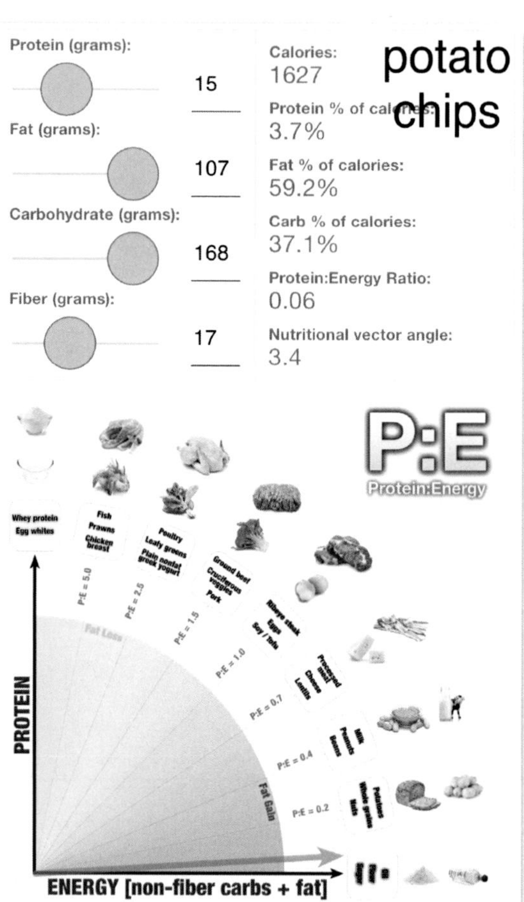

Our four pounds of food (salmon, eggs, potatoes, and yogurt) contained 186 grams of protein — and a RIDICULOUS amount of satiety. If you ate this much food, you will NOT be hungry. Contrast that to only 0.8 pounds of doughnuts—which is only four large raised glazed doughnuts —which only contain at total of 22 grams of protein. It is quite likely that four hours after eating the doughnuts you are literally hungrier than if you ate NOTHING AT ALL. The potato chips are even worse; it only takes a measly 10 ounces (0.6 pounds) of potato chips to hit 1600 calories. Worst of all, these chips only contain a shockingly low 15 grams of protein—prepare to be EXTREMELY hungry in just a few hours.

M.E.A.L. Diet

for rapid fat loss

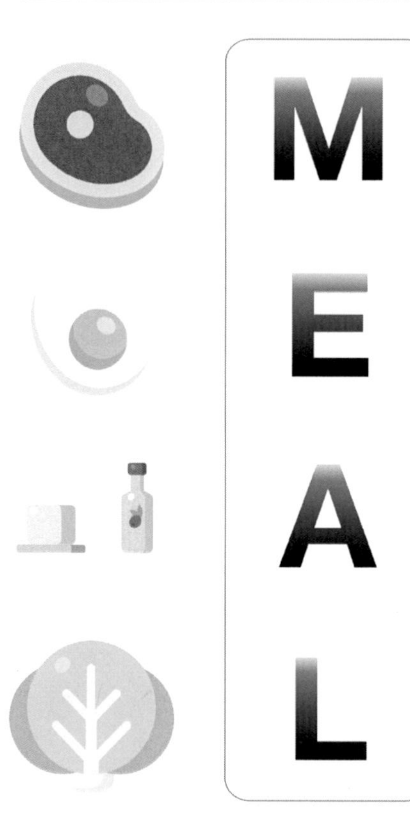

Meat
any animal product

Eggs

Added
fats for cooking

Leaves
non-starchy vegetables

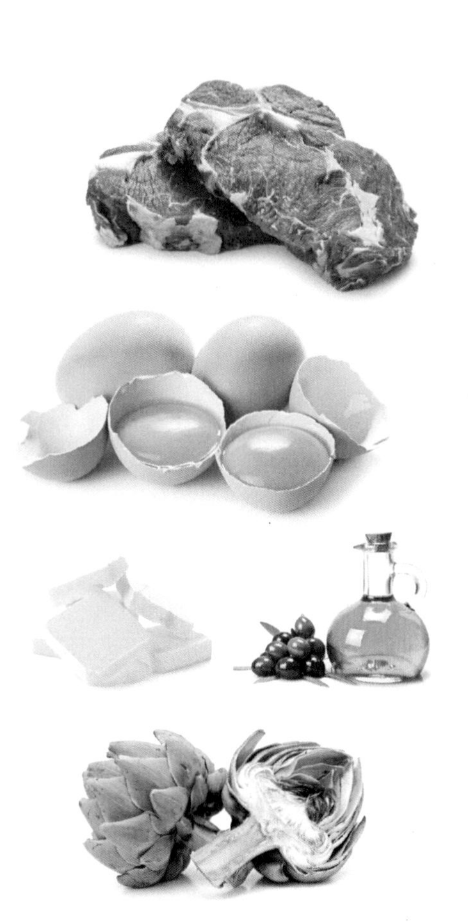

If you are just looking for the simplest fat loss plan imaginable, try our 'M.E.A.L.' acronym.

THE P:E DIET — HIGH LEVEL SUMMARY

Wow—we're impressed that you're still reading! But we know that we have covered a lot of ground here, so at this point we want to stop and do a brief recap of the highlights. The next ten pages will quickly review the main points thus far.

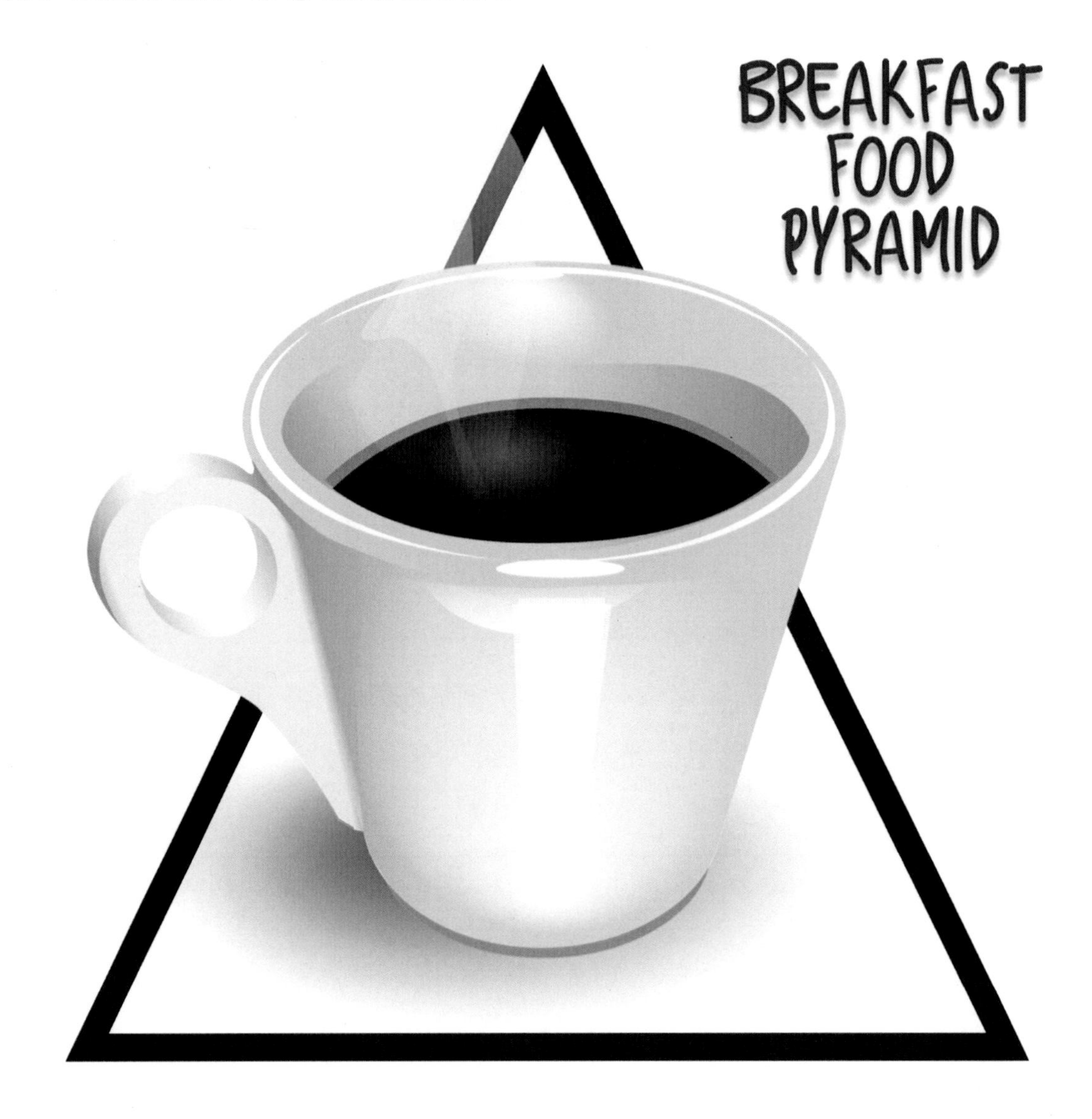

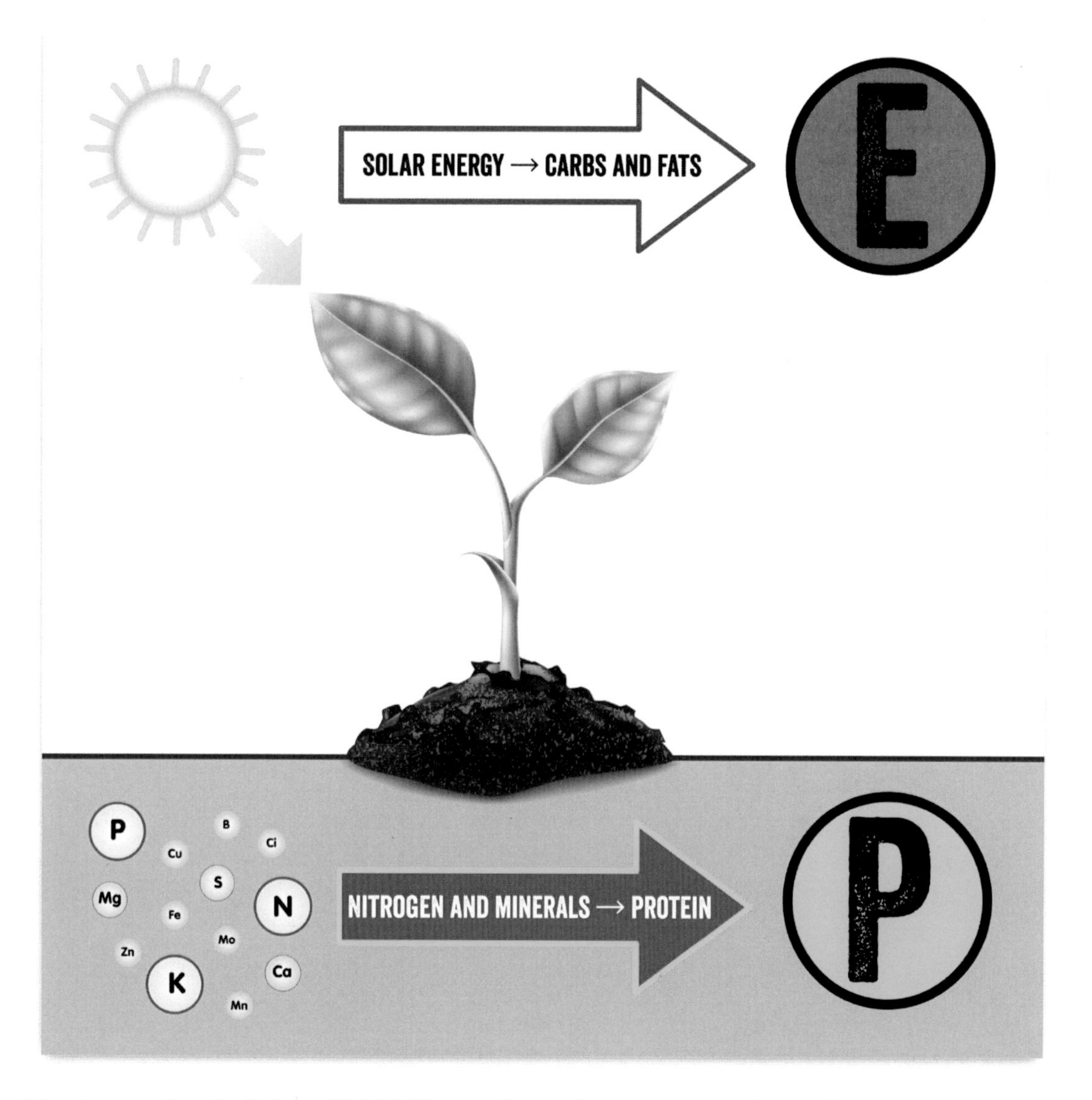

Plants create all dietary ENERGY, storing solar energy as CARBS and FATS. Plants create all dietary PROTEIN, using nitrogen and other minerals from the soil. Animals receive both of these by eating plants (or other animals that have eaten plants).

2/10

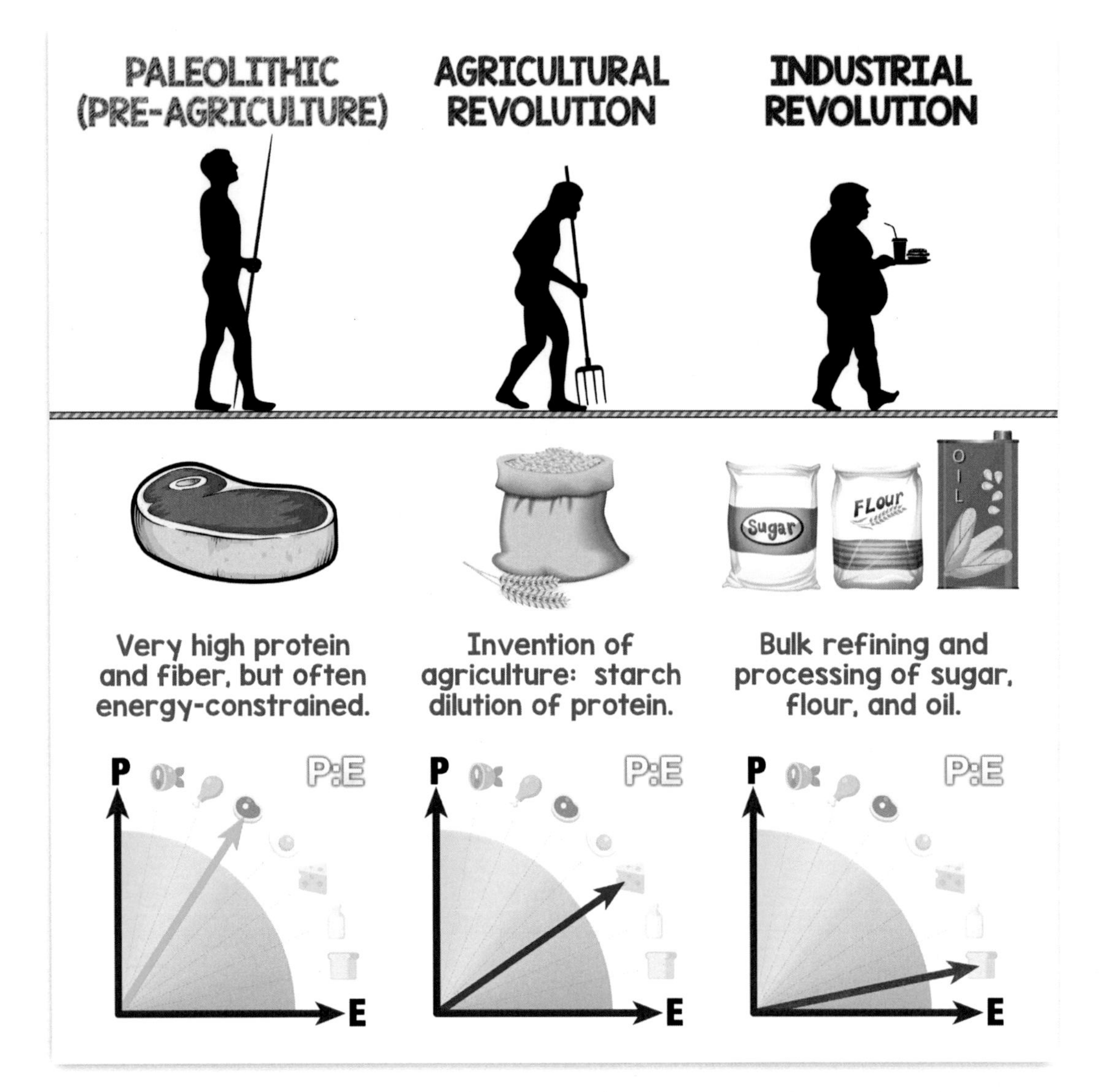

We humans have always attempted to use technology to feed ourselves. We learned how to increase the amount of dietary energy in our environment by domesticating plants and animals. We invented agriculture, then bulk refining and processing.

3/10

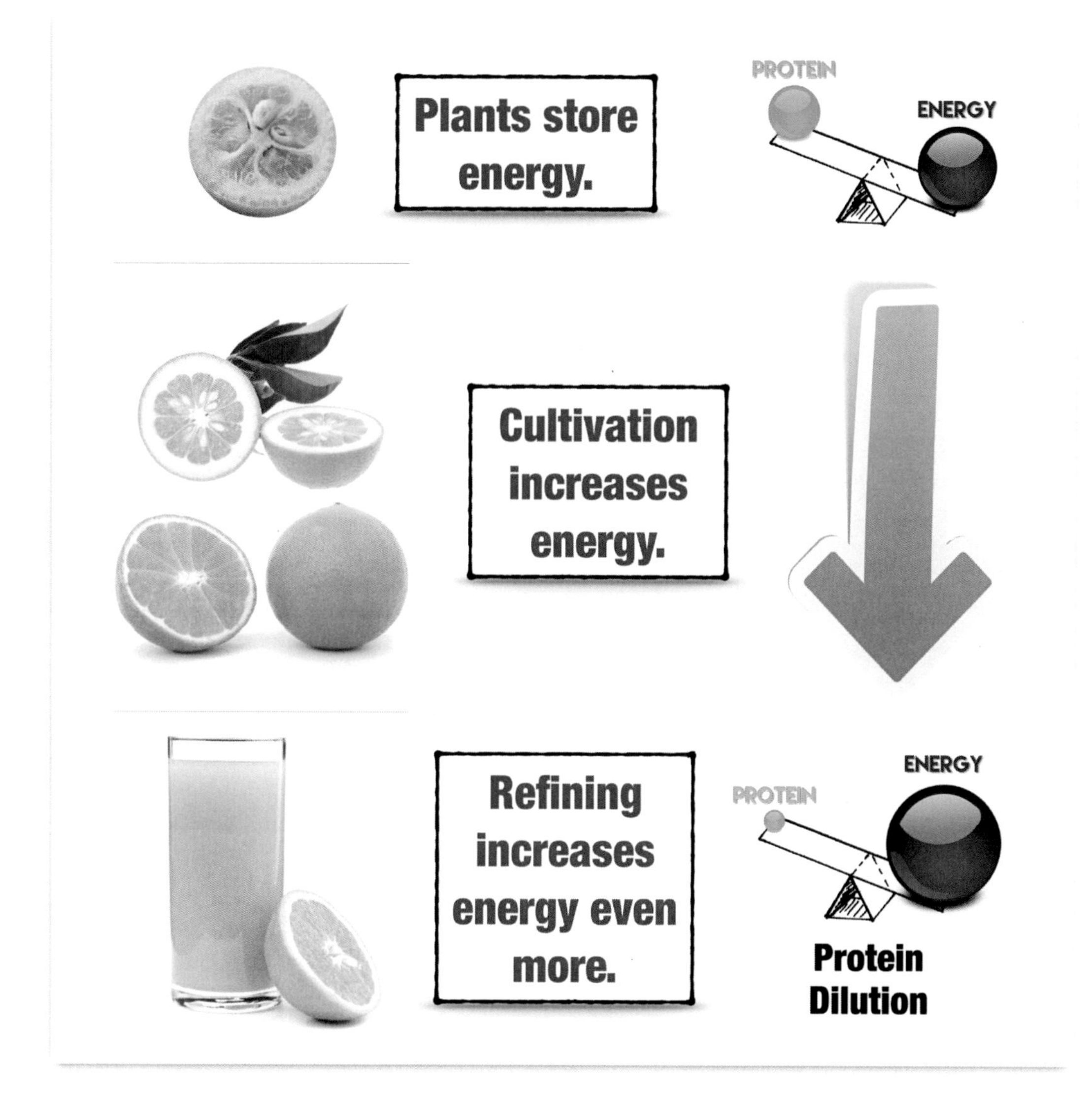

We are hardwired to obtain the highest possible dietary energy from our environment with the least amount of energy expenditure. Our agricultural and food production practices are designed to provide the maximum amount of energy possible.

4/10

PROTEIN : ENERGY

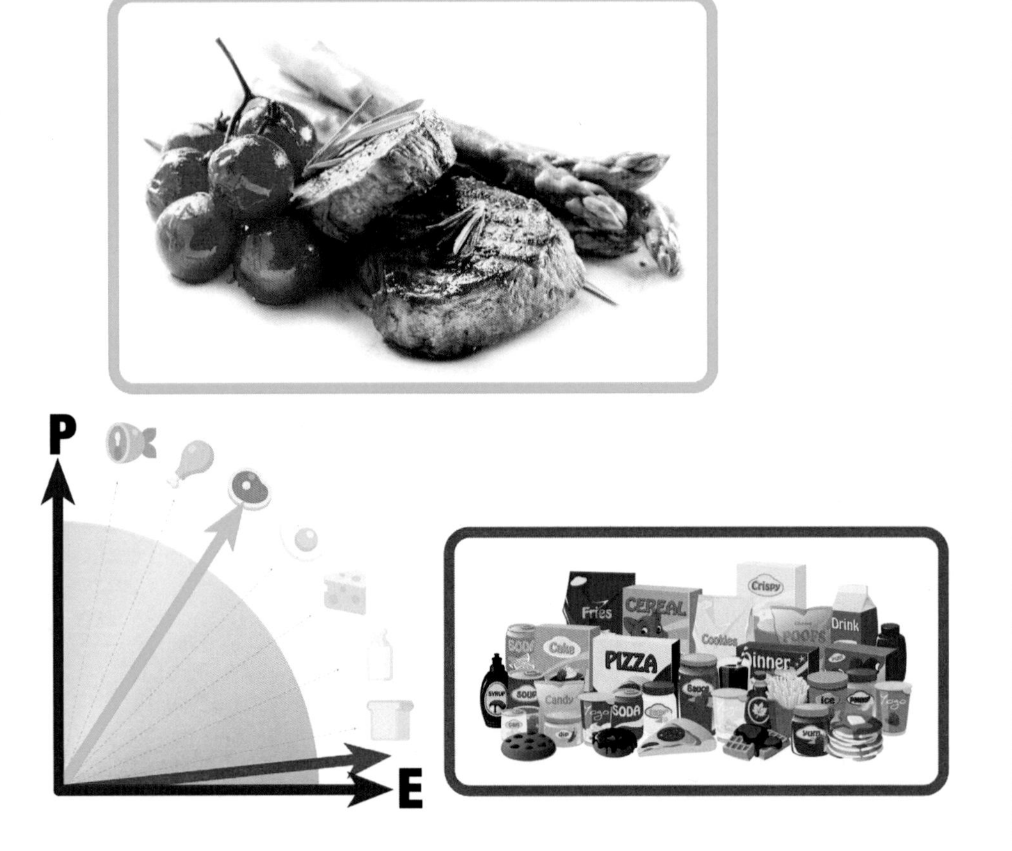

Cheap and plentiful empty carb and fat energy calories have so severely diluted the protein and minerals in the human food supply that we have to massively overeat non-protein energy (carbs and fats) just to get enough protein for survival and satiety.

5/10

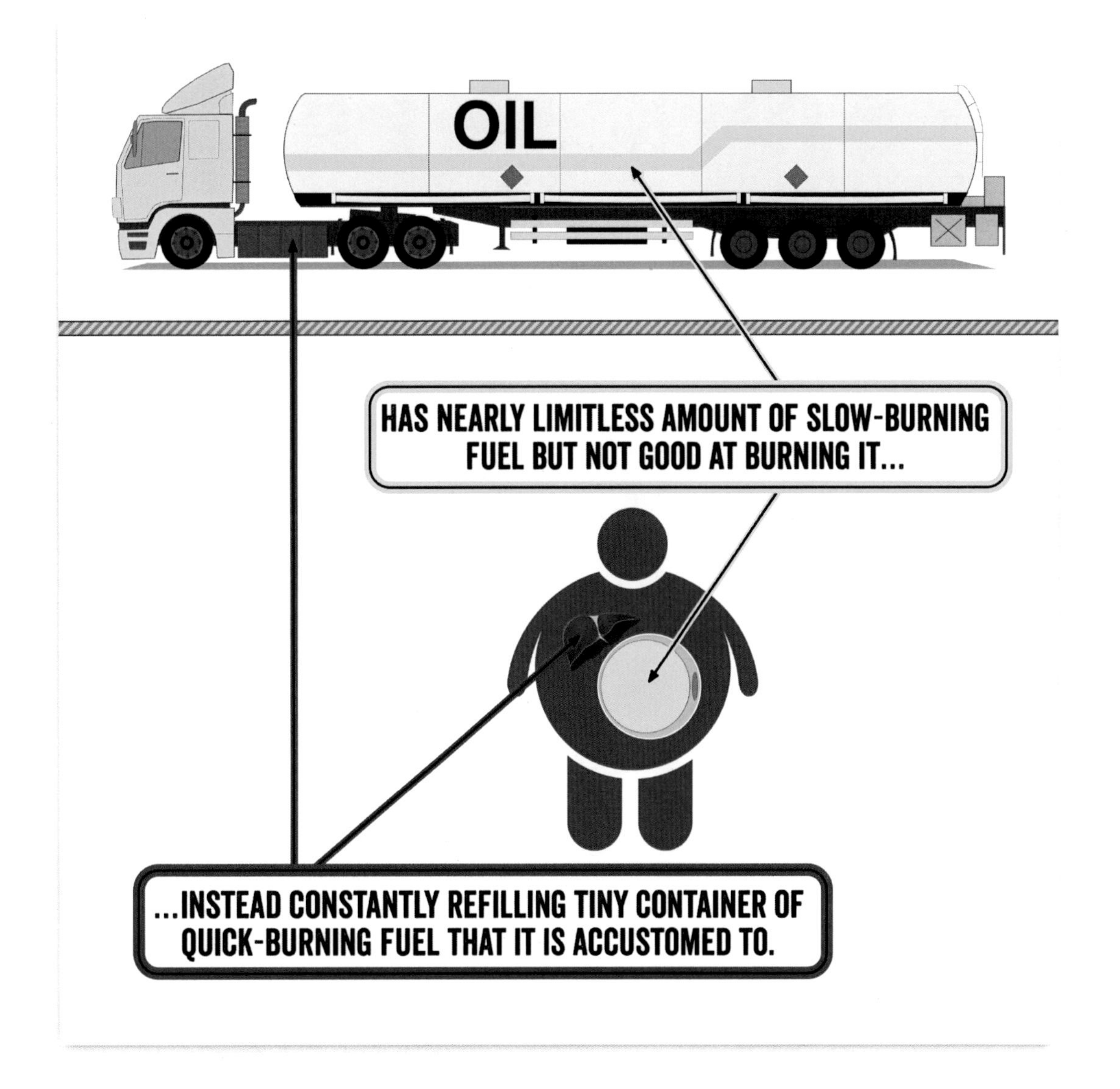

We eat carbs with such high frequency that we lose the ability to run our metabolism normally on stored body fat. This loss of 'fat adaptation' leads to frequent hunger, frequent eating, glucose dependence, and excess storage of dietary fat as body fat.

CARBS + FAT

This combination is rarely found in nature.

These foods produce drug-like dopamine reward in the brain and are highly addictive.

You can create obesity in any omnivore mammal with these junk foods.

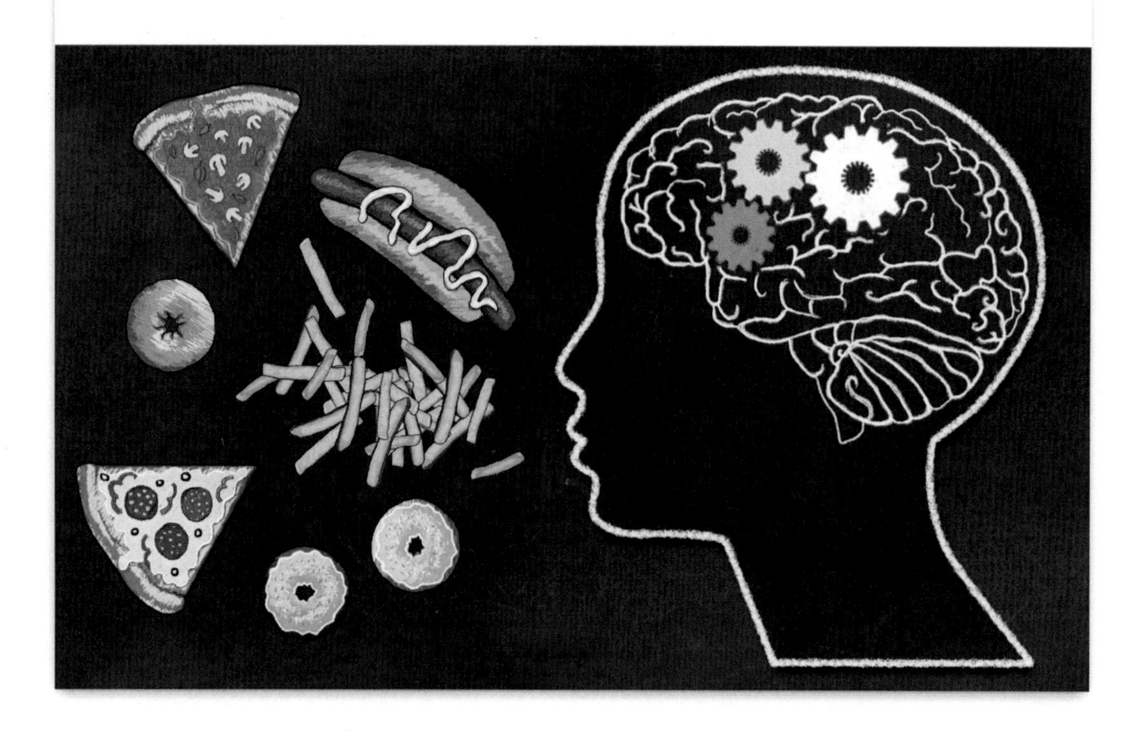

We are now addicted to the food reward of carbohydrates and fats together, a combination that was designed to drive seasonal overeating when energy was plentiful so that we could survive seasonal reduction in available dietary energy.

7/10

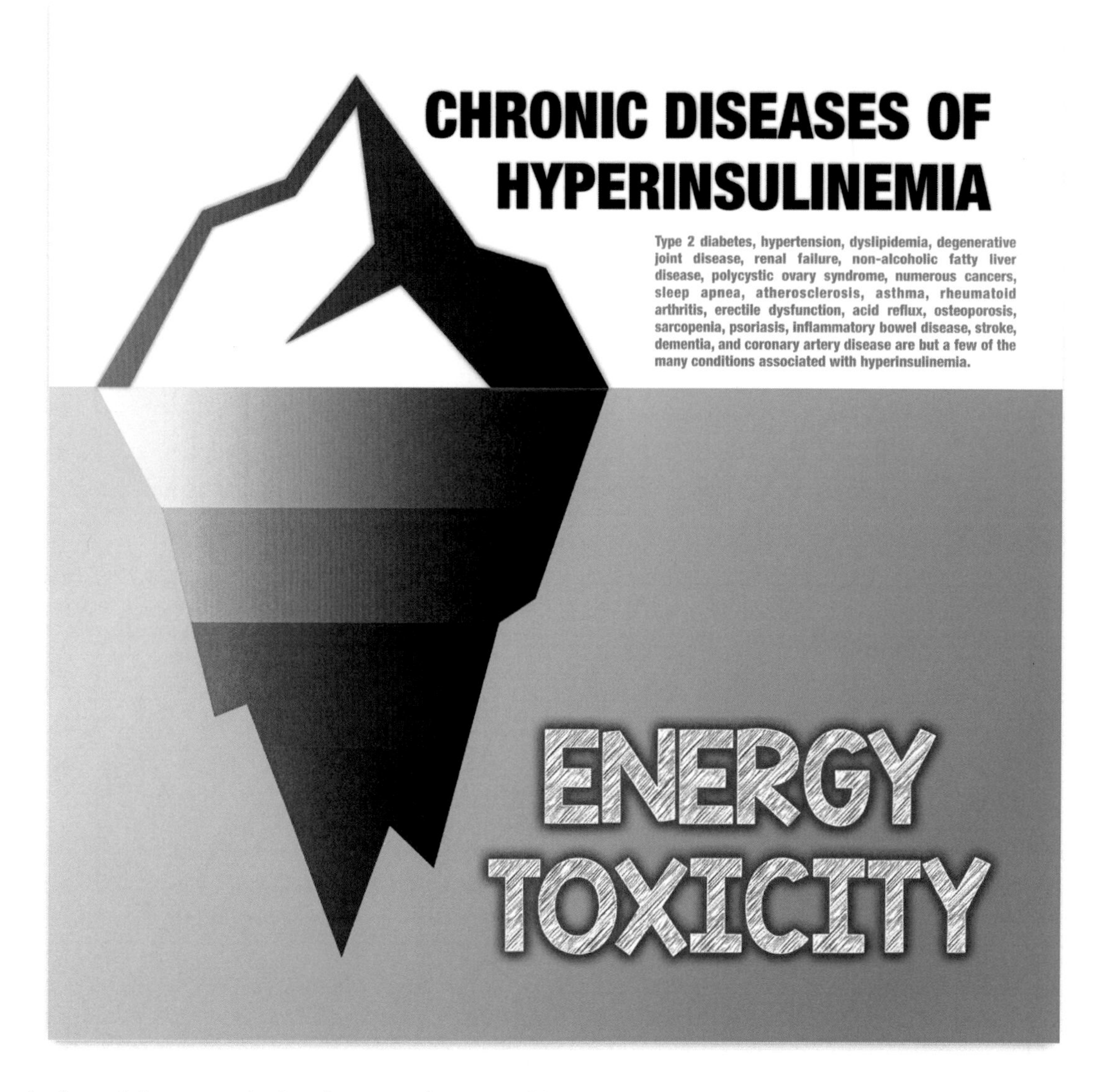

The majority of the population is now damaged by the energy toxicity that results from chronically exceeding your energy storage capacities. This has created a tsunami of chronic degenerative diseases—truly the greatest epidemic in all of human history.

8/10

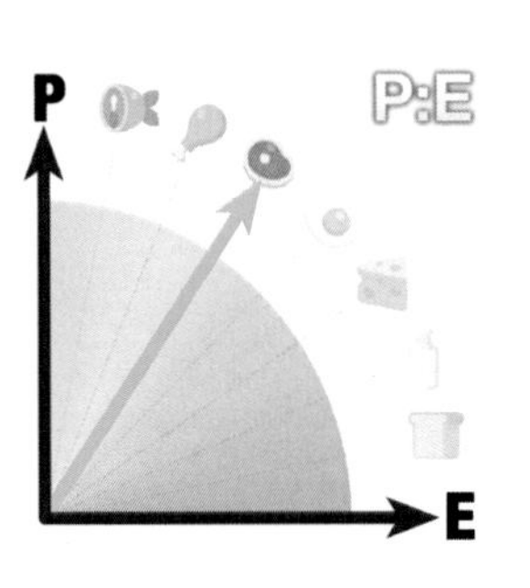

1. **MAXIMIZE SATIETY.**

TARGET PROTEIN AND MINERALS FOR HIGHEST NUTRIENT DENSITY.

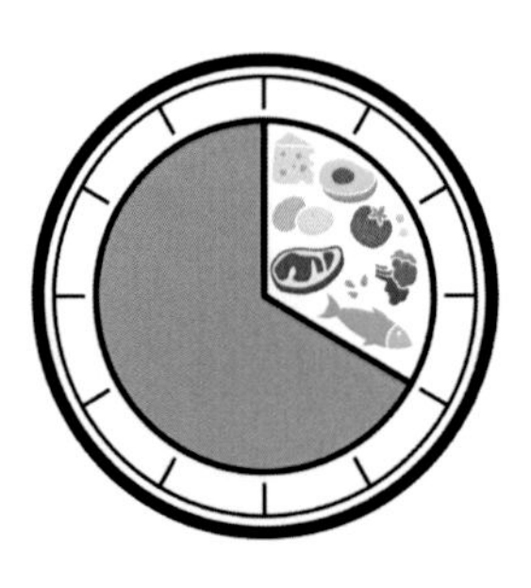

2. **MAXIMIZE FAT ADAPTATION.**

USE INTERMITTENT FASTING WITH LOW CARBOHYDRATE FREQUENCY.

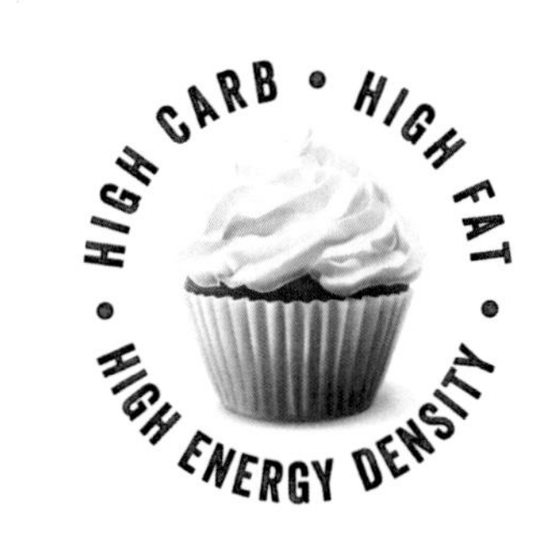

3. **AVOID THE TRIFECTA.**

HIGH CARB + HIGH FAT + HIGH ENERGY DENSITY = OVEREATING.

The solution to energy toxicity? Target nutrient density (protein and minerals) over energy density (carbs and fats). Reduce carbohydrate frequency to improve fat adaptation. Avoid the overeating that results from high energy density carbs + fat.

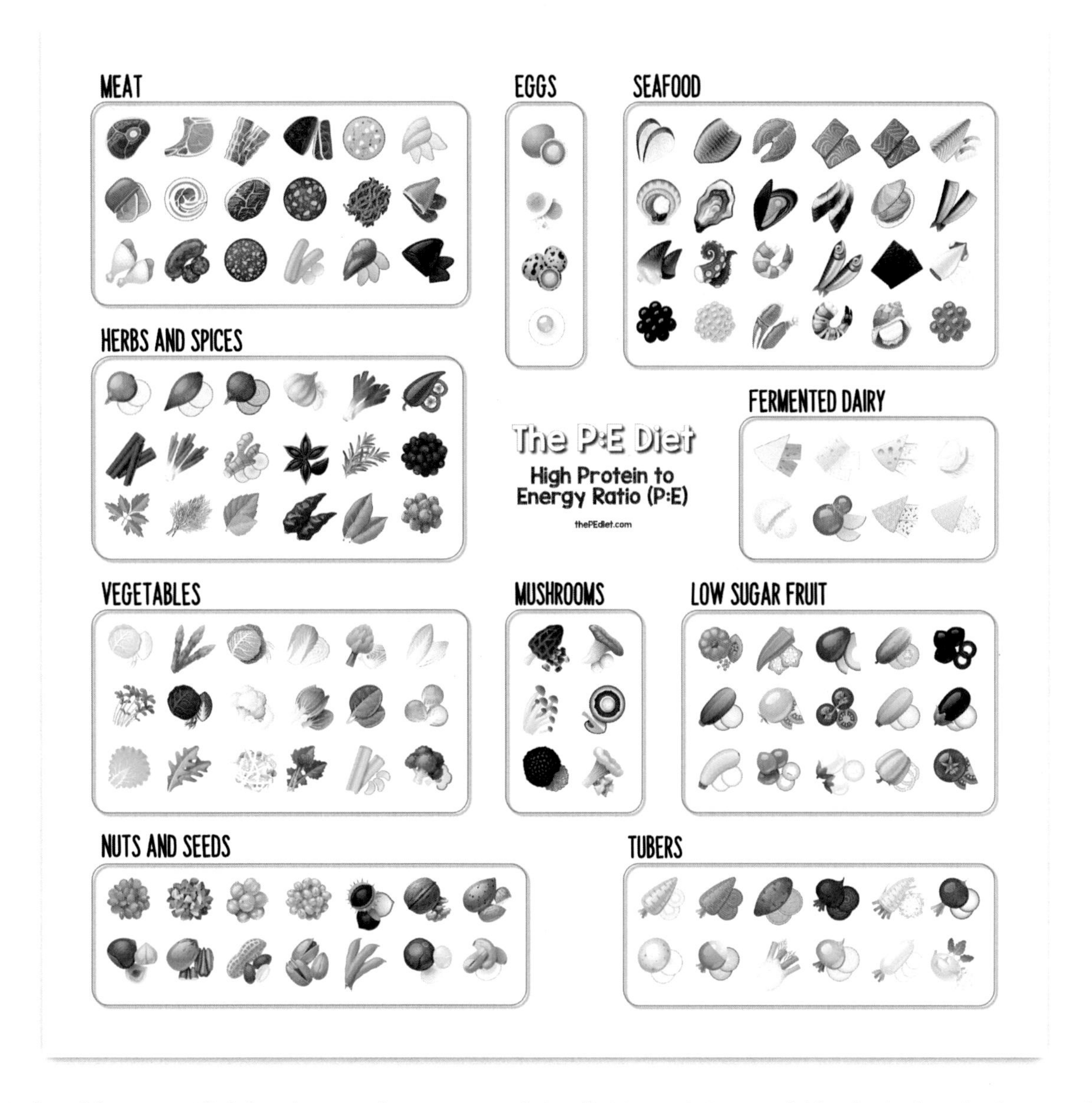

What should you eat? A basic species-appropriate diet template would include foods that are high in protein, fiber, and minerals—while being low in refined and concentrated carbs and fats (energy).

10/10

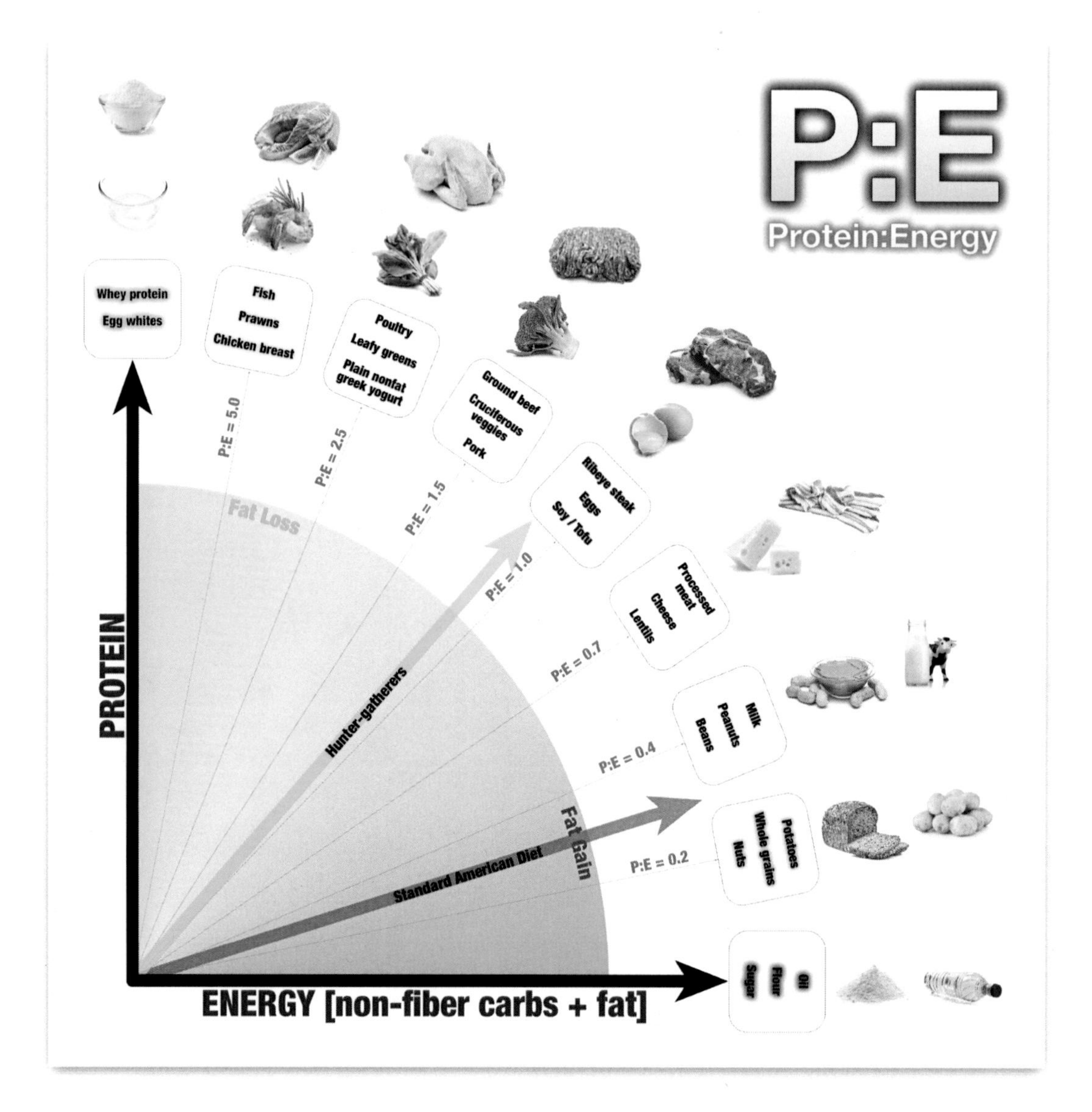

The P:E ratio is a simple metric that allows you to evaluate various foods and make small incremental substitutions to your food choices, in order to improve the overall protein to energy ratio of your diet. This will improve body composition and health.

You made it through our summary! Ok, let's move on and talk a little bit about COOKING!

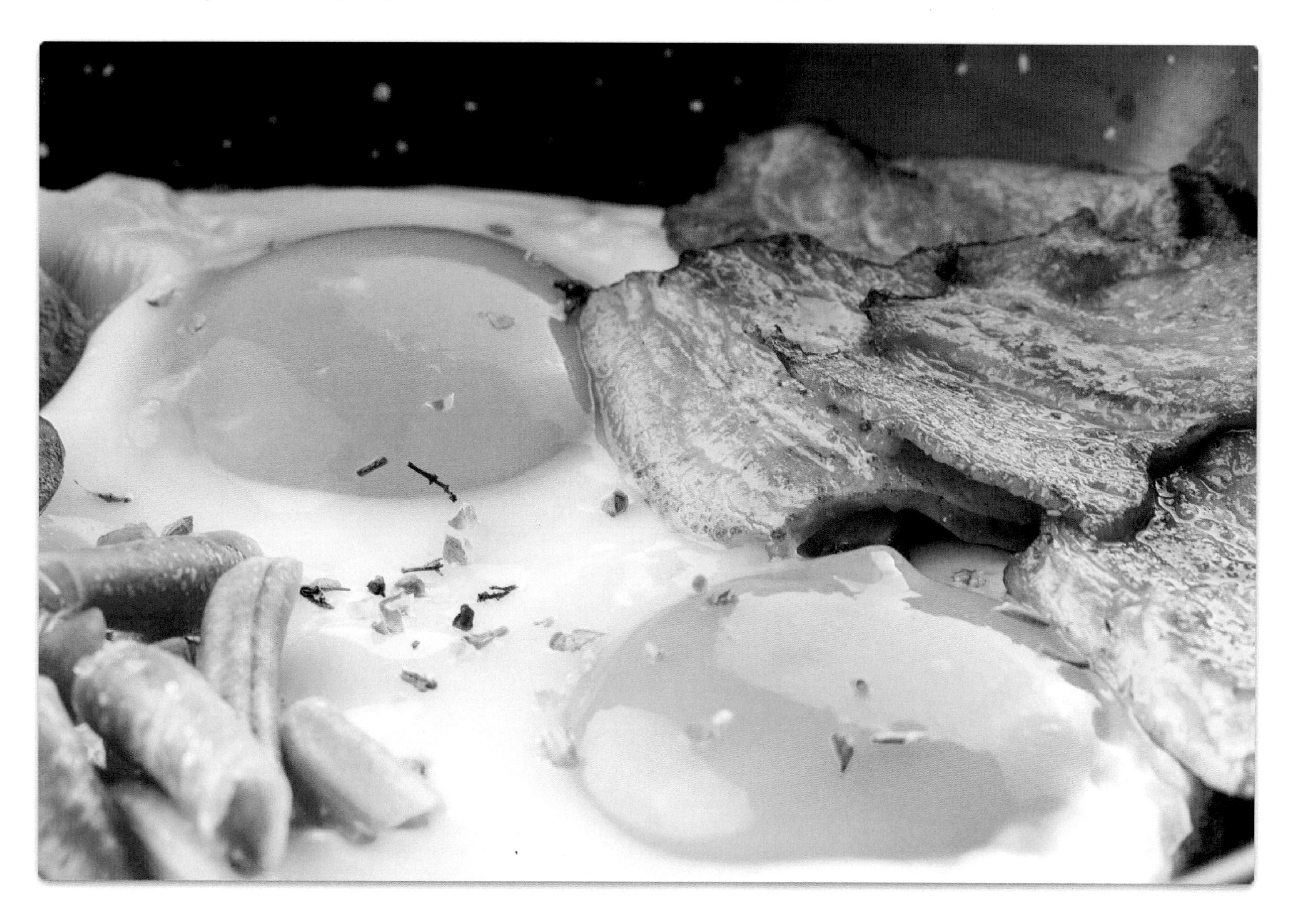

COOKING

90% of Americans don't like to cook, and today it is easier than ever to go through your entire life without cooking a thing. Unfortunately, this has been an unmitigated disaster for our health. The reality is that everyone who is in the business of selling food is trying to profit as much as possible—from small local restauranteurs, all the way up to the Big Food companies that manufacture packaged 'food'. And when you are trying to profit from selling food, the less protein you give people the better. You can see this everywhere around you. Want to Super Size your fries and soda? These empty calories, mostly sugar and oil, will cost you almost nothing. But the amount of meat on that burger is tightly controlled down to the gram, and believe us, you are not getting anything extra there. The fact that protein is the most expensive macronutrient, by a wide margin—while empty calories from sugar and oil are cheap—has been a huge economic driver of obesity and diabetes.

The very best way to fight back against all of this? Buy and cook your own food.

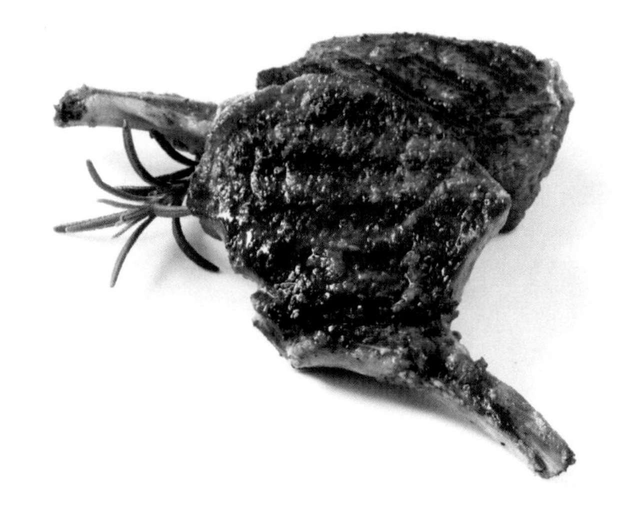

Hopefully everyone reading this is already a gourmet chef, and we are just preaching to the choir. But many of us find cooking quite daunting, if not impossible! But like anything else in life, cooking is only difficult until you learn how. And since the majority of us are suffering from the chronic diseases of poor diet, learning to cook just might save your life.

Learning to cook is all about learning to cook PROTEIN—and yes that does dovetail quite nicely with the over all theme of this book. The good news is that almost all of the proteins that you encounter can be cooked with just a few simple techniques! As with all of the information in this book, we want to give you the 20% of knowledge that will allow you to cook 80% of the foods you will encounter.

First of all, let's start with the equipment you will need. Buying equipment is expensive and daunting, but this is probably a shorter list than you would have guessed, and many of these items will last a lifetime.

COOKING ESSENTIALS:

1. **Cast iron skillet**. This is probably the single most important thing you could own for cooking protein.
2. **Chef's knife.** You really only need one good knife and you can use it for everything.
3. **Cutting board.** Bigger is better.
4. **Cast iron pot (dutch oven).** Used for braising.
5. **Mixing bowl.** Ideally non-reactive and heavy (stainless steel is good). The bigger the better.
6. **Non-stick skillet.** Ideally something safe like ceramic. For cooking delicate proteins like eggs and fish.
7. **Spatulas.**
8. **Sheet pan.** For oven roasting.
9. **Tongs.** For flipping steak, etc.

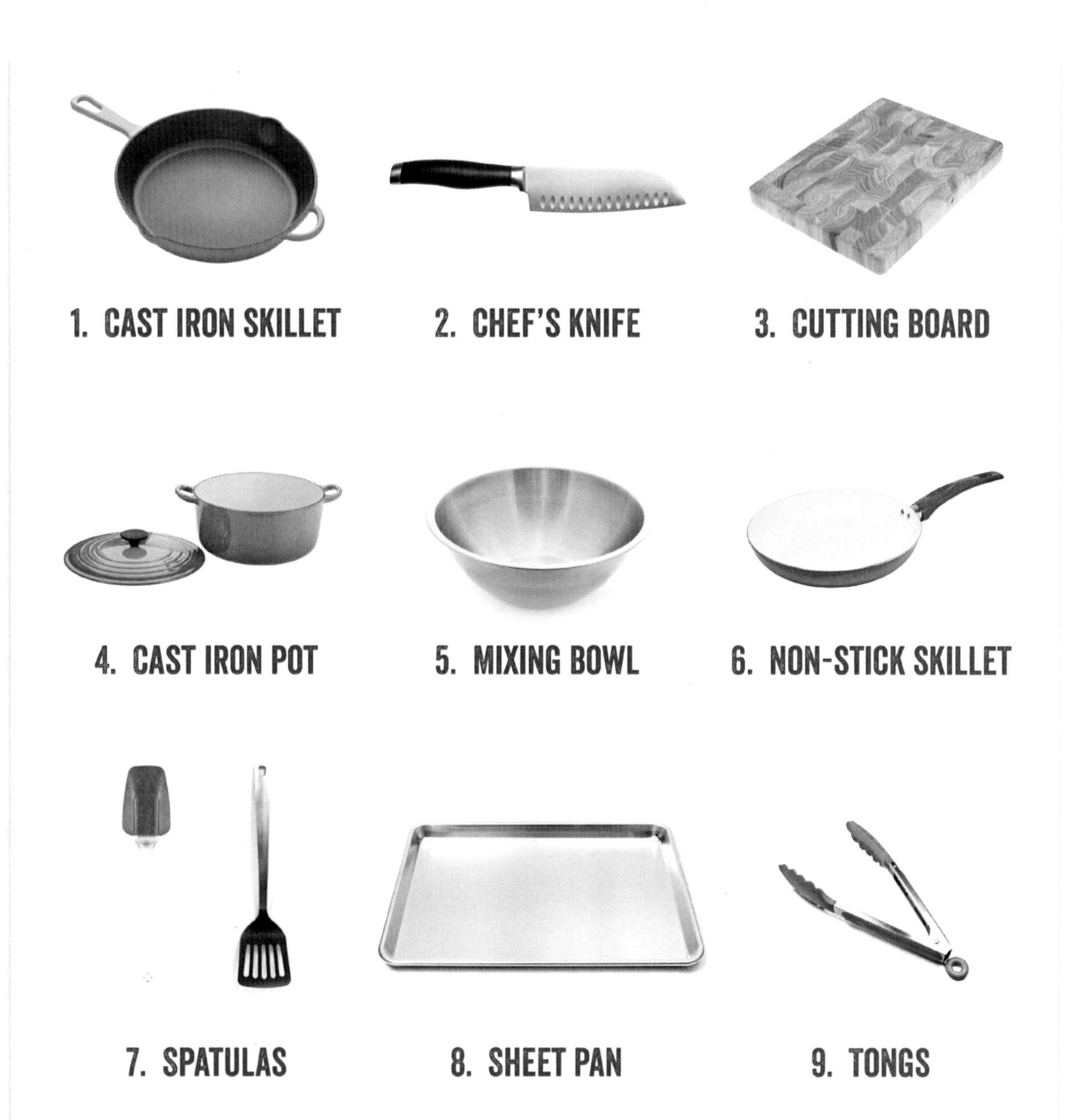

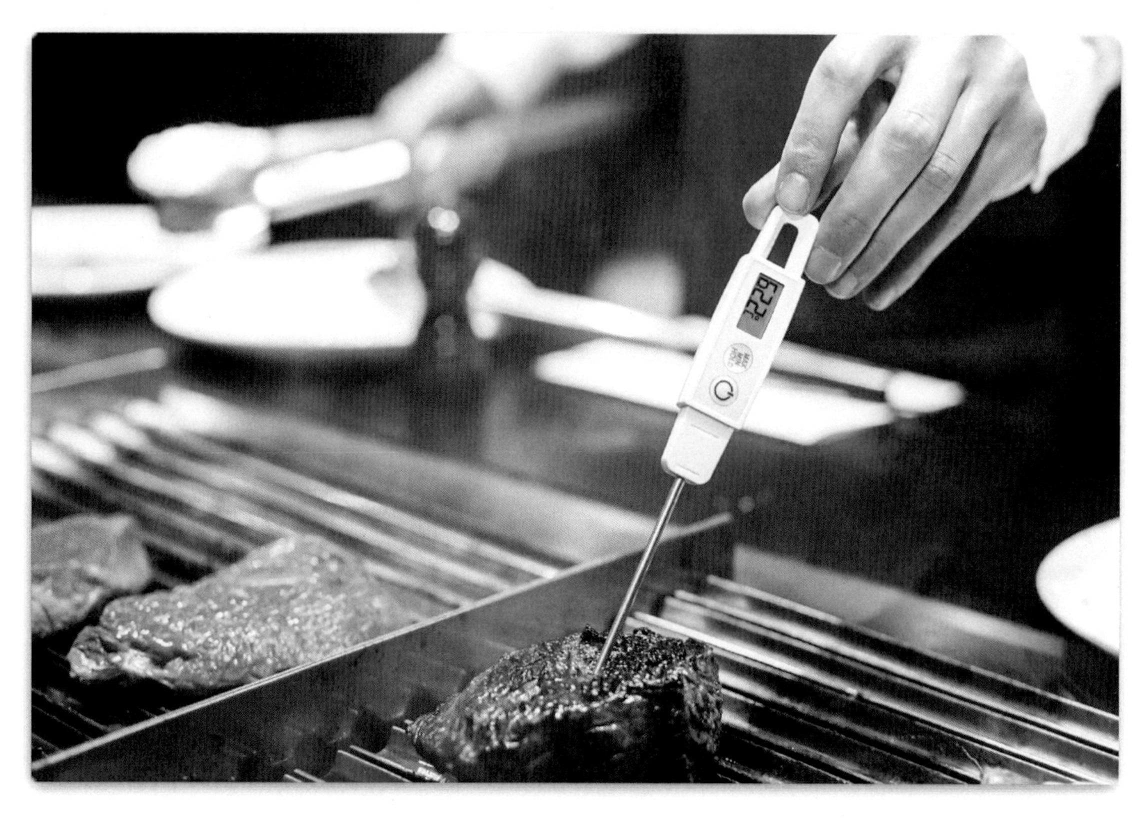

Want steaks that are cooked to perfection, and poultry that is done but not overcooked? Invest in an instant-read temperature probe.

If we had to add one more item to the list of equipment you might want to have for cooking protein, it would be an instant-read thermometer probe, like the one pictured here. This will allow you to cook the perfect steak, and make sure that poultry is at a safe temperature without being overcooked.

The basic template for cooking foods on The P:E Diet? Center your meal around a high-quality, properly-raised animal protein. Then throw in some non-starchy veggies as a side dish.

We will go through the five most common strategies for cooking proteins:

1. **Pan-sear.**
2. **Sauté.**
3. **Braise.**
4. **Roast.**
5. **Grill.**

In order to cook any protein, you will need some SALT to season it. Someone could probably write another entire book on why kosher salt is your very best choice for cooking, but in the interests of time we are just going to ask you to trust us. You will also need some sort of fat to cook most proteins in; our favorites are butter, ghee, and fruit oils such as avocado and olive oils. Because of its incredibly high smoke point, avocado oil is our very favorite (with ghee as a close second). As always, avoid any industrial seed oils like the plague (corn oil, vegetable oil, etc).

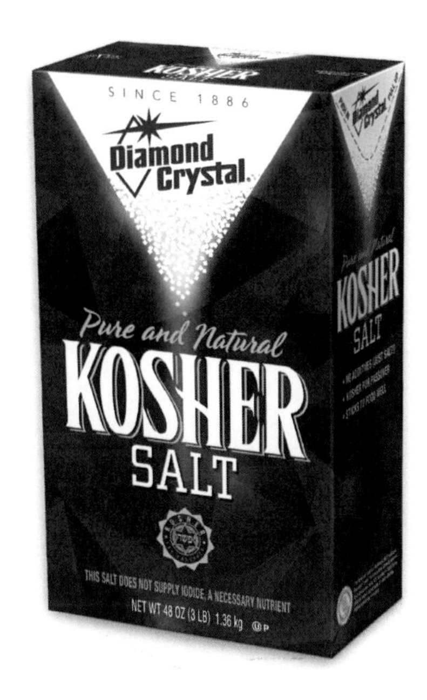

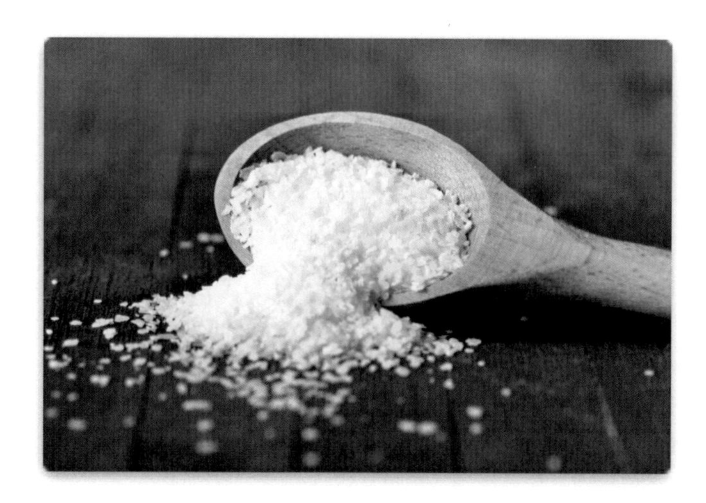

Kosher salt, such as the Diamond Crystal brand shown here, is your best salt for cooking. The reasons why are beyond the scope of this book, so you might have to take our word for it!

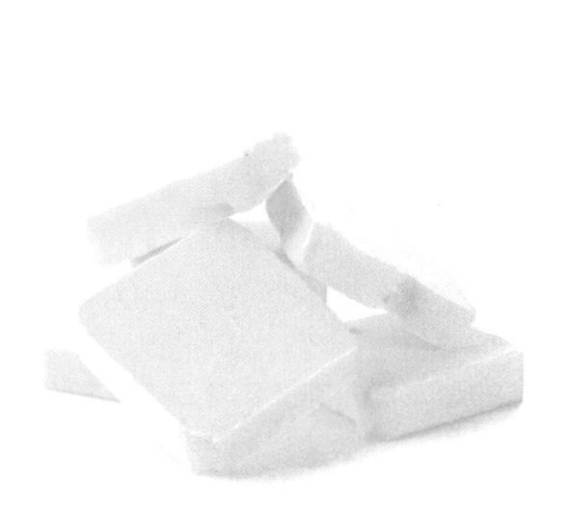

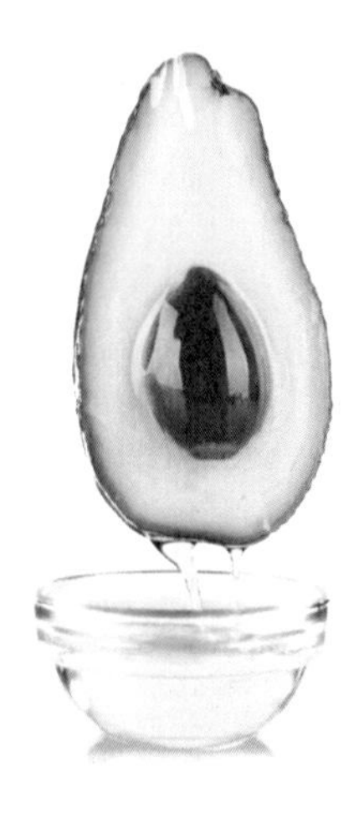

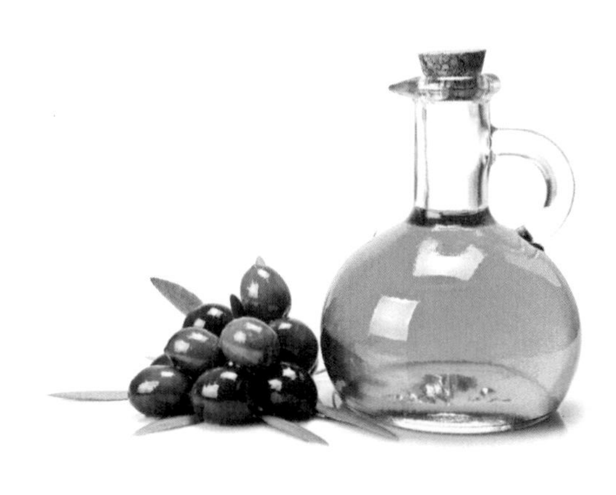

Avocado oil might be one of our favorite fats for cooking, due to its incredibly high smoke point. Ghee (clarified butter) would be a close second! If using lower temperatures, olive oil and regular butter are also good.

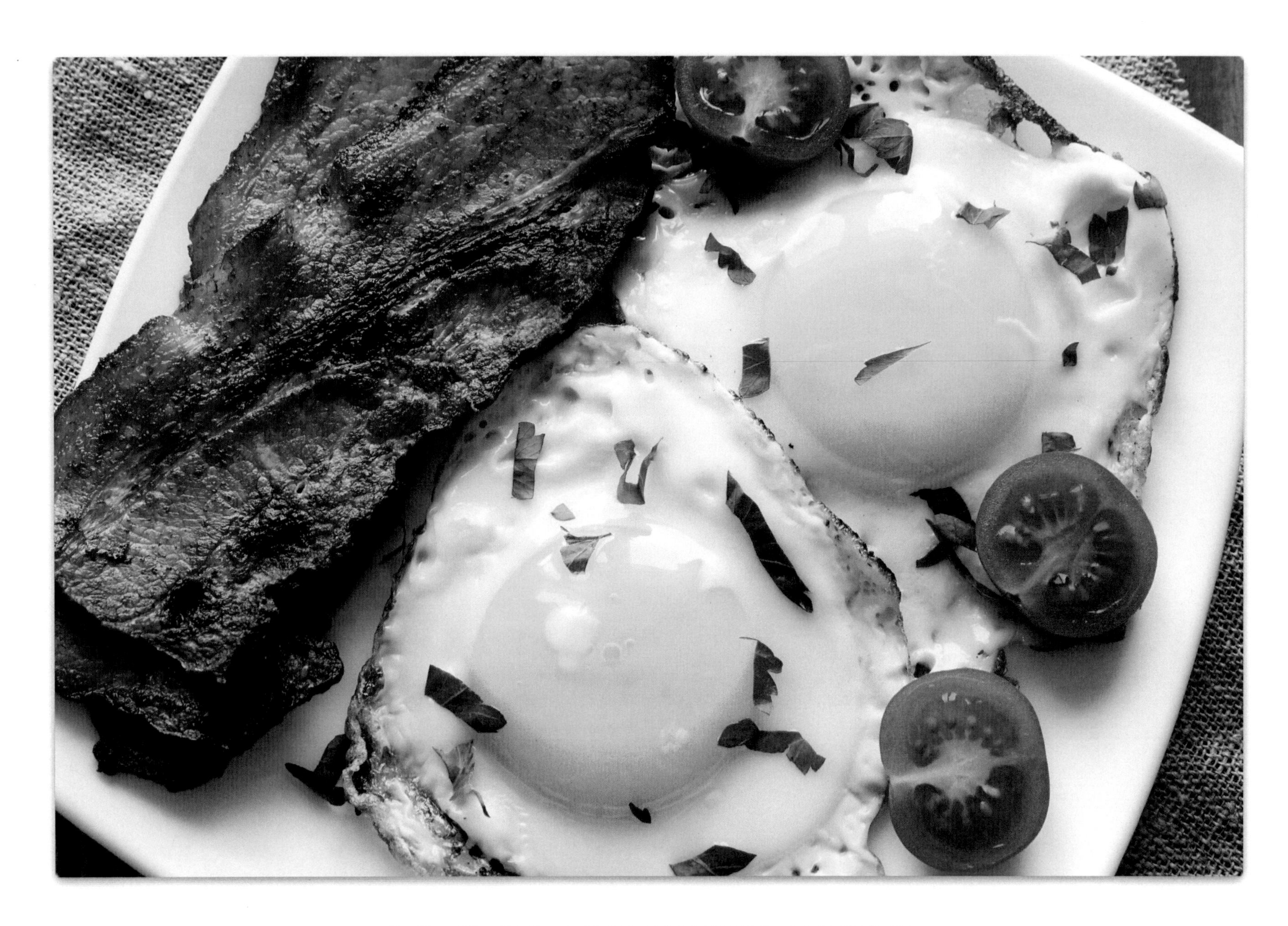

Cooking skills will last you a lifetime, and you can use them every single day.

PAN-SEARING

Pan-searing is probably our favorite method of cooking proteins. All you need for pan-searing is a piece of protein that is no thicker than roughly two inches, a nice hot pan, a fat with a high smoke point (avocado oil or ghee are your two very best choices), and a light dusting of kosher salt. Everything else is purely optional. Pan-searing is fast and easy —what's not to love? Cast iron is daunting for a lot of people, but because it is heavy it has a ton of 'thermal mass', which means it gets really hot and stays really hot—this helps you put a really great sear on your steaks or whatever protein you have selected. Start by heating the pan over medium high heat for a couple minutes, then add a few tablespoons of oil. When the oil starts to shimmer, you are ready to go. Gently place your protein in the pan and press it down so it makes good contact with the hot surface. Leave it there for at least a few minutes undisturbed, so it forms a really nice crust which will naturally release from the cast iron instead of sticking. When it looks like you have cooked the bottom half of your protein, flip it over and repeat on the other side. After cooking, remove your protein from heat and allow it to rest for a few minutes, then enjoy!

If your protein is thicker than 2 inches, you can 'butterfly' it, or cut it in half in a transverse direction, making two identical steaks that are each half as thick.

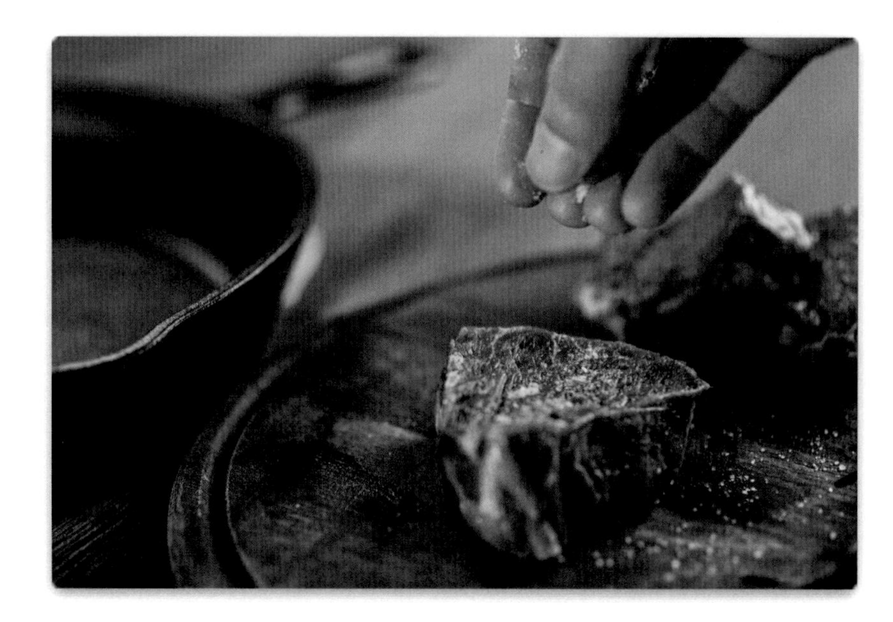

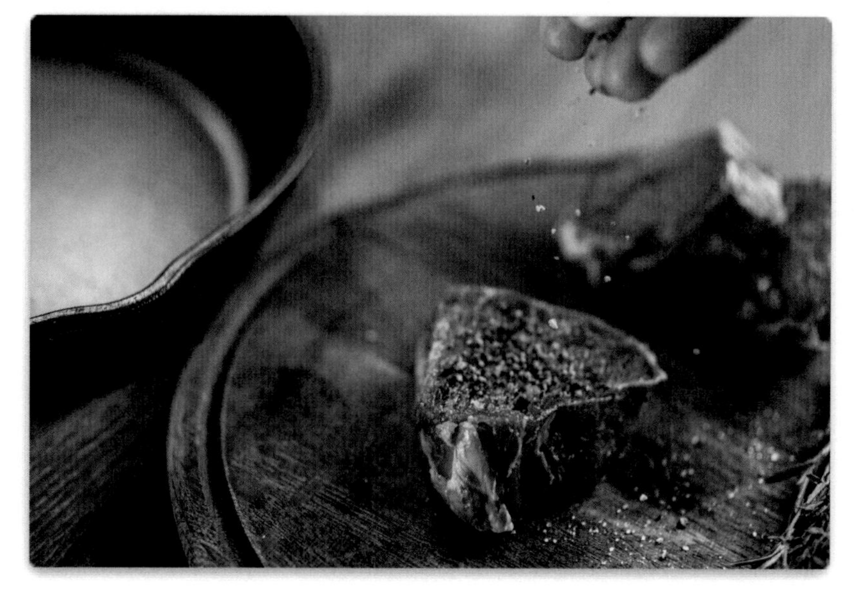

All you really need to season beef for pan-searing is a generous sprinkle of kosher salt. If you are feeling crazy, add some fresh cracked pepper as well!

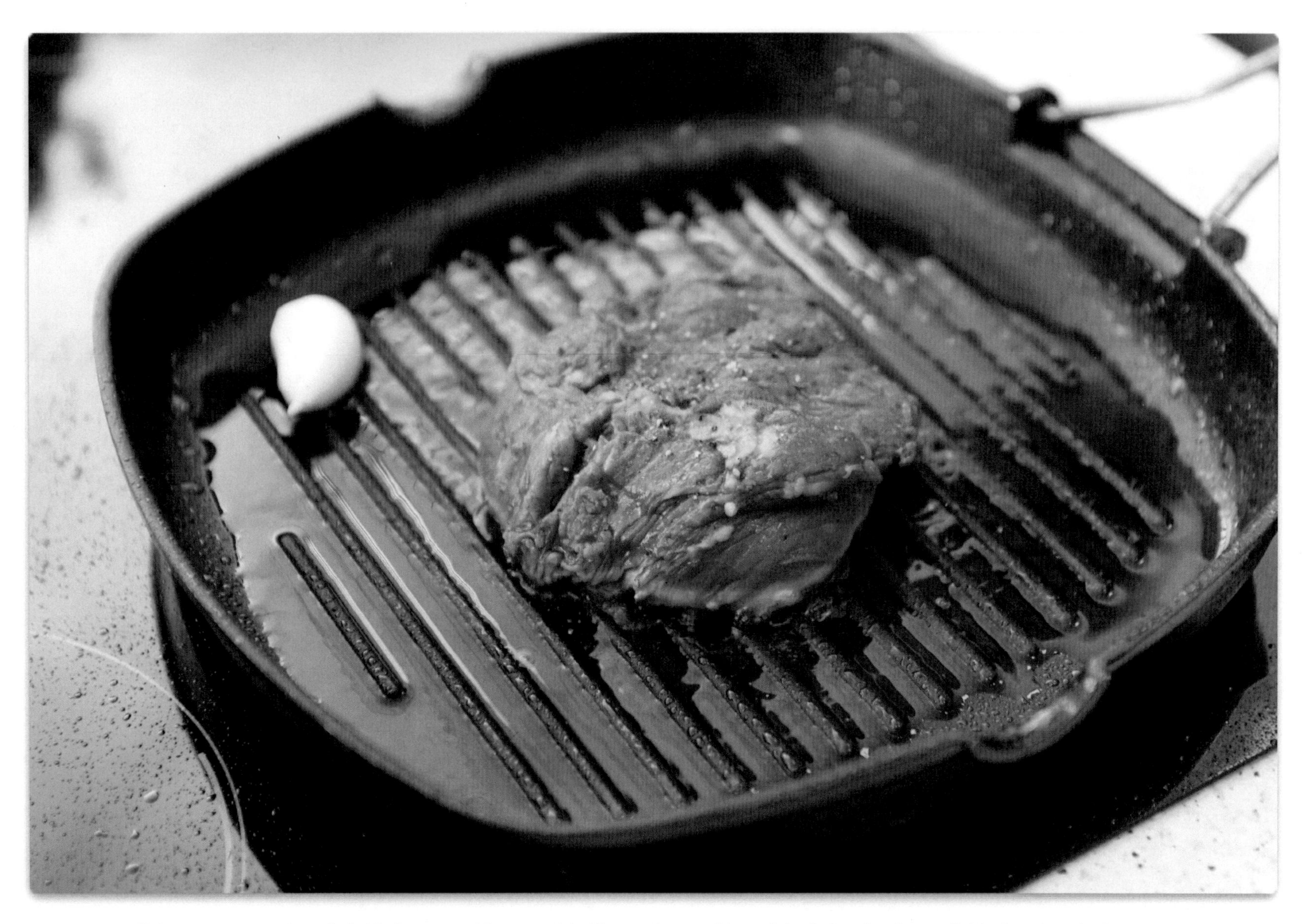

Make sure your pan is really hot before you add your protein. You want some shimmering of oil and perhaps a light wisp of smoke from your cooking fat (but not much). Leave the protein undisturbed for at least several minutes, so it forms a nice crust and your protein naturally releases from the pan before you turn it over. You might want to use your exhaust fan because this can make some smoke!

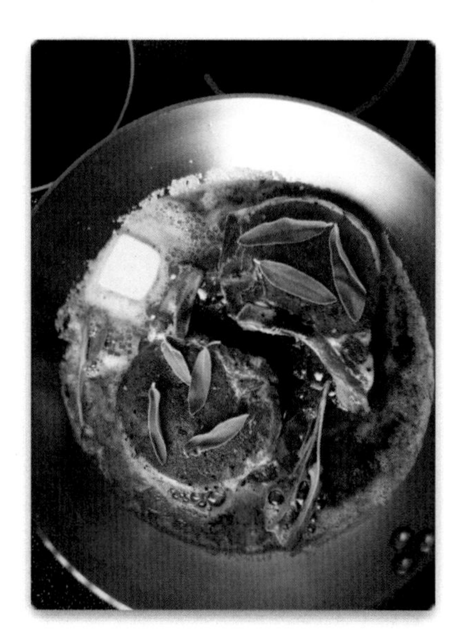

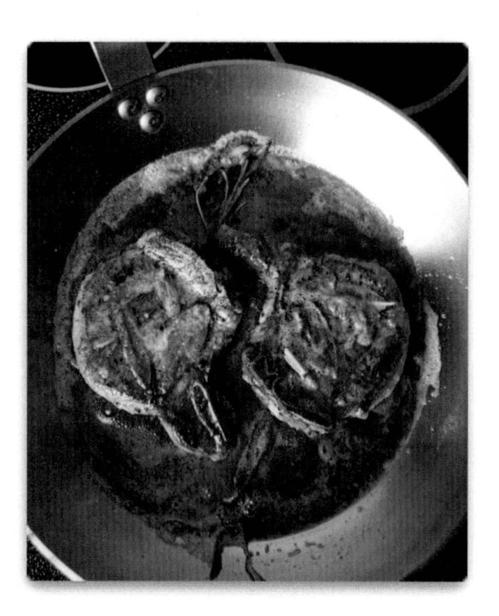

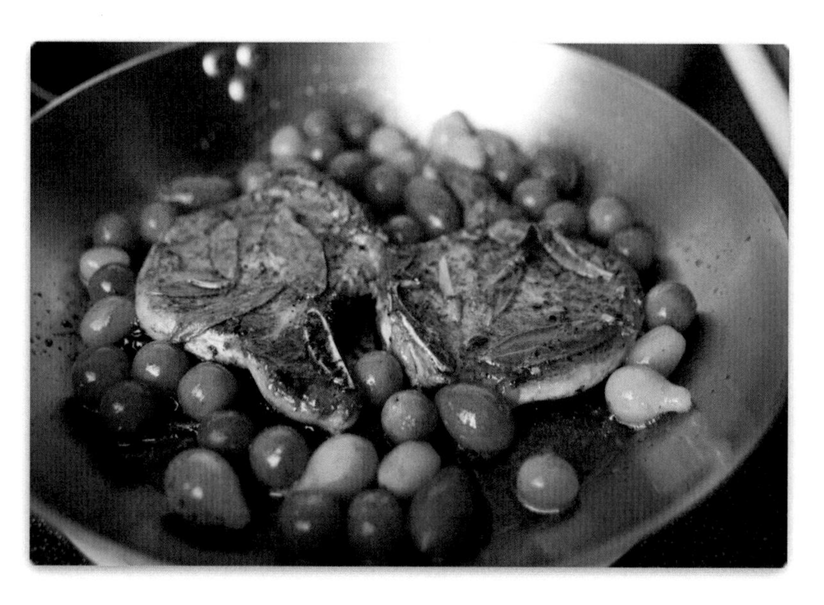

Pork chops are great for pan-searing, and have an excellent protein to energy ratio as well.

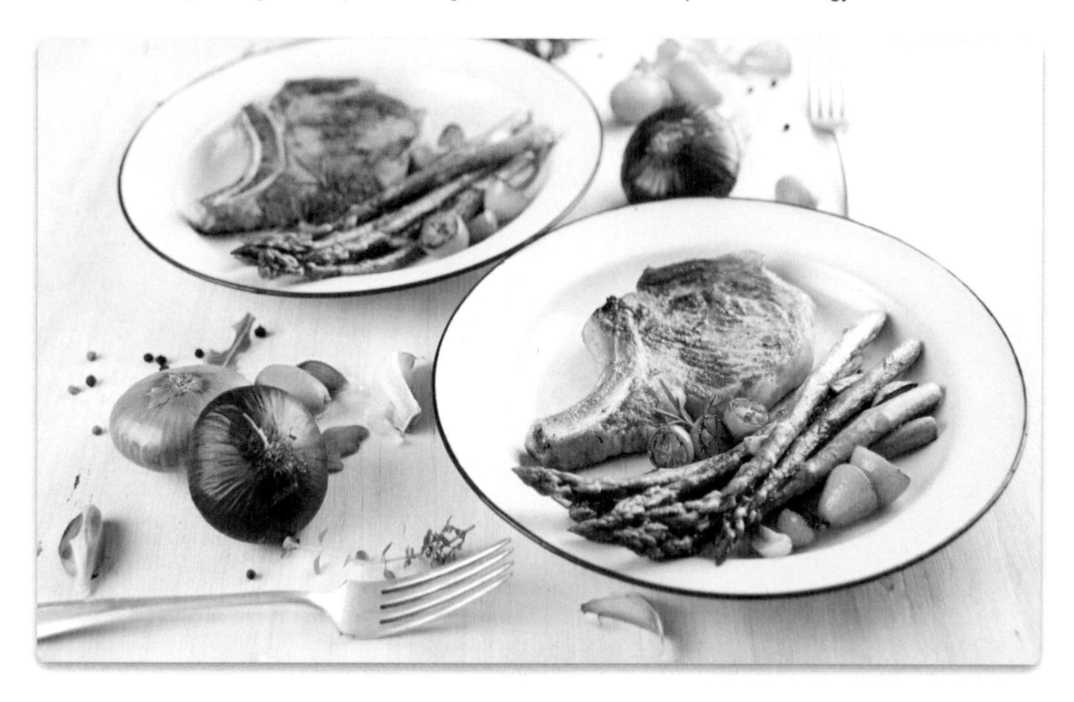

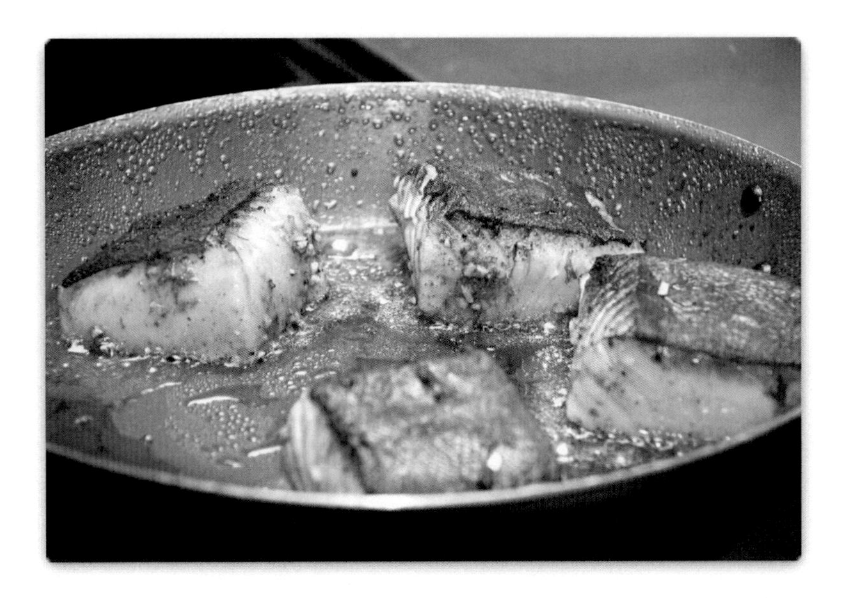

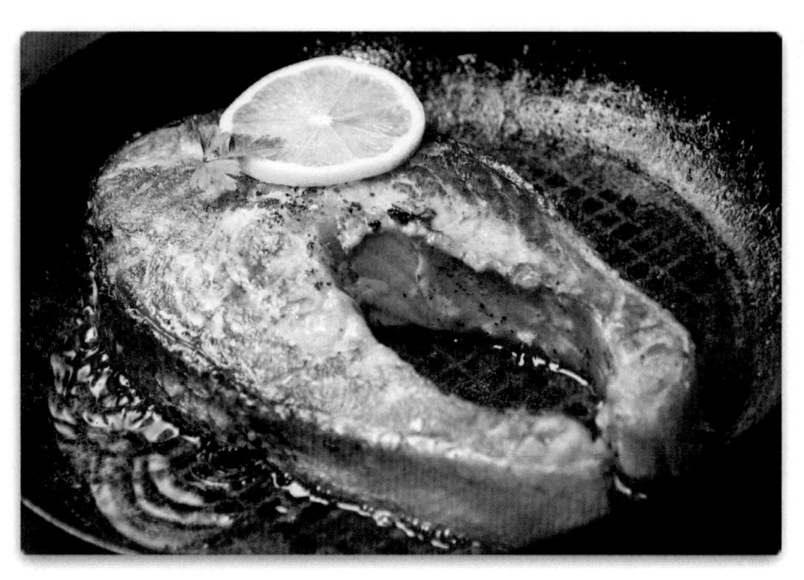

Fish is one of our favorite proteins for pan-searing. Fish also has the highest P:E ratio of any food, plus omega-3 fats and a ton of minerals. As fish is a very delicate protein and prone to sticking, you might want to use your ceramic non-stick skillet when cooking fish.

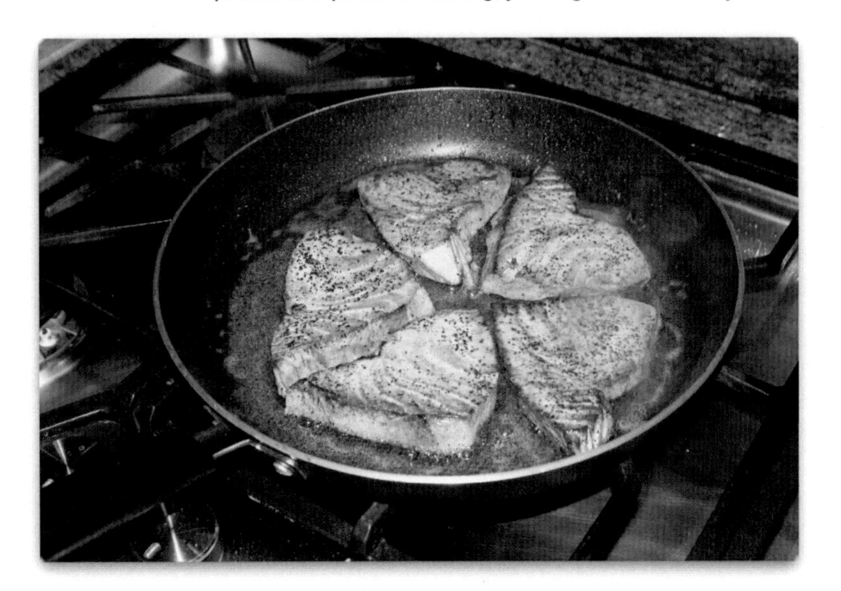

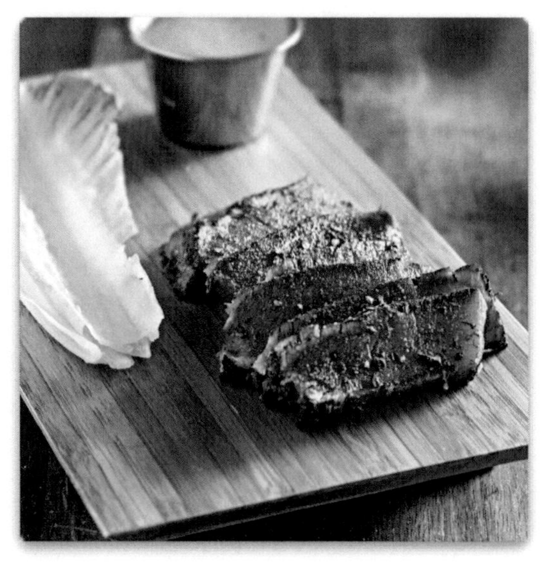

Tuna steaks pan-sear in almost no time—but even faster is searing just the outside of some sushi-grade tuna!

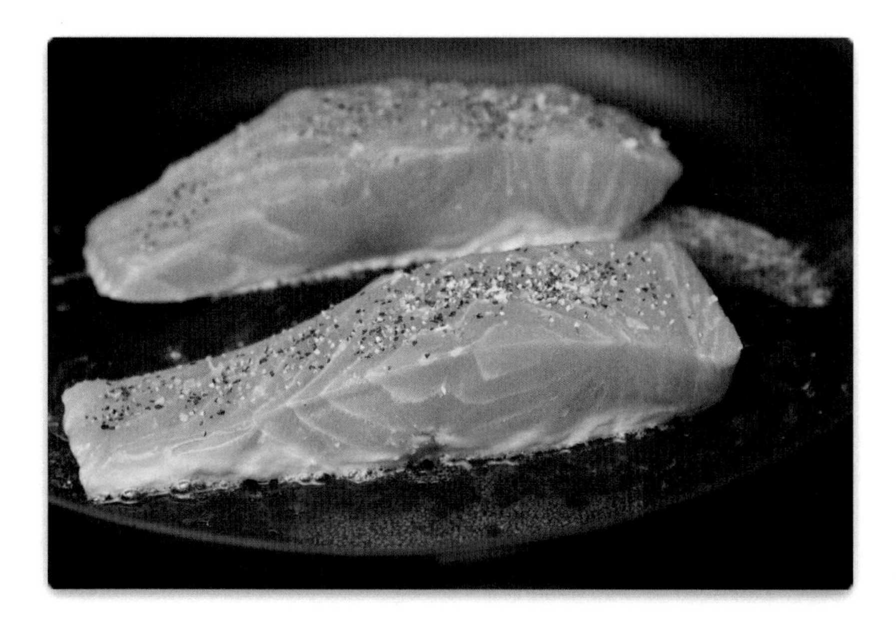

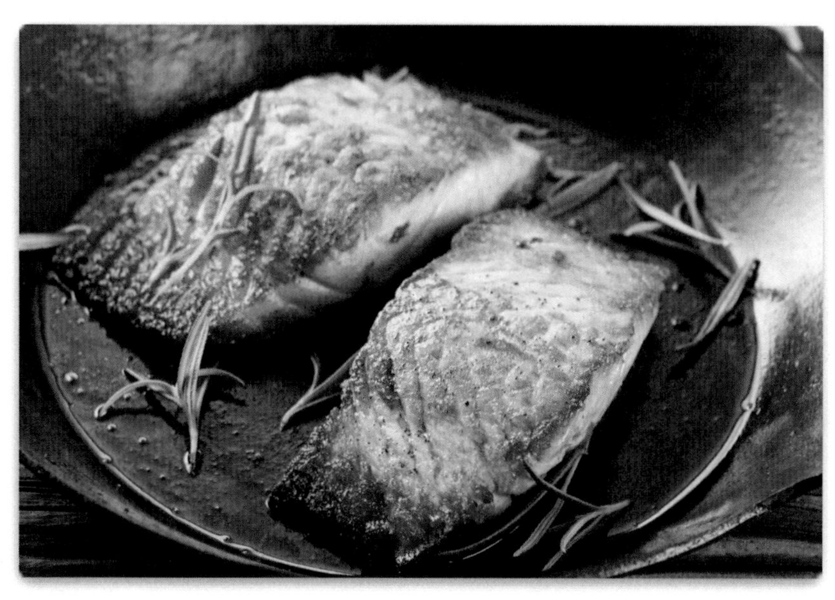

Cooking a restaurant-quality salmon fillet is amazingly easy. Heat your pan to medium and add some oil or ghee. Season the salmon with salt (and pepper if you are feeling it), then place the salmon in the pan, skin-side down. Leave it undisturbed for at least four minutes, until you see an opaque color about halfway up the thickness of the side of the fillet (which indicates that it is cooked). Turn the fish and cook for another three minutes or so, until it is fully opaque.

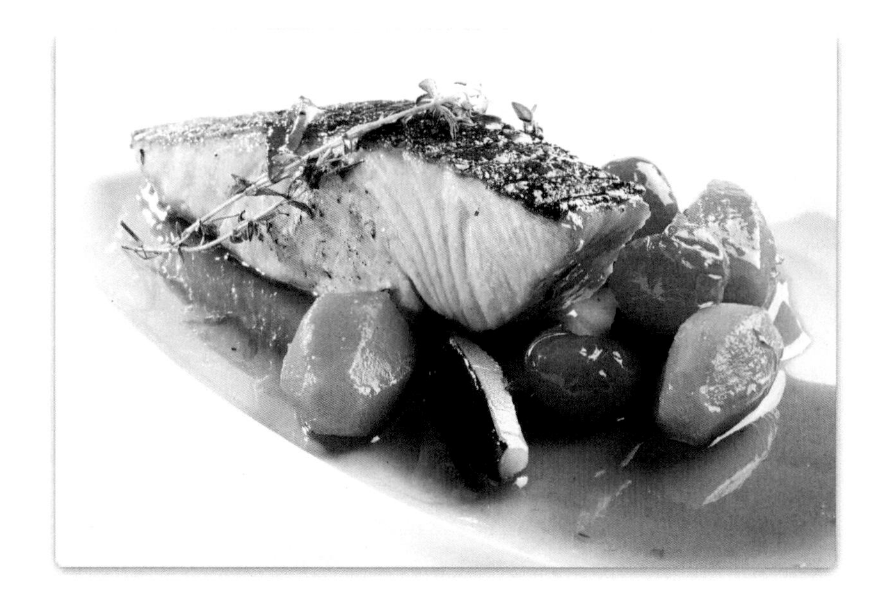

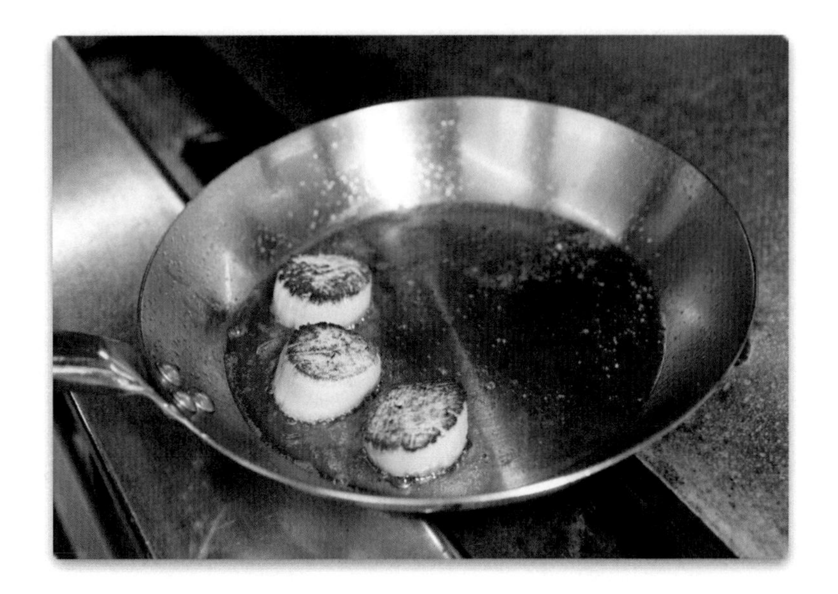

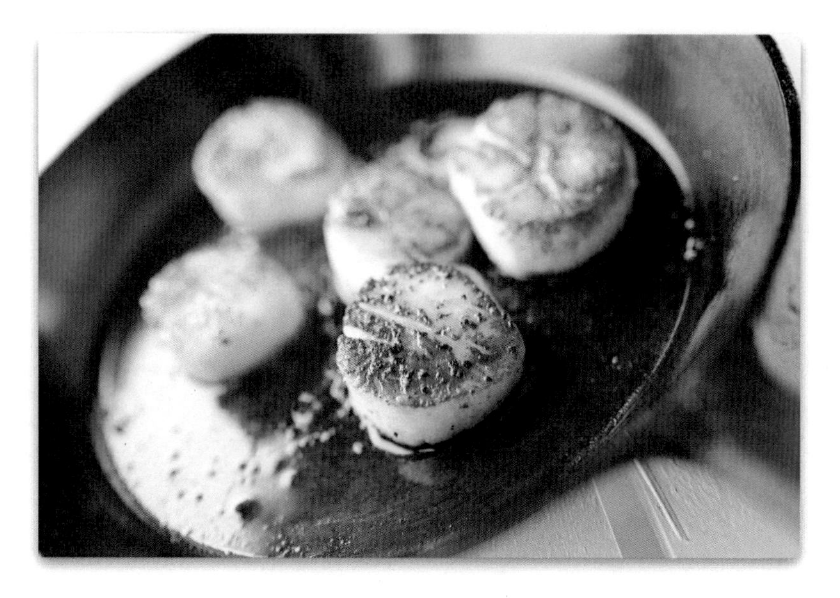

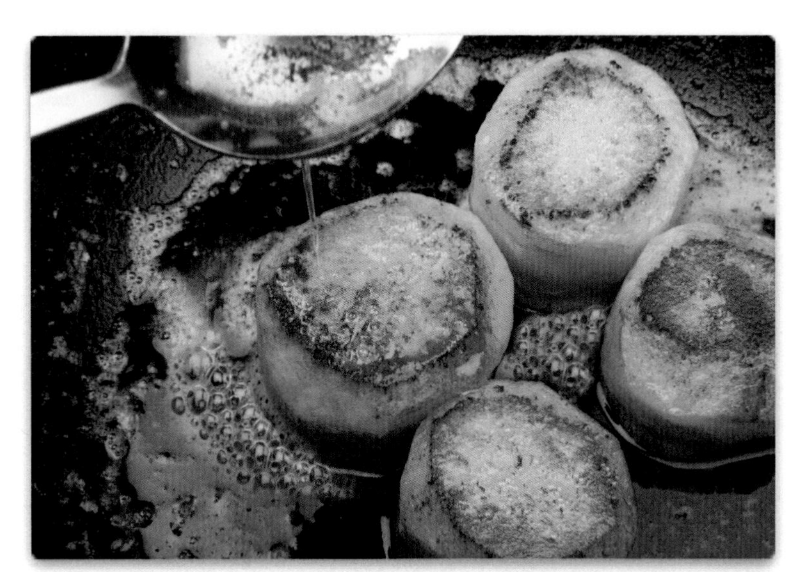

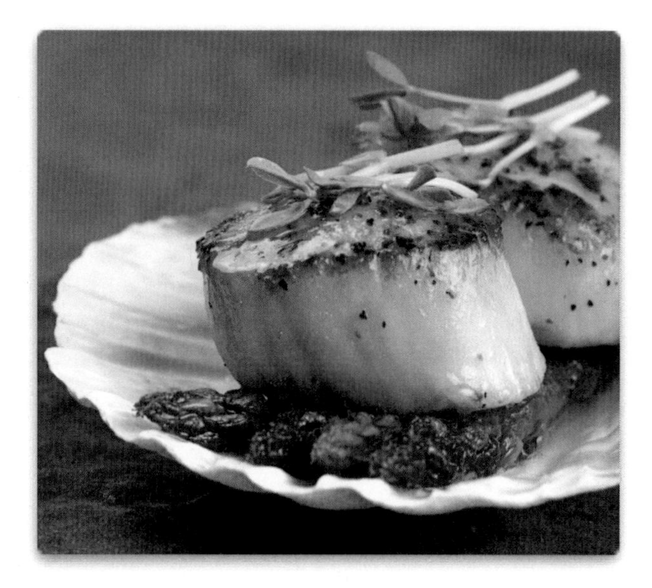

Scallops are highly nutritious and have impressive health benefits. They have an insanely high protein to energy ratio, and are an excellent source of several trace minerals, including selenium, zinc, and copper. They are also an excellent source of omega-3 fatty acids. As if that wasn't enough, they are also delicious and you can pan-sear them in almost no time at all!

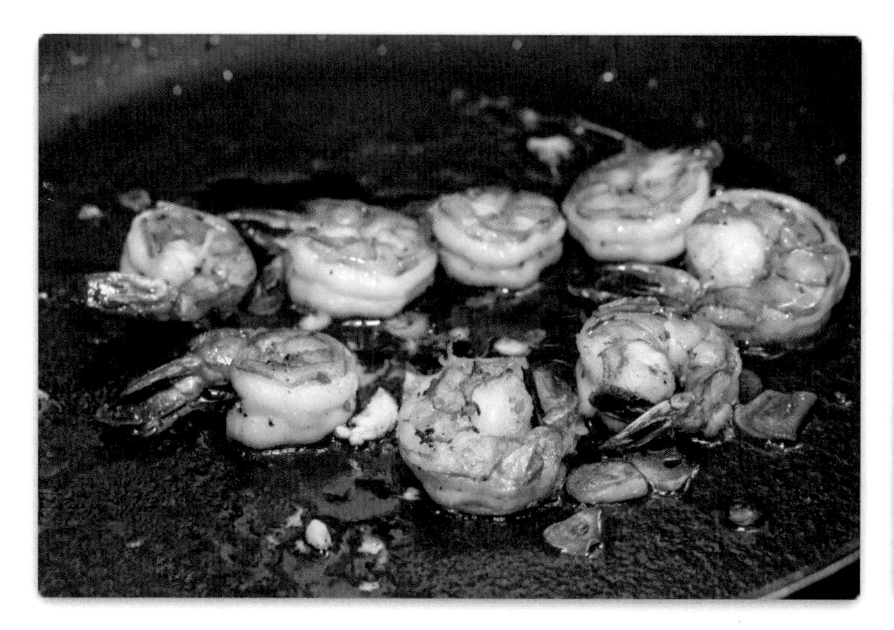

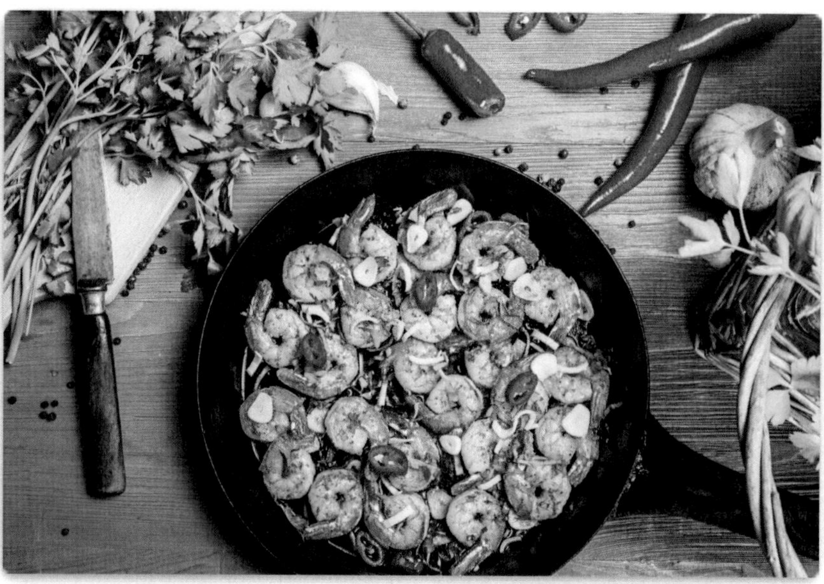

Shrimp is another delicious seafood with an amazing protein to energy ratio and plenty of nutrients, including iodine and omega-three fats. You can pan-sear shrimp in just two minutes per side! Add any spices you want, including garlic, lime, cilantro, or hot peppers for more flavor.

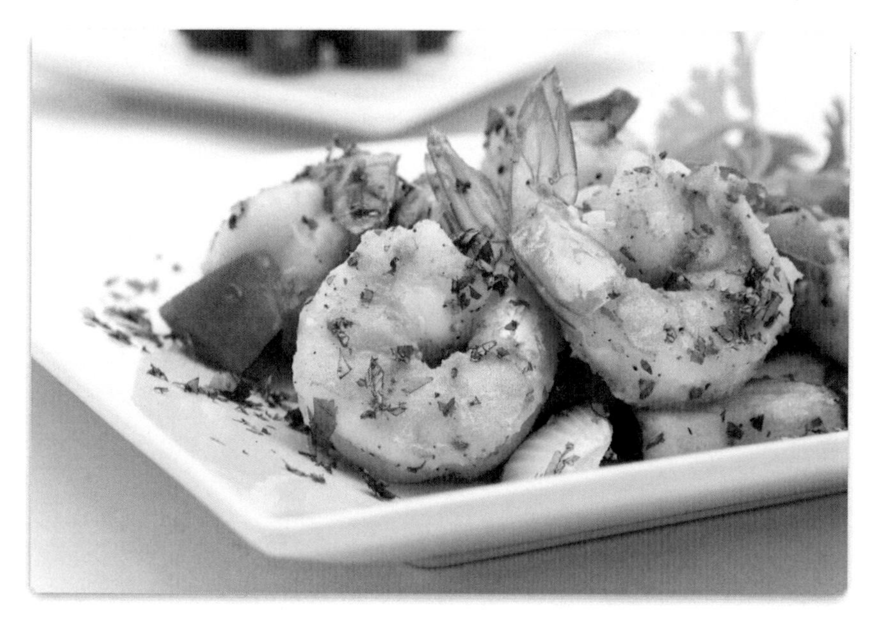

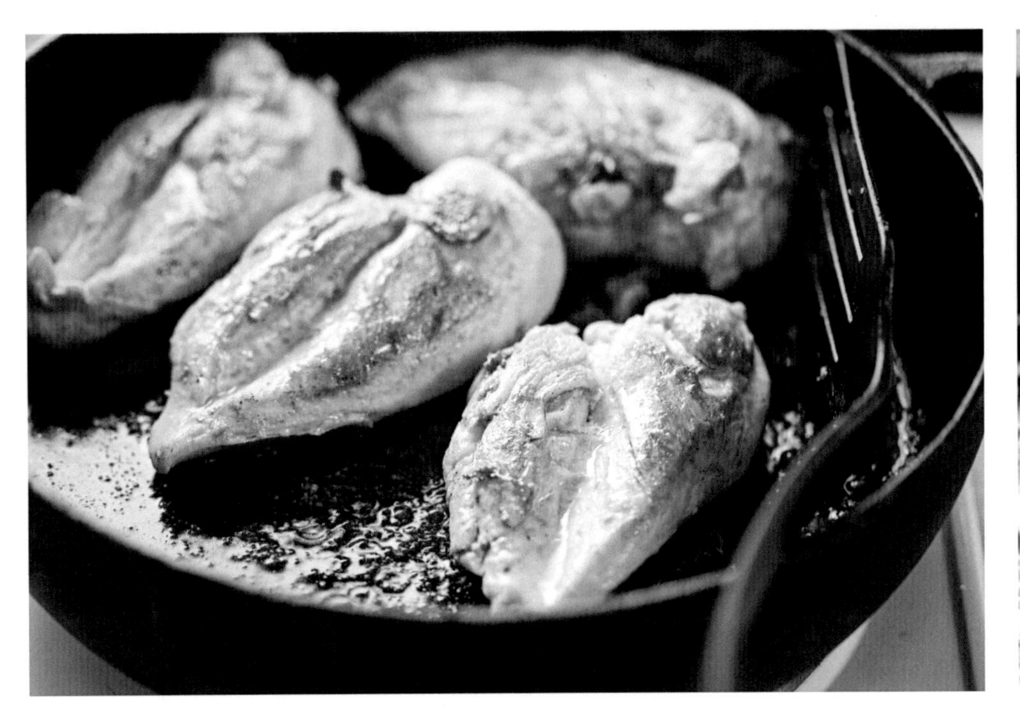

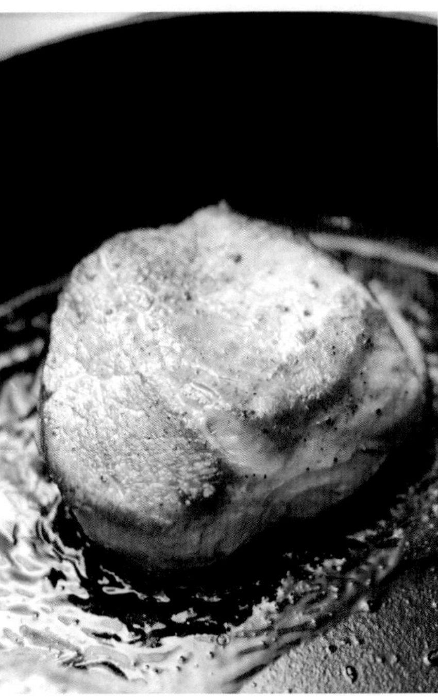

Chicken breasts have a spectacular P:E ratio, and are perfect for pan-searing. Because they are a bit thicker, you want to cook these at a lower temperature for a little bit longer. Try a heat slightly lower than medium and cook for nine minutes on the first side, then six minutes on the second side. Similar to cooking fish, you can watch an opaque line slowly going up the side of the chicken breast, indicating that it is cooked, and you will typically flip the chicken breast over when the line goes halfway up the side. You might want to use your thermometer probe to make sure the center is perfectly cooked, until you get the hang of it and you can cook a perfectly done chicken breast without it.

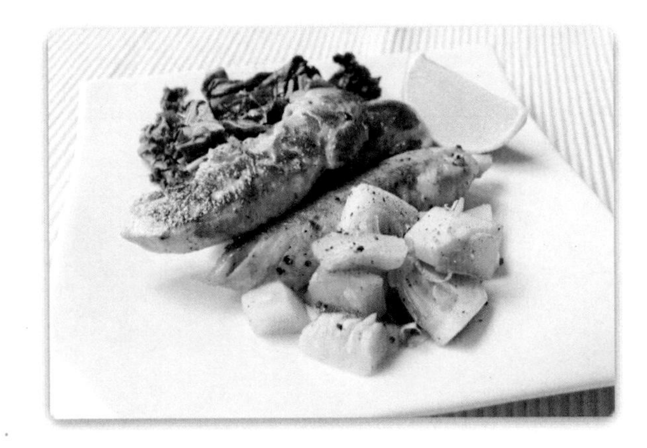

SAUTÉING

Sautéing is pretty much identical to pan-searing, except it involves cooking smaller pieces of food. Use this technique for bite-sized pieces of meat or ground proteins (ground beef, lamb, chicken, turkey, or pork). This technique might involve more prep work (cutting up meat), but it allows you to throw in chopped up flavor vegetables. Alliums, such as onions, leeks, shallots, and garlic are fantastic using this technique.

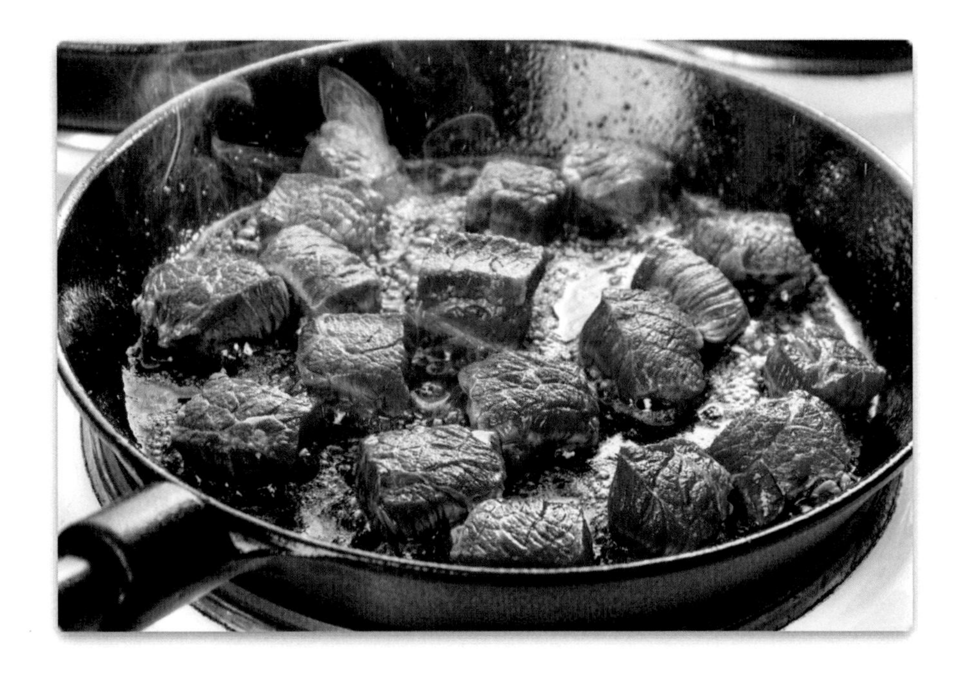

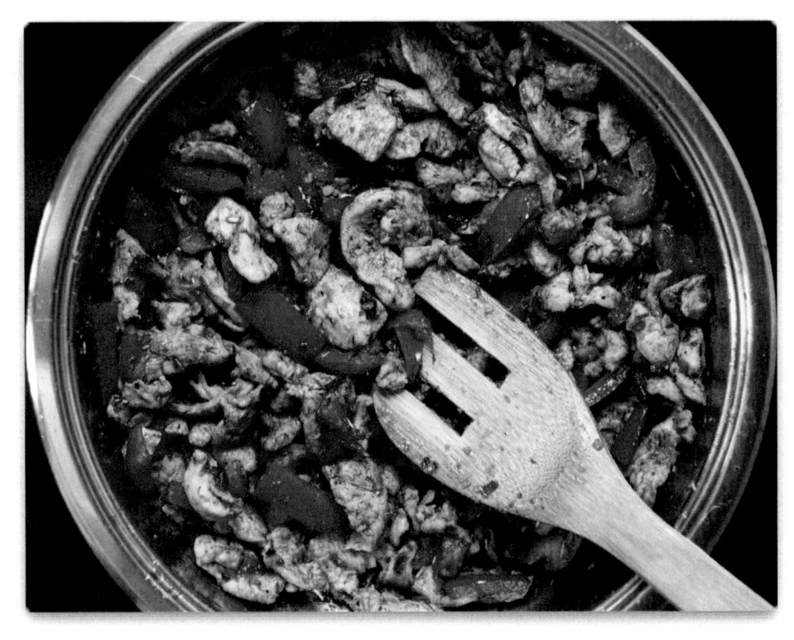

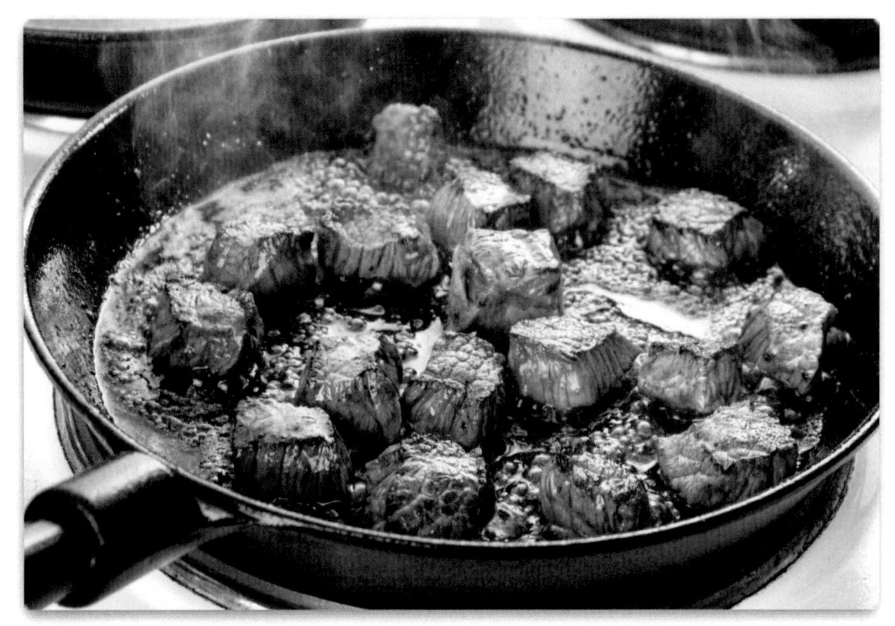

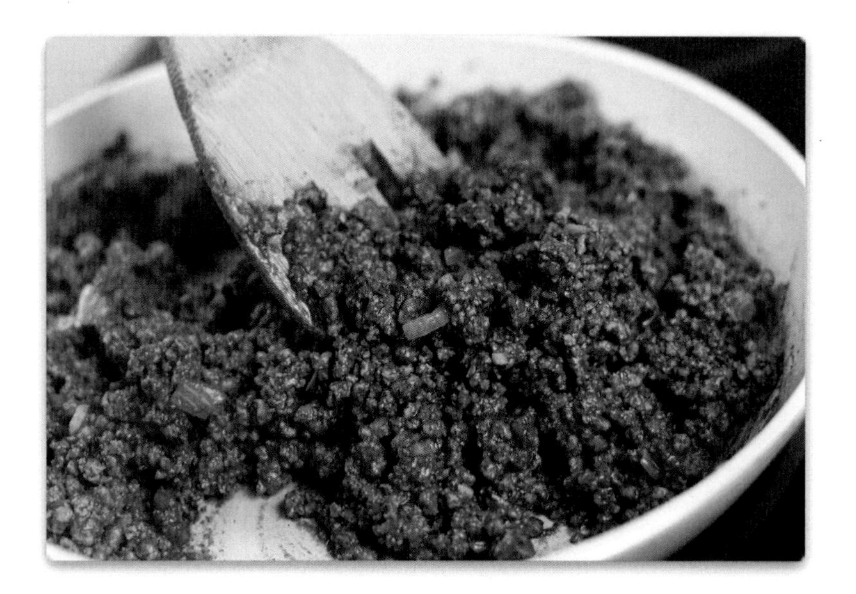

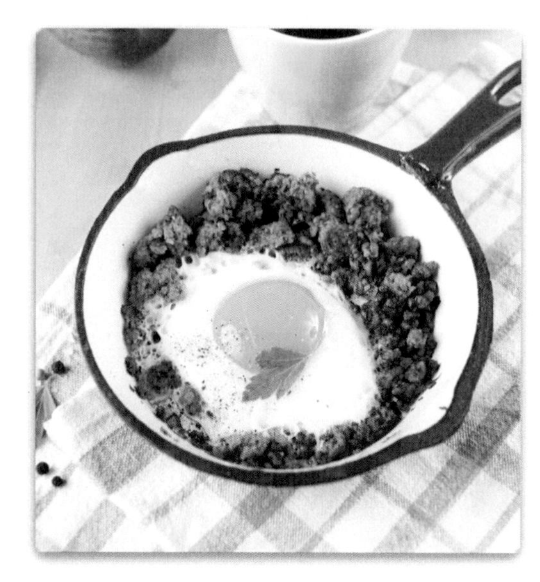

Ground proteins, like ground beef, ground pork, and ground turkey are quick and easy to cook! Season with some garlic and onions, plus any other spices you want. Cumin, chili pepper, oregano, and paprika are all excellent.

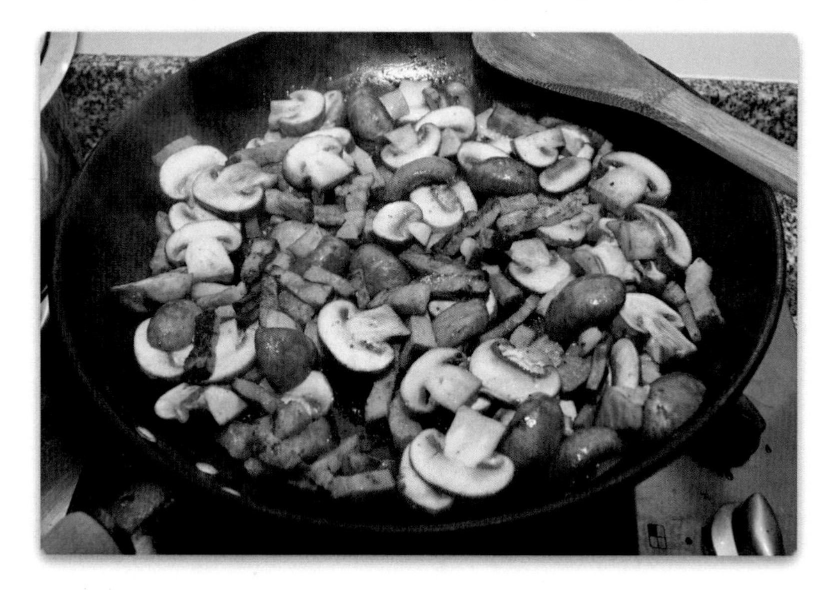

Sautéed mushrooms are an amazing side dish.

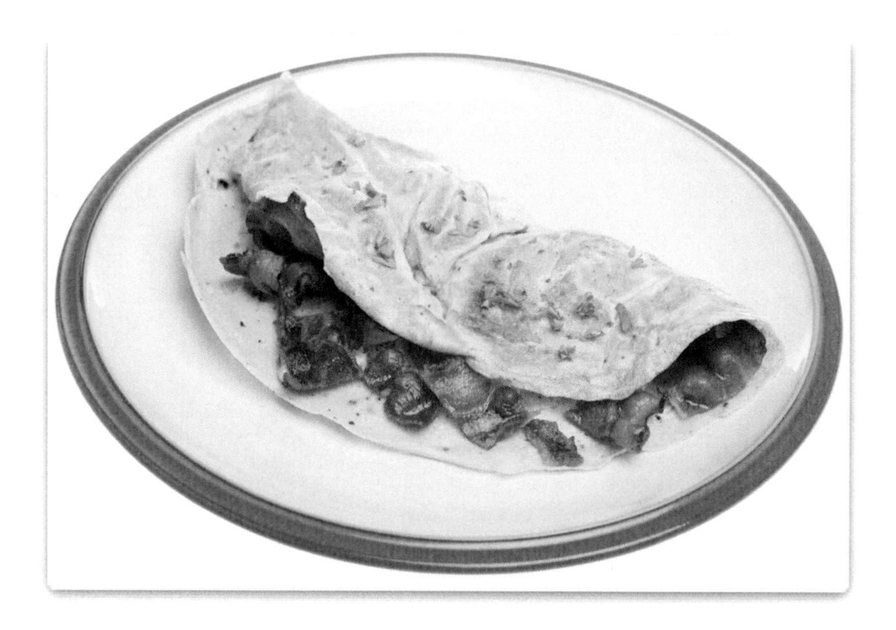

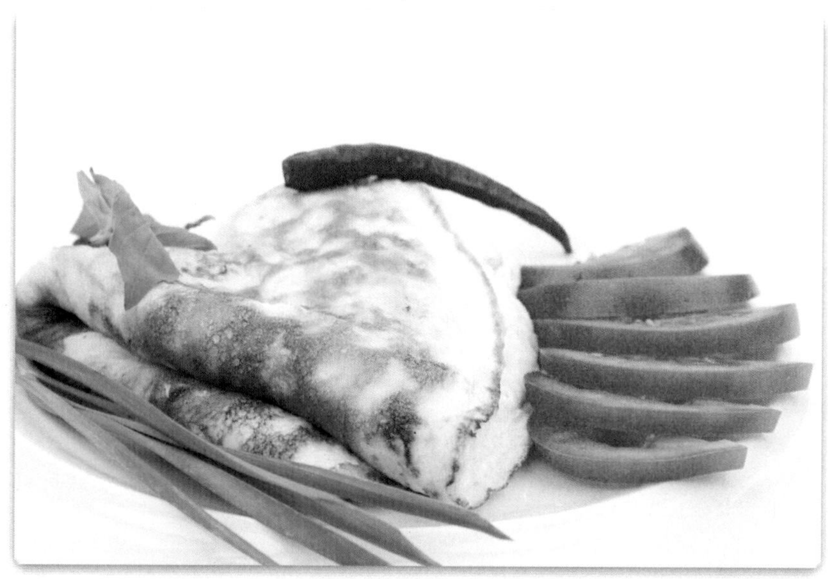

Omelettes and scrambled eggs are basically sautéed, and eggs are an amazing food with an incredibly high nutrient density.

Cooking a perfect omelette is tricky at first, and if you don't know how we would recommend spending five minutes on YouTube—you will pick up the necessary skills in no time!

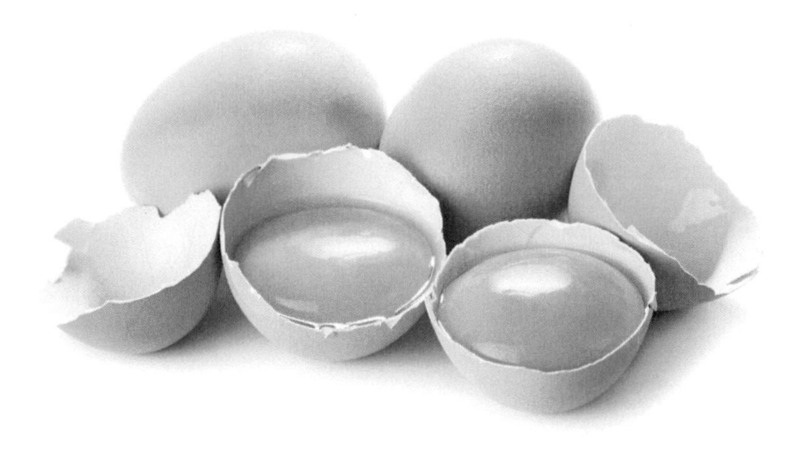

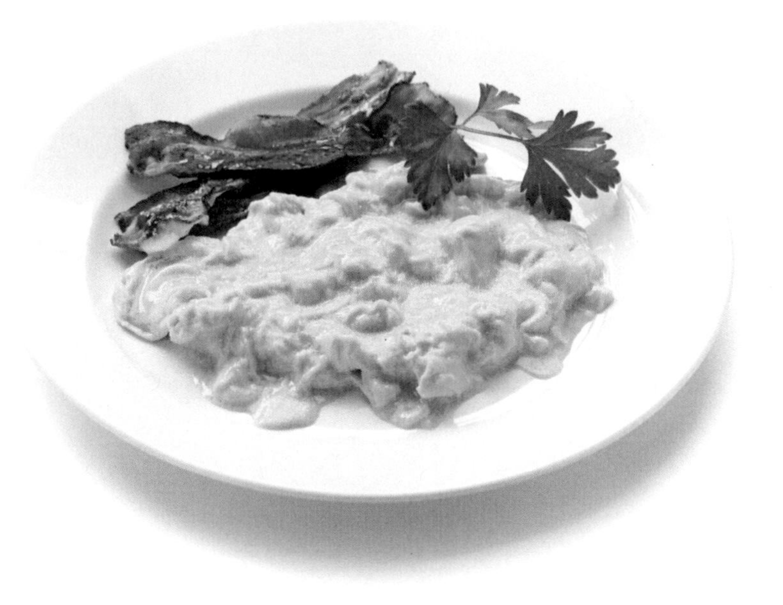

BRAISING

Braising starts out identical to pan-searing because you add your protein to a heavy cast iron pot over high heat to brown the meat's surface and enhance its flavor. The difference is that you are using a larger and thicker protein that would never cook all the way through with pan-searing. Instead, you sear all the surfaces of your protein over high heat, then add some liquid and finish cooking the meat in a COVERED pot over lower heat for a much longer period of time. Braising relies on time and moisture to break down the tough connective tissue (collagen) that binds muscle fibers in meat together, making it an ideal way to cook larger and tougher cuts of meat. Slow cooking (crockpots, etc) are basically forms of braising.

All braises follow the same basic steps. Here is the basic template for braising anything. Start with a large inexpensive cut of meat. Chuck, shank, brisket, short ribs, bottom round—any of these are great. Heat a small amount of avocado oil in a heavy dutch oven (enameled cast iron is excellent) over high heat. When the oil is very hot, add the meat and brown for a minute or two on all sides, flipping with tongs. Remove the meat and set it aside. Lower the heat to medium. For bonus flavor, you could throw in some aromatic vegetables like chopped onions, carrots, celery, and garlic at this stage and sauté a few minutes—but this step is optional. Deglaze the pan with a cup or two of some flavorful liquid such as any kind of broth, scraping the tasty burned bits from browning off of the bottom of the pot (this adds a ton of flavor). Return the meat to the pot along with some sort of acidic ingredient like diced tomatoes, a splash of wine, or a few tablespoons of vinegar—the acid helps break down the tough connective tissues in the meat.

Now it is time to cover the pot with a tight-fitting lid and simmer the meat for 1 to 5 hours, depending on the size of your protein—typically about an hour per pound. You can either simmer it on the stovetop over medium-low heat (enough heat to keep the water just below the boiling point, with some very gentle bubbling but nothing resembling a full

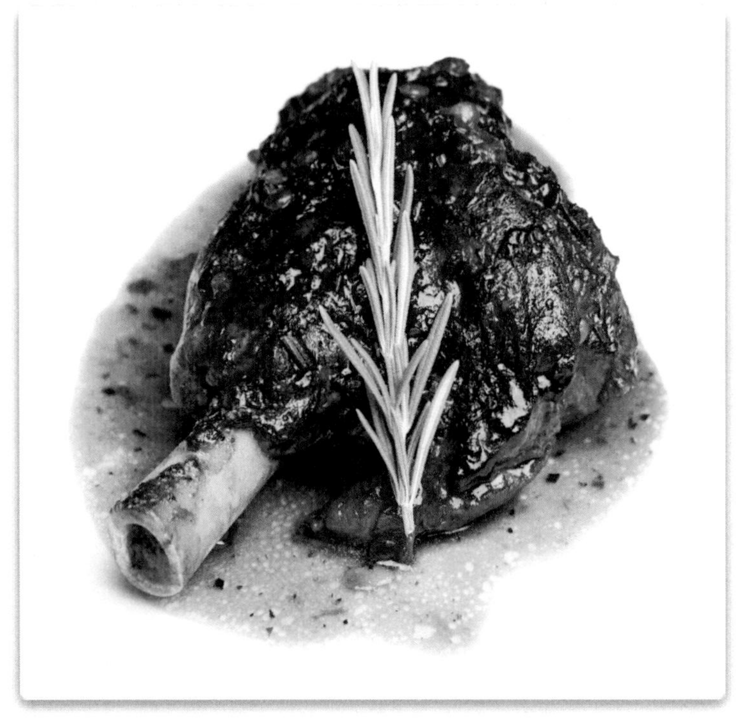

aggressive boil), or put it in the oven set to 300°F, which will have the same effect. You will know when your meat is cooked because it will be fork-tender. Remove the protein from the pot to rest it for a few minutes, and in the meantime, boil the remaining liquid in the pot over high heat on the stove to thicken it until you have a less watery consistency and you can use this as a sort of gravy.

You can also throw some root vegetables into your braising pot just prior to the slow-cooking simmer—carrots are the most popular, but you could also try beets, kohlrabi, potatoes, radishes, rutabaga, sweet potatoes, or turnips.

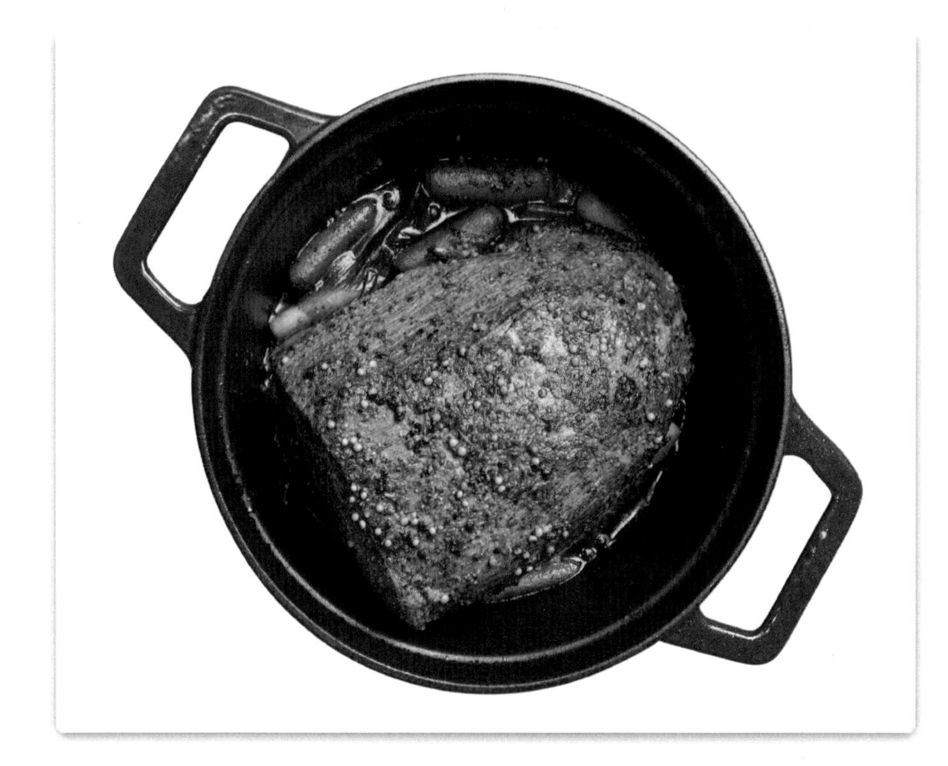

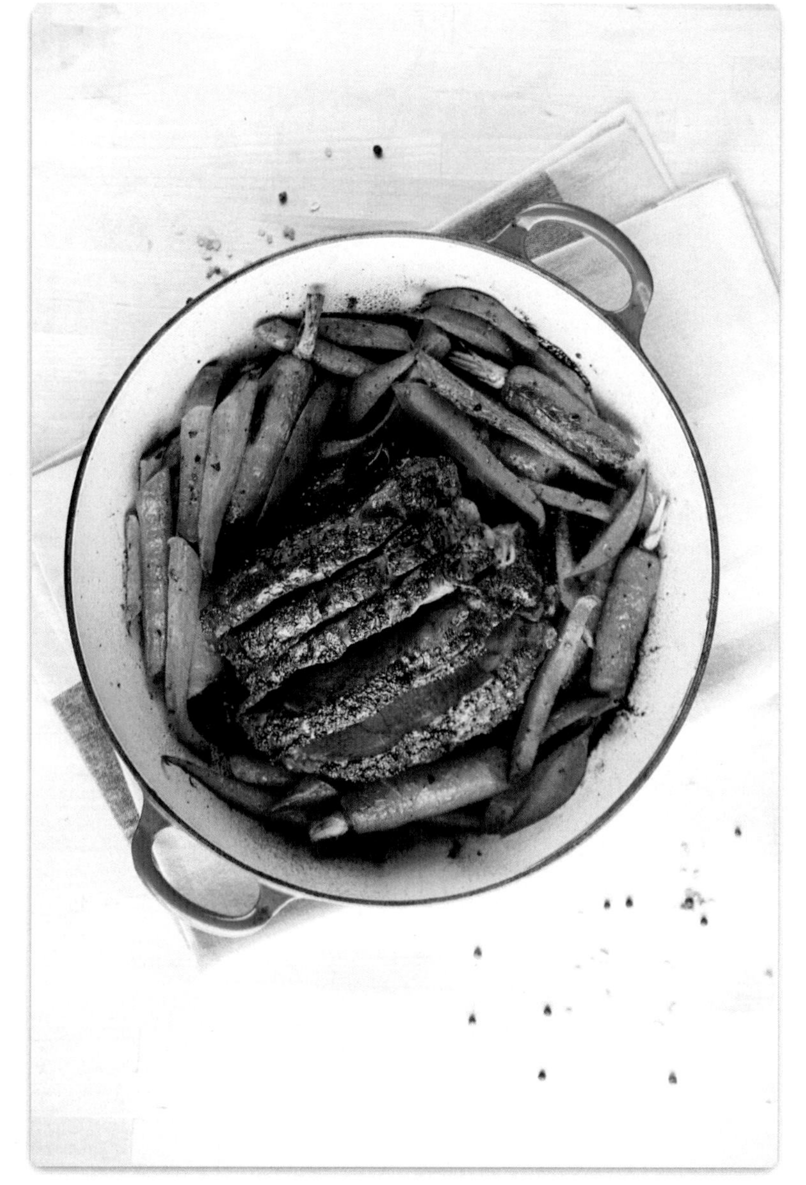

ROASTING

Roasting is a dry heat oven cooking method that might just be the easiest technique of all. To roast, all you need is a baking sheet of some sort, and a hot oven. Some ovens are hotter than others, but you generally want to roast in the 400 to 450°F range (you could probably set your oven for 425°F and throw away the knob). The first thing you need to learn how to roast is BACON! Yes, place bacon on your baking sheet and throw it into your hot oven for 15-25 minutes (all ovens run hotter or colder so keep a close eye on your bacon and the exact time for your oven may vary). Voilà—the fastest and easiest and most convenient and least messy bacon of your entire life!

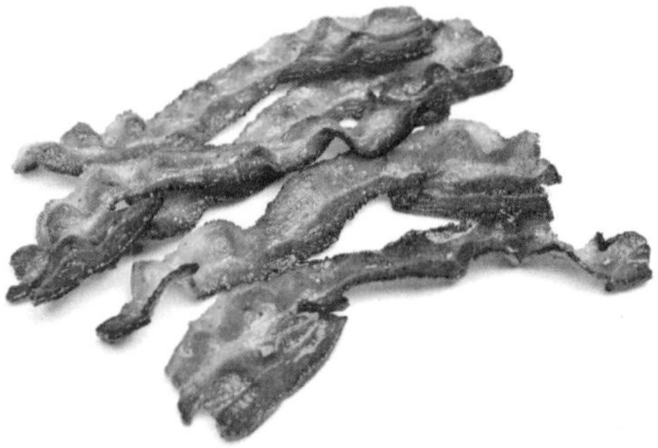

Roasting is a great technique for poultry but you can also roast pork loin, fish, vegetables, or beef using a roasting technique. For larger cuts, such as a whole chicken or a rib roast, you will definitely want to use your probe thermometer to check the internal temperature for doneness.

Roasting is a fantastic technique for certain vegetables, such as root vegetables, broccoli, Brussels sprouts, zucchini, summer squash, onions, cauliflower, bell peppers, mushrooms or really almost anything you can think of. Cut vegetables into even-sized pieces, based on density: a high-density root vegetable such as a potato should be cut into smaller pieces and a lower density vegetable such as broccoli should be cut into larger pieces, as both of these will then finish cooking at the same time. After you have cut up your vegetables, slick them with a small amount of fat (again, avocado oil is probably your very best choice) and spread them out

on your baking sheet. Use parchment paper if you are as lazy as we are and you want the easiest cleanup afterwards. Sprinkle your veggies with kosher salt and throw them into your preheated oven (again, 425°F would be a pretty good universal temperature) for 15-35 minutes. You will have to keep a close eye on these the first time you cook them because we

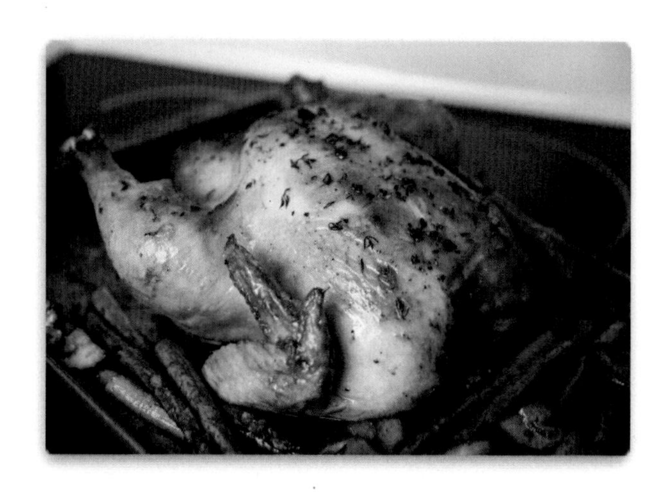

have no idea how hot your oven really gets and cooking times here can be highly variable!

Our favorite roasted vegetable? Hands down this would be Brussels sprouts. Cut these in half and place the cut sides down on baking sheet—the browning and caramelization that this produces is absolutely amazing!

If you want, you can also roast an entire sheet pan meal, complete with a protein and vegetables together—just pair a thin protein (chicken breast, shrimp, fish, etc) with cut-up vegetables so they both finish cooking at the same time. For more ideas, simply Google 'sheet pan dinners' and you will see what we are talking about here!

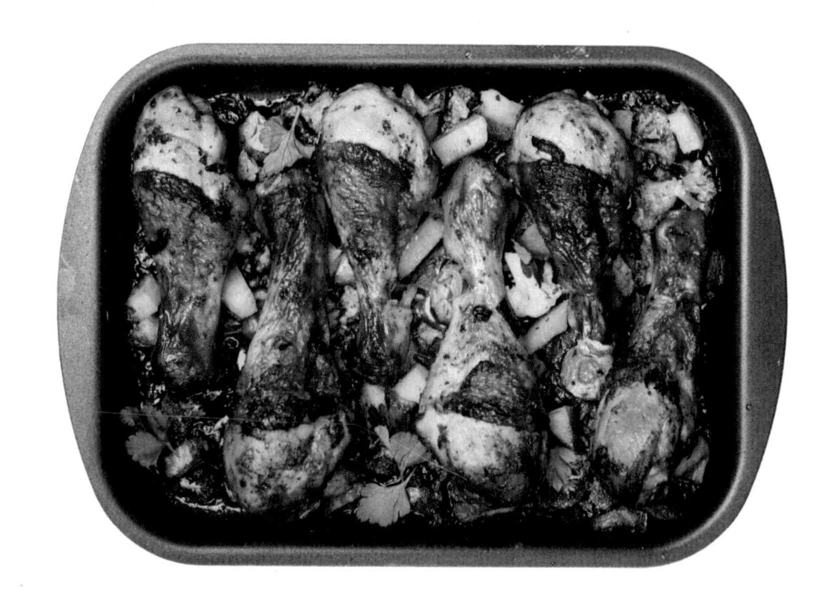

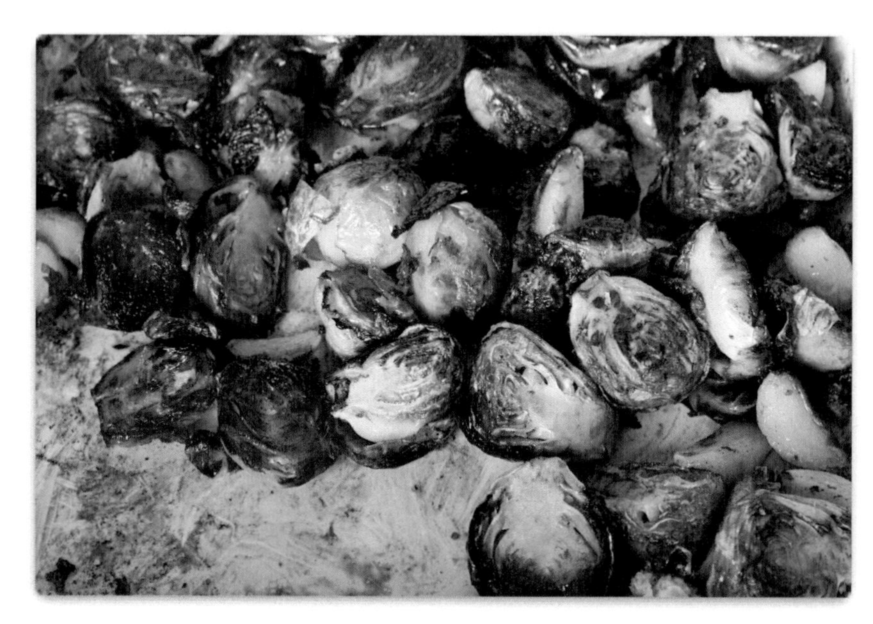

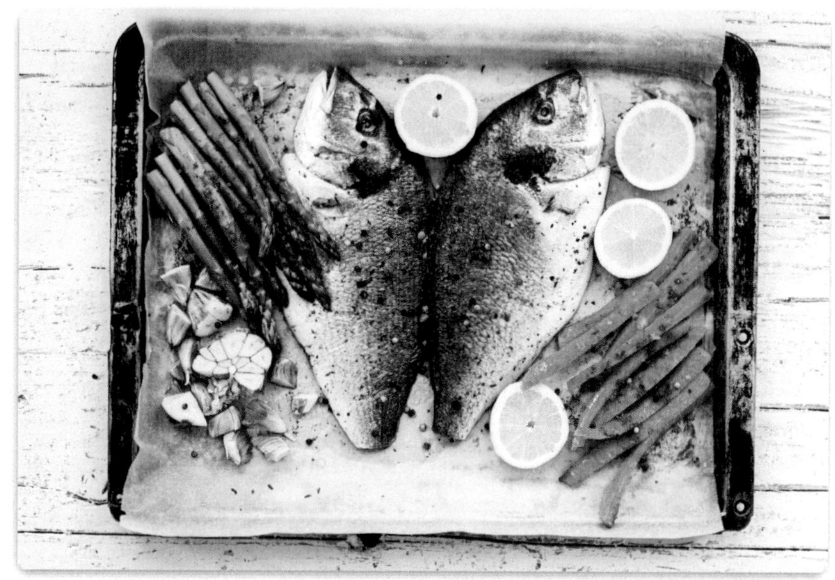

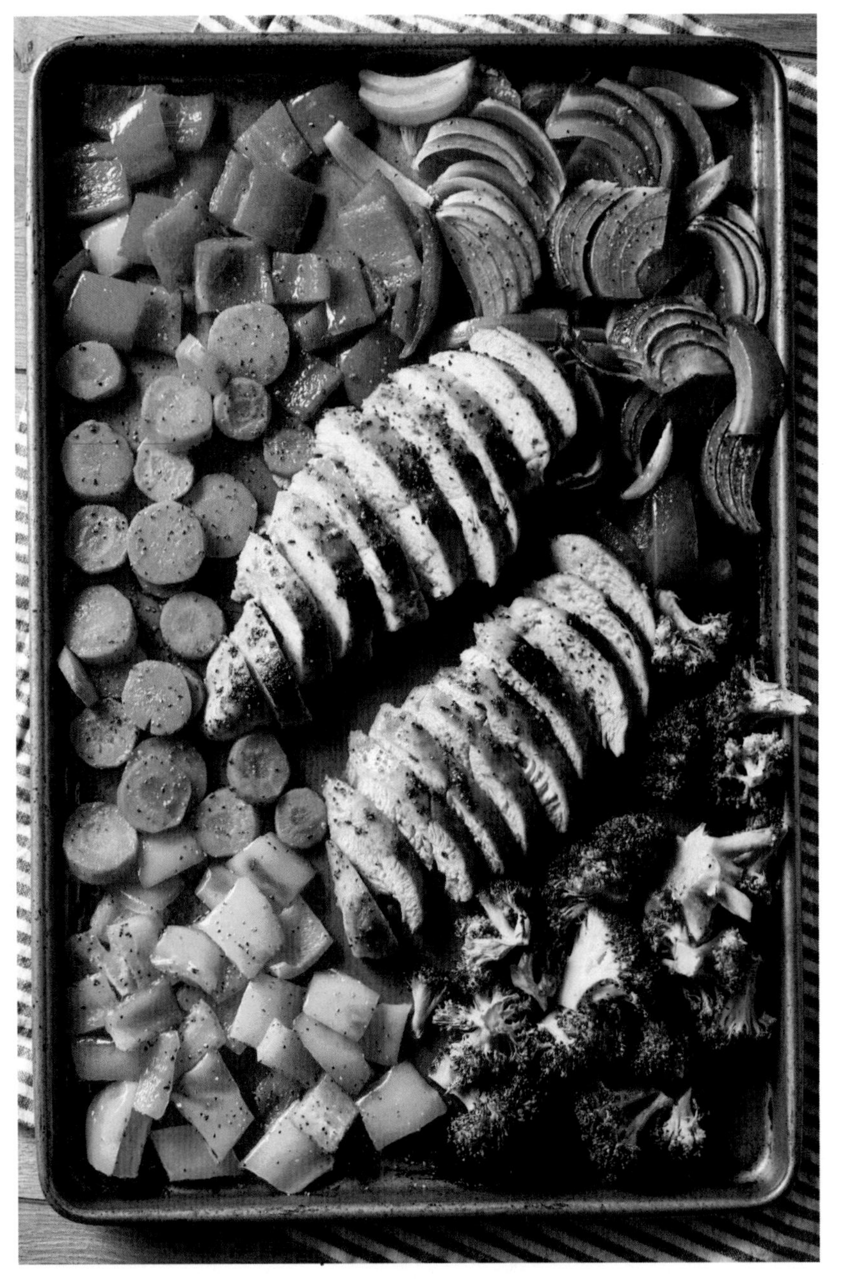

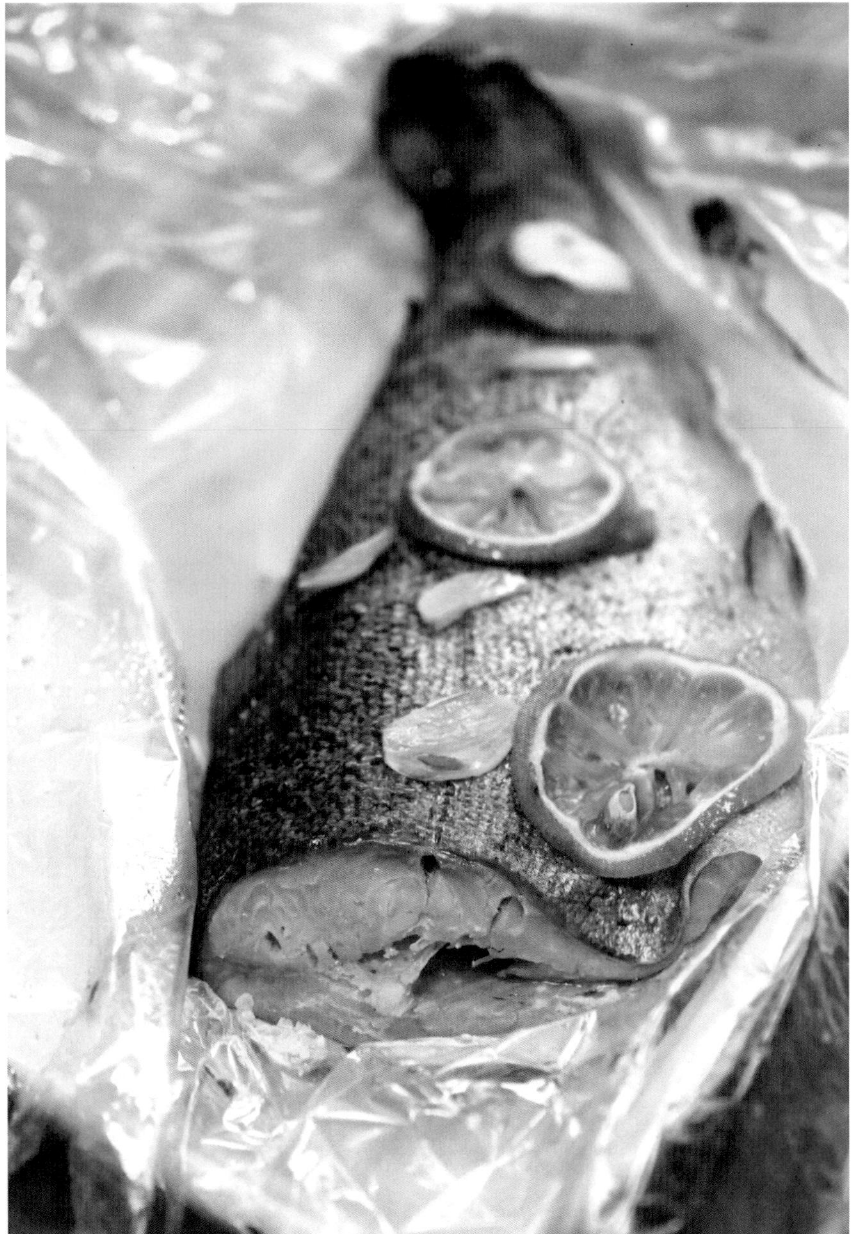

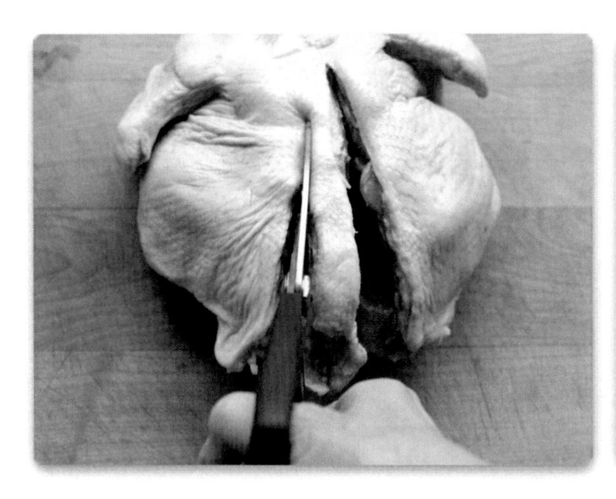

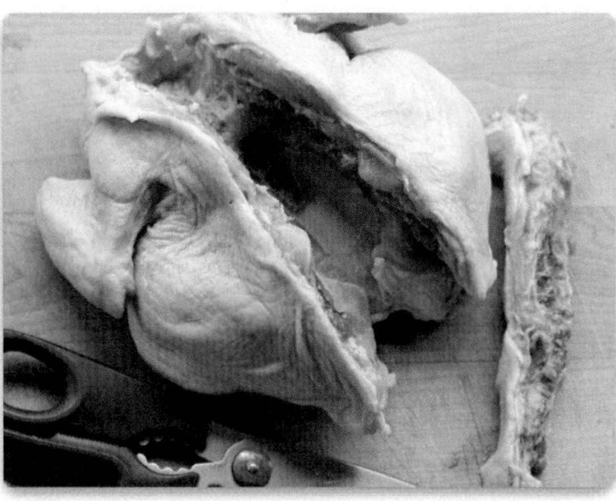

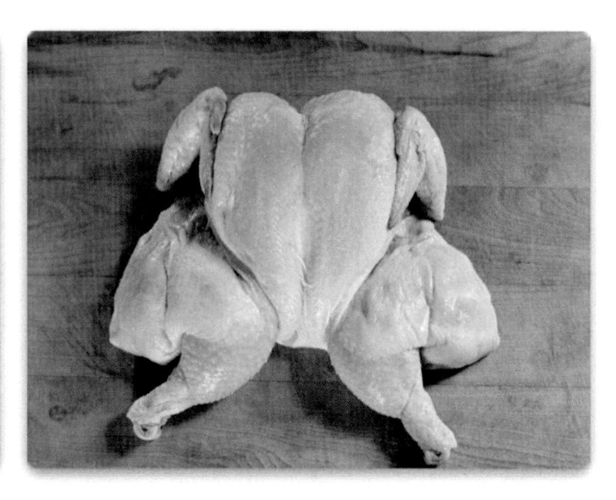

One of our favorite roasted proteins? Butterflied chicken! Flattening the chicken in this fashion causes it to roast faster and more evenly, and also leaves you with crispier skin. You will need a good pair of poultry shears, although in a pinch you can use any good sharp heavy kitchen shears or even those inexpensive trauma EMT shears that can cut a penny in half (you know the ones). Start by cutting out the backbone by cutting along its length on either side. Flip the chicken over, breast side up, and press down firmly on the breastbone to break it, flattening the bird. Lightly coat with avocado oil, then salt and any spices you want. Throw it on your baking sheet and toss it into your oven at your favorite roasting temperature (typically 425°F, but anything that starts with a '4' is probably good). This usually takes about 40 minutes to cook but you should use your temperature probe the first few times, since you really don't know what your oven is going to produce. Aim for a temperature of 165°F in the meatiest part of the thigh (not touching any bones). Let the bird rest a few minutes, then carve and enjoy!

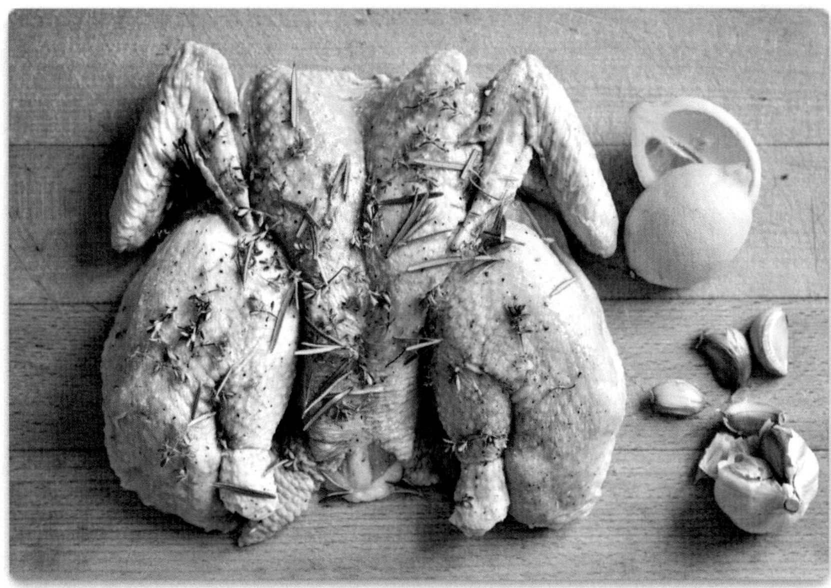

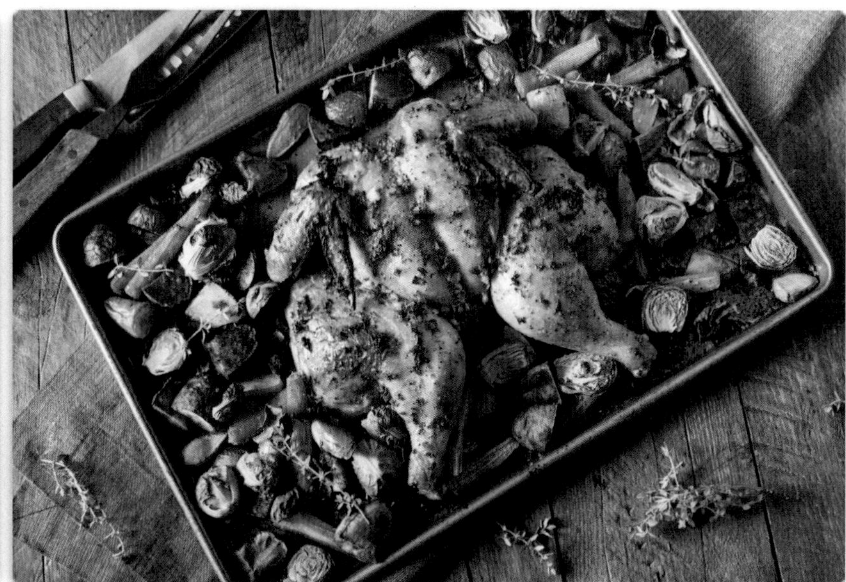

GRILLING

Cooking meat over an open flame is a ritual of religious proportions for every single culture on earth. Nothing else transcends race and language and unites homo sapiens together in such a universal manner. But grilling is more than just a sacred art in every corner of the globe—it is also one of the simplest ways to cook some of the very most amazing food.

Think of grilling as identical to pan-searing minus the exhaust fan and most of the clean-up! How to grill properly would easily take an entire book this size, but let's just say you owe it to yourself to invest the time and money into buying a good grill and then learning how to master it. These days, anyone can spend some time on YouTube and walk away with most of what you need to know.

The basic approach is the same as pan-searing. Get the grill nice and hot, then throw on some well-seasoned (with kosher salt, naturally) protein. Cook for a few minutes (variable based on temperature of the grill and thickness of your protein), then flip and cook the other side.

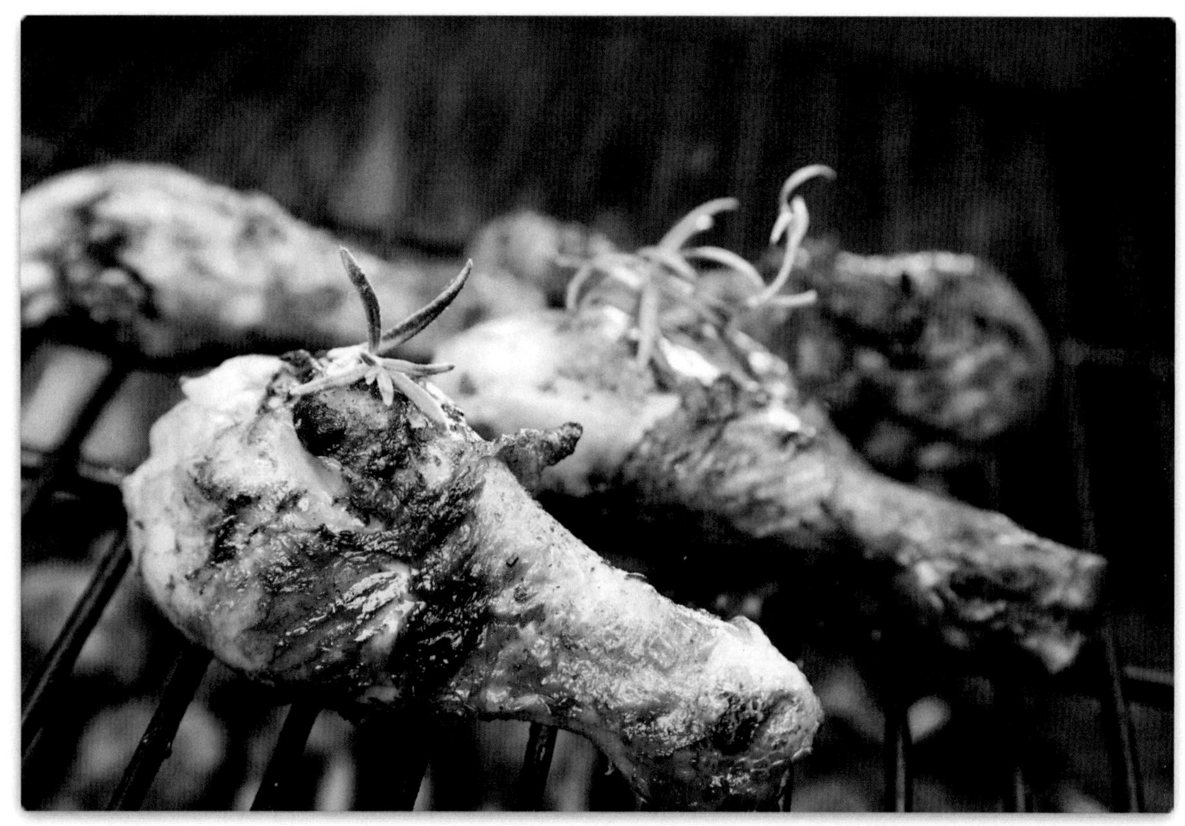

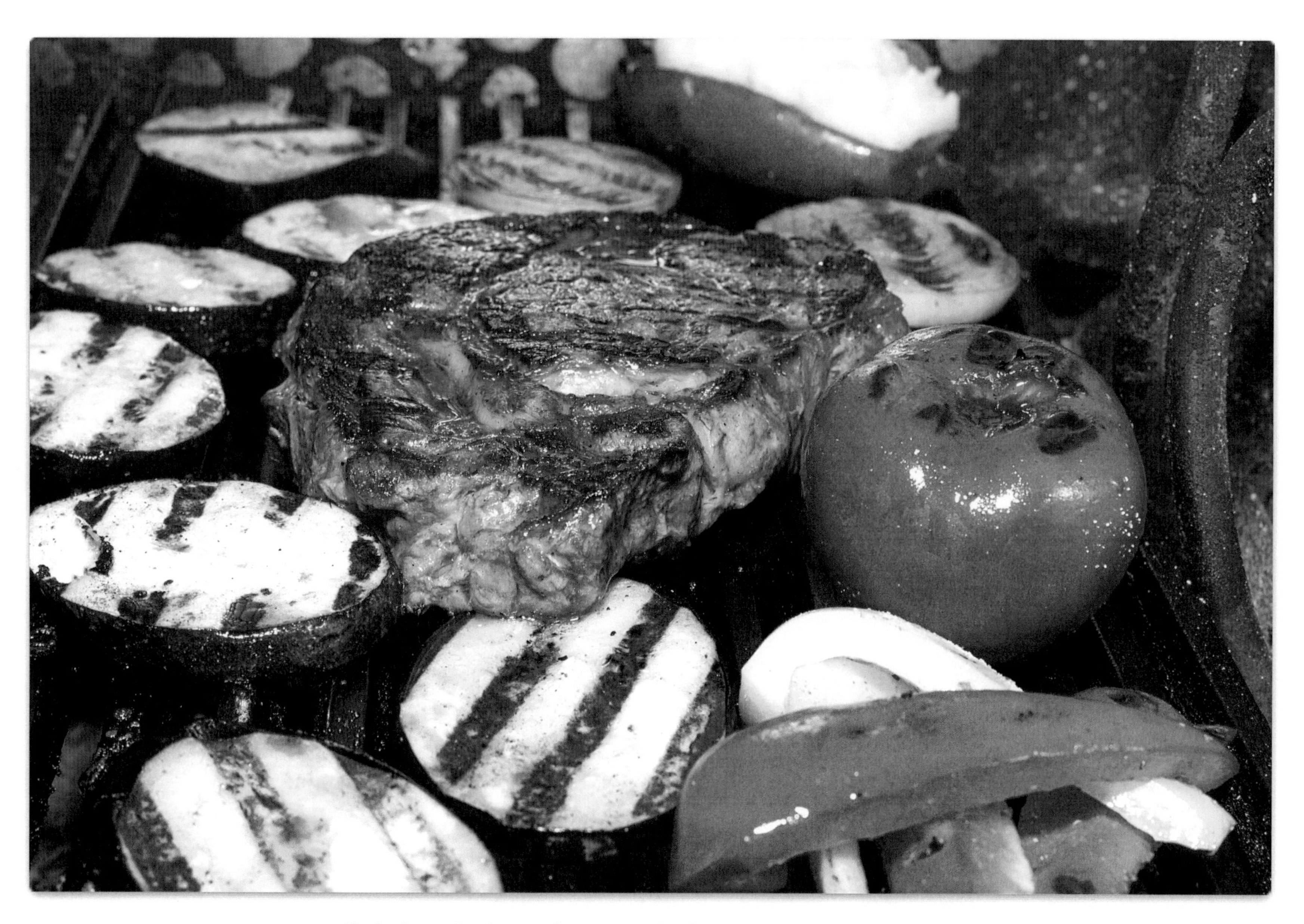

The basic template is meat plus some veggies. Peppers and zucchini grill very nicely!

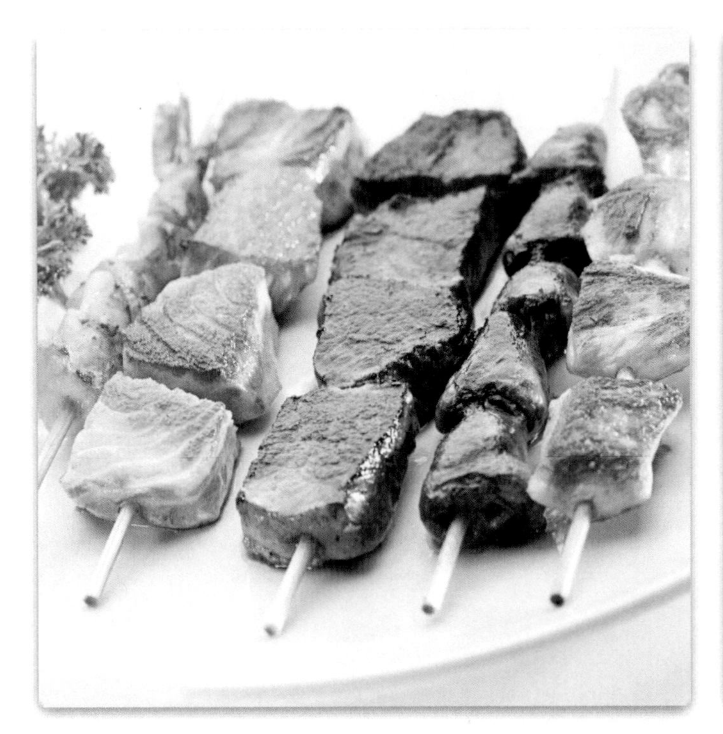
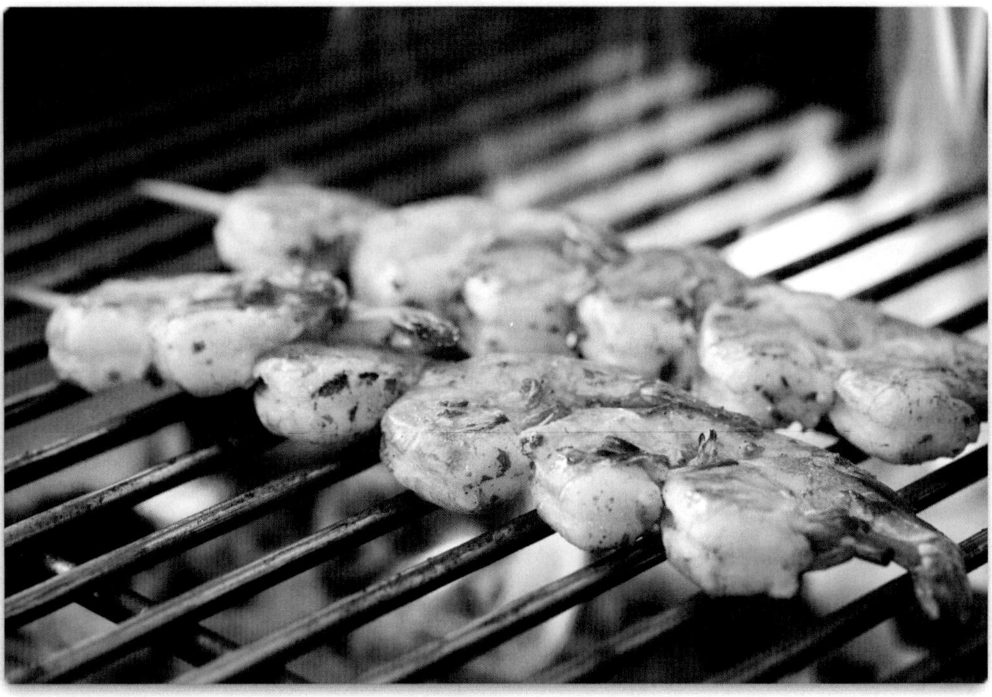

Kabobs are a great way to grill almost any kind of meat or vegetable. Cut food into even sizes and grab some skewers!

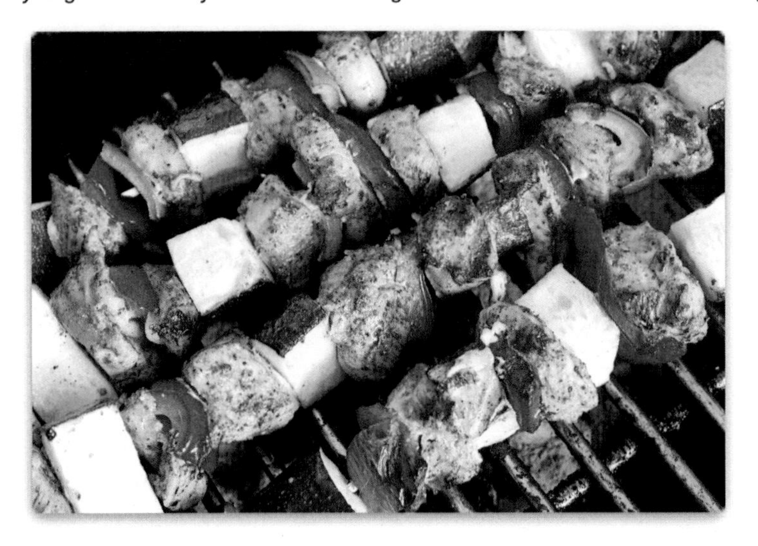

SIDE DISHES

A lot of people try to overcomplicate cooking. All you REALLY need is a high-quality protein, and everything else is optional. So don't feel the need to create some gourmet masterpiece with every meal. You also don't need a ridiculous number of side dishes or anything exotic. The main template is a nice properly raised, well-seasoned, perfectly cooked piece of protein, and then some sort of simple accompaniment. Your two fastest and easiest sides are either a vegetable (including a salad) or a low sugar fruit such as tomatoes or cucumbers or peppers. A bit of color makes your meals more appetizing (and likely healthier). Add a splash of acid such as lemon juice or vinegar (sherry vinegar is our favorite) to really liven up your taste profile.

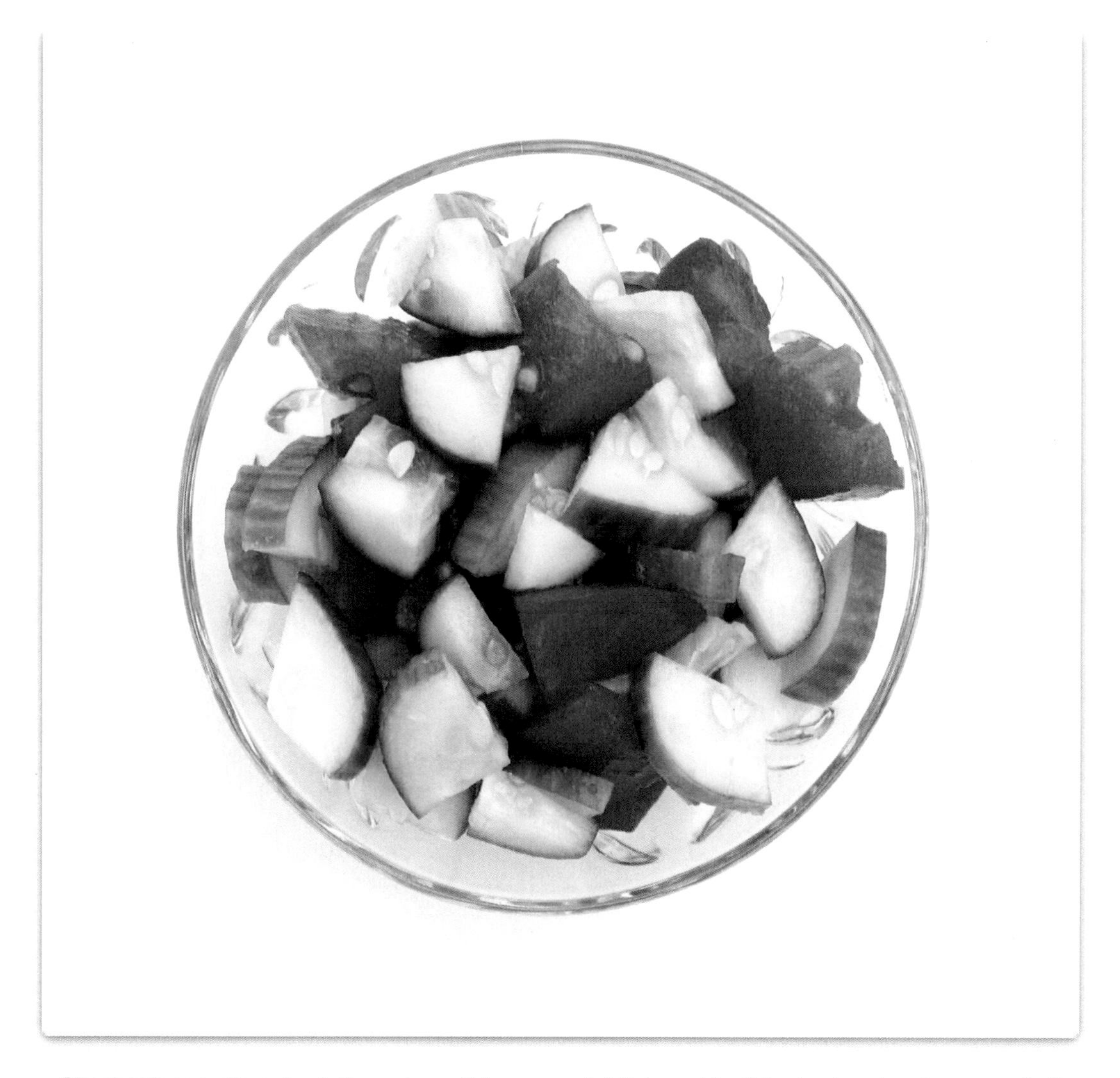

Simplest is sometimes best. For an incredibly easy and delicious side dish, simply cut up low sugar fruit such as cucumbers and tomatoes. Add a splash of acid—our favorite is sherry vinegar, but in a pinch you could use whatever vinegar you have. A squeeze of lemon or lime juice works as well!

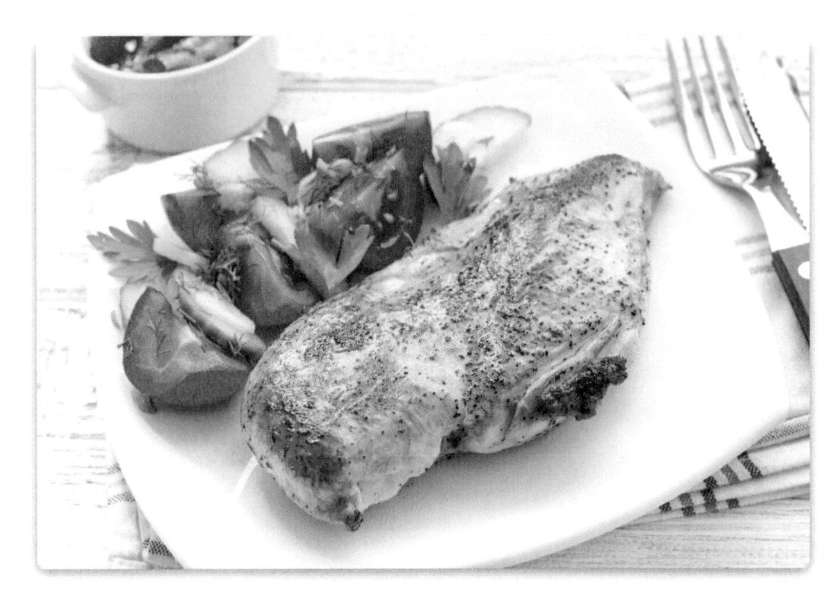

Low sugar fruit like tomatoes and cucumbers make an instant side dish.

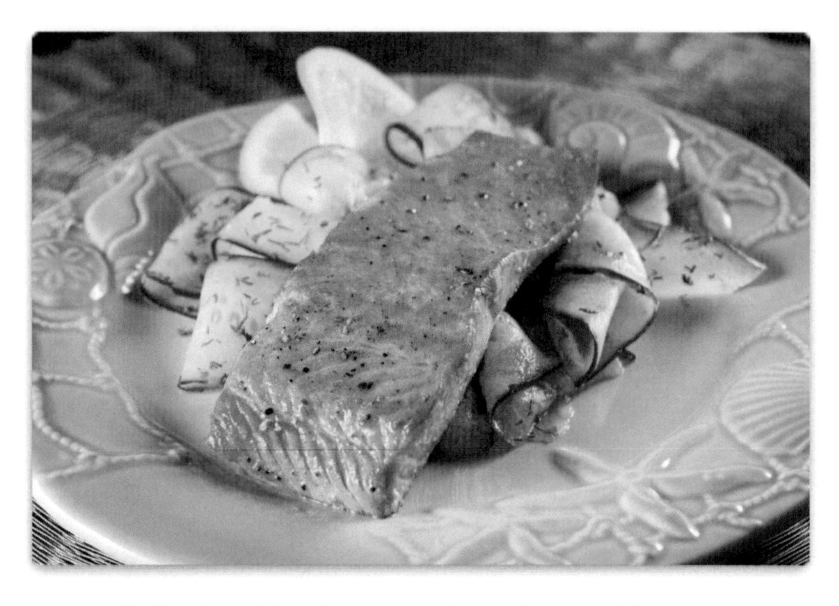

Feeling fancy? Attack your cucumber with a vegetable peeler!

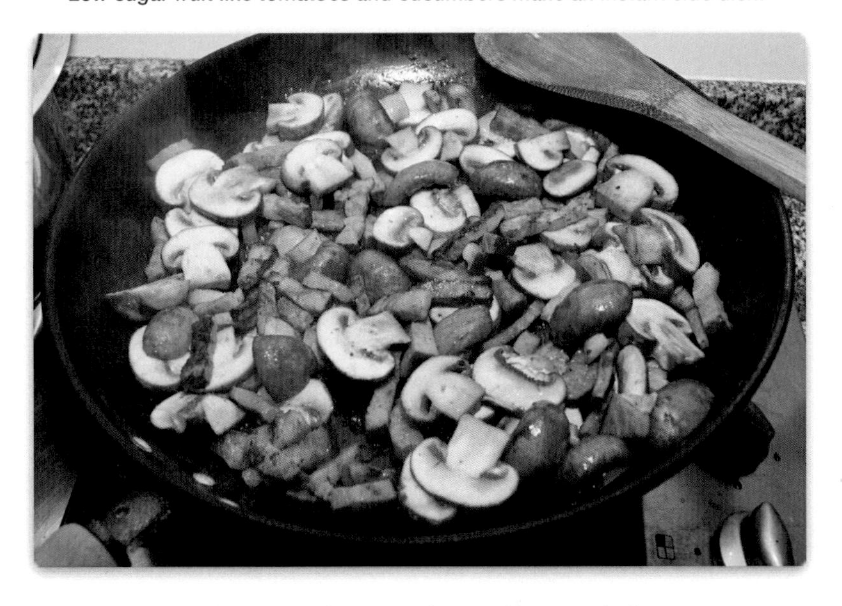

If you have time to cook something, sautéed mushrooms are an EXCELLENT side dish!

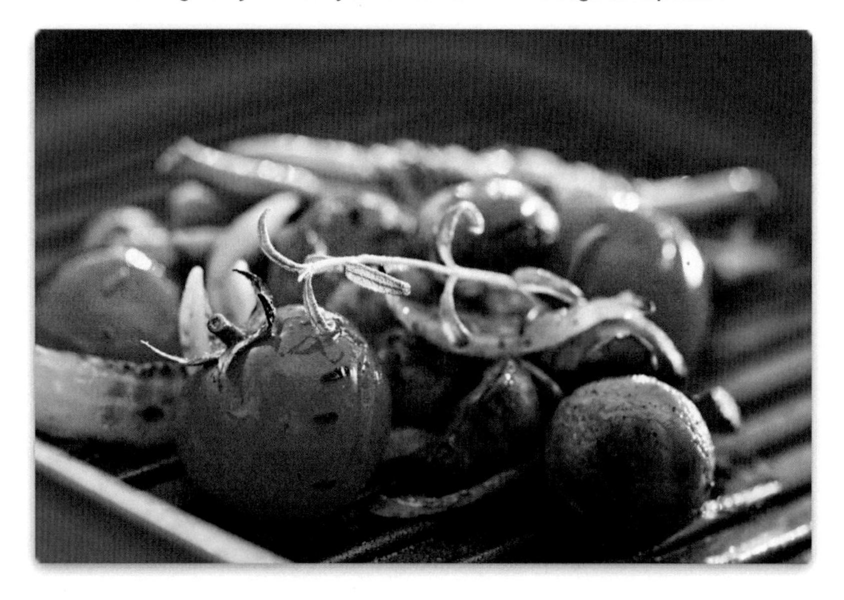

In addition to mushrooms, you can sauté onions, cherry tomatoes, or pretty much any vegetable or low sugar fruit you want!

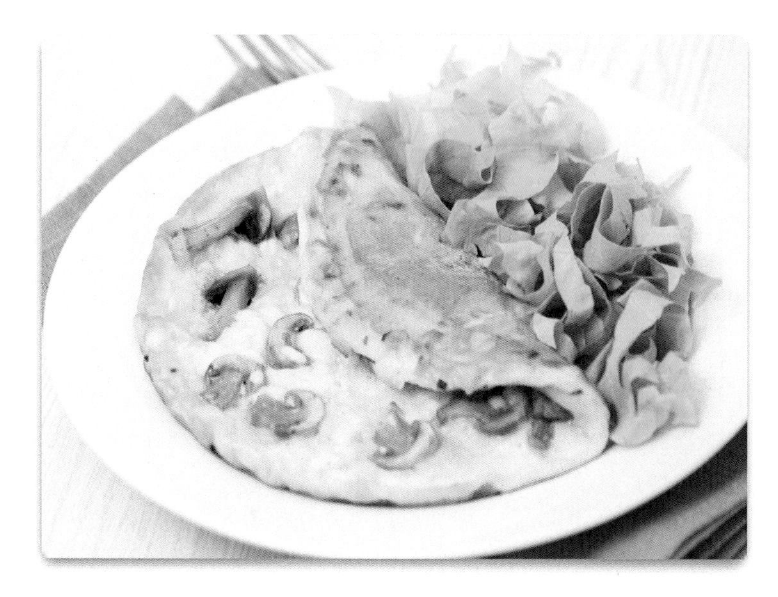

Even just plain lettuce could make your meal more interesting. But once again, you might want to add a splash of sherry vinegar.

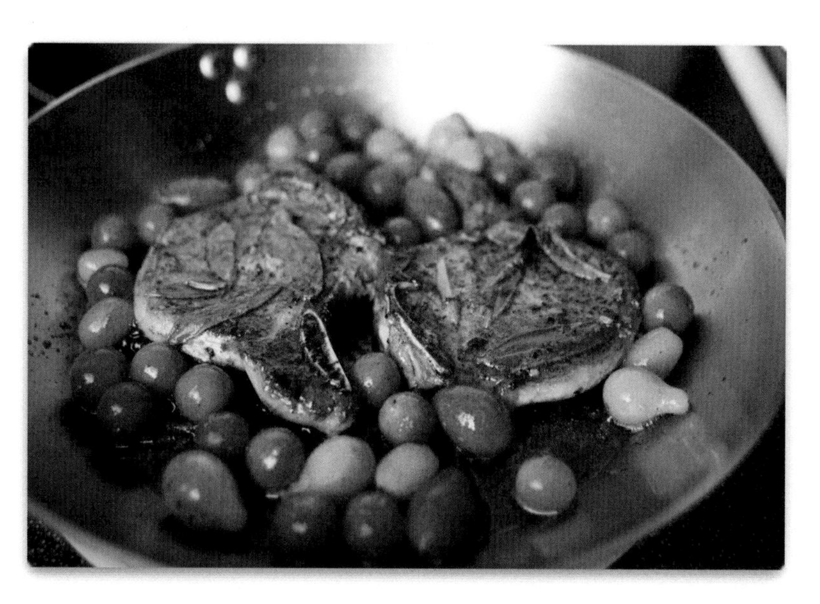

Cherry tomatoes cook in no time and add a nice dimension and some color to any dish.

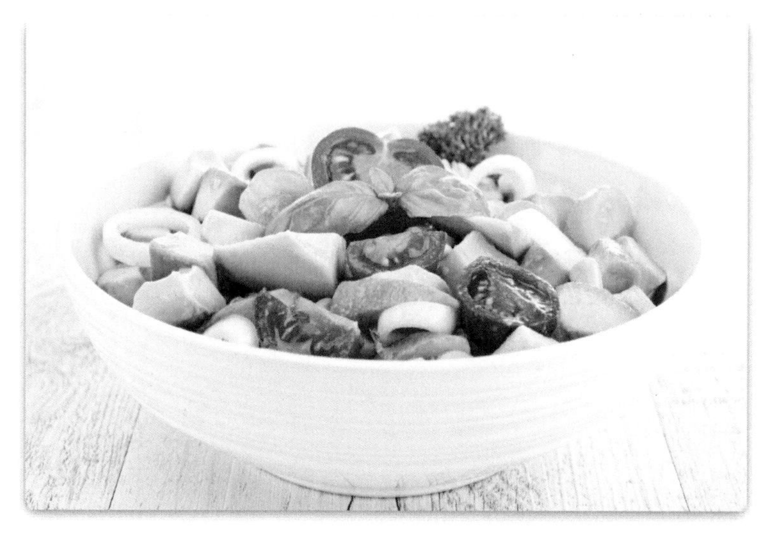

More low sugar fruit: avocado plus cherry tomatoes. Take this simple salad to the next level with a splash of sherry vinegar, a sprinkle of salt, and a little sliced allium (onions, shallots, leeks, scallions, chives, etc).

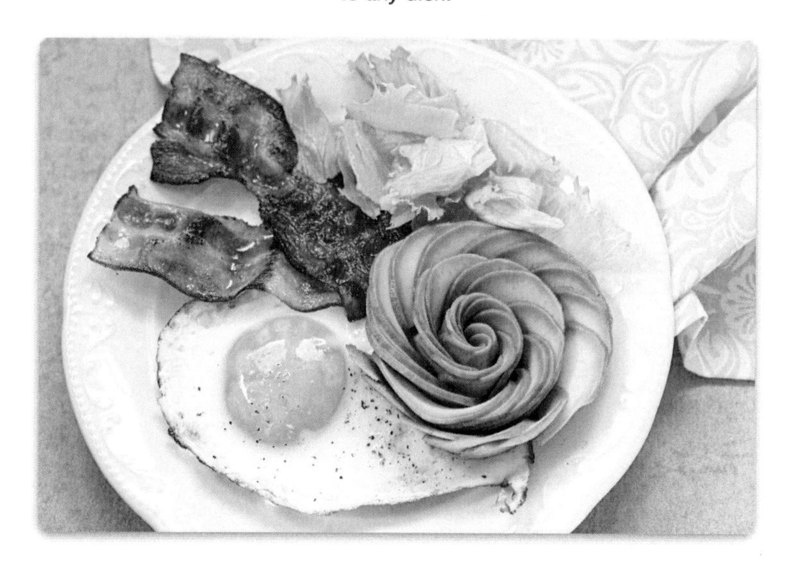

In a pinch, just throw in some slices of avocado and you're done!

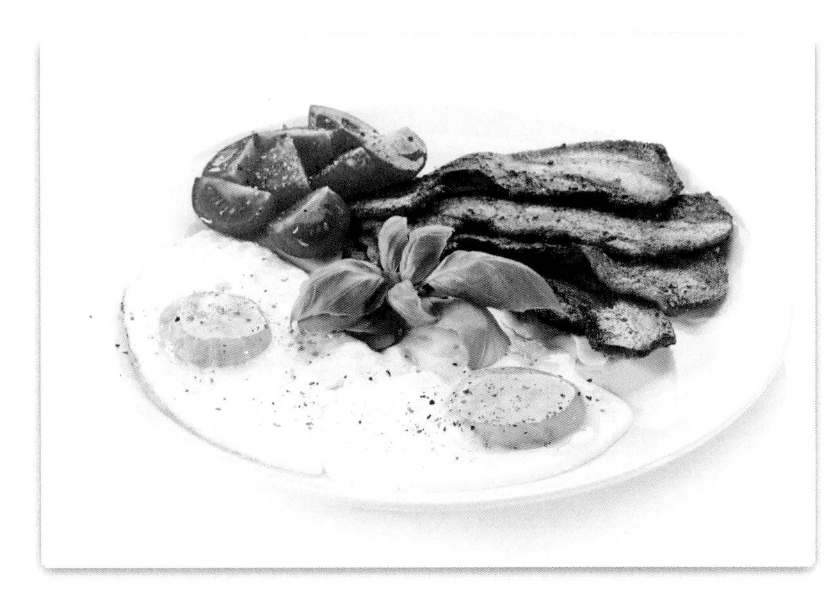

Just a sliced tomato and a sprig of basil? Yes—this works!

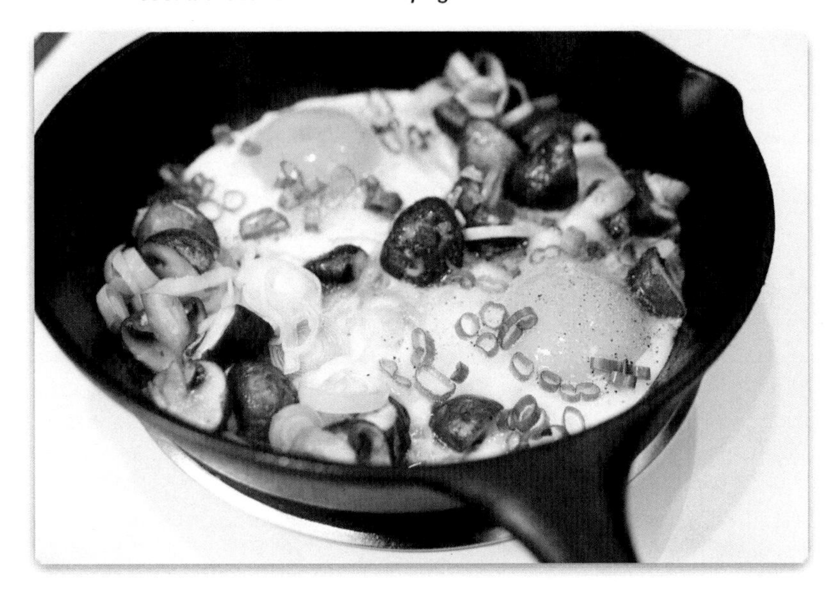

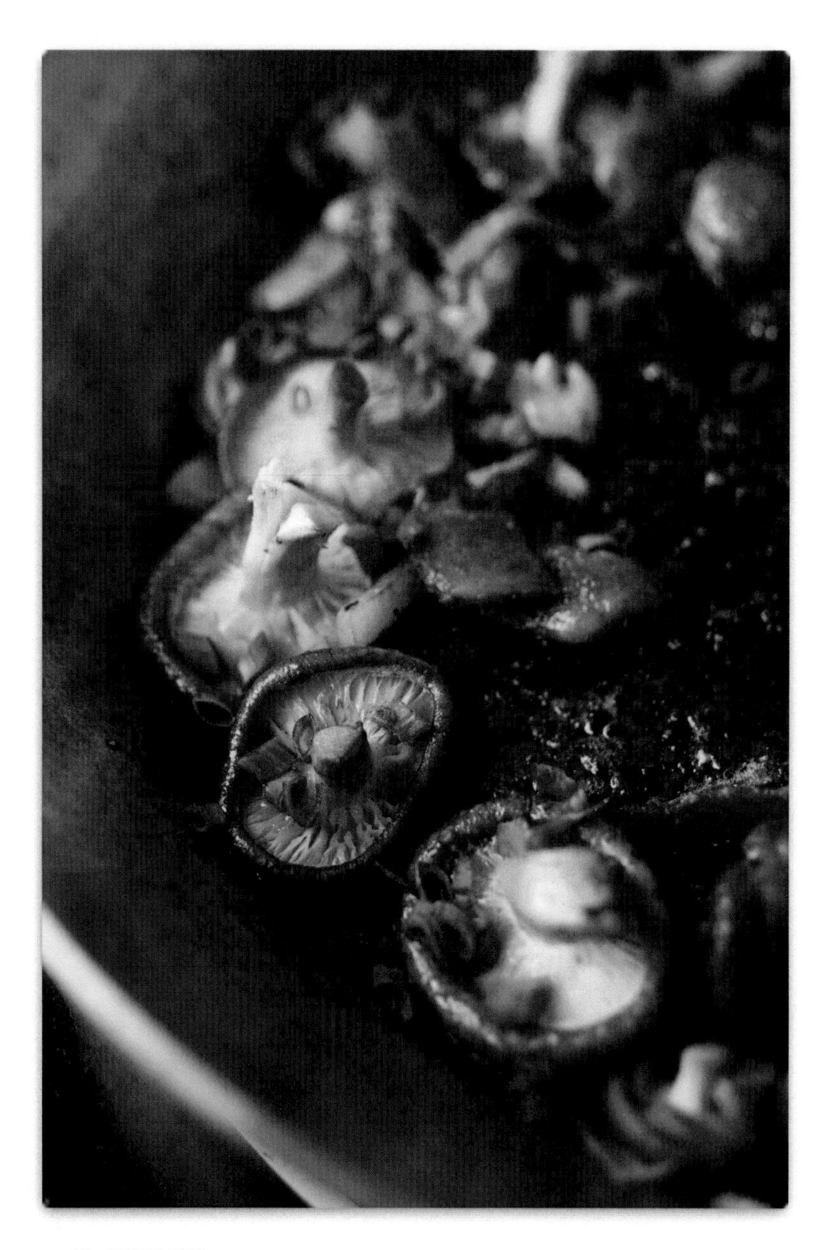

Sautéed mushrooms and scallions go with ANYTHING.

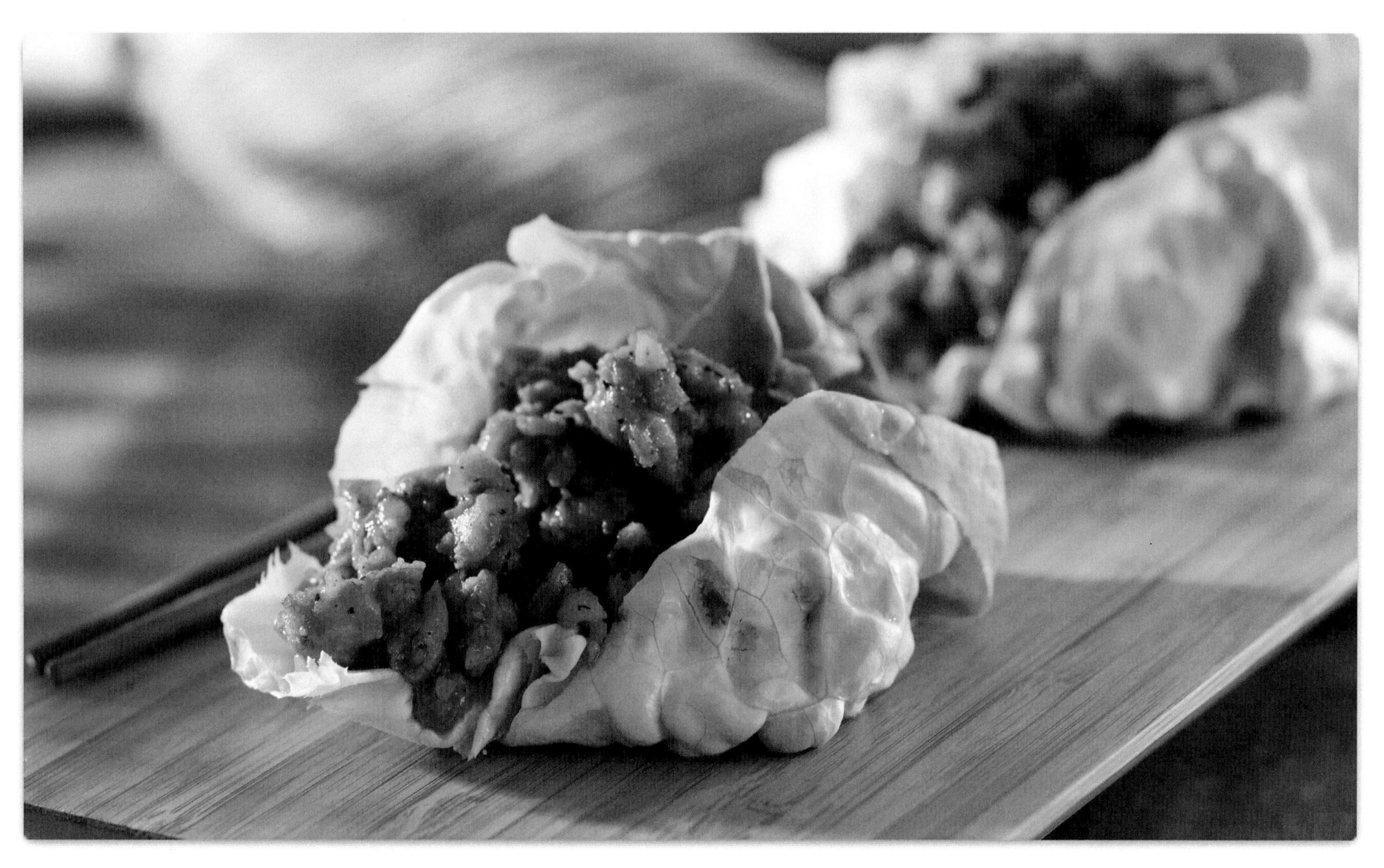

Wrap something in lettuce (in this case, sautéed ground chicken with some onions and a splash of soy sauce) and you don't even need another side! Is this cheating? Yes. Do we care? No.

NON-COOKING IDEAS

We get it. You don't always feel like cooking anything at all, nor do you always have time. In these situations, it really helps to have some proteins around that you can throw together in virtually no time. Try to keep things on hand like hard boiled eggs, cooked chicken breasts, sliced deli meat, canned salmon, and higher protein lower fat cheeses (try a mozzarella or Swiss from skim milk—these have an excellent P:E ratio and still taste spectacular).

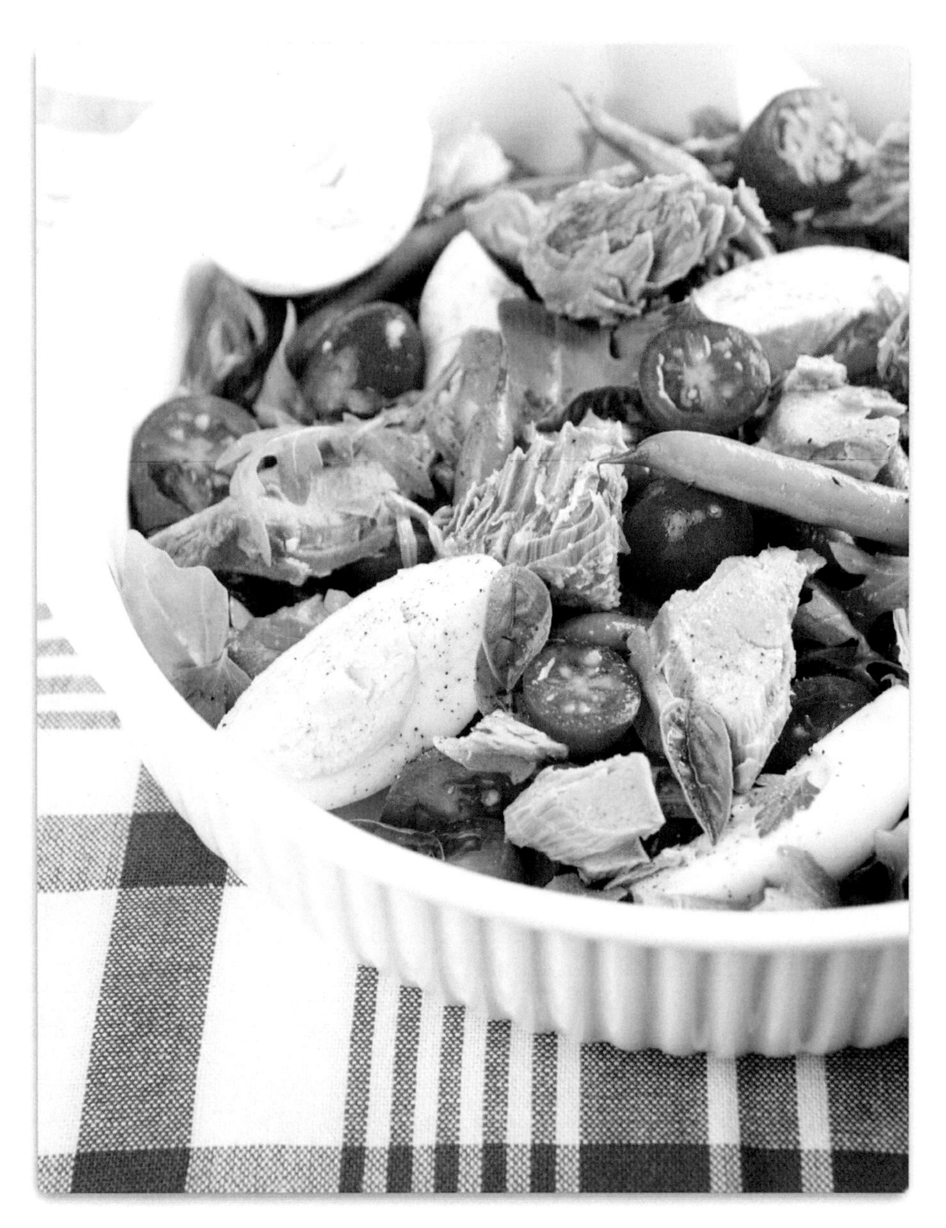

With canned salmon and hard boiled eggs on hand, you can make a quick high protein salad in no time at all.

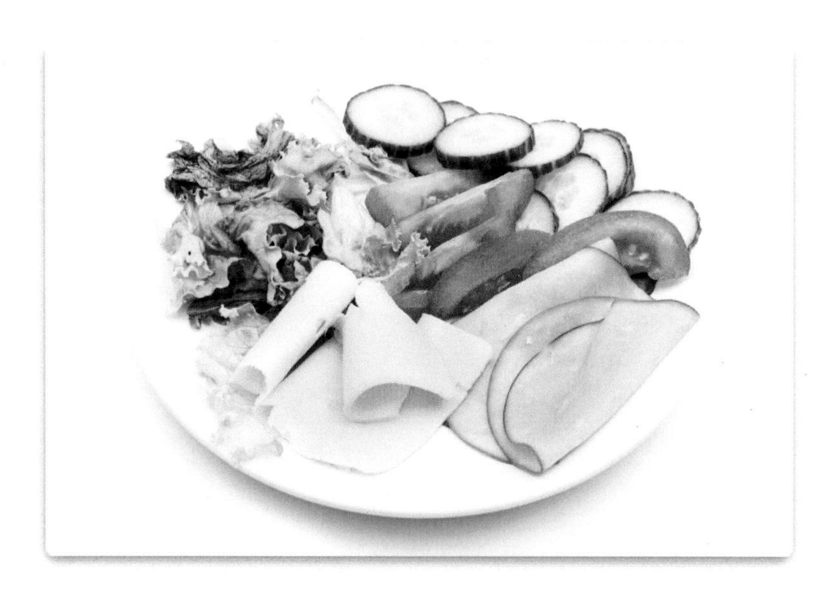

Try slices of deli meat and cheese. Low fat Swiss cheese has higher grams of protein than fat.

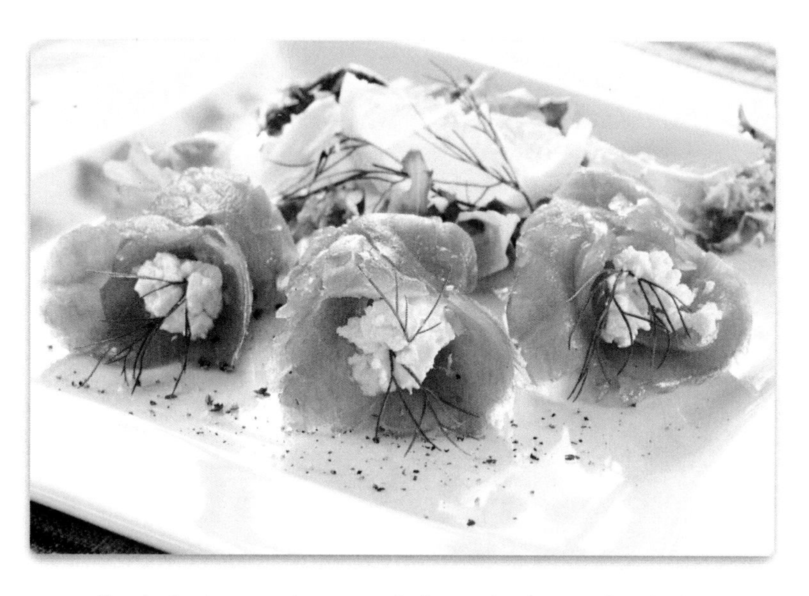

Smoked salmon and some goat cheese. Looks amazing, tastes amazing, is ridiculously healthy, and takes 30 seconds to make.

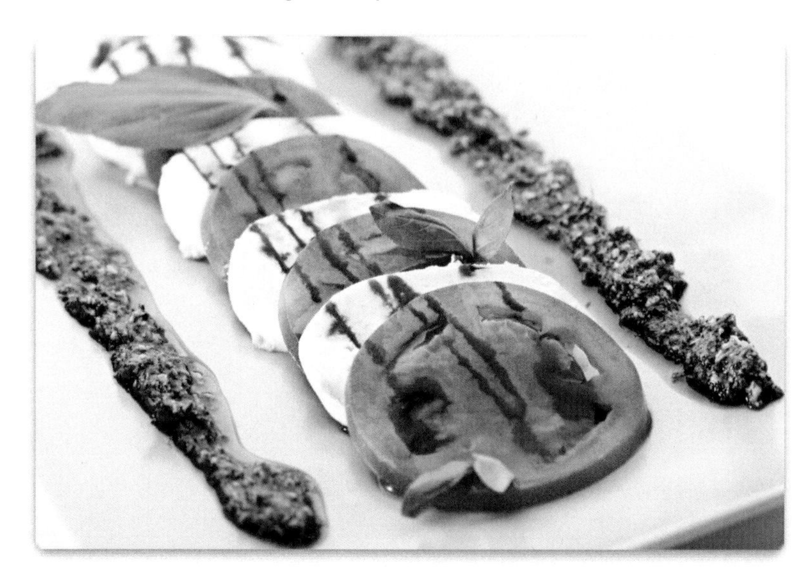

Fresh mozzarella has a great P:E ratio. Add slices of tomato, a little basil, and a drizzle of olive oil and balsamic vinegar.

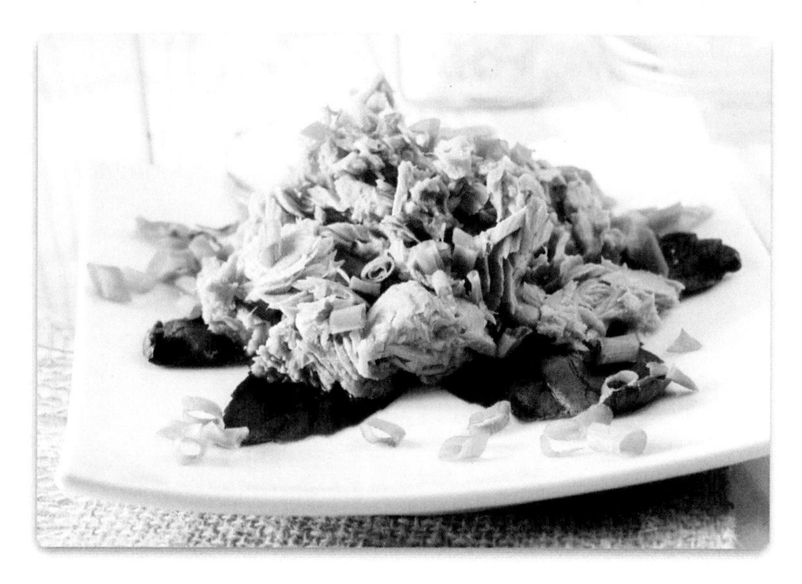

Even a can of tuna becomes more appetizing if you chop up some scallions for crunch and color and flavor.

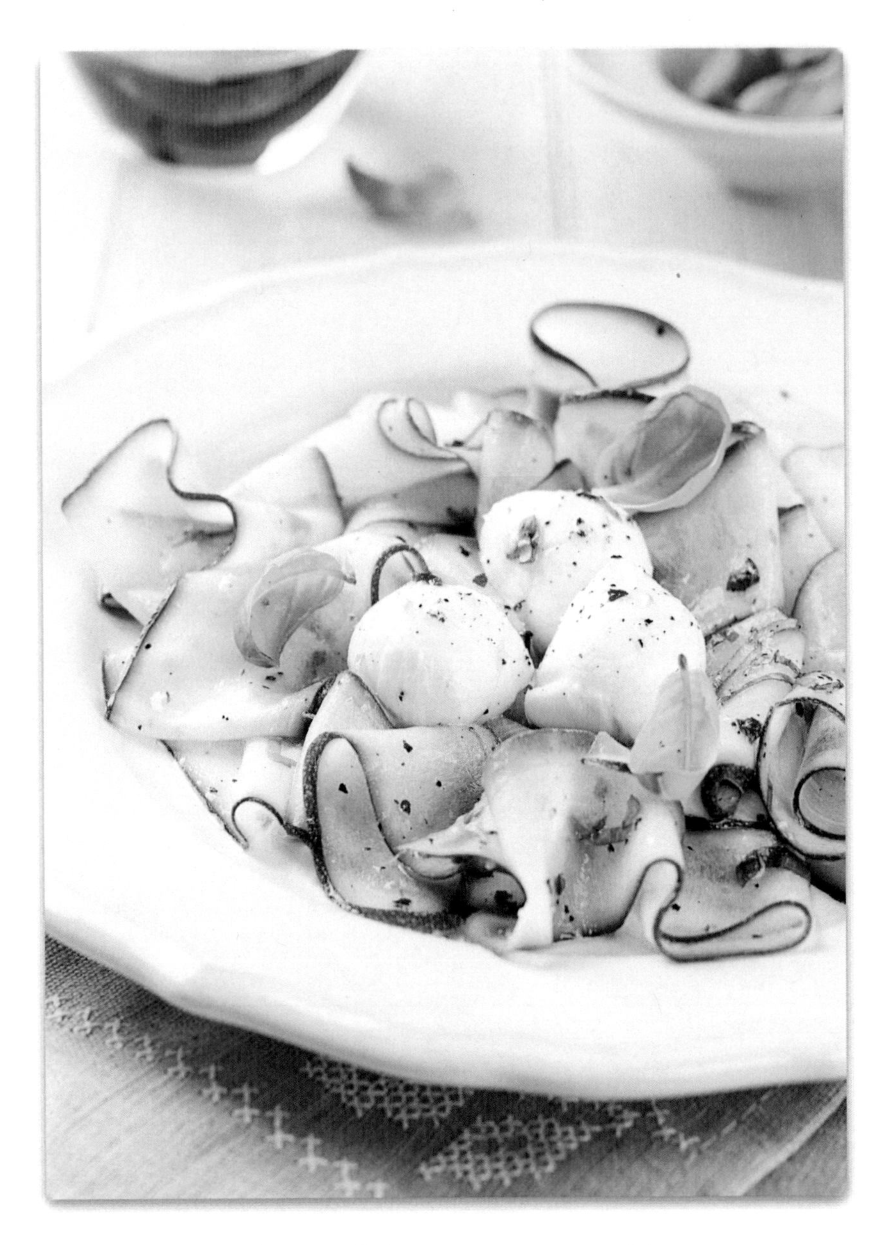

Fresh mozzarella is a great emergency protein.

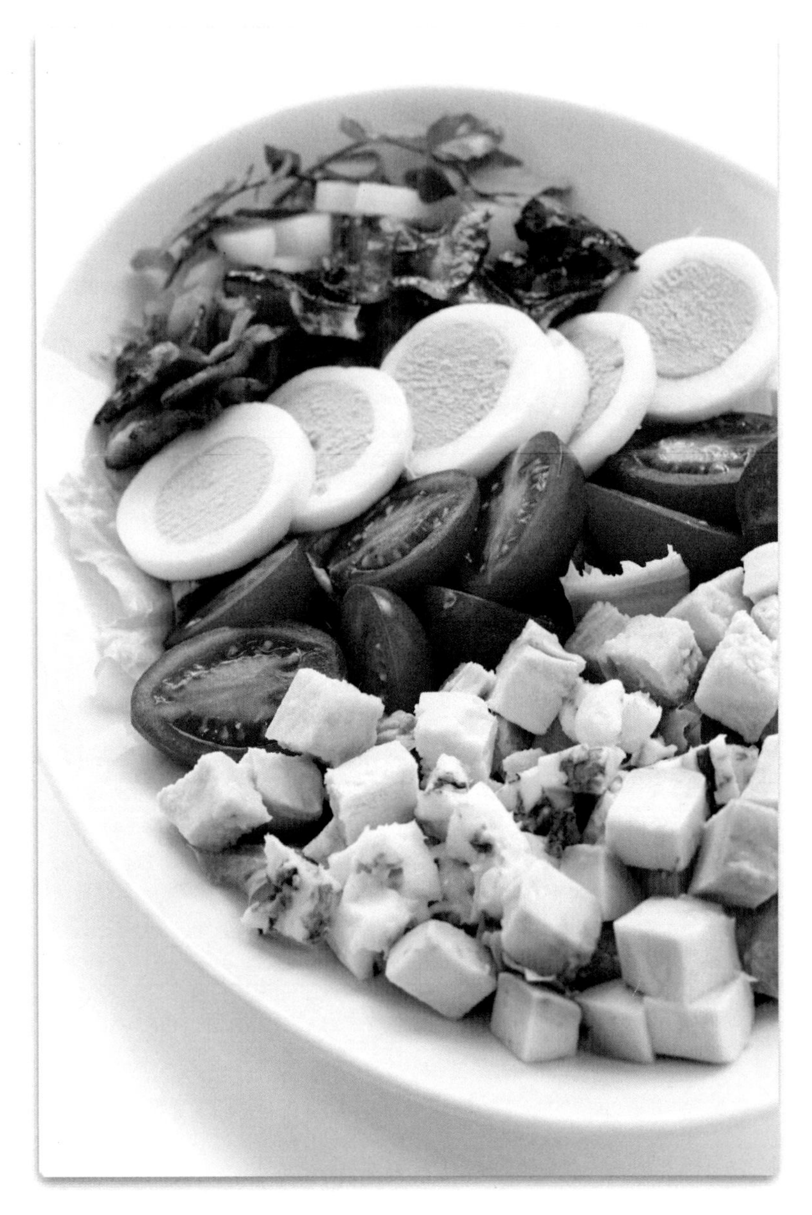

If you have some leftover chicken breasts and hard boiled eggs in your refrigerator, you can make a Cobb salad in no time.

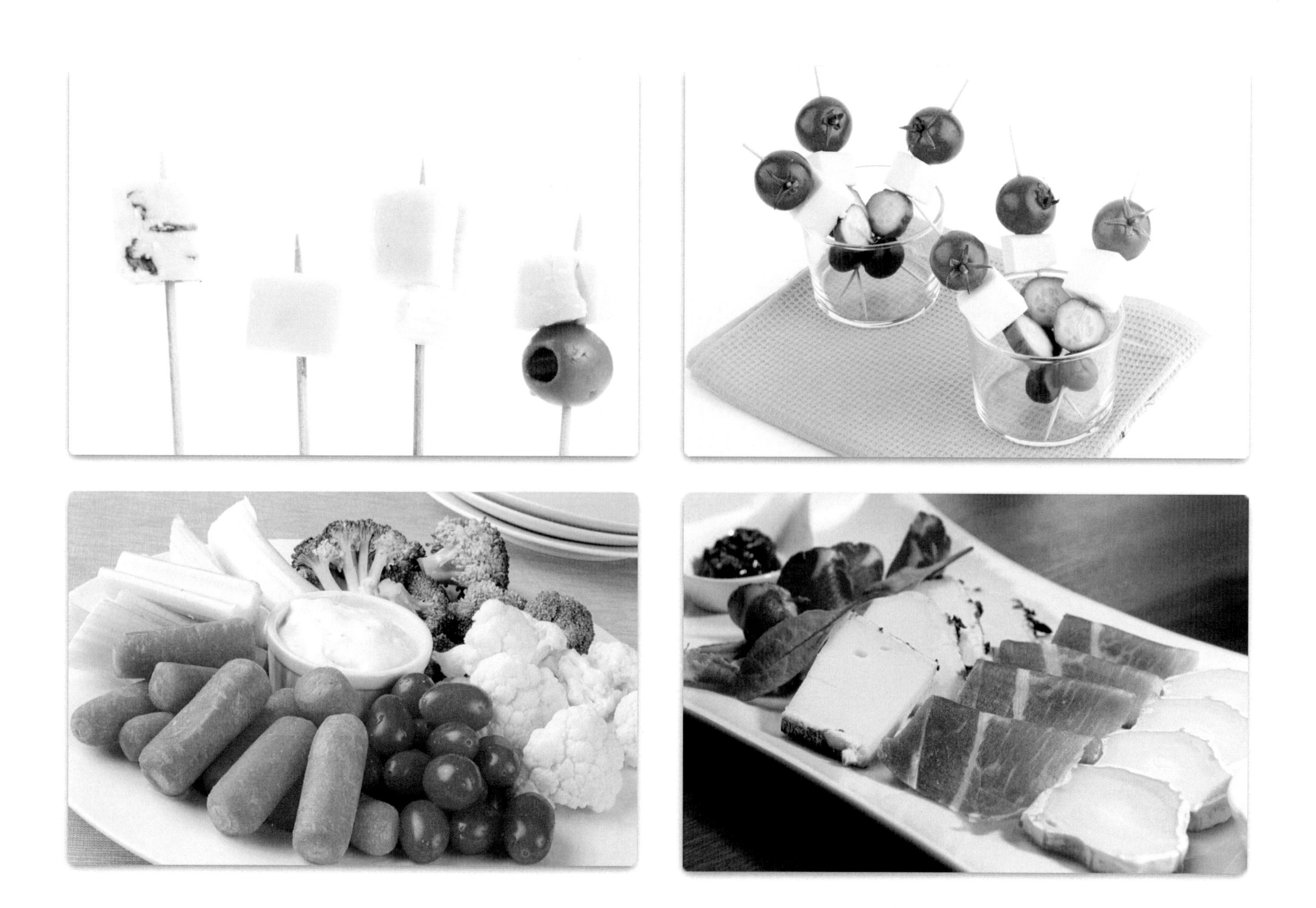

Crudités, charcuterie, and assorted cheeses are always an option!

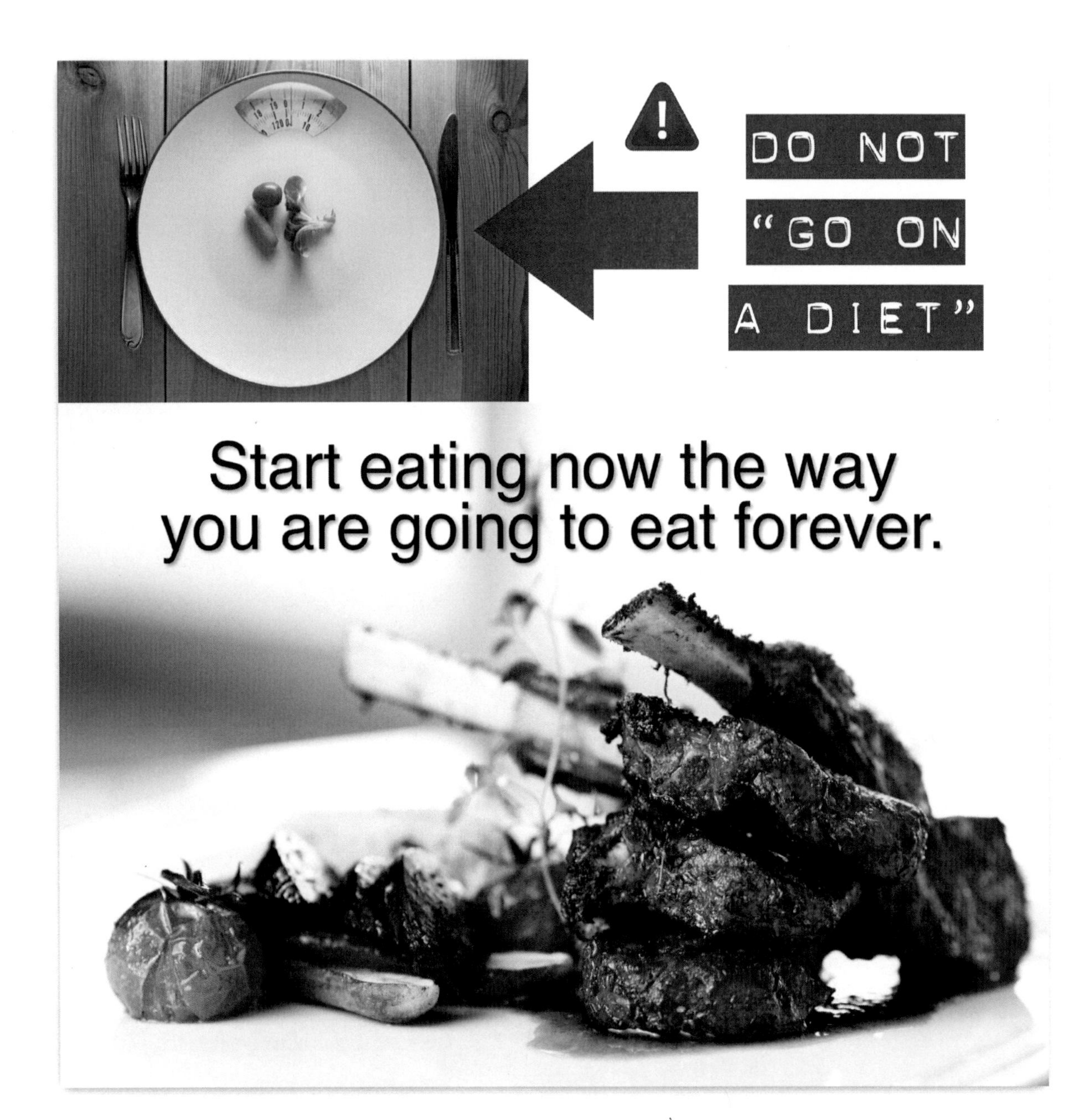

Eating is a lifelong endeavor, not something with a 'stop' date. Make sure you enjoy the process!

RECIPES

For those of you who want some specific recipes, we have included a few on the following pages. Please feel free to change these in any way to your liking! This is part of the beauty of cooking your own food.

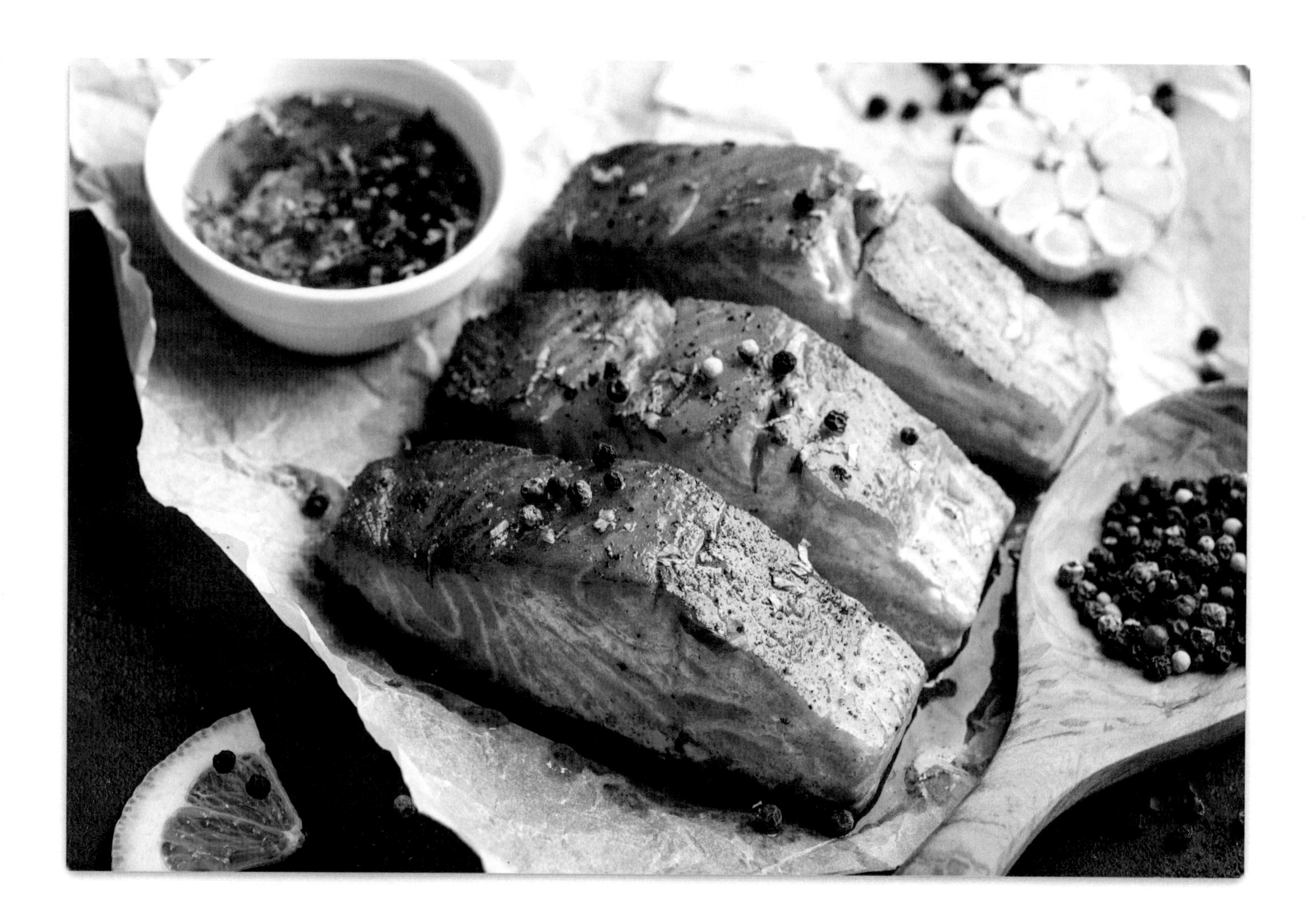

RECIPE: ROASTED SALMON

Ingredients:

- 10 oz wild-caught Alaskan salmon
- 2 tsp olive oil
- 1 tsp Tarragon leaves
- 1 tbsp chopped chives

Directions:

1. Preheat oven to 425°F. While oven is preheating, chop chives.
2. Rub salmon with olive oil and season with salt and pepper. Roast, skin side down on a foil-lined baking sheet in upper third of oven until fish is cooked throughout—roughly 12 minutes.
3. Cut salmon in half crosswise then plate. Season salmon with herbs.

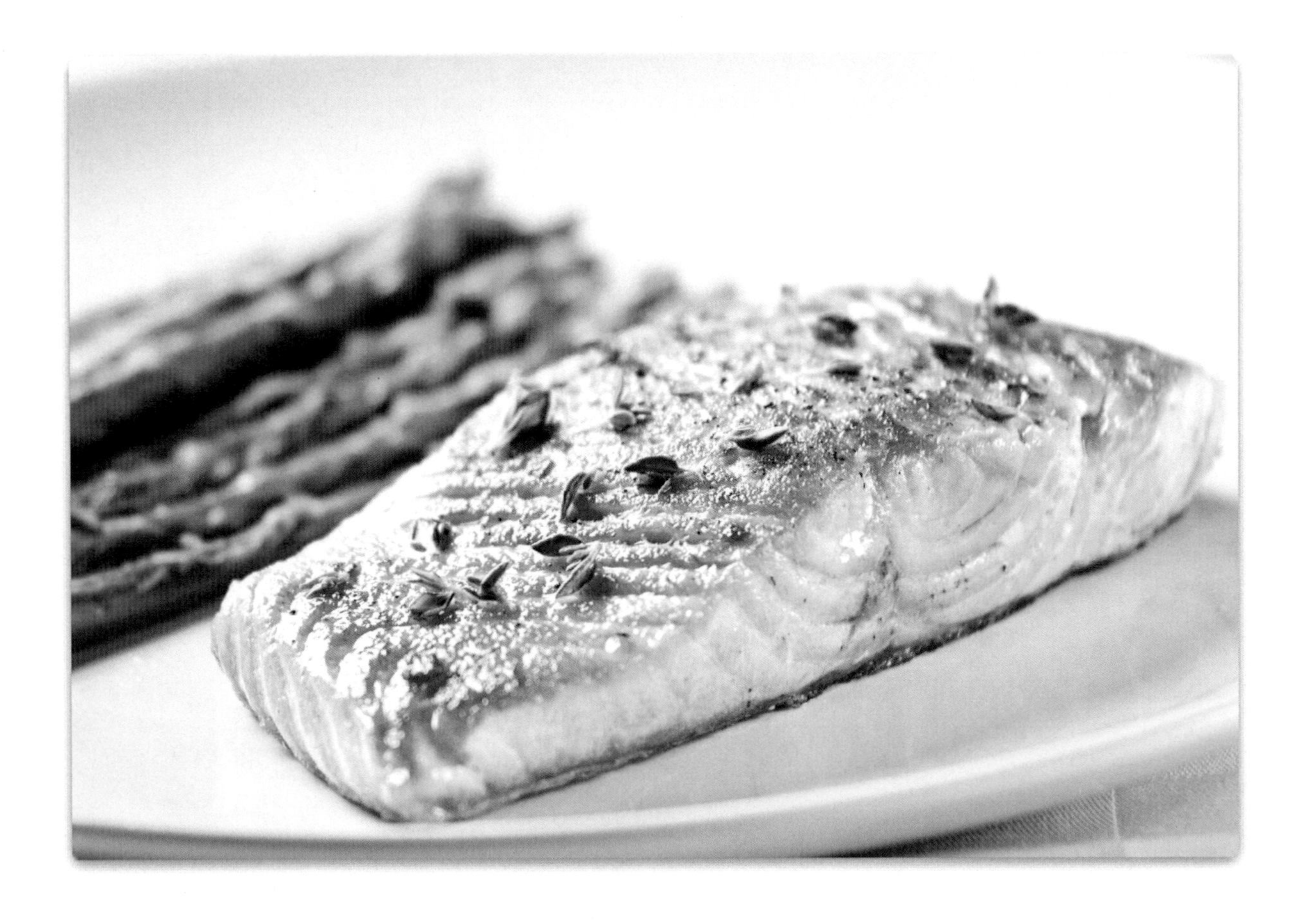

RECIPE: NEW YORK STRIP STEAK

Ingredients:

- 8 oz New York strip steak
- 1 tsp salt
- 1/4 tsp pepper
- 1 tsp olive oil

Directions:

1. Season the steak on both sides with salt and pepper. Rub both sides with olive oil and set aside.
2. Heat frying pan over high heat for 3-4 minutes. Place steak in the pan and let cook for 3-4 minutes, until dark crust begins to form on the bottom.
3. Using tongs, flip the steak and let cook for another 3-4 minutes, until medium rare. To check the steak, press with a fork. It should be firm on the outside and give in the center. With a thermometer, it should read 125°F—130°F.
4. Transfer steak to cutting board and let cool for 5 minutes before plating.

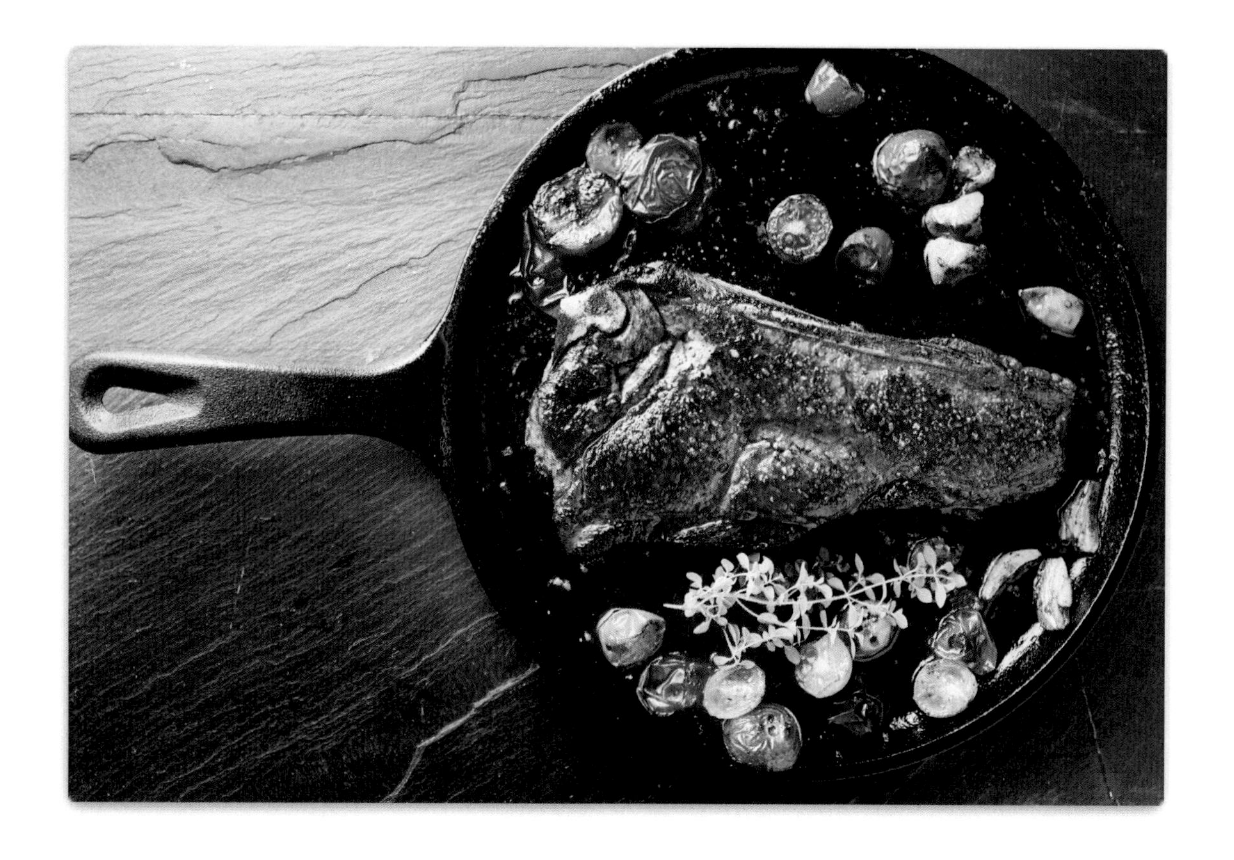

RECIPE: CHEESY EGG OMELETTE

Ingredients:

- 3 large eggs
- 1 dash salt
- 1/2 cup shredded mozzarella cheese
- 1 dash pepper
- 1/2 tbsp butter

Directions:

1. Whisk three whole eggs and season with salt and pepper.
2. Heat non-stick pan on medium low heat. Add grass-fed butter and allow to melt.
3. When butter is melted, add egg and begin to swirl pan until egg evenly covers the pan.
4. Add cheese to half of omelette. Fold over the other side and allow the cheese to melt for around one minute.
5. When omelette is finished, gently slide onto plate.

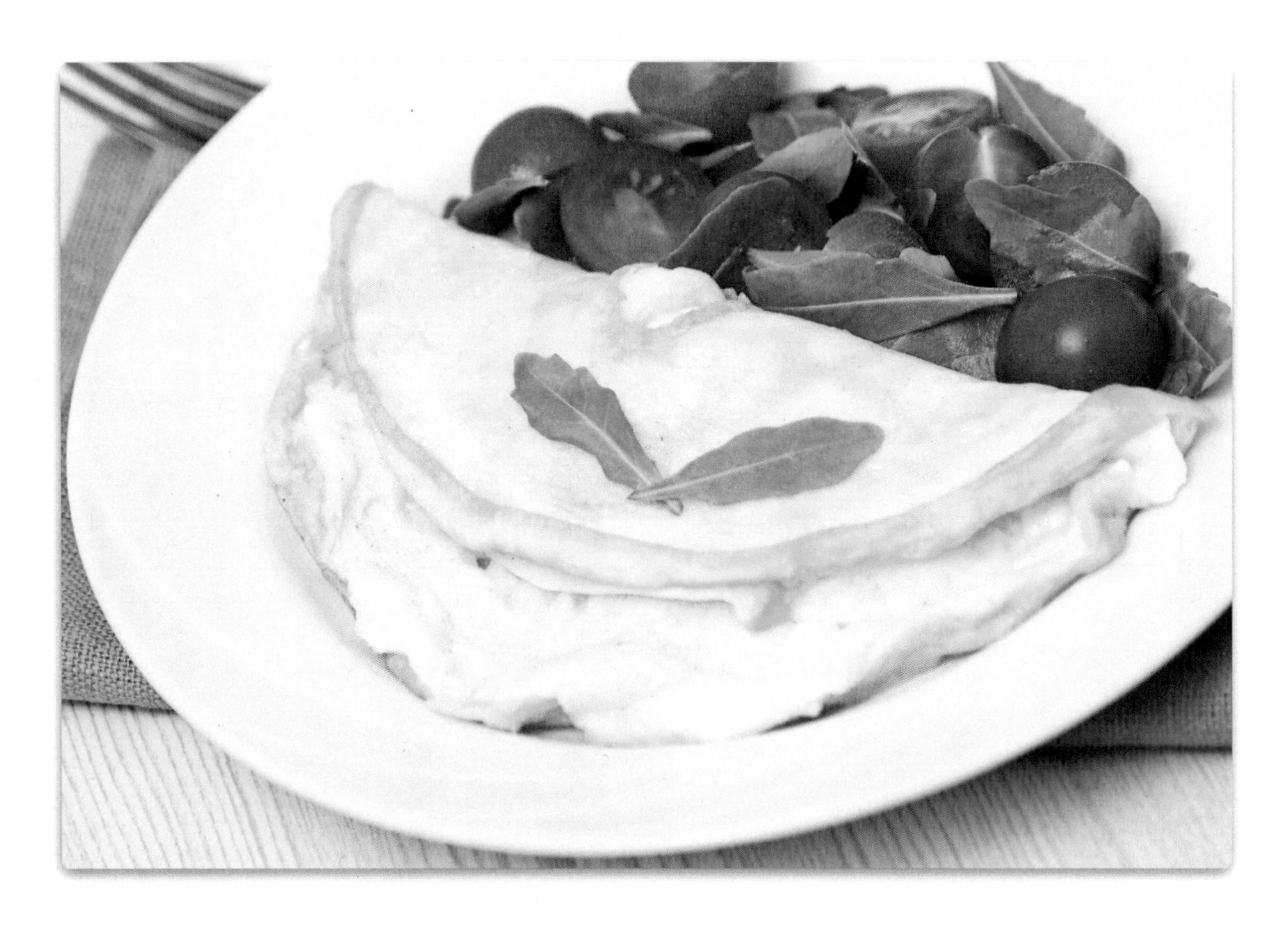

RECIPE: FETA-STUFFED HAMBURGERS

Ingredients:

- 1 lb ground beef
- 1/8 tsp Worcestershire sauce
- 1/4 tsp parsley
- 1 dash salt
- 1 dash pepper
- 1/4 cup crumbled feta cheese

Directions:

1. Preheat grill for medium heat, and lightly oil the grate.
2. Knead together the ground beef, Worcestershire sauce, parsley, salt, and pepper in a bowl. Form the mixture into 8 equal sized balls; flatten to make thin patties. Place about 1/4 cup of feta cheese onto each of four of the patties. Top each of the patties with cheese with one of the patties without; press the edges together to seal the cheese into the center.
3. Cook on the preheated grill until the burgers are cooked to your desired degree, 5-7 minutes per side. An instant read thermometer should read 160°F.

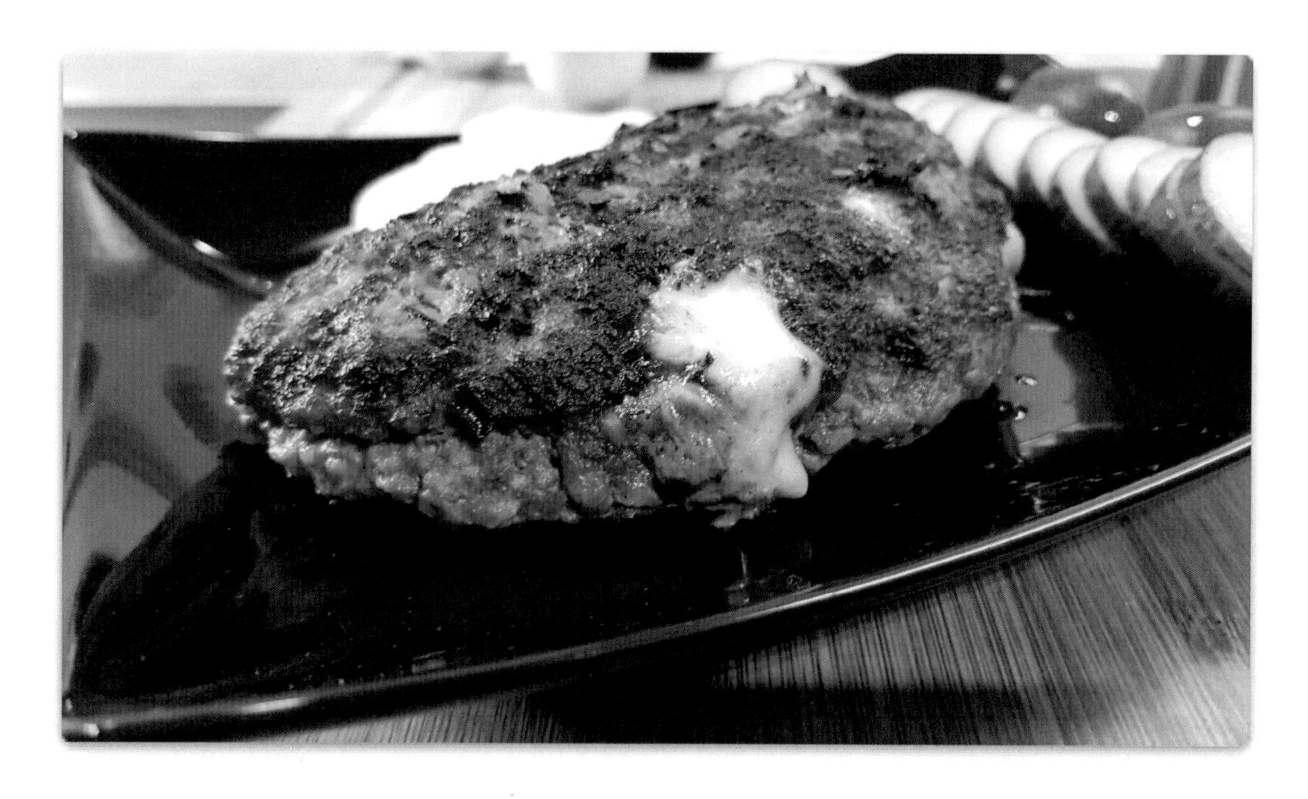

RECIPE: ASPARAGUS WITH PARMESAN

Ingredients:

- 1/2 tbsp butter
- 10 stalks of asparagus
- 1/4 cup parmesan cheese
- 1 dash salt
- 1 dash pepper

Directions:

1. Melt butter in skillet over medium heat. Add asparagus stalks and cook, stirring occasionally for around 10 minutes to desired firmness.
2. Drain excess fat and sprinkle with Parmesan cheese, salt and pepper.

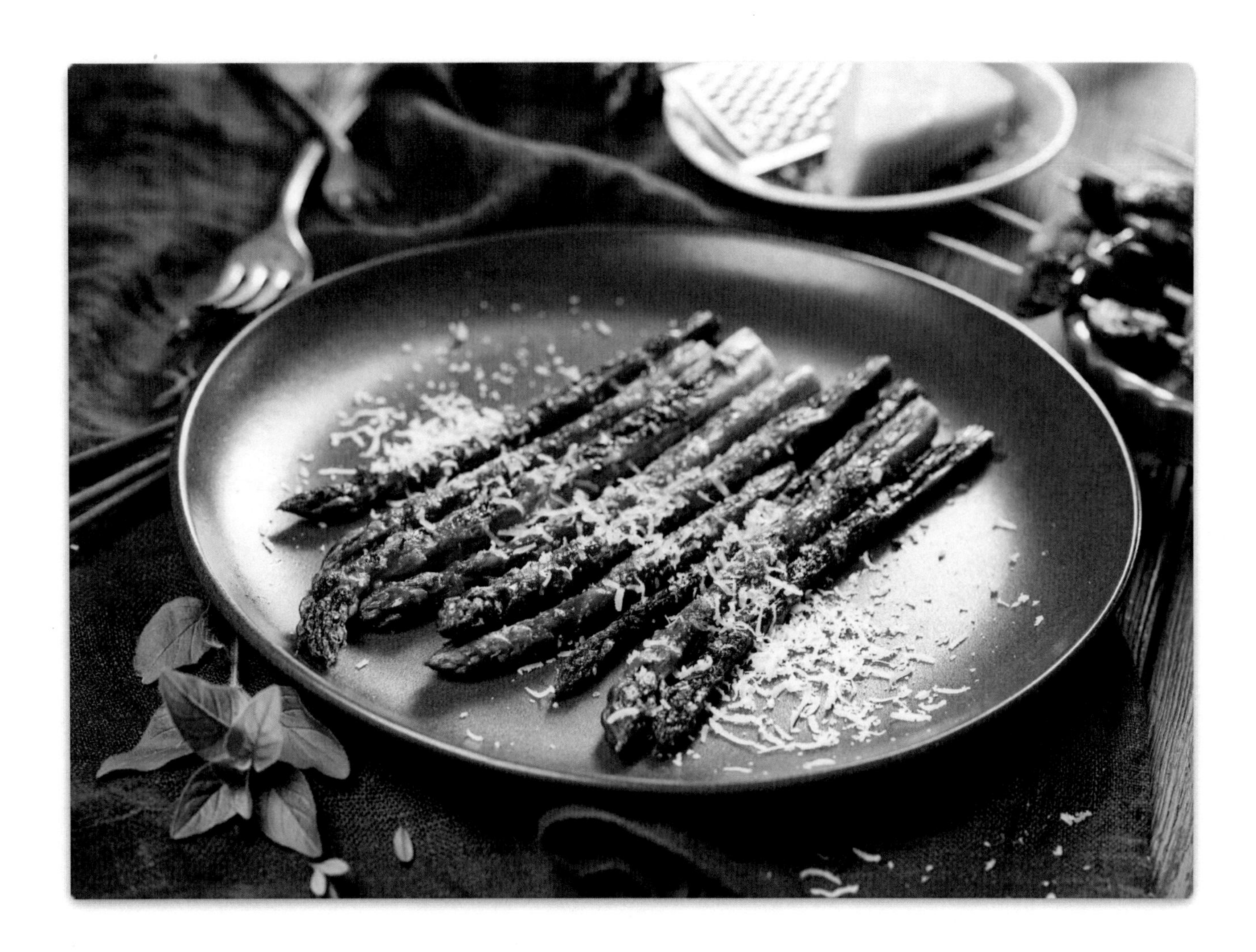

RECIPE: SMOKED PAPRIKA CHICKEN

Ingredients:

- 1 tbsp paprika
- 1/2 tsp garlic powder
- 1/2 tsp parsley
- 1/2 tsp salt
- 1.5 tbsp olive oil
- 2 boneless, skinless chicken breasts

Directions:

1. In a bowl, combine smoked paprika, garlic powder, dried parsley, salt, and olive oil to create a smooth paste. Brush each chicken breast with an even layer of the paprika paste. Let stand for at least 20 minutes to allow the flavor to infuse into the meat.
2. Set the oven to broil and place a rack in the upper third of the oven. Place the chicken breasts on a foil-lined baking sheet. Place the chicken under the broiler for 7-8 minutes, until a crust begins to form around the edges. Flip the breasts and cook them under the broiler for another 7-8 minutes, until cooked throughout.
3. Once cooked, let the breasts rest for a minute or two before serving to allow the juices to evenly distribute through the meat. Sprinkle with chopped parsley and serve.

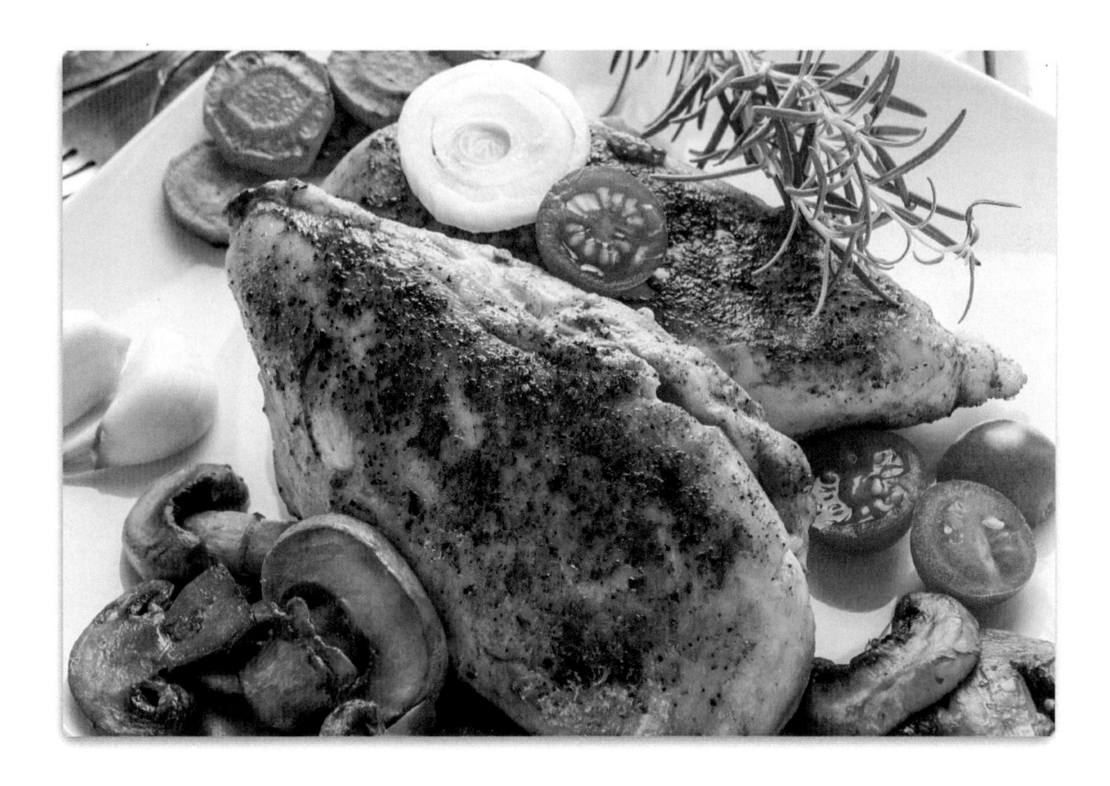

RECIPE: BEEF AND SPINACH MEATBALLS

Ingredients:

- 16 oz ground beef
- 1 cup spinach
- 1 cup chopped onions
- 1 tsp garlic
- 1 tbsp cumin
- 1 dash salt
- 1 dash pepper
- 1 tbsp olive oil
- 1 tbsp parmesan cheese

Directions:

1. Set oven to 400°F.
2. Mix ground beef, chopped raw spinach, red onions, garlic, and spices. Mix thoroughly using hands until spinach is completely mixed into the meat.
3. Form meatballs of roughly the same size. Place meatballs on an oil lined baking sheet and roast in the oven for 10-15 minutes.
4. Garnish with light cheese and serve.

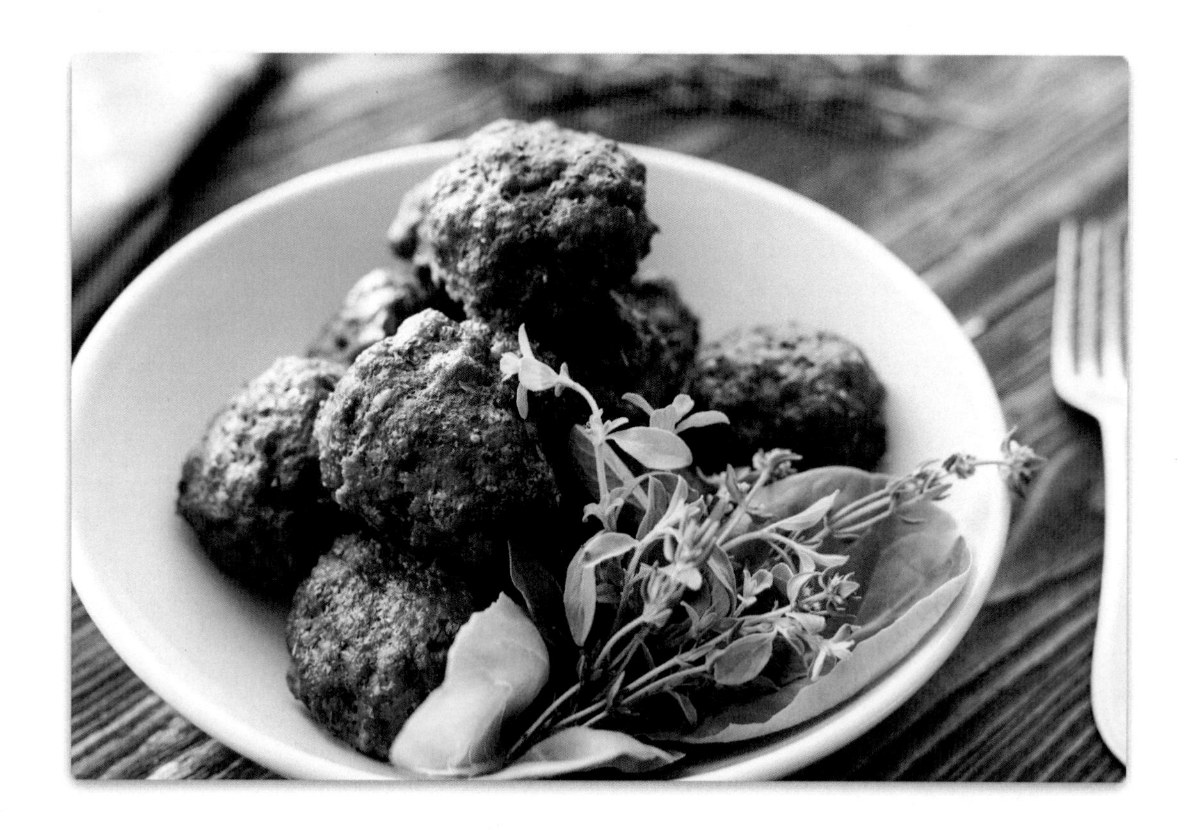

RECIPE: LEMON PEPPER CHICKEN THIGHS

Ingredients:

- 2 lbs chicken thighs
- 5 tbsp butter
- 2 tbsp lemon juice
- 1 dash lemon pepper
- 1 dash pink salt

Directions:

1. Preheat oven to 400°F.
2. Season chicken thighs with salt and lemon pepper.
3. Heat 2 tbsp butter in oven-proof skillet over medium heat. Add chicken and cook for 5-6 minutes until crispy.
4. Flip chicken thighs over and transfer skillet to oven. Roast for 15-20 minutes.
5. Transfer skillet back to stove. Plate chicken. Add remaining butter and lemon juice to pan on medium high heat and mix into sauce.
6. Pour sauce over top of chicken.

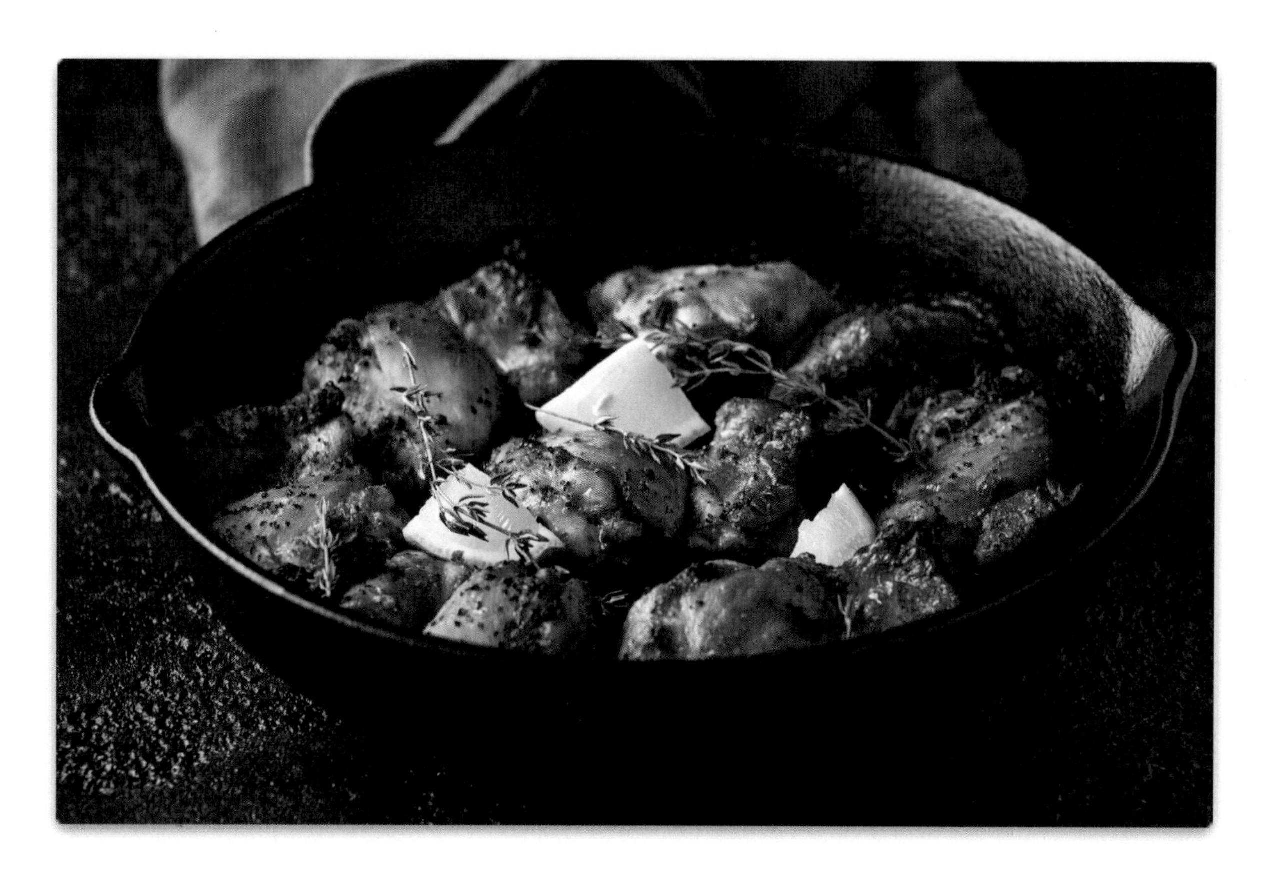

RECIPE: ROASTED AND DRESSED ZUCCHINI

Ingredients:

- 6 small zucchini
- 1/4 tbsp avocado oil
- 1 dash salt
- 1 dash pepper
- 1/2 tbsp red wine vinegar

Directions:

1. Preheat oven to 400°F. Wash zucchini and pat dry. In a baking dish, toss zucchini with the avocado oil, salt, and pepper.
2. Roast zucchini for 15 minutes until soft.
3. Once roasted, dress with a few splashes of red wine vinegar.
4. Add more avocado oil and salt if desired.

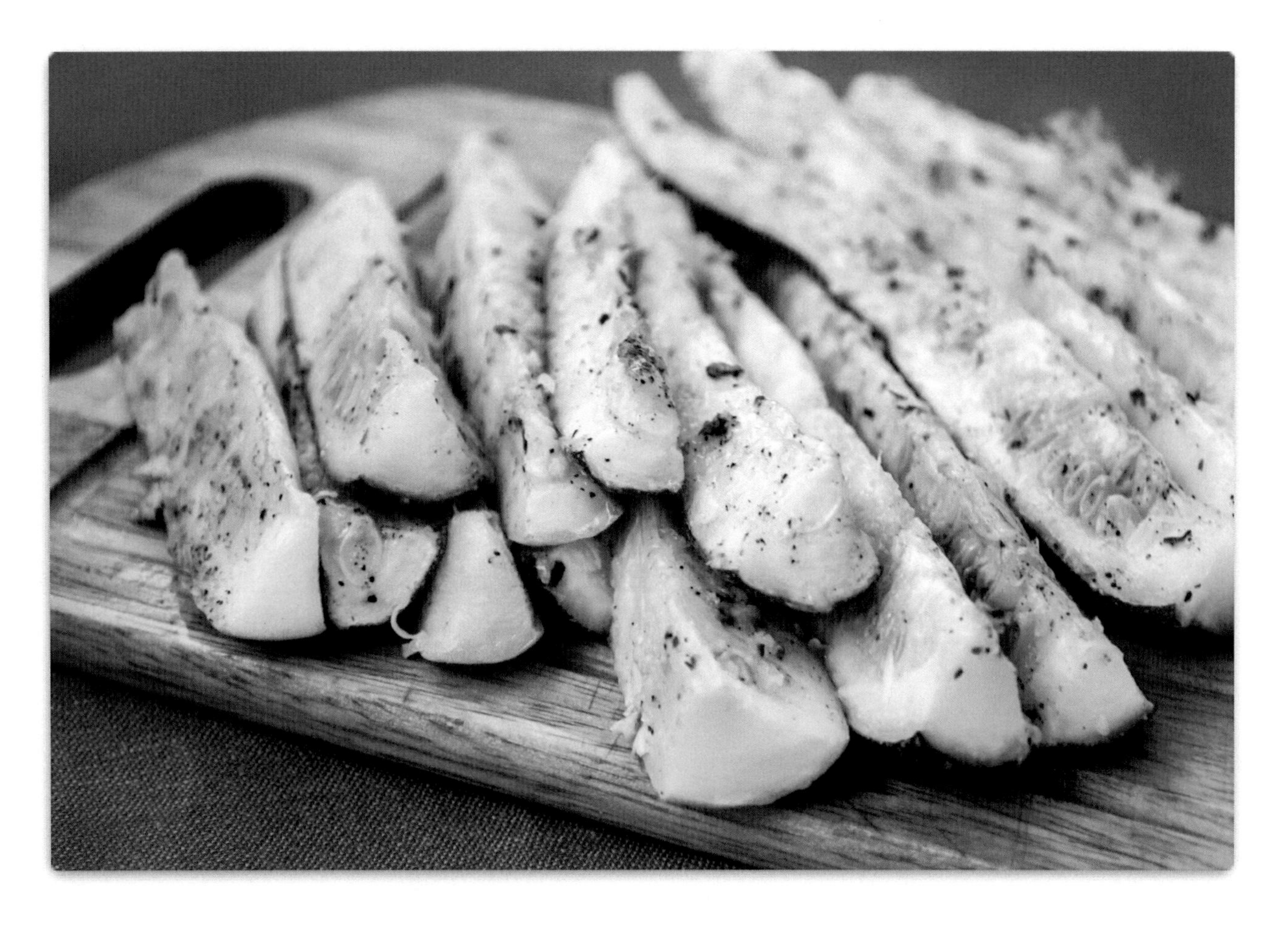

RECIPE: CHOCOLATE GREEK YOGURT

Ingredients:

- 6 oz 2% Greek yogurt
- 1 small packet stevia
- 1 tsp cacao powder

Directions:

1. Mix stevia and cacao powder in Greek yogurt to create a chocolate pudding dessert.
2. Enjoy!

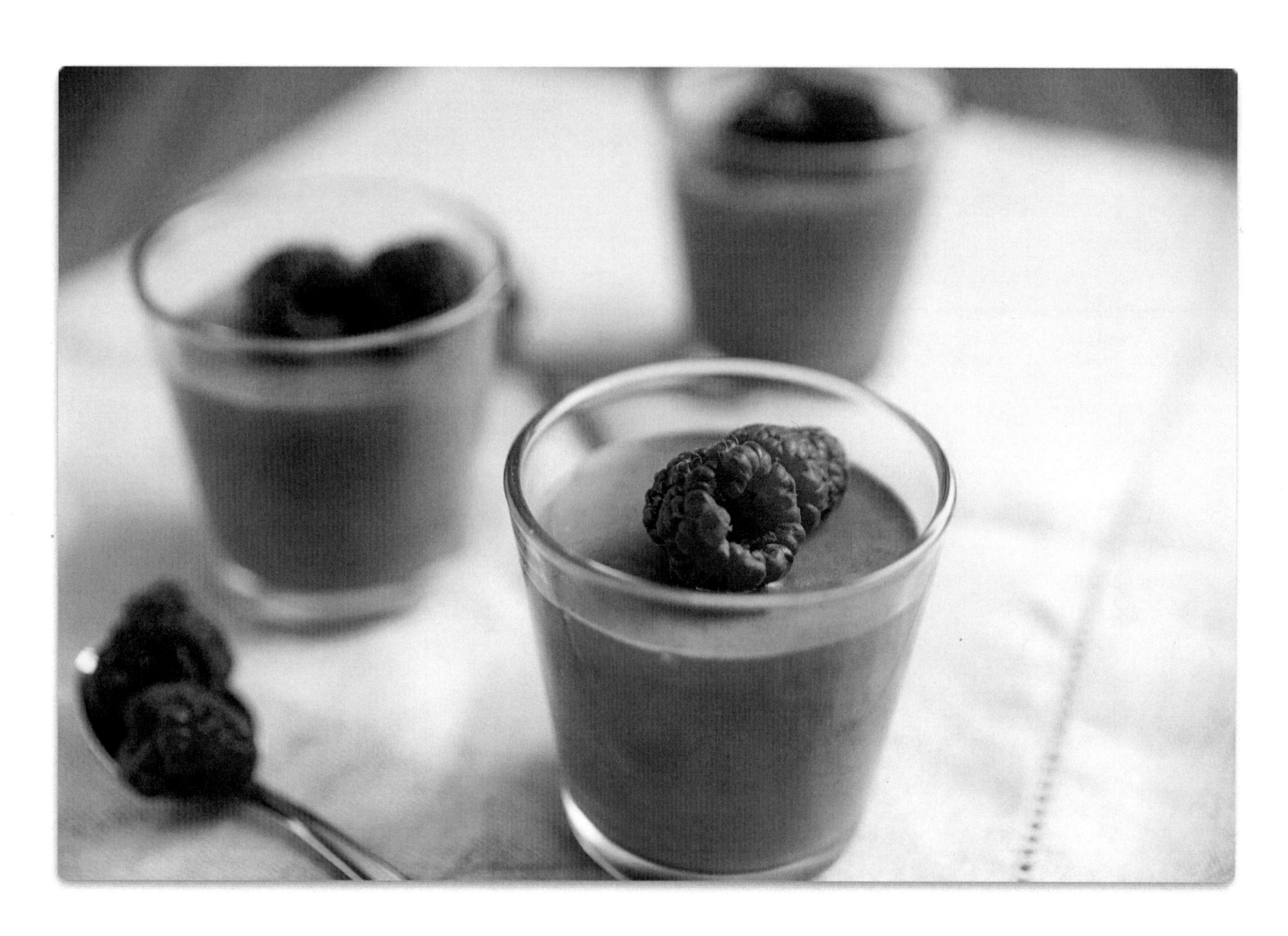

SAMPLE MENU

The following pages give just one small example of what a week of The P:E Diet might look like. This sample menu is built around a 16:8 intermittent fast, skipping breakfast and eating lunch and dinner in roughly an 8 hour window, with a snack in between your two main meals. If you find that an 8 hour eating window is too small, definitely feel free to start with 12 hours and reduce from there as tolerated. This sample menu is intentionally very low in net carbohydrate, and if you are not yet fat-adapted you might need to add in some carbs at the end of your eating window, in the form of tubers or fruit or grains. Potatoes, apples, and oatmeal would be examples of high fiber low energy density carbohydrate sources which might be ideal if you do find that you need to eat up to 100 grams of carbohydrate at the end of the day to achieve adequate satiety with this meal plan. You can maximize your fat adaptation by keeping these carbohydrates as low in quantity as possible and also by lowering their frequency as much as possible—for example, only once per day, at or near the end of your eating window, and always after eating adequate protein.

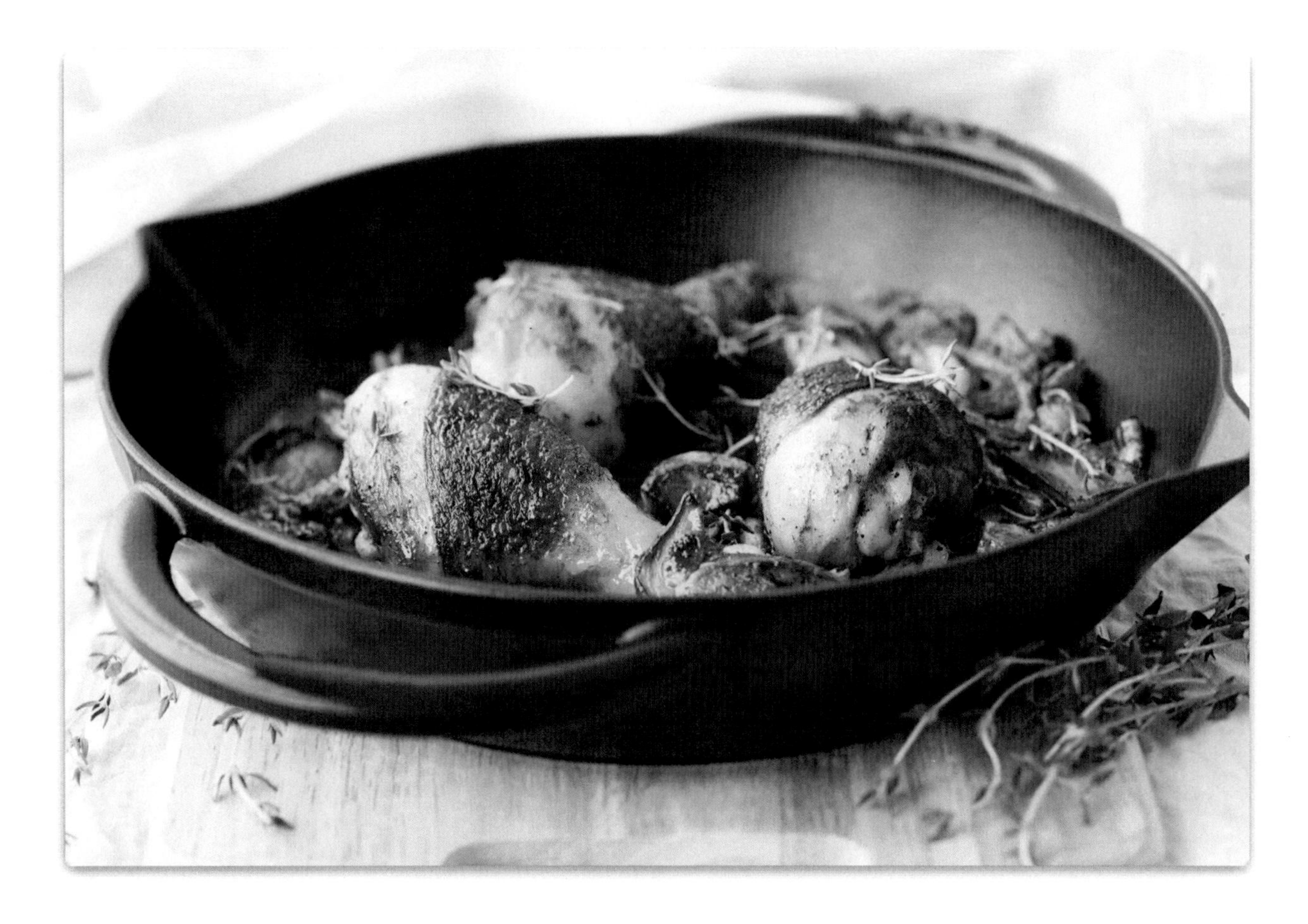

SAMPLE MENU: DAY ONE

MORNING: COFFEE WITH CREAM

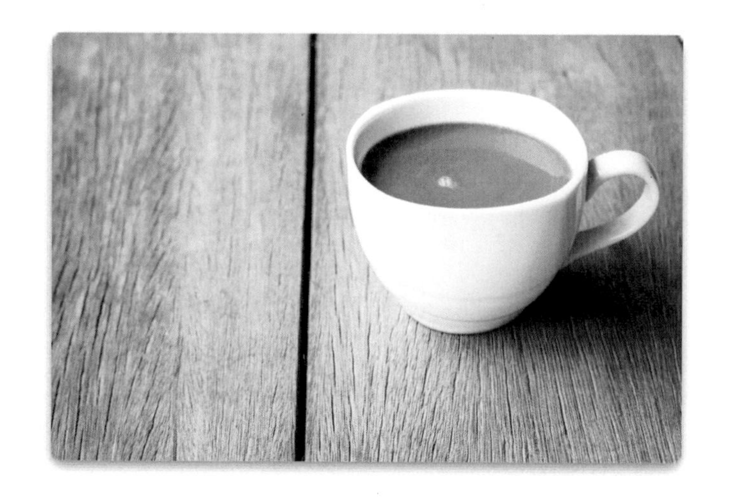

LUNCH: GRILLED CHICKEN

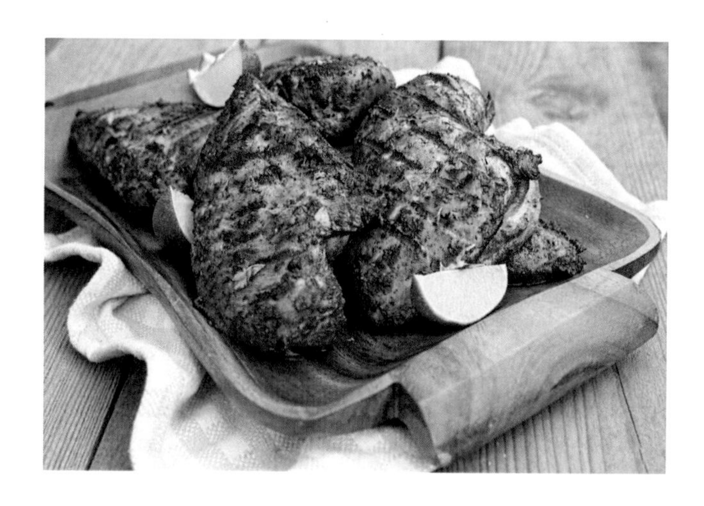

SNACK: RAW VEGETABLES

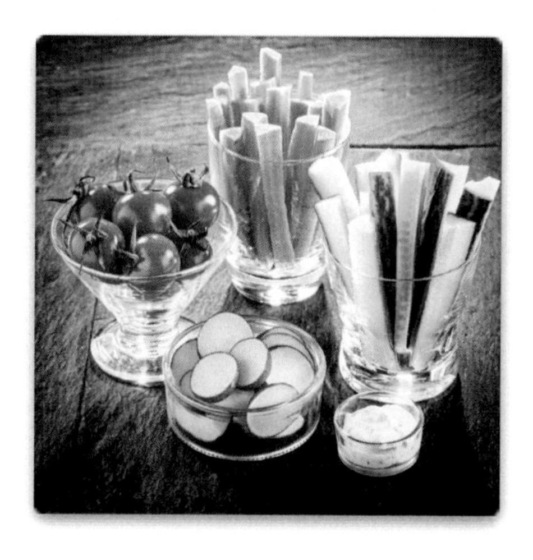

DINNER: T-BONE STEAK WITH ASPARAGUS

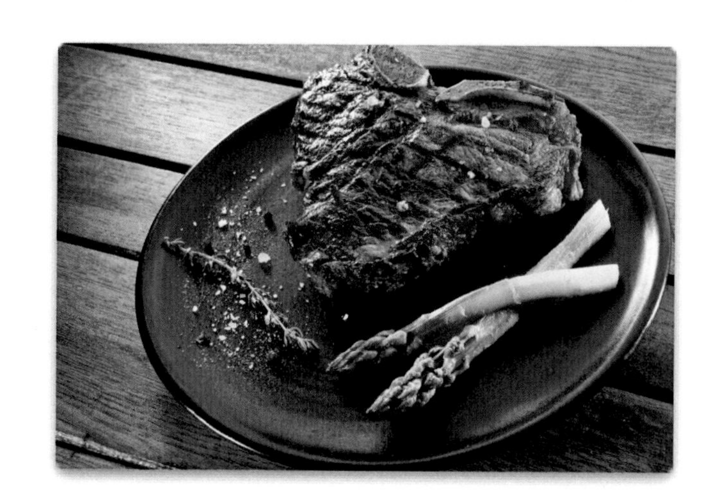

SAMPLE MENU: DAY TWO

MORNING: BONE BROTH

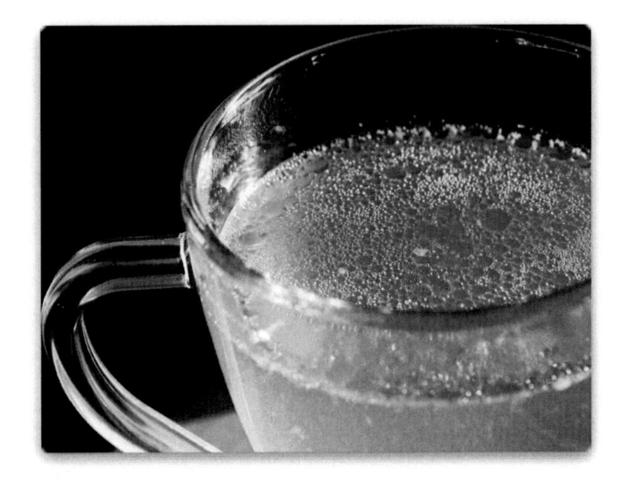

LUNCH: SALMON FILLET WITH ASPARAGUS

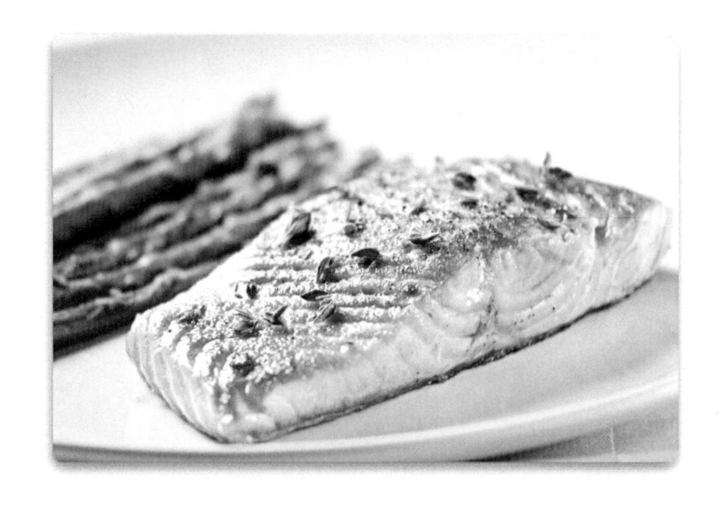

SNACK: HARD-BOILED EGGS

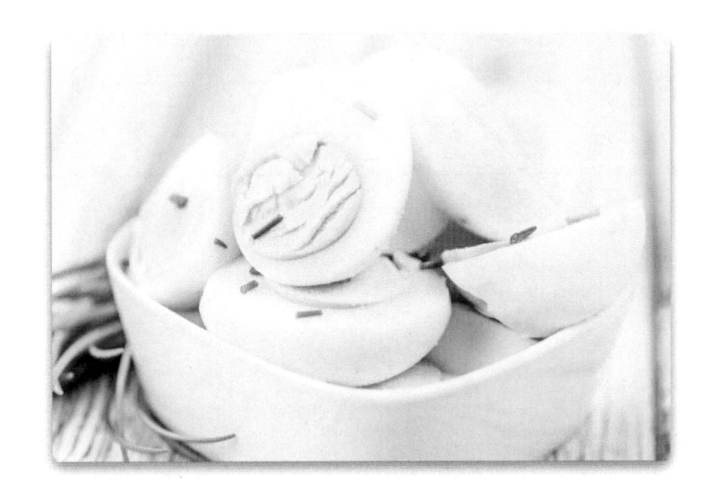

DINNER: SLOW-COOKER POT ROAST

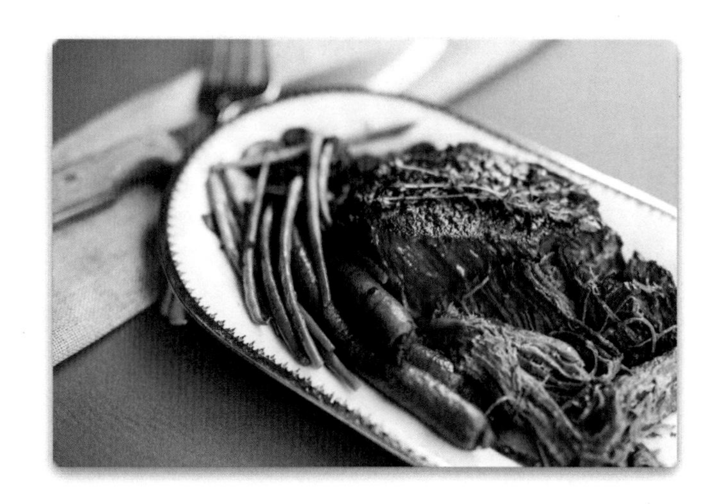

SAMPLE MENU: DAY THREE

MORNING: BLACK COFFEE

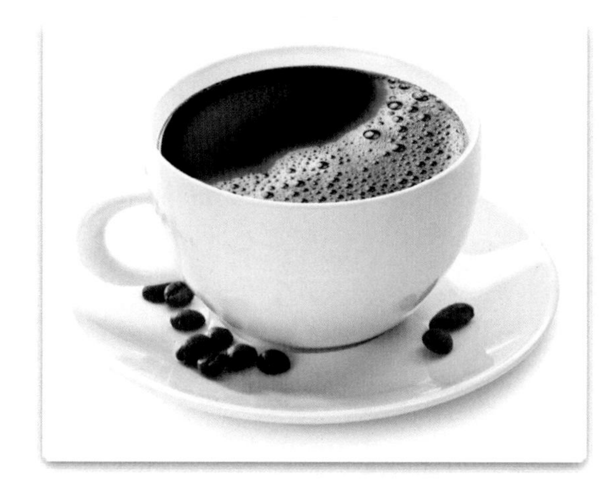

LUNCH: TURKEY BACON AND EGGS

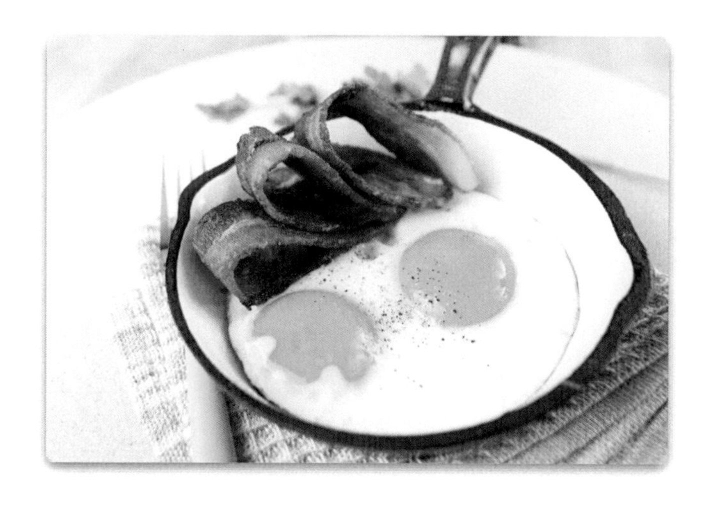

SNACK: SARDINES IN OLIVE OIL

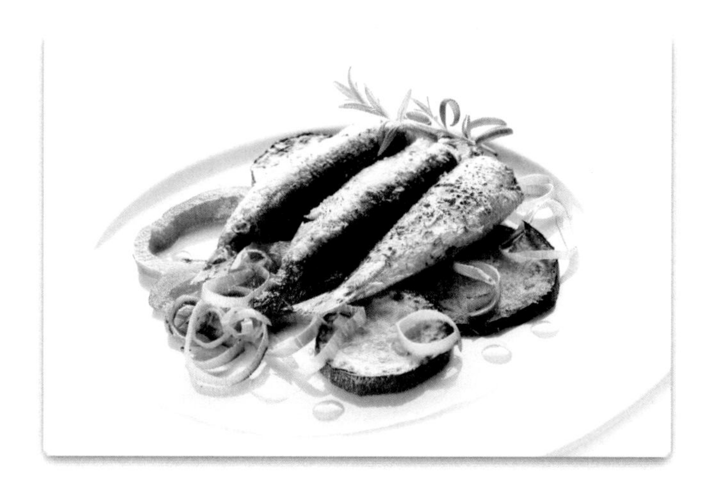

DINNER: SEARED LAMB CHOPS

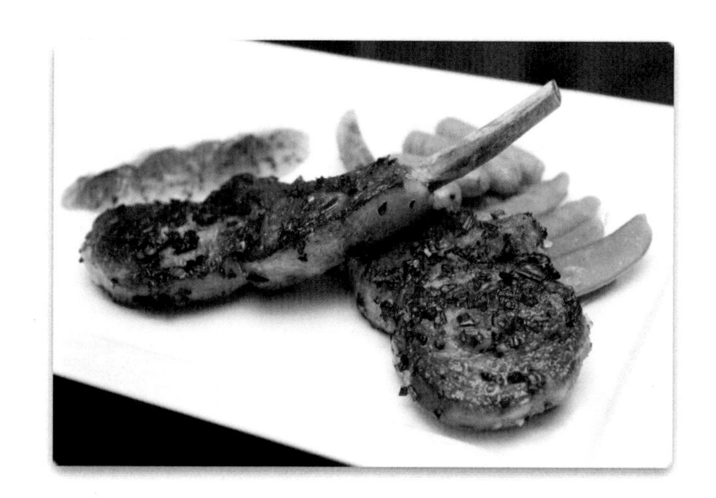

SAMPLE MENU: DAY FOUR

MORNING: EARL GREY TEA

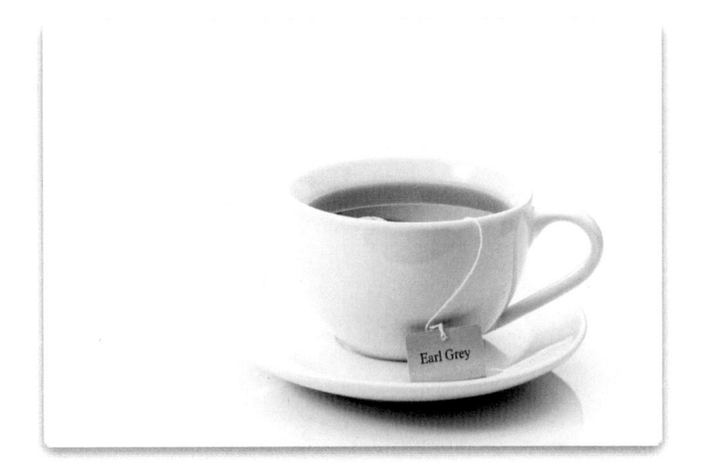

LUNCH: COBB SALAD

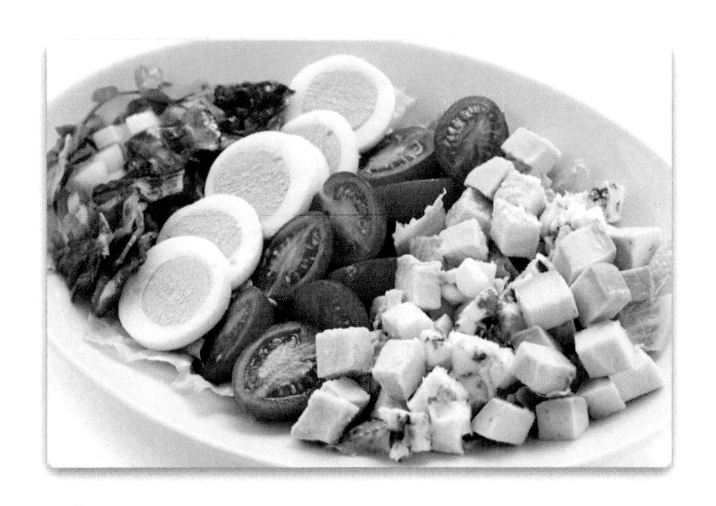

SNACK: SALAMI AND CHEESE

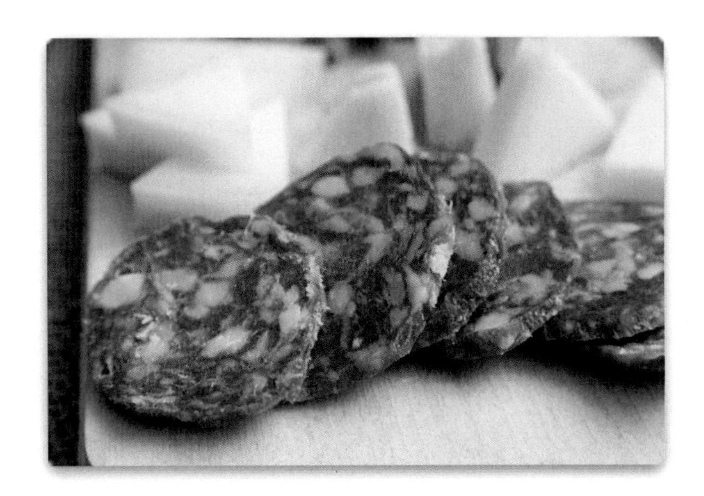

DINNER: CHICKEN WINGS

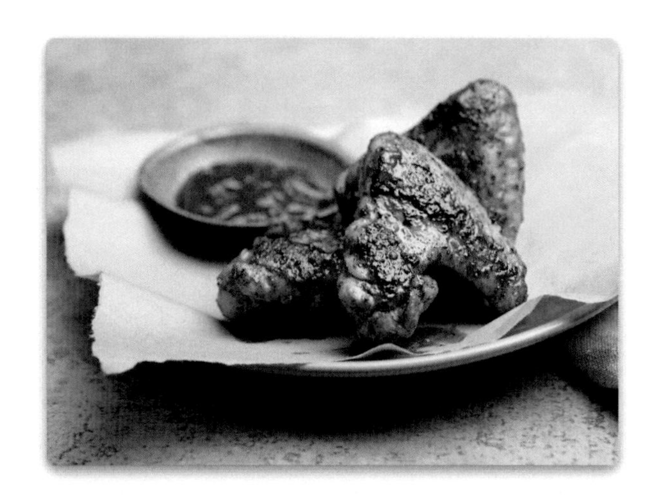

SAMPLE MENU: DAY FIVE

MORNING: AMERICANO

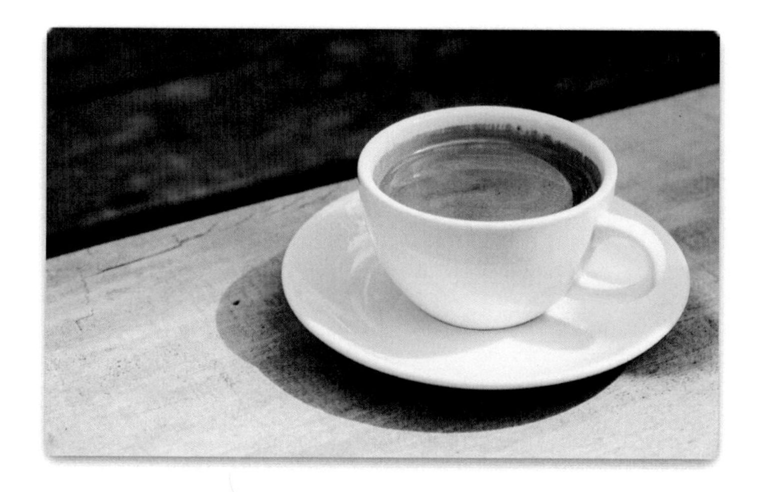

LUNCH: NEW YORK STRIP STEAK

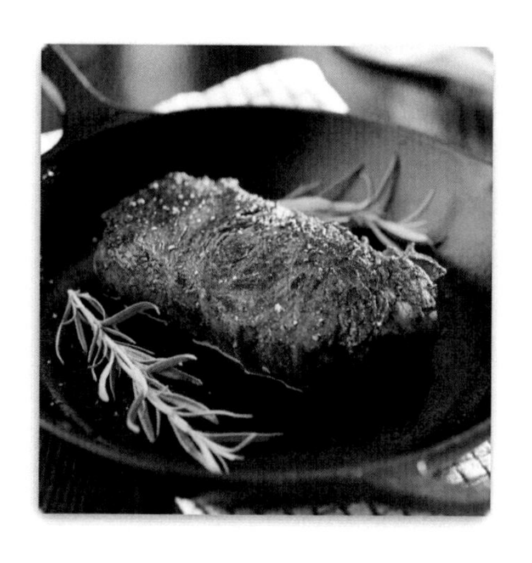

SNACK: GREEK YOGURT

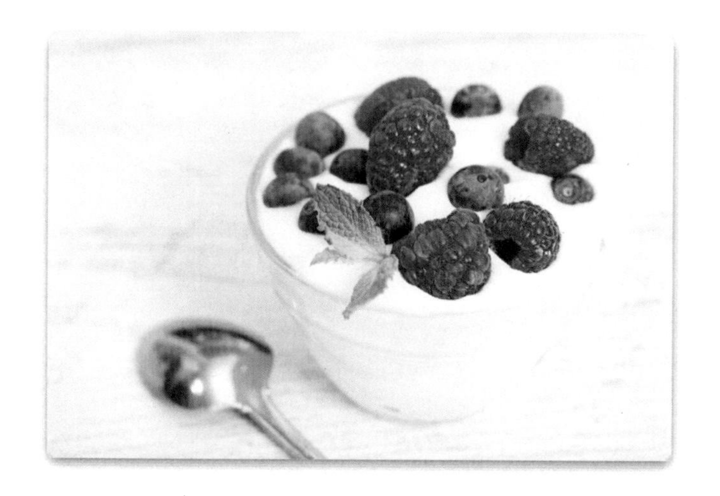

DINNER: ROAST TURKEY, VEGETABLES

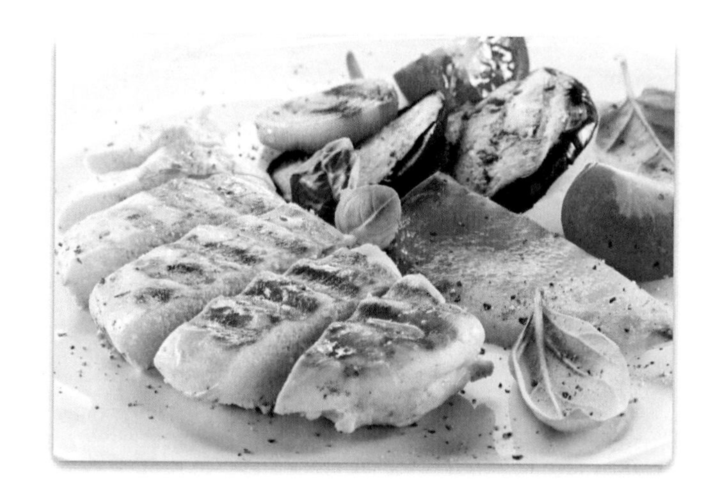

SAMPLE MENU: DAY SIX

MORNING: COFFEE WITH CREAM

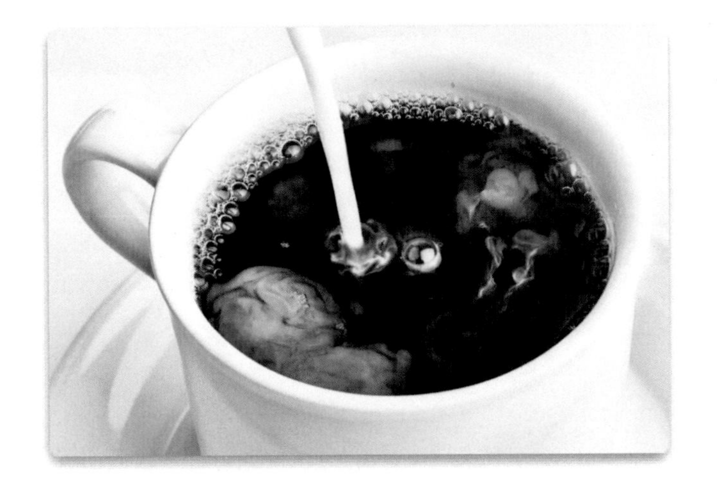

LUNCH: BEEF BURGERS, COTTAGE CHEESE

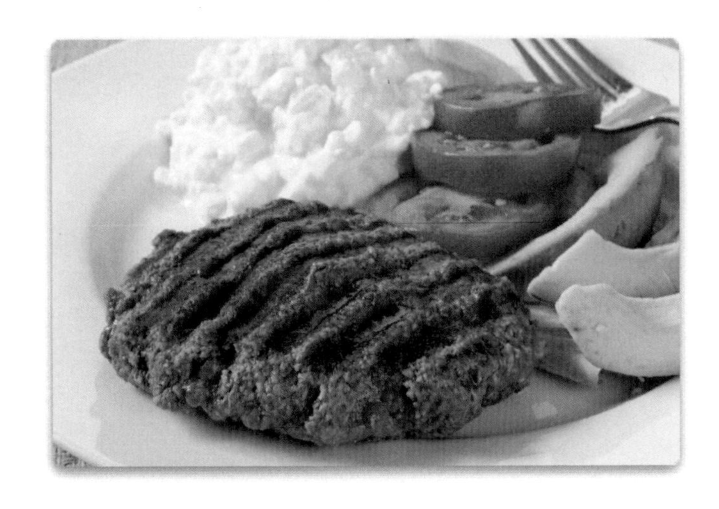

SNACK: SUGAR-FREE BEEF JERKY

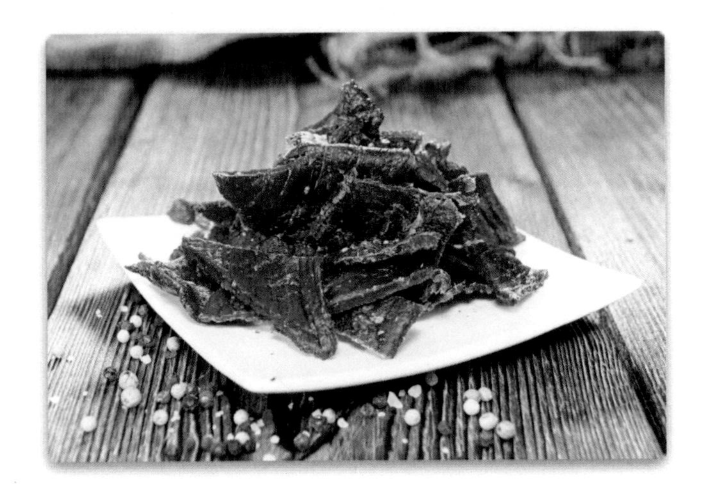

DINNER: LIVER WITH ONIONS

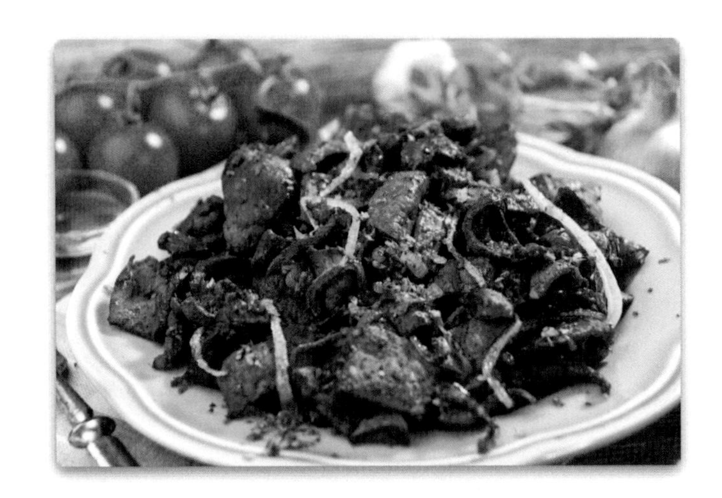

SAMPLE MENU: DAY SEVEN

MORNING: DIET SODA

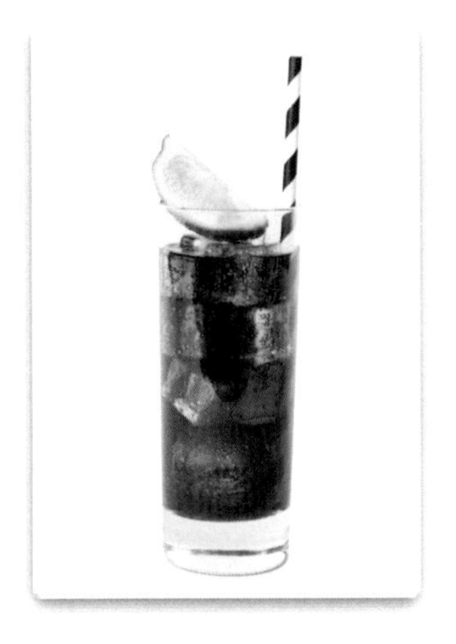

LUNCH: BACON-WRAPPED SALMON

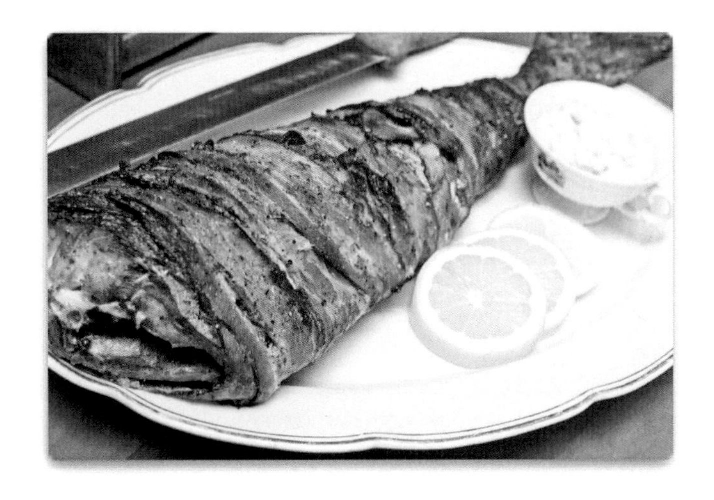

SNACK: OYSTERS WITH LEMON

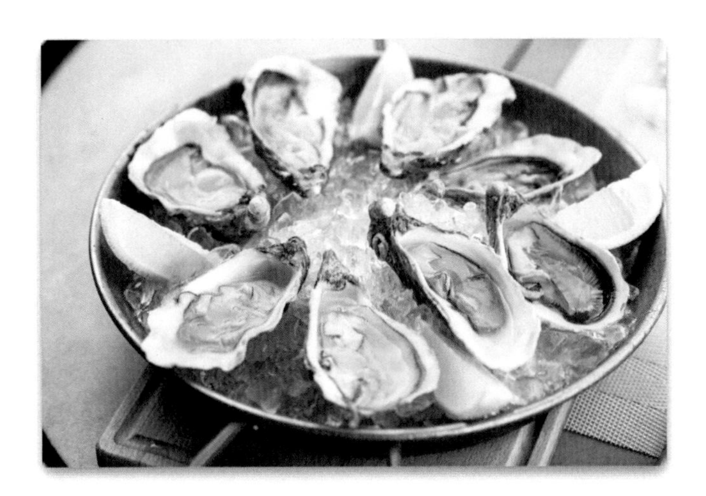

DINNER: SMOKED SALMON OMLETTE

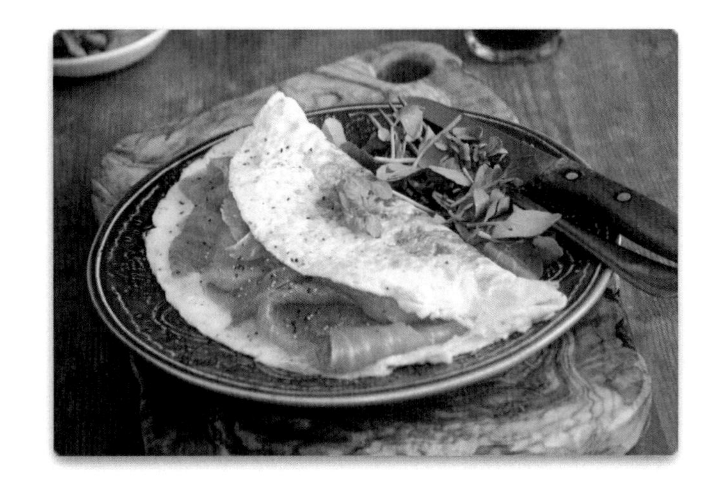

EXERCISE

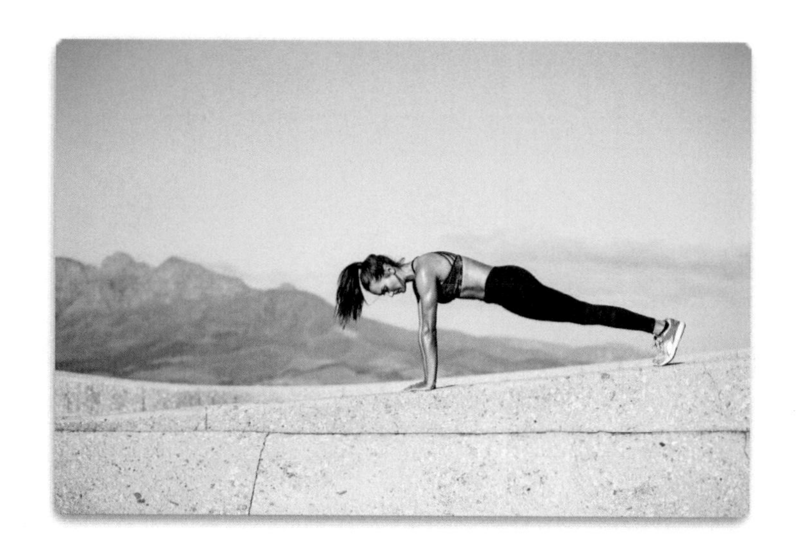

WHAT IS EXERCISE?

Exercise has a singular purpose: self-improvement. If done correctly, exercise provides a stimulus to your body that leads to positive adaptation. The adaptations to exercise are numerous, and can include increased muscular strength and size, improved stamina, improved cardiovascular fitness, an increase in metabolic rate, improvements in glucose metabolism, and increased fat oxidation. Diet is important, but you will never reach your health and body composition goals without proper exercise! So you might as well dive right in.

You can't out-train a bad diet.

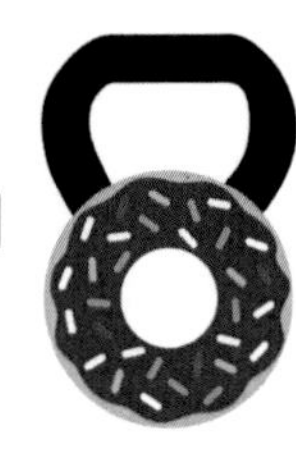

You also can't out-diet ZERO TRAINING.

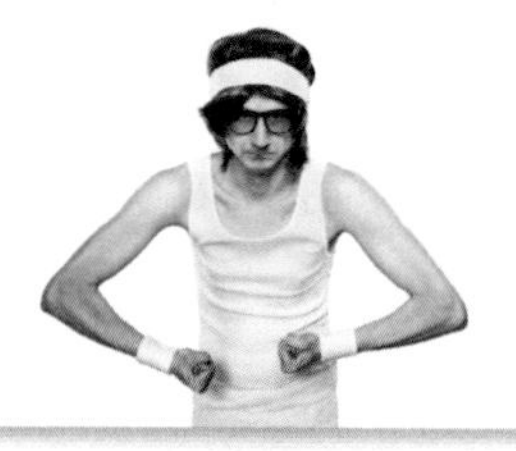

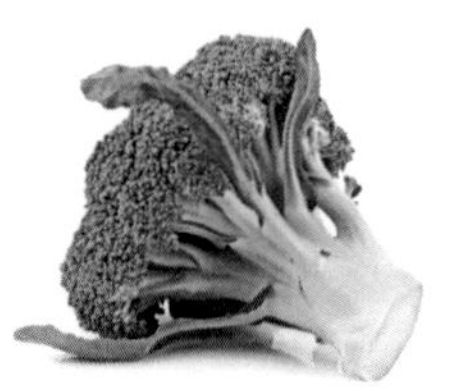

INTRO TO 'DEMAND TRAINING'

Your body is the most amazing survival machine ever imagined. Humans will adapt to endure their environmental conditions in a near-infinite number of ways. Your brain and body are constantly remodeling to best conform to the highly unique set of circumstances that you are exposed to. Your genetics demand of your body only one thing: stay alive in order to reproduce.

Some of these environmental adaptations we are quite familiar with, because they are visible and everyone has experienced them. If you never go outside and then you lay in the sun all day, get ready for a painful and damaging sunburn. But spend an hour in the sun every day all summer, and your body will respond by increasing the pigmentation of your skin, protecting you from burning. Dig ditches all day and expect some horrific blisters on your hands. But dig one ditch per day for a few months, and you will be protected by some world-class callouses on your hands.

The reality is that your body is constantly adapting to your surroundings in an attempt to maximize your survival. Thankfully this is almost always to your benefit. But occasionally, things don't go exactly the way you would want.

Take, for example, lack of exercise. Imagine for a moment that you were accidentally hit in the head with a stale croissant in some sort of freak bakery aisle accident and you spent the next few weeks or months in a coma. Your body responds to the disuse of your muscles and bone. Lean mass, like bone and muscle, is metabolically quite expensive, and a large portion of your basal metabolic rate, or the amount of calories it takes just to stay alive, is partitioned to the maintenance of your lean mass. A crucial survival tactic employed by your body is maximum energy efficiency—because from an evolutionary point of view, your body never knows when your next meal is going to turn up. So your body assumes it is doing you a huge favor by reabsorbing the protein and minerals from chronically unused lean mass, lowering your caloric requirements in the most miserly fashion possible, and hopefully keeping you from dying of starvation in the process.

In a way, we are all 'bodybuilders', and our bodies are constantly responding to our activity or LACK of activity in a precise fashion that is designed to maximize our survival. If you have more or less muscle mass than you used to, we can almost always trace that back to an environmental response of some sort.

Lean mass equals strength and longevity. The more lean mass you have, the better. Your entire goal, for both aesthetics and health, should be achieving the highest lean mass you can—while maintaining the lowest fat mass possible (without starving yourself). The question is, how exactly do we accomplish this?

Muscle, like callouses on your hands, is a functional tissue that responds to the environment in an adaptive way. And because it is metabolically quite expensive and your body is some sort of caloric Ebenezer Scrooge, you have to CONVINCE your body that extra muscle tissue is one hundred percent mission critical to your survival. But your muscles don't speak English, so there is only one way to deliver the message: Demand Training™ [ok not actually trademarked haha].

Imagine that you decide that you need more exercise, so from now on, you are going to walk three hours every single day. Yeah we know, that's dumb—but work with us here for a second. As a result of walking three hours every day, your body will never be convinced that it has to be any stronger, or any larger, or have any more muscle mass. Your body WILL adapt, however, in order to keep you alive. You will get VERY efficient with your gait and you will be able to walk in a way that you use the very least amount of energy possible. You will also get some really good callouses on your feet to protect your skin from all that friction. And you will probably lose lean mass on your [unused] upper body in an attempt to conserve energy to ensure your survival. You will get to the point where you can walk 3 hours and only burn 100 calories. If these are the things you want, then by all means, go hit the treadmill.

Now imagine instead for a moment that you suddenly decide to sprint up a mountain at your highest possible speed. After about 30 to 60 seconds of this, your heart rate will be the highest it has ever been and you will be sucking so much wind that you will feel like you're about to die. Eventually you will pretty much collapse on the ground and it will take you 10 minutes just to recover. But guess what: you just sent a message to your body. What was the message? HOLY S*** WE ALMOST DIED.

Your body has no idea what happened. For all your body knows, you were being chased by a polar bear and you narrowly escaped with your life. The only thing your body understands is that it gave you EVERY SINGLE BIT of muscular and cardiovascular output that it had, and it STILL WASN'T GOOD ENOUGH TO KEEP YOU ALIVE. You demanded so much energy output from your body that it completely failed. And in this case, failure means you don't get to pass on your genetic code. This kind of failure is COMPLETELY UNACCEPTABLE to your body. And so right there and then, your body makes a solemn vow: we have to be BETTER, or next time we really are going to die.

The adaptations to exercise are so slow that they really are imperceptible—to both you and everyone else. But believe us, they ARE happening. Every day you go outside and attempt to run up the same mountain, with the highest possible speed, for as long as you possibly can, until you hit failure. And slowly, after days and weeks and months, things start changing. Your leg muscles get larger and stronger. Your cardiovascular fitness improves. Your speed and distance both gradually increase. Pretty soon you are running halfway up the mountain before you collapse. And eventually, maybe even years down the road, you finally run all the way up to the top. At that point, you are an amazing sprinter, and the difference between your initial sprinting capacity and your current ability is mind-boggling.

Demand Training is a way of communicating to your body. You are DEMANDING an adaptation, in order to ensure your survival. But the communication signal needs to be loud and clear. And you can only send this signal by maximizing the INTENSITY and EFFORT of your activity. The goal is to produce the HIGHEST amount of muscular force for the LONGEST amount of time possible, until you reach the highest level of failure discomfort that you can tolerate.

Built in to Demand Training is the concept of 'progressive overload'. What is progressive overload? Allow us to explain.

Imagine that you decide that you are going to do 20 push-ups every day for the rest of your life. At first, you struggle to even do 10 push-ups. But after a month or so you gradually work up to 20 per day without too much trouble. You feel yourself getting slightly stronger, and you even notice a bit more muscle when you look in the mirror. After a few months however, 20 push-ups feels like nothing. Keep doing this for a couple of decades, and half a million push-ups later you are absolutely no stronger or more muscular whatsoever—you are just really efficient at 20 push-ups and can do these while only expending maybe 5 calories or something like that.

Now imagine for a moment that you decide that instead of picking an arbitrary number, like 20, you are going to do one set of push-ups every day ALL THE WAY TO FAILURE. At first you struggle to get to 20, but then every day you push yourself all the way to failure and beyond. On the 21st rep you are struggling with 10/10 exertion, sweating, short of breath, and pushing for your life, but you still go all the way to absolute failure. As weeks and months go by, something amazing happens. You go from 20 push-ups a day to 30, then 40, then 50. You add a lot of visible muscle, and you feel strong as hell. This is progressive overload—every time, you are pushing yourself as far as you possibly can, and your body continues to respond to the signal of failure.

Pushing your muscles to the point of NOT BEING ABLE TO MOVE sends the biggest message to your body of all. From the evolutionary place your body comes from, the inability to move means certain instantaneous death. Maybe you are being crushed by a boulder, or eaten by a sabertooth tiger, but either way you're toast. So working your muscles all the way to complete failure—to the point of not even being able to move a single millimeter—is like grabbing a bullhorn and screaming at your body "WE ARE GOING TO DIE BECAUSE YOU ARE NOT STRONG ENOUGH!!!" Afterwards, your body completely freaks out and responds by adding MORE MUSCLE and LARGER MUSCLE, so that next time you can not only create larger tension in your muscles (strength), but you can also sustain this tension for a longer period of time.

The secret to Demand Training is carefully and deliberately placing the VERY HIGHEST TENSION you can possibly generate in your muscles, and sustaining this tension for the VERY LONGEST AMOUNT OF TIME you possibly can, all the way to failure. Maximizing time under tension, with maximum effort and intensity, sends the very loudest signal to your body that it needs to adapt—you are DEMANDING it. In response, your muscles will gradually become larger—providing you with the muscular strength and endurance to survive what your body perceives as an environmental threat to your very survival.

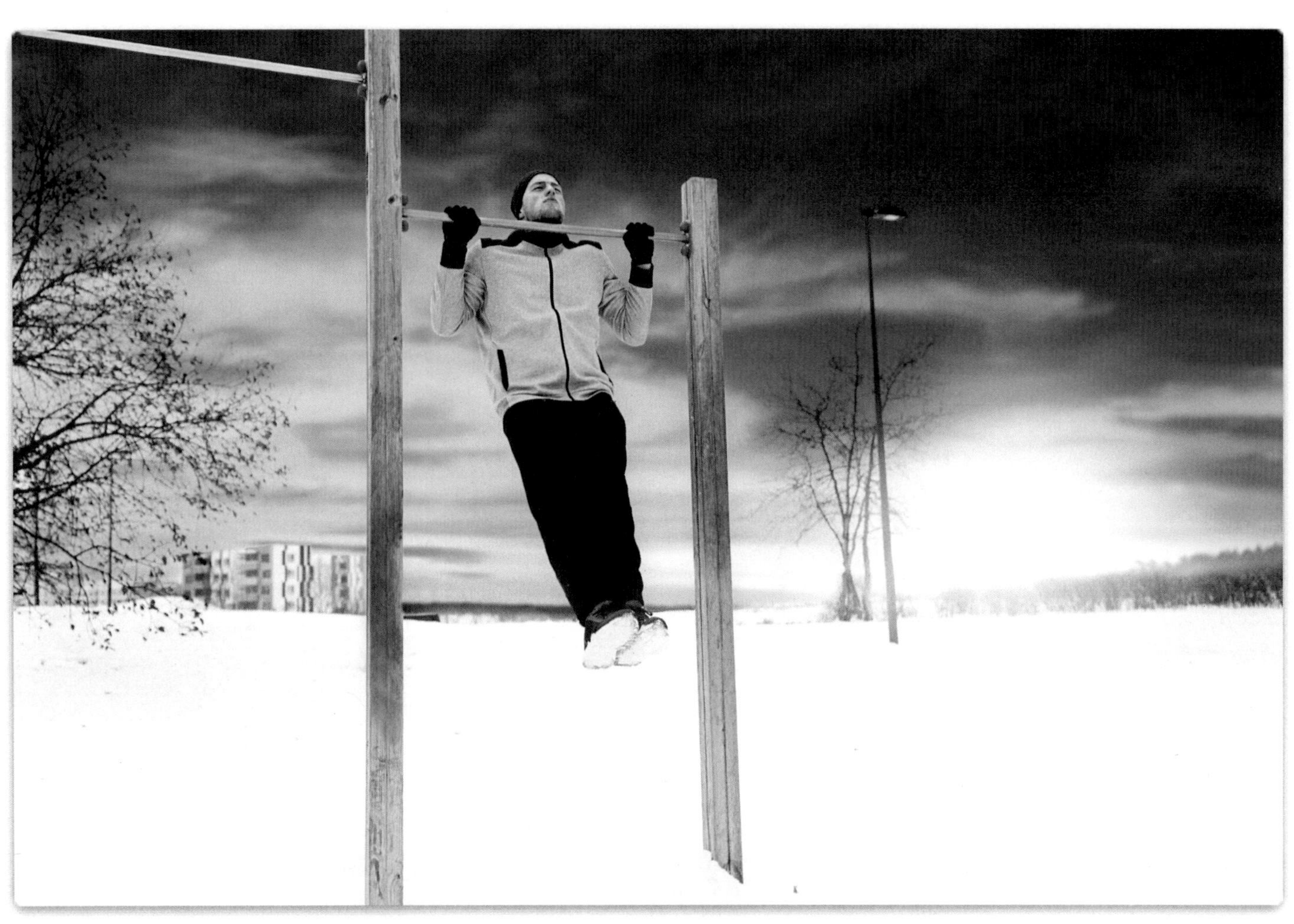

Pull-ups are the king (or maybe queen) of upper body pulling exercises.

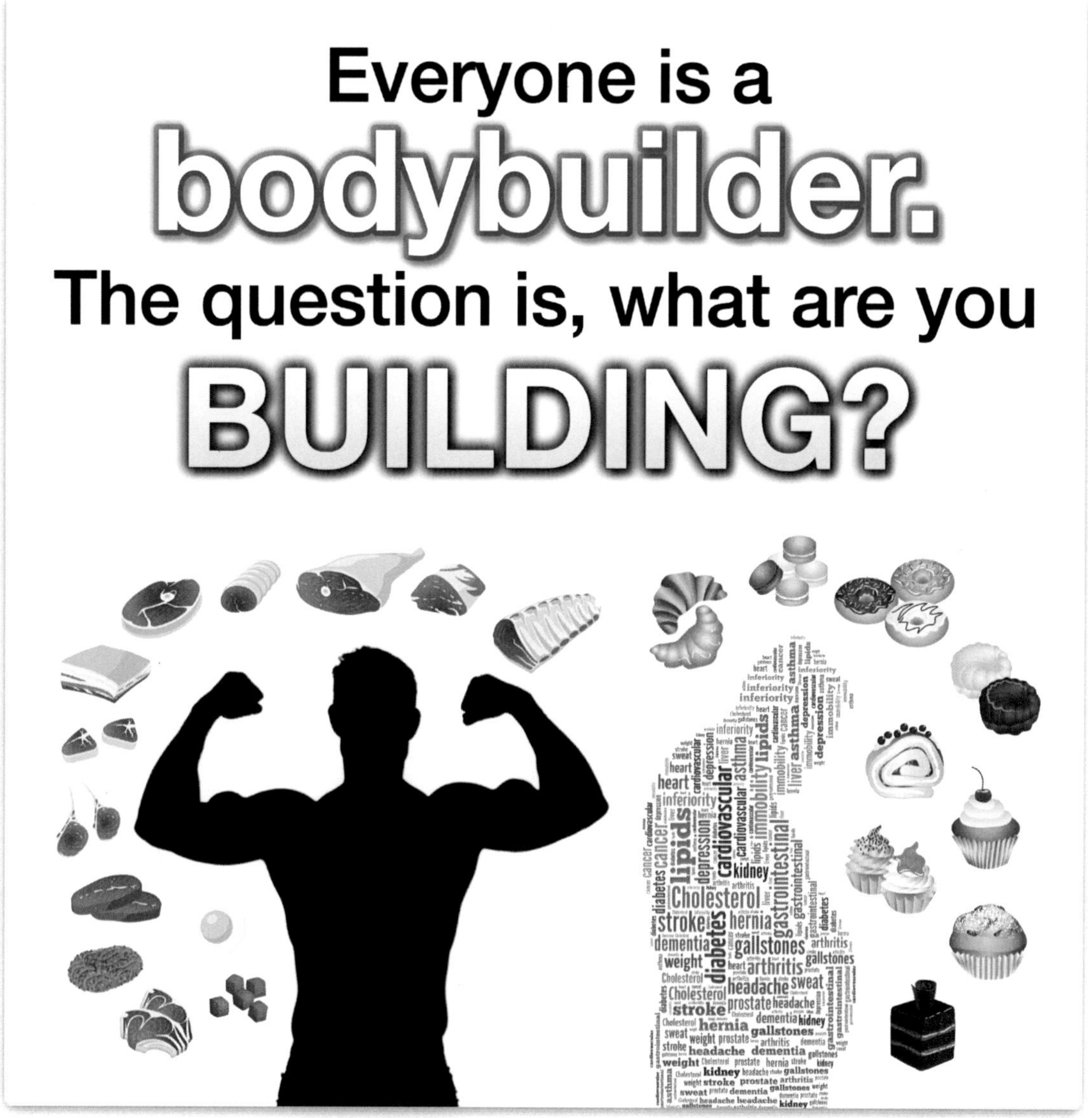

Everyone is a

bodybuilder.

The question is, what are you

BUILDING?

You really are building your body daily. Your body is just doing its job and reacting to the diet and exercise environments you create. Take control! Protein and high-intensity training build lean mass (muscle and bone), while non-protein energy (carbs and fats) build fat mass. Choose wisely!

FAT EXITS YOUR BODY VIA MITOCHONDRIA.

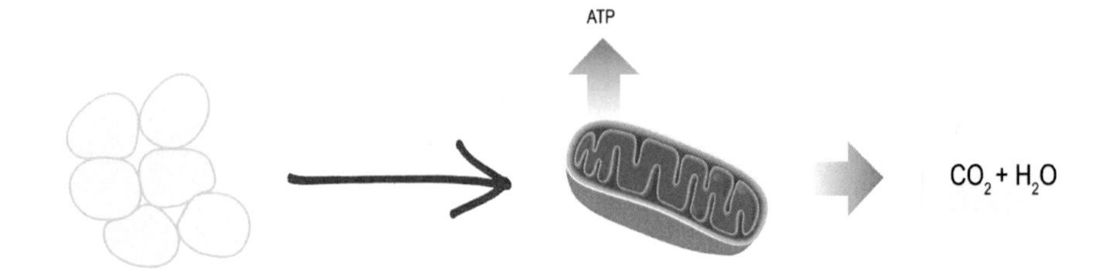

TRAINING DOUBLES YOUR MITOCHONDRIA.

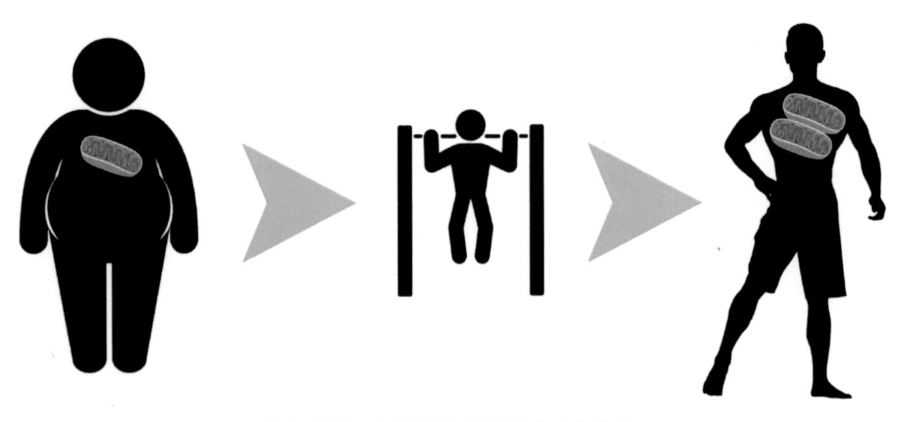

ANY QUESTIONS?

Exercise dramatically improves your capacity for burning fat and is crucial for optimum body composition and metabolic flexibility.

RESISTANCE VERSUS CARDIO

There are two basic types of exercise: resistance, and cardio. In Demand Training, resistance is defined as working a particular set of muscles in the body, such as the muscles involved in upper body pushing and pulling movements, in a deliberate fashion designed to produce maximum time under tension. Cardio, however, involves larger whole-body movements that lead to cardiovascular limitations prior to the absolute failure of any particular muscle group.

For example, doing push-ups in a slow and deliberate fashion, with perfect form, for absolutely as many as you possibly can—and then still holding the push-up position until you collapse on the ground—would be proper RESISTANCE training of the 'pushing' muscles of your body. But jumping up and down as high as you can until you were so short of breath that you absolutely have to stop and rest would be 'CARDIO'. Similar to resistance exercise, proper cardio would demand the very highest level of energy output that your body can manage, for the longest amount of time you can sustain it.

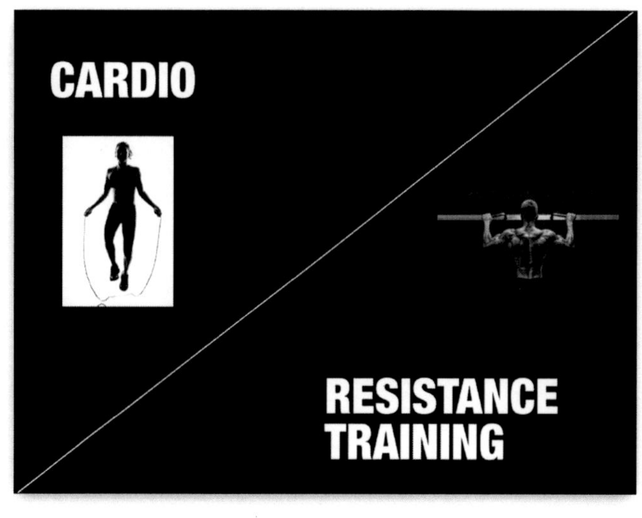

Good examples of Demand Training cardio would be sprinting as fast as you can for as long as you can. Or doing squat jumps as high as you can for as long as you can (good luck doing more than 30 seconds of either of these). You could go all out on a spin bike or rowing machine as well—both excellent ways for maximum power output.

Don't forget the first rule of exercise: don't get hurt. So you want to pick movements that are absolutely not going to result in an injury. If you are doing cardio and you want to pump out the very highest amount of energy you can for the longest amount you can, we highly recommend rowing machine sprints, squat jumps, or just sprinting on safe and level terrain. Be careful and stay within your coordination limitations—you want to challenge your power output ability, not necessarily your agility (save that for sport-specific training). When it comes to resistance exercise, bodyweight movements are extremely safe, as are weight machines in the gym. When performing resistance moves, be sure to use slow and deliberate form and technique to reduce the chance of injury. The goal is to make the exercise as difficult as possible by using perfect form, rather than piling on a ton of weight and then using poor form (much more likely to result in an injury).

RESISTANCE EXERCISE

There are three basic movement patterns: push, pull, and squat (legs). Any full body Demand Training workout will involve at least three different exercises—one for each of these movement patterns. The most basic workout would be push-ups, pull-ups or rows (any sort of 'pulling' motion, depending on level of ability), and finally squats or lunges (or other leg movement).

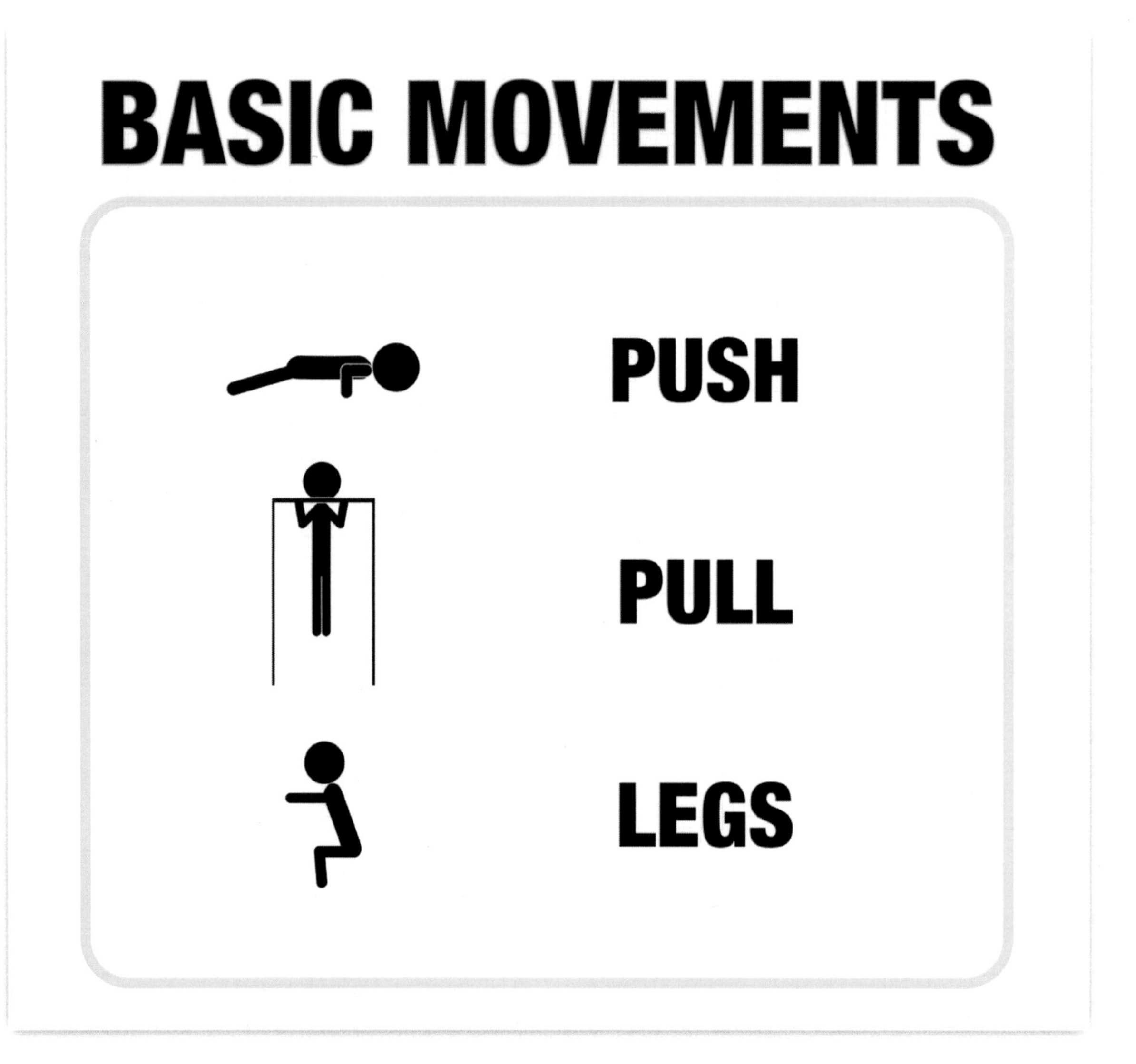

PUSH

The classic bodyweight push movement is the push-up. As with all bodyweight exercises, there will be a HUGE amount of variability between individual capabilities. If you are severely out of shape you might have to start with the easiest progression of all—a wall push-up. You want to find a difficulty level that allows you to do at least 5 repetitions ('reps') with perfect form, but ideally with a high enough difficulty level that you hit failure by the time you hit at most 10 repetitions. So let's say that starting out you can only do five wall push-ups. Every day you would do these to failure, and eventually you work up to 10 wall push-ups. Congratulations, now it is time to graduate to the next difficulty progression: push-ups on a bench. Again, you might be back down to five of these, and it could take you a while to work up to ten. Next would be knee push-ups. After 10 knee push-ups, you would perform regular push-ups on your toes, but with only a half of the range of motion. Gradually you work up to 10 regular push-ups. Next is diamond push-ups (with hands touching each other near center of chest), and eventually you get to the hardest level of all: a one-arm push-up. This move is so incredibly difficult that almost nobody can perform it. So let's just say that push-ups will remain challenging for your entire lifetime.

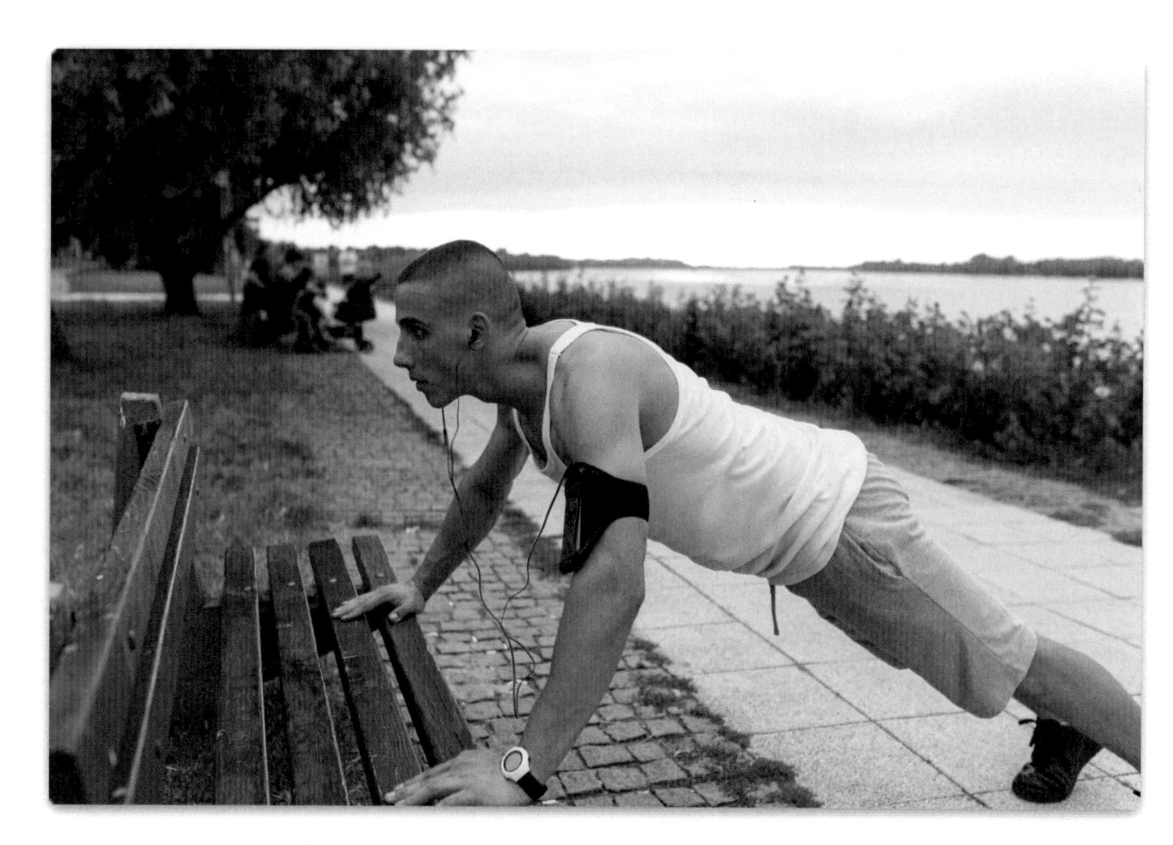

If you can't do a push-up, start with either a wall push-up or a push-up on an elevated surface, like a bench.

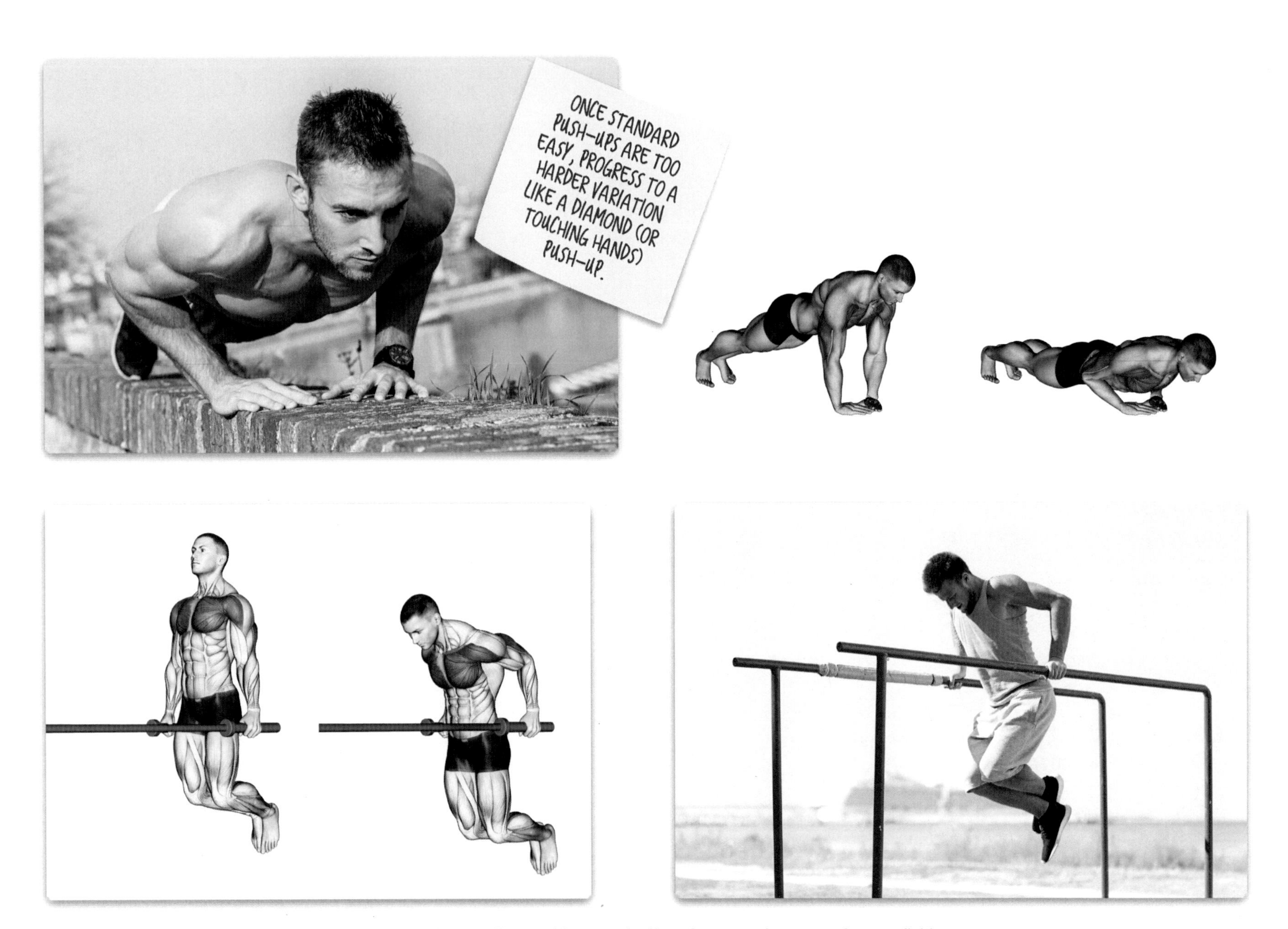

Dips are another excellent pushing exercise if you happen to have some bars available.

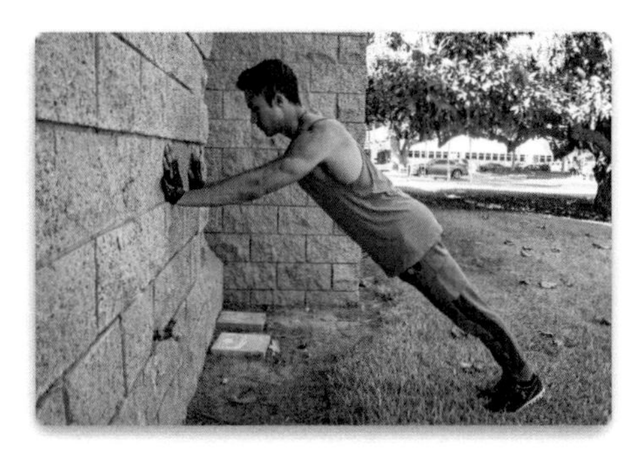
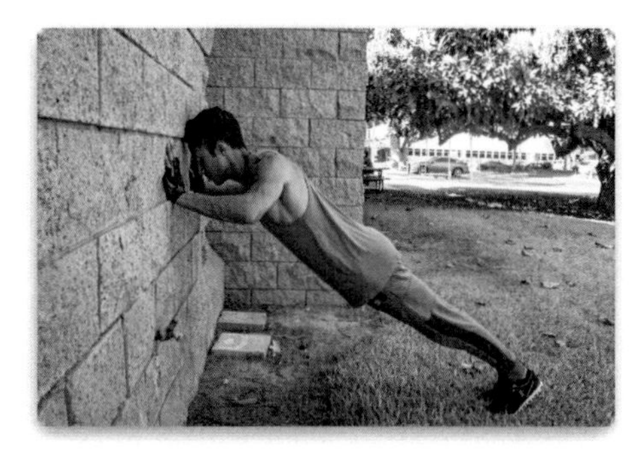

The very easiest pushing movement is a wall push-up. Make these as easy as you have to, based on your angle to the ground, but keep your body rigid and aim for good form at all times.

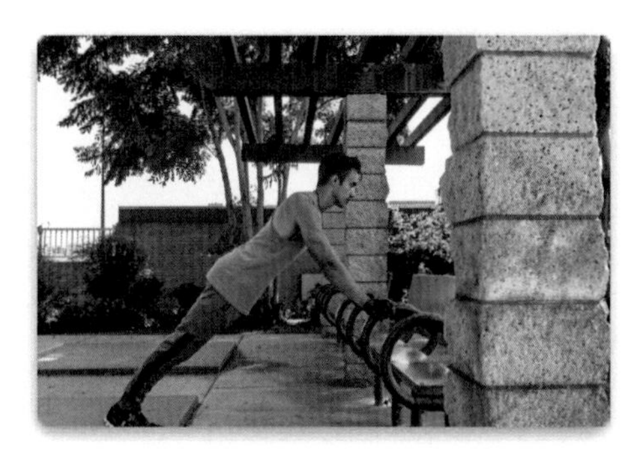
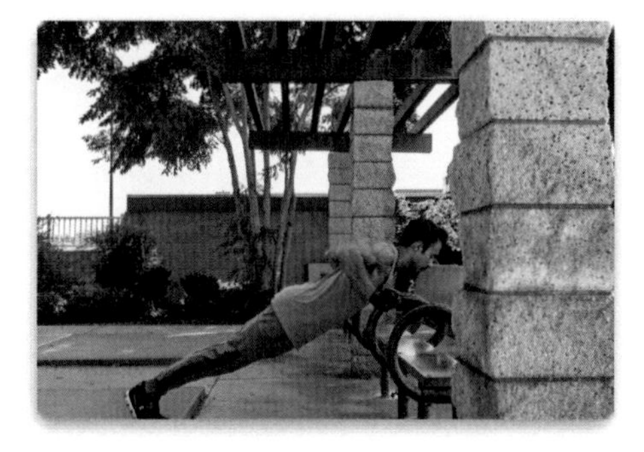

Once you have mastered wall push-ups and can do 10 of them with perfect form, try push-ups on an elevated surface (like this bench).

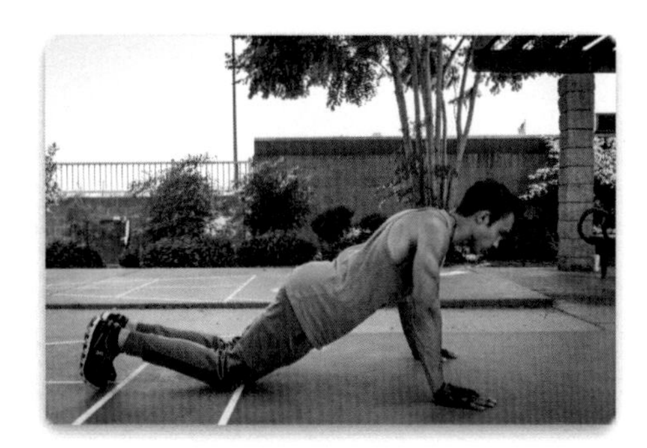
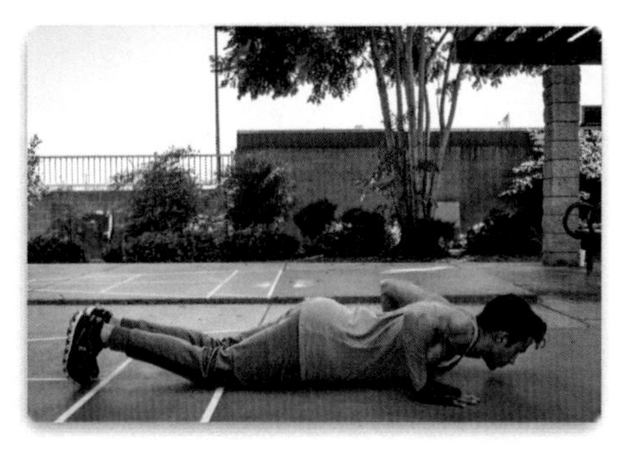

After you can do 10 of the elevated surface push-ups with perfect form, you have graduated to knee push-ups. Keep working on these until you can do 10 with perfect form.

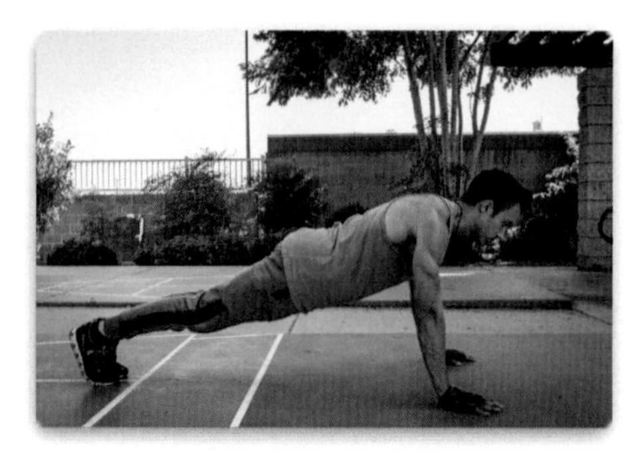
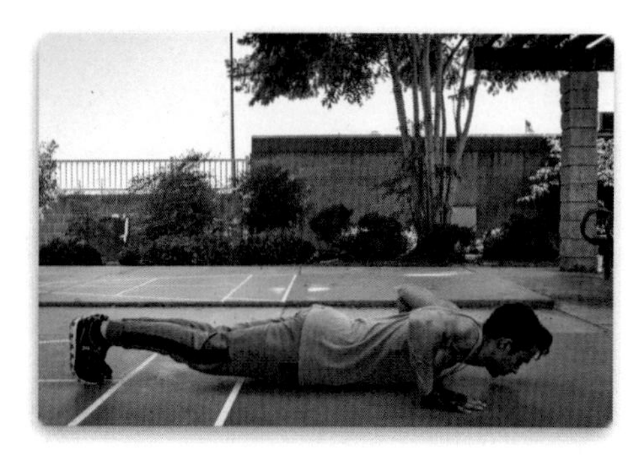

Next up is the full perfect form push-up, on your toes. Start out with limited range of motion if you have to at first, but eventually you want to get all the way down to the ground with each rep.

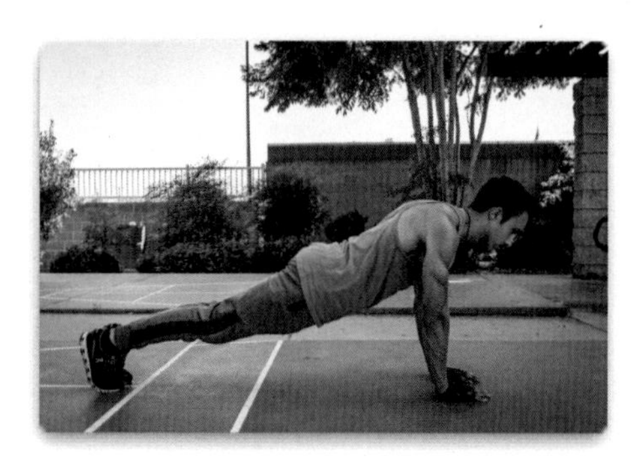
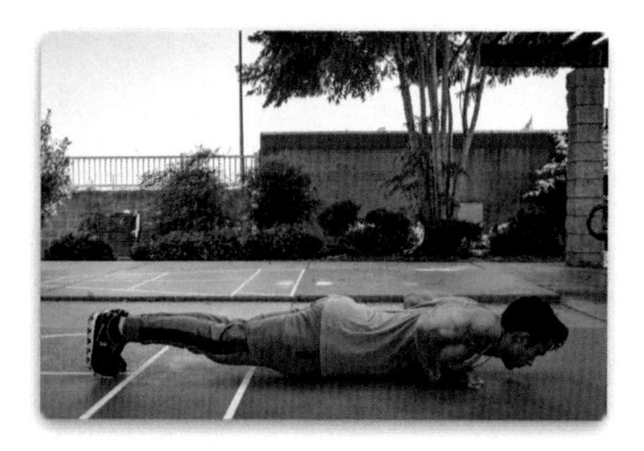

So you can do 10 perfect form full range of motion push-ups on your toes? Make things more difficult with the next progression: diamond pushups, with your hands touching in the center of your chest.

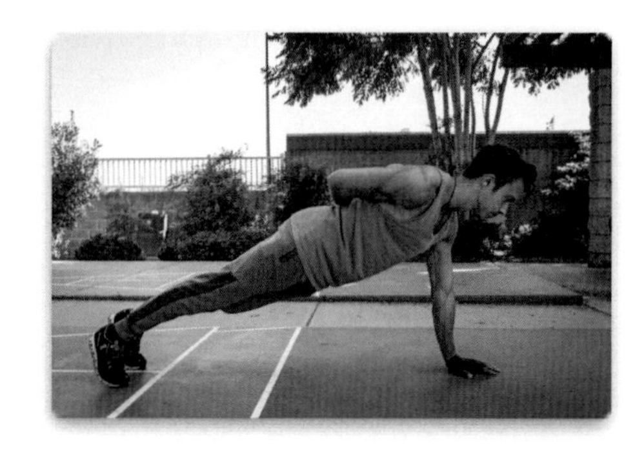
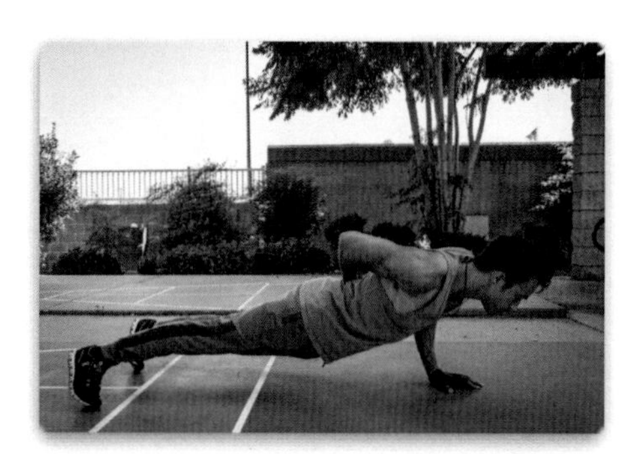
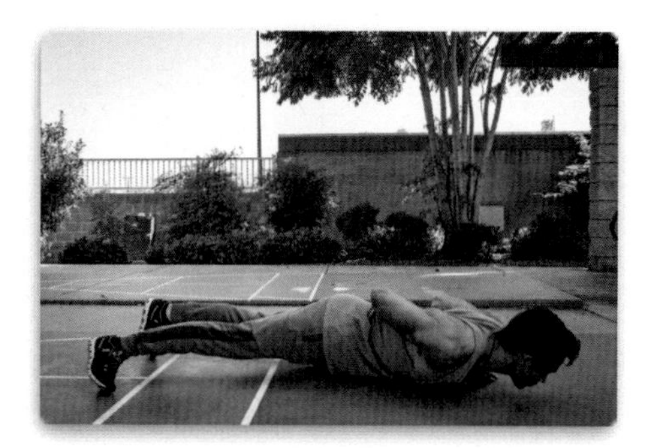

The ultimate bodyweight pushing exercise is the one-arm push-up. Start with a limited range of motion, or "half" one-arm push-ups, and gradually work on increasing your range of motion over time. Don't be discouraged if it takes forever to get one of these — very few humans can do this!

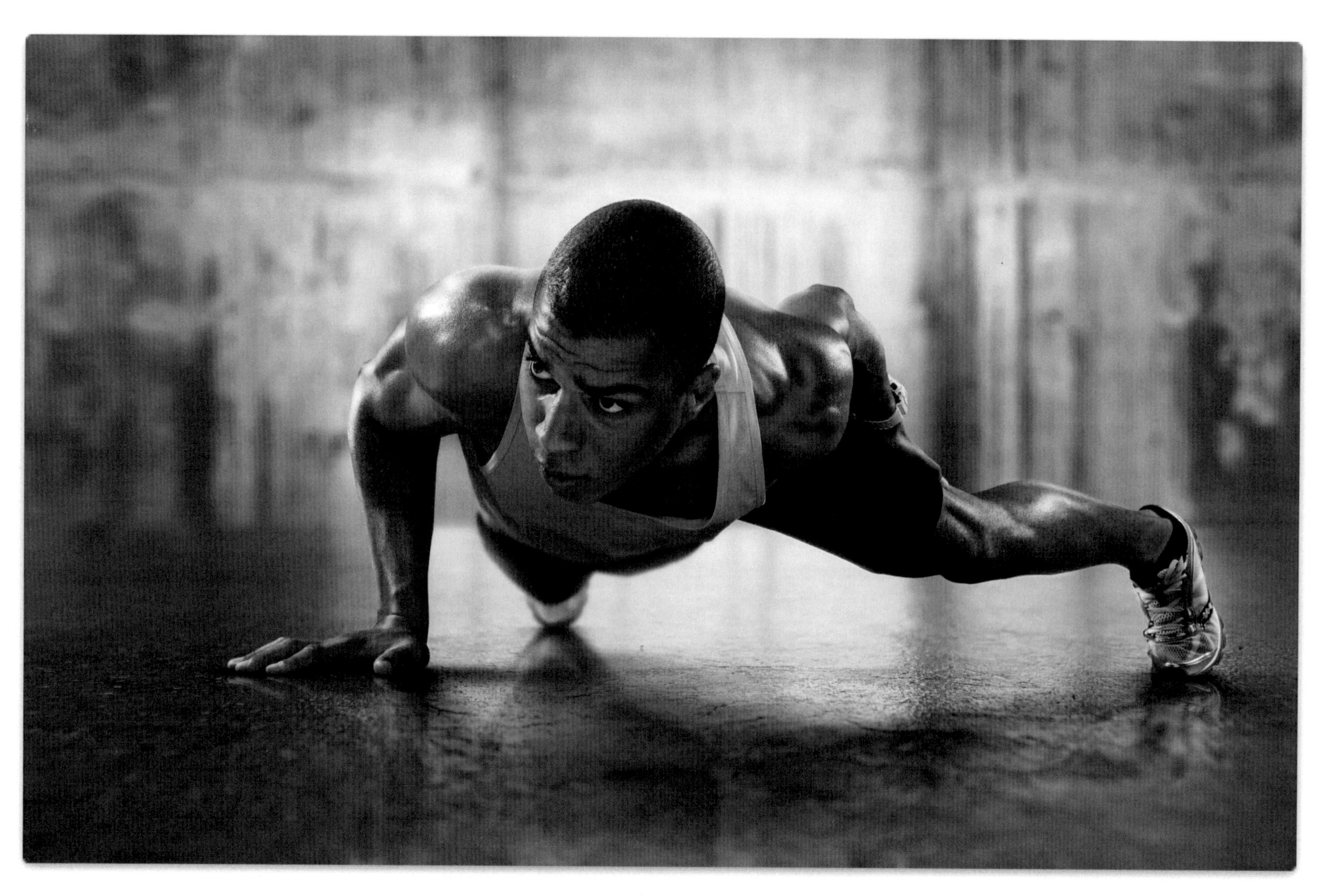

The one-arm push-up is the ultimate bodyweight pushing exercise.
This is why bodyweight progressions will last you a lifetime.

PULL

Next up is pulling exercises. Similar to pushing movements, there are a number of individual muscles that comprise your 'pulling chain', but it doesn't matter—all your body knows is that you are PULLING as hard as you possibly can, and using any and all muscles that could possibly assist with this movement. The classic pulling exercise is the pull-up, but most of us are not capable of doing even one full bodyweight pull-up. So a good starting point is some sort of 'suspension trainer'. This could either be a TRX or a cheap set of rings or any sort of bar that you can pull from. Start by doing 'rows', which are a pulling move on a suspension trainer at a 45 degree angle to the floor so that you are only pulling half your body weight. You can make this infinitely easier or harder by adjusting your angle, so this is a very nice way to progress. Try to use slow perfect form, and pick an angle that allows you to hit maximum intensity within 5 to 10 reps. After you can reach 10 reps, it is time to make them more difficult somehow. After you can do 10 full bodyweight rows with your body completely horizontal, you want to start working on your pull-ups. A good starting point here is 'negative' pull-ups. Start in the 'top' position of the pull-up (with your chin over the bar) and let yourself down (a 'negative' pull-up) as slowly as possible, aiming for maximum muscular failure on your way down by going as slow as you possibly can. Eventually you will be strong enough to start pulling your body up. It might take you as long as a year or two in order to work all the way up to just one single pull-up, but don't give up. You are getting way stronger no matter what, even if you never get all the way to pull-ups. Your only competition here is yourself, and the goal is to be the strongest version of yourself that you can achieve.

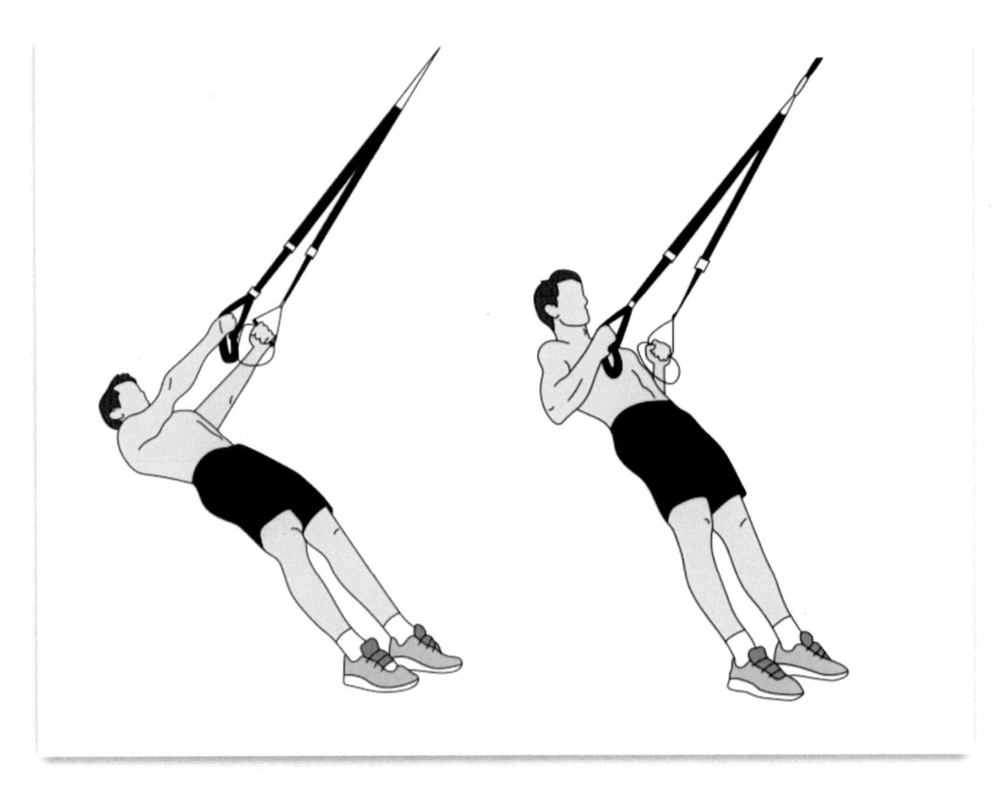

A suspension trainer is a great way to get started with bodyweight pulling exercises.

Just in case you wondered, the ultimate pull-up progression is the one-arm pull-up, which almost nobody can perform. So don't worry that you are going to run out of progression in the bodyweight pulling department any time soon!

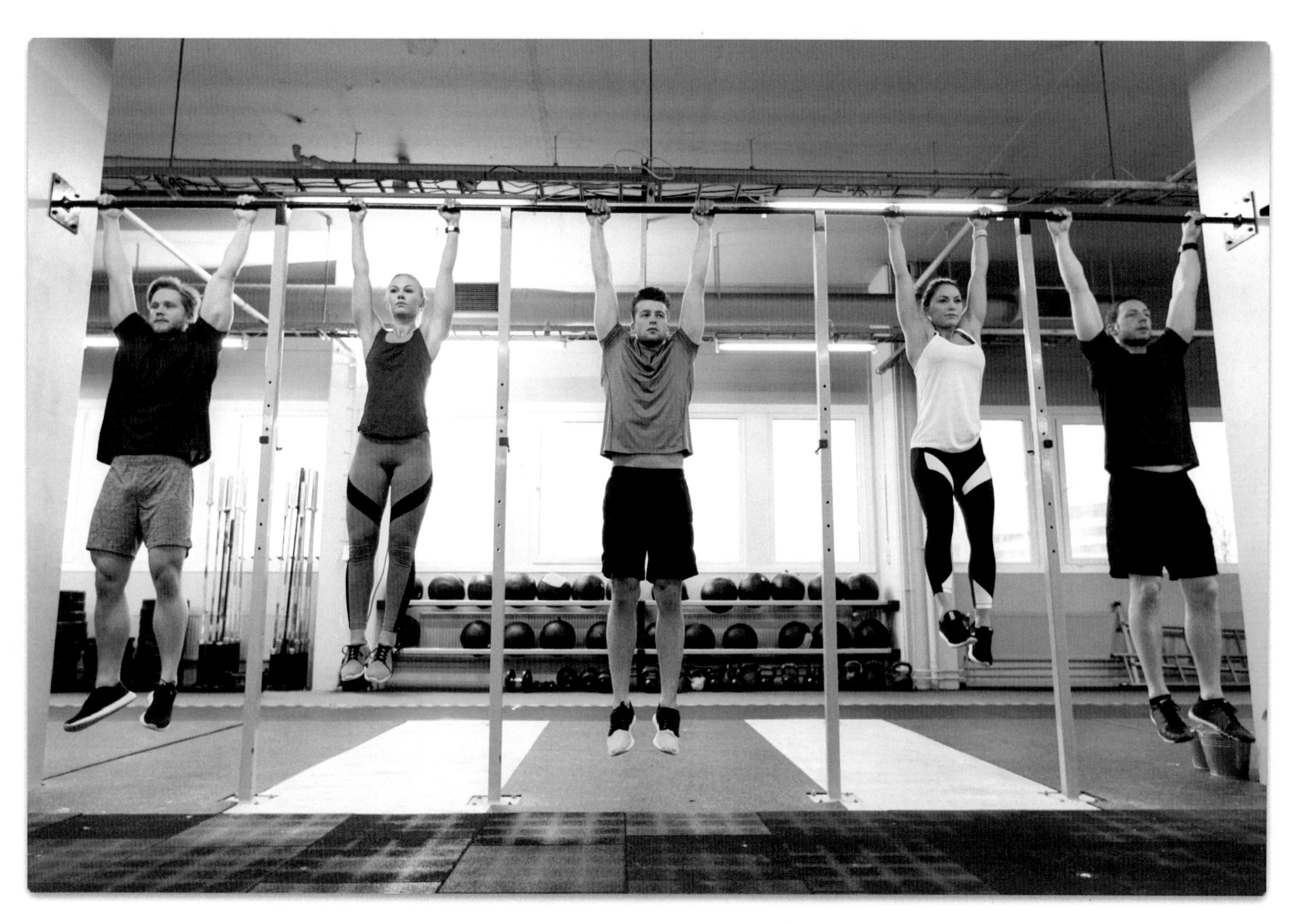

If you can't do a pull-up, start by hanging in the bottom position of a pull-up for as long as possible.

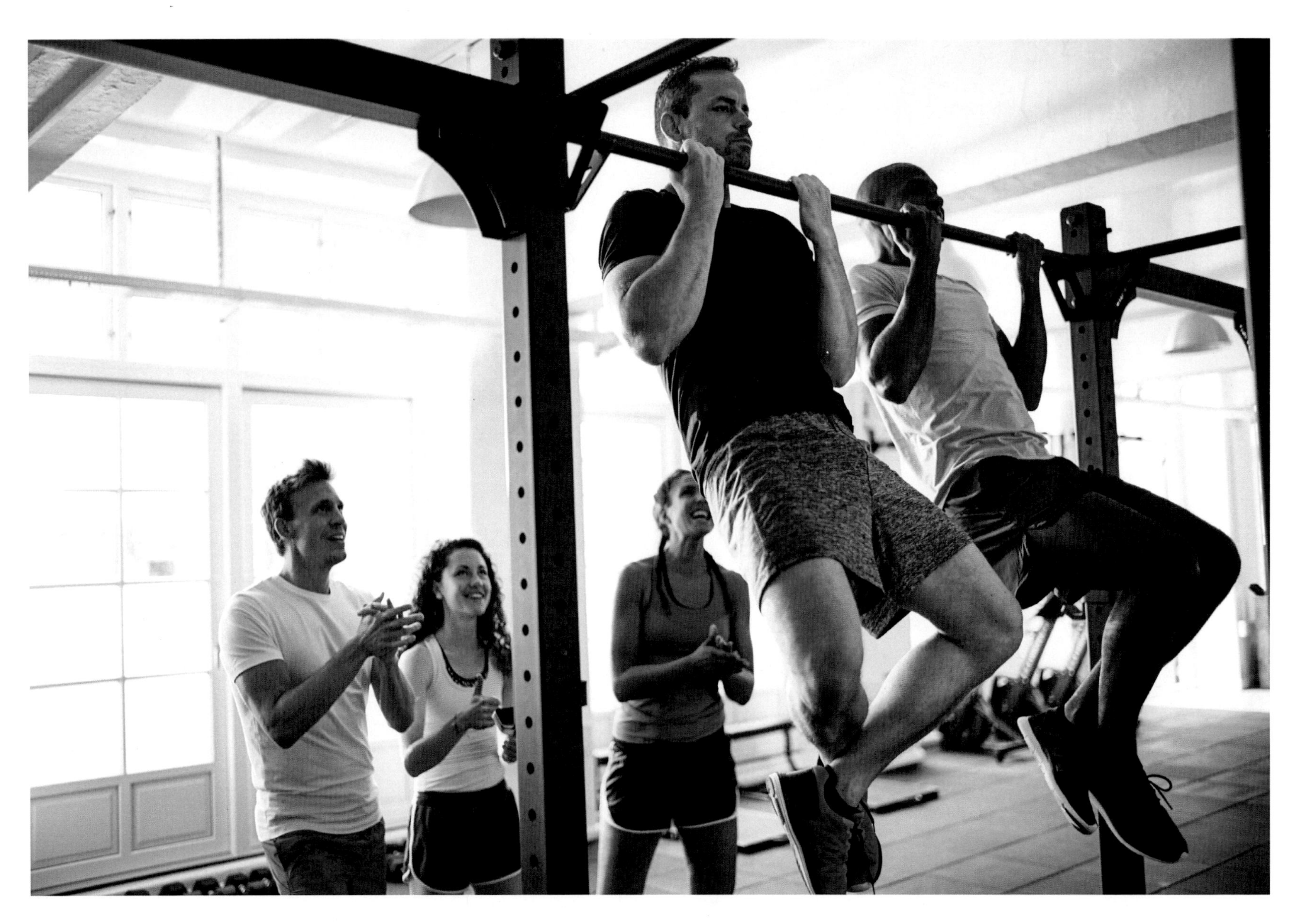

You can work up to a full pull-up gradually by holding a 'flex hang', or the top part of a pull-up, for as long as possible. You can also progress this by doing slow pull-up 'negatives', where you start in a flex hang and then lower yourself as slowly as possible.

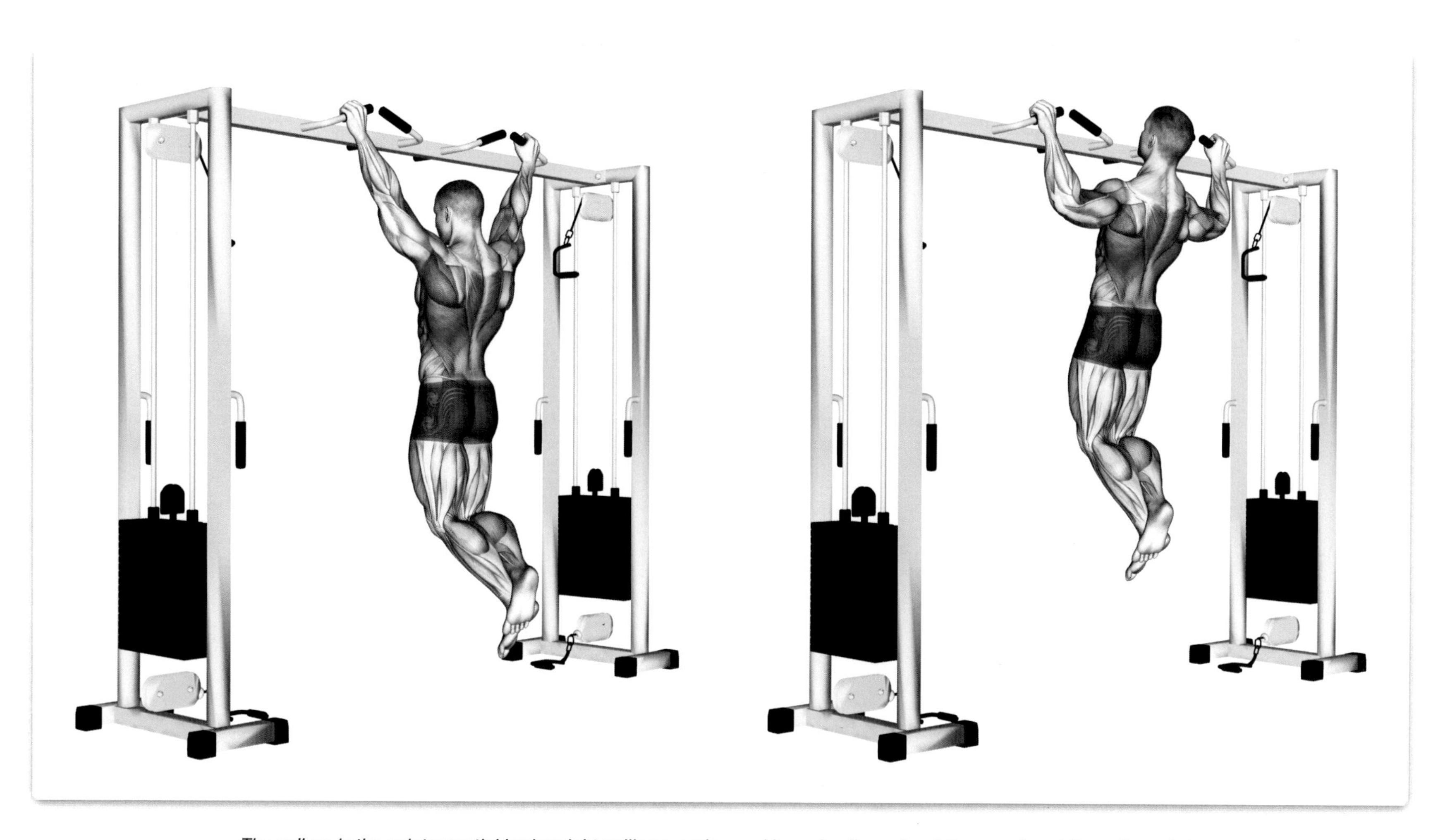

The pull-up is the quintessential bodyweight pulling exercise, and it maximally works all the muscles of the pulling chain.

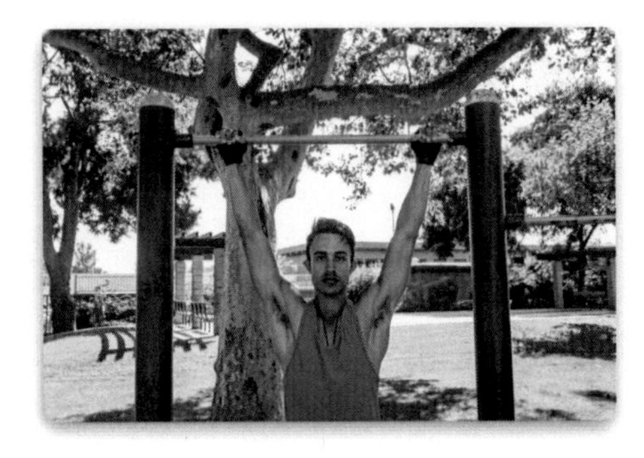
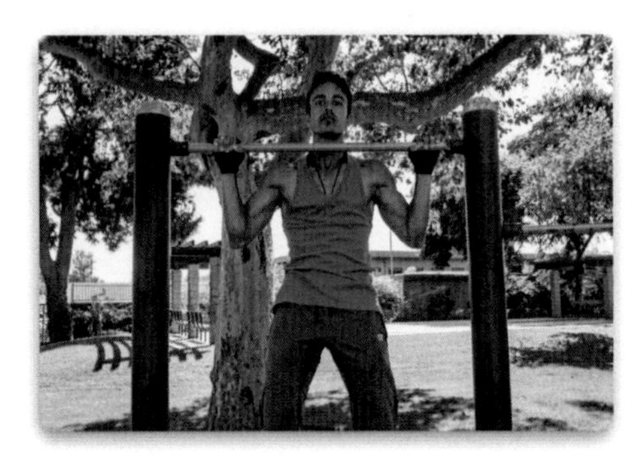
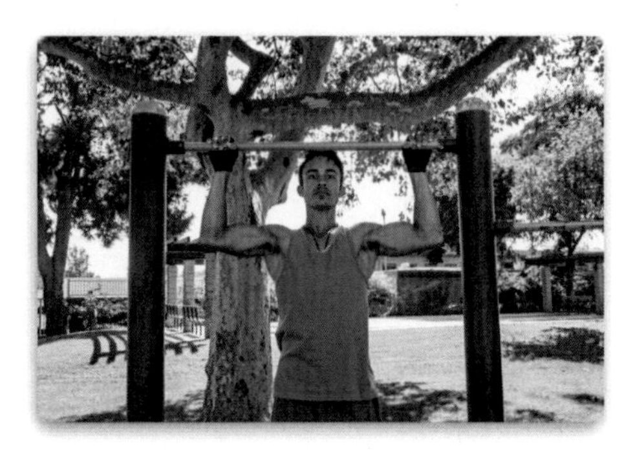

If you can't do a pull-up, start by hanging at the bottom of the movement for as long as possible. Then try a 'flex hang', or hanging at the top of the movement for as long as possible. Then try doing pull-up 'negatives', by starting at the top and lowering yourself as slowly as possible.

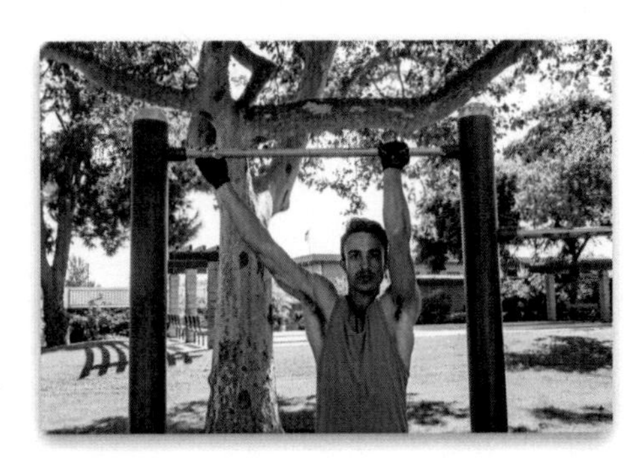
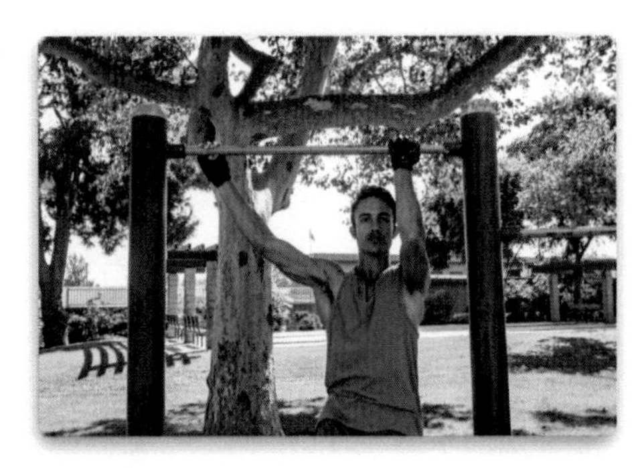
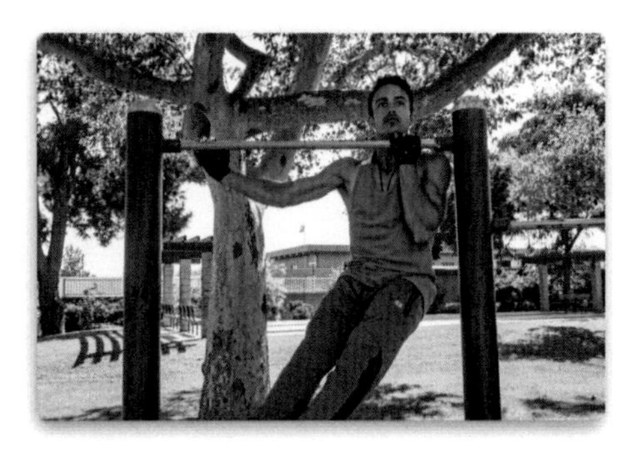

If you have mastered regular pull-ups and you can do ten perfect form reps with no difficulty, start working towards a one-arm pull-up or chin-up (pictured here). The first step is placing most of your weight on one arm at a time with these asymmetrical chin-ups.

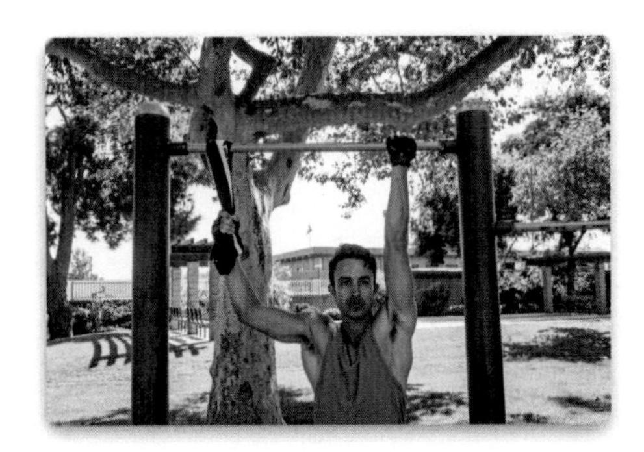
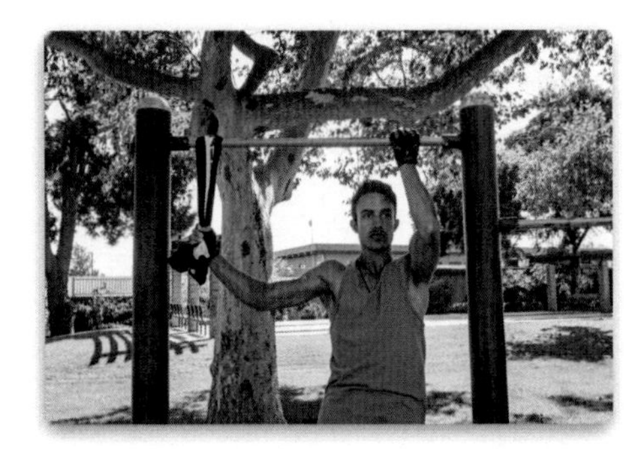
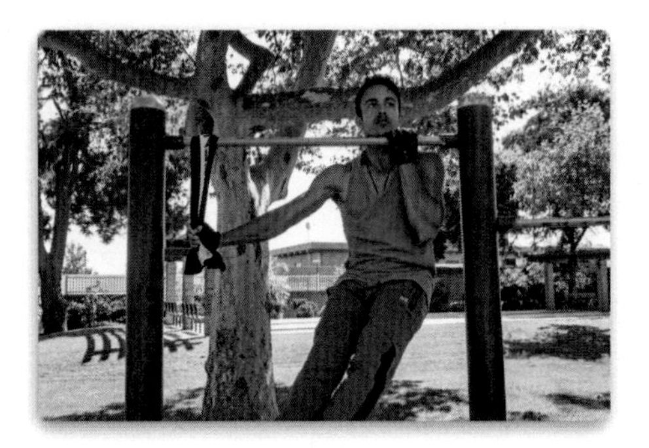

The next progression towards a one-arm chin (OAC)? Gripping a towel or a rope over the bar with the assisting arm, which makes things even more challenging for the arm that you are focusing on. The lower the grip with the assisting arm, the higher the difficulty.

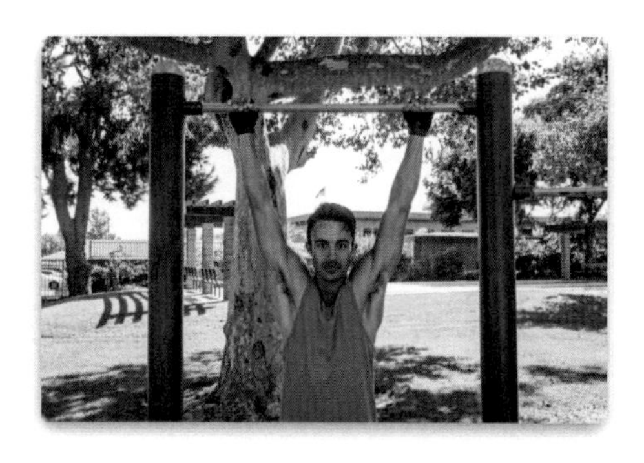
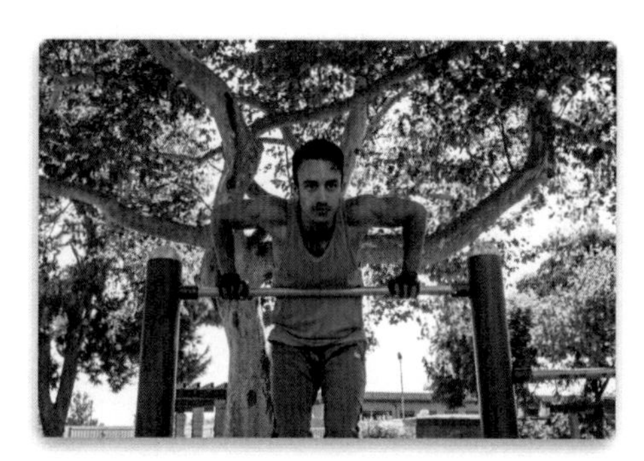
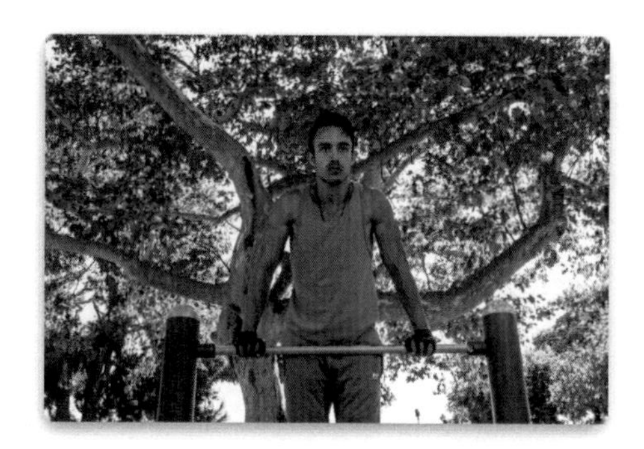

The muscle-up is a very advanced bodyweight move which is incredibly difficult—but it is an amazing exercise that involves both pulling and pushing, maximally working all of the muscles of the upper body at the same time. No other single upper body exercise is this powerful. Most people have to train for these for months to years, so you won't run out of bodyweight training goals anytime soon!

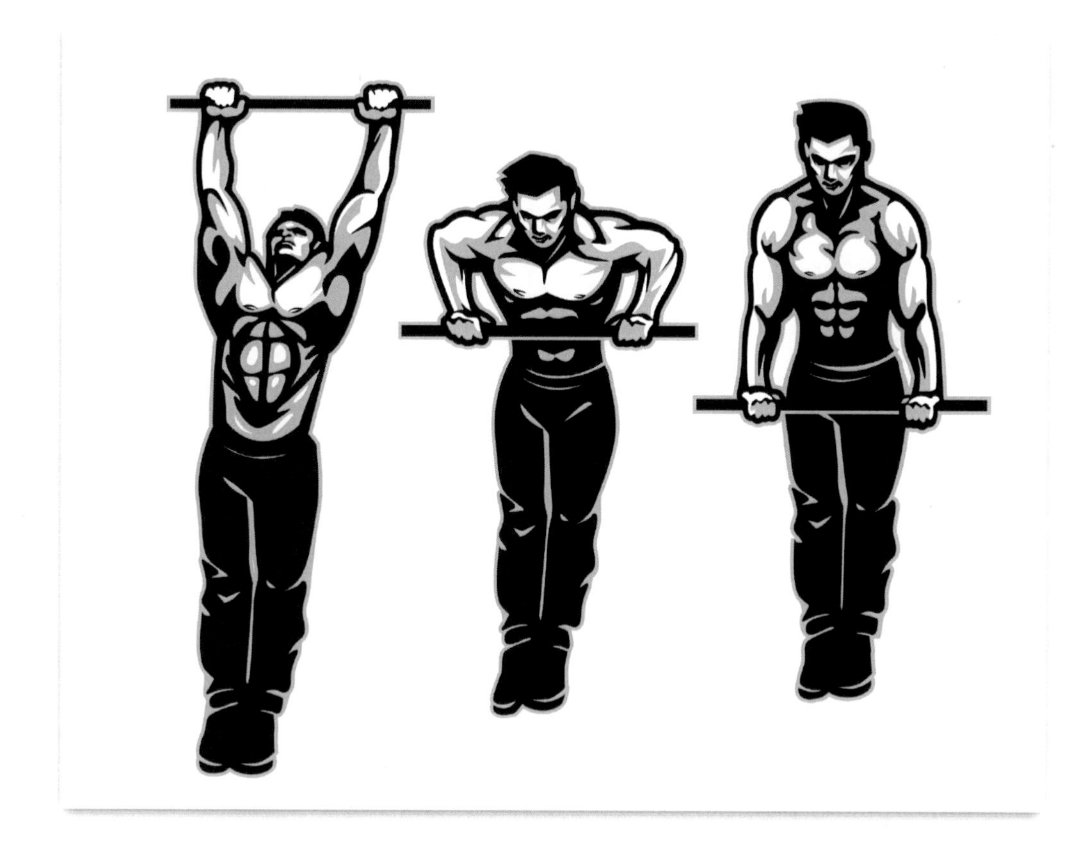

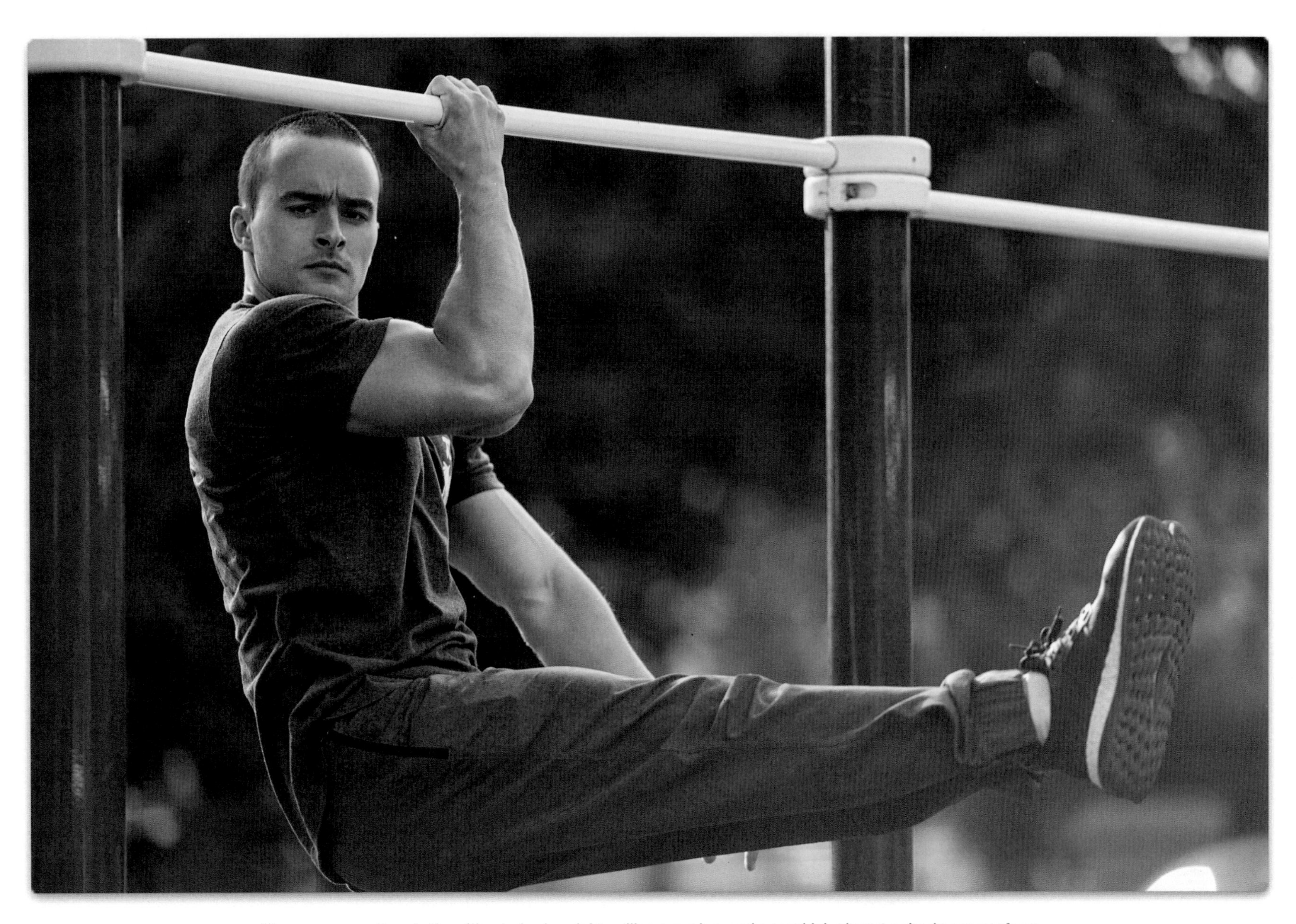

The one-arm pull-up is the ultimate bodyweight pulling exercise, and one which almost nobody can perform. Let's just say you have plenty of room for progression with bodyweight exercises.

LEGS

Your legs really just perform one basic movement: pushing your body away from gravity. Squatting, lunges, and jumping are all compound leg movements that involve a ton of muscles as well as flexing your hip, knee and ankle at the same time. But again, all your body knows is that it is using your legs to push against gravity as hard as possible. So you can do wall sits, bodyweight squats, or single leg lunges to work your legs. The problem with an ordinary two-legged bodyweight squat is that it is fairly easy so most of us can do more than 10 of them without a ton of difficulty. You can make these more challenging a number of ways. First of all, you could do a SLOW bodyweight squat. Go down into the low part of the squat VERY slowly, targeting about 30 seconds going down. Then hold the bottom of the squat for 30 seconds. Then take 30 seconds to go back up as slowly as possible. Repeat until you hit complete failure—and believe us when we say that this won't take very long!

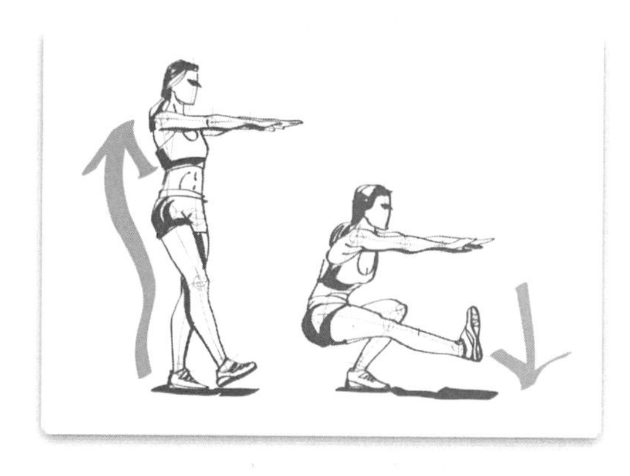

Single-leg pistol squats are the ultimate progression of bodyweight leg exercises.

Eventually you might graduate to the most difficult bodyweight leg move of all: the single-leg pistol squat. This highly advanced move may very well take years for most to work up to—and that is just to do ONE of them. By the time you can do 10 pistol squats on each leg, you are pretty much an elite human and your legs are strong as hell.

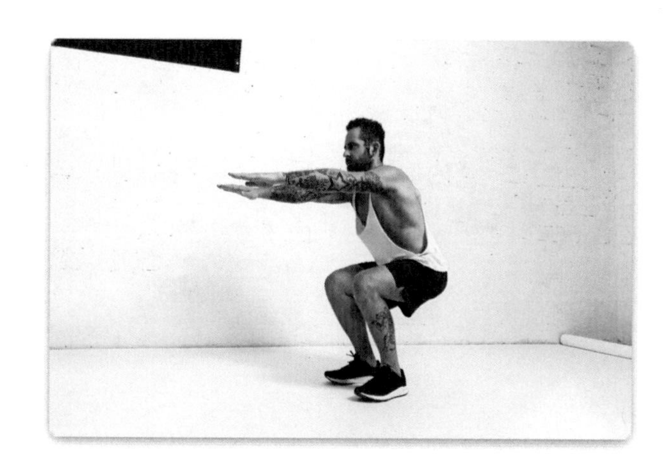

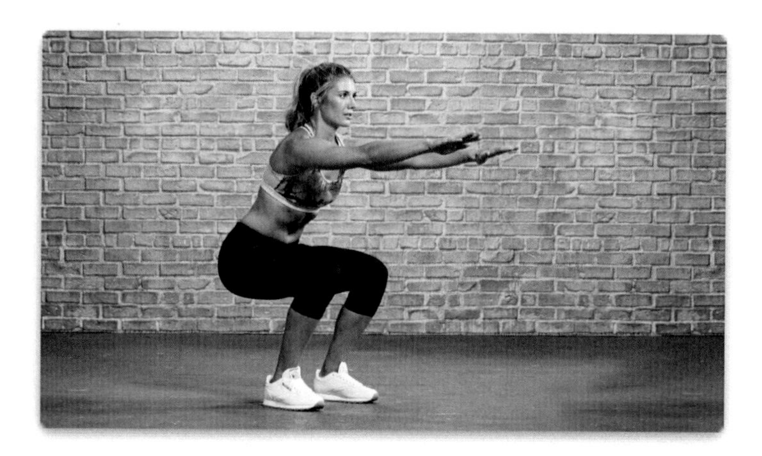

Bodyweight squats are the starting point for leg exercises.

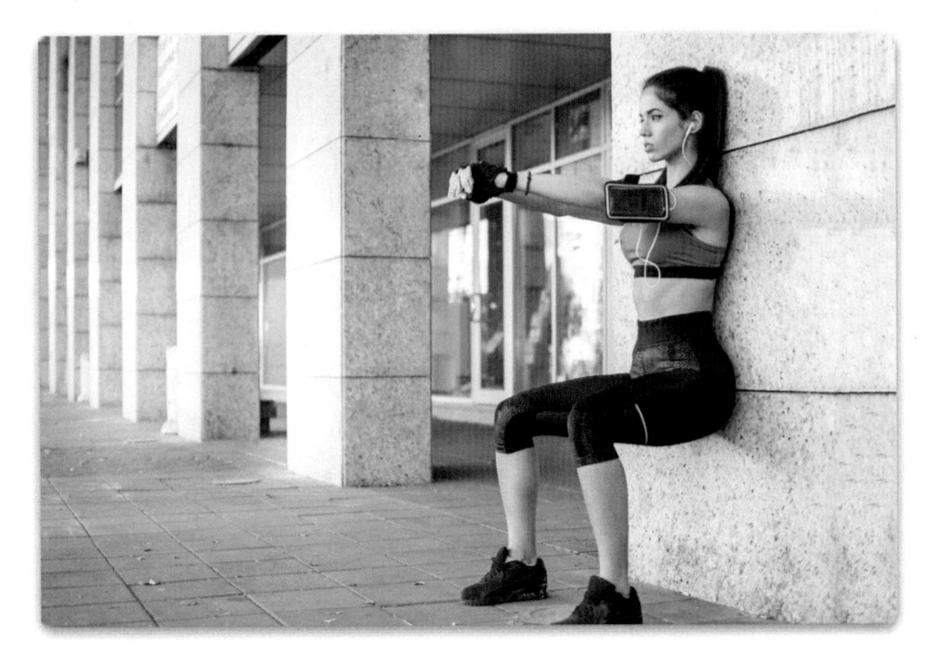

Holding a wall sit is a great isometric exercise for your legs.

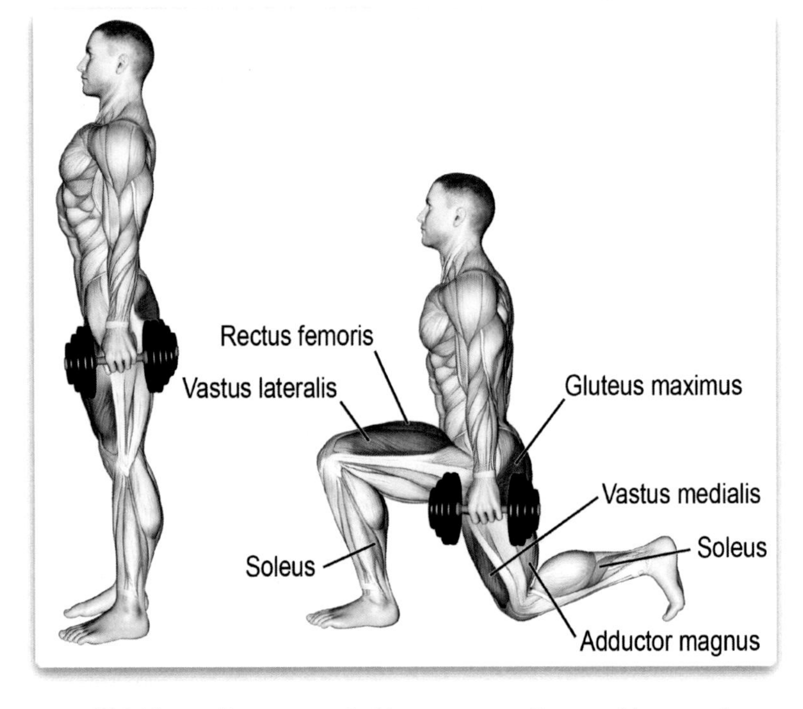

Weights aren't necessary, but lunges are another good leg exercise.

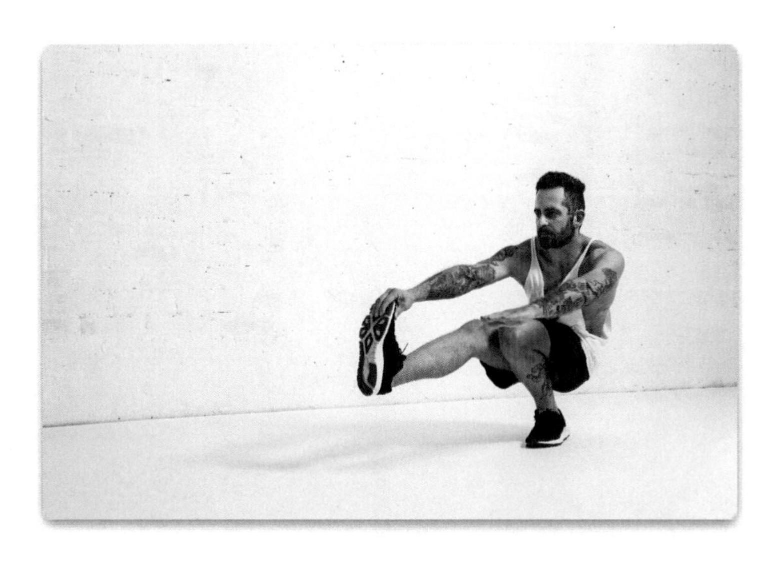
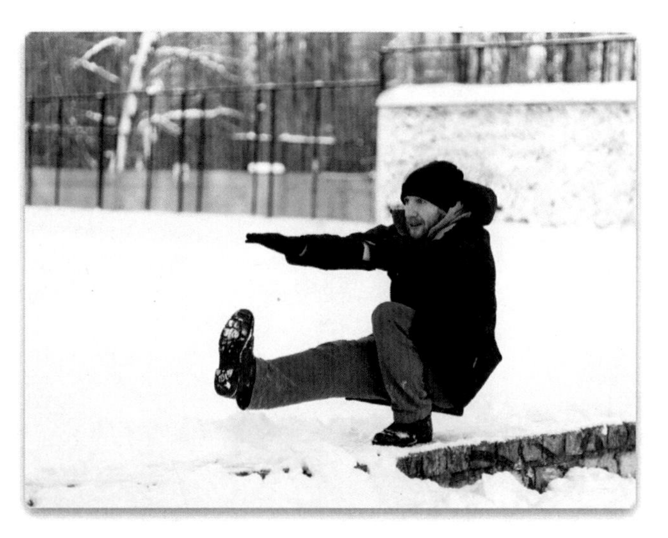

It usually takes months or even years to work up to these single-leg pistol squats.

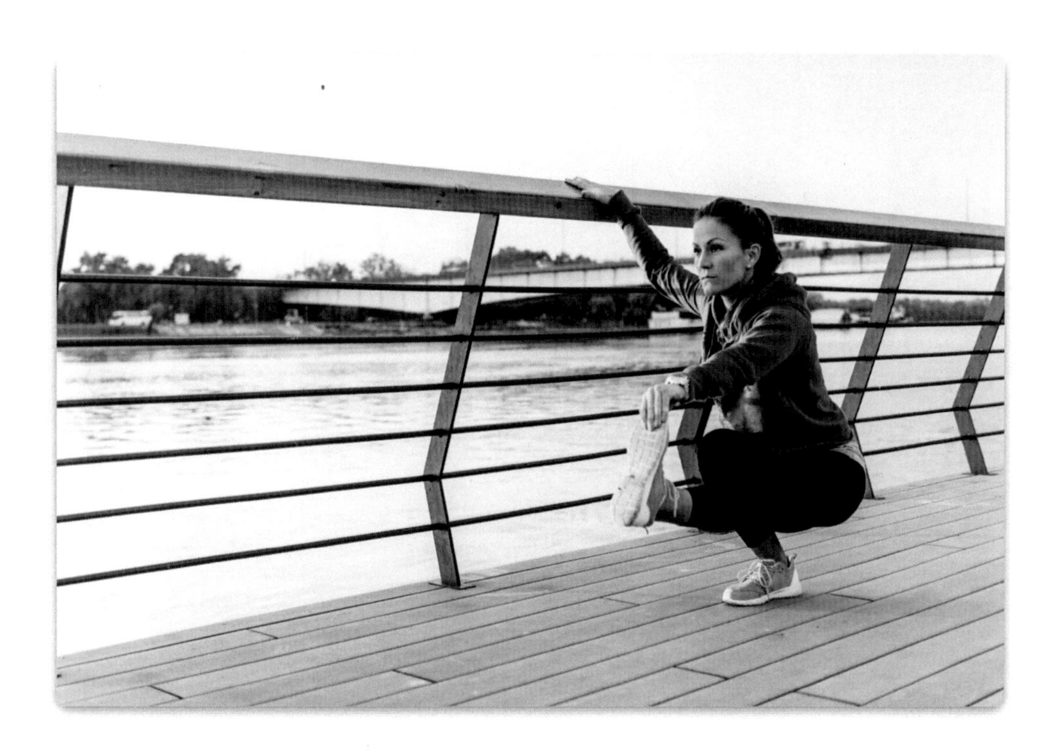

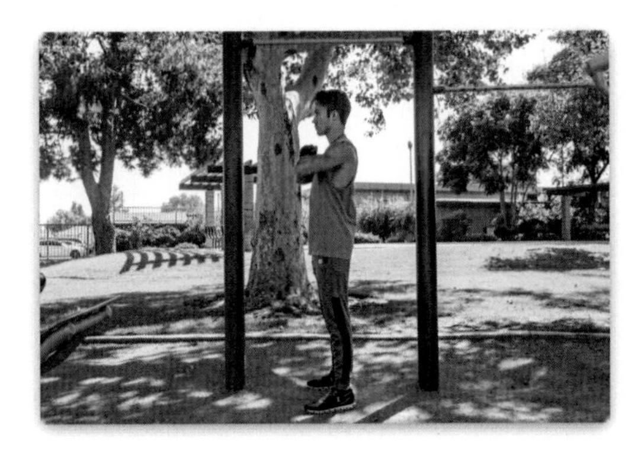

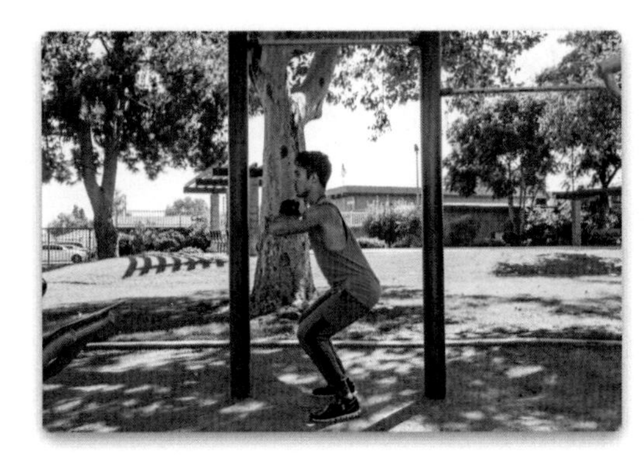

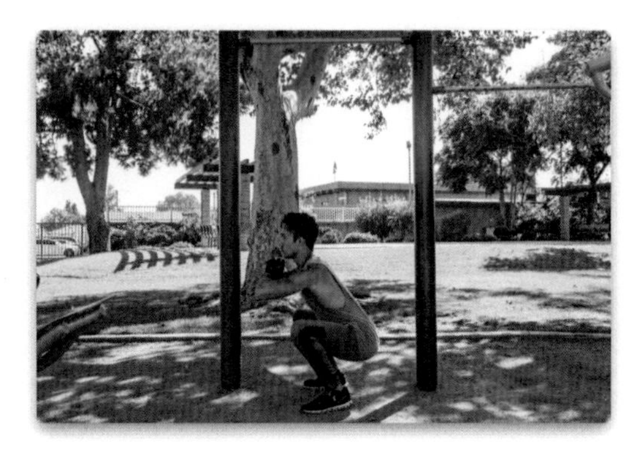

The starting point for leg exercises is the bodyweight squat. To add difficulty, be sure to use a full range of motion and aim for perfect form, with chest high. Still too easy? Try the super slow version (~30 seconds down, hold at the bottom for ~30 seconds, then ~30 seconds going back up—repeat to failure).

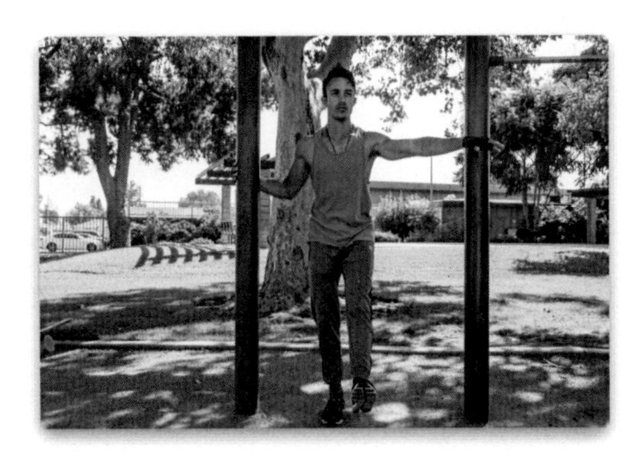

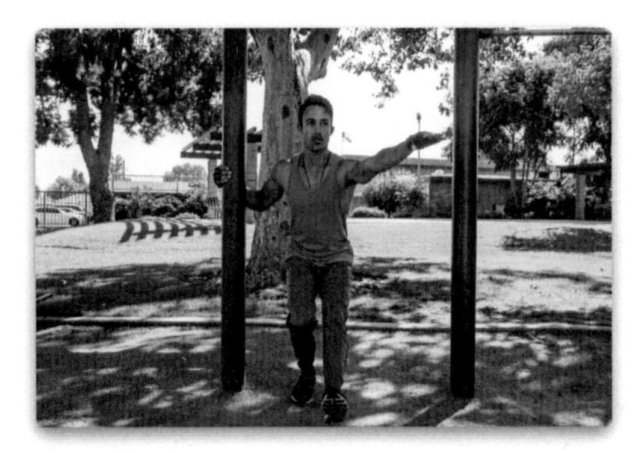

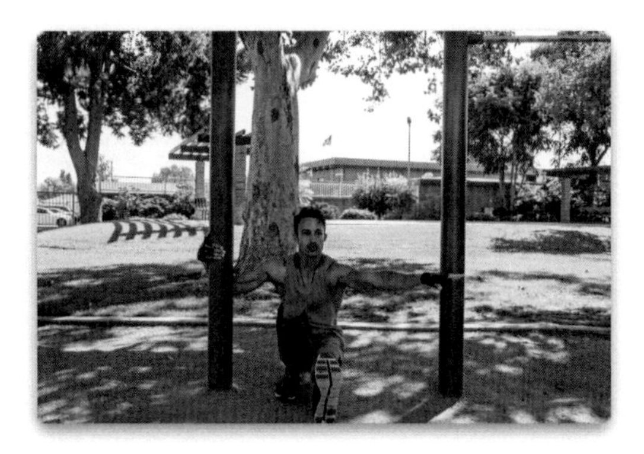

Eventually it will be time to double the difficulty by using one leg at a time with the 'pistol squat', or single leg variation. These are very challenging and most people have to gradually work up to these over months or even years! Progress these VERY slowly so you don't risk injuring your knee (or anything else). Start with partial range of motion, plus holding onto a solid object for support.

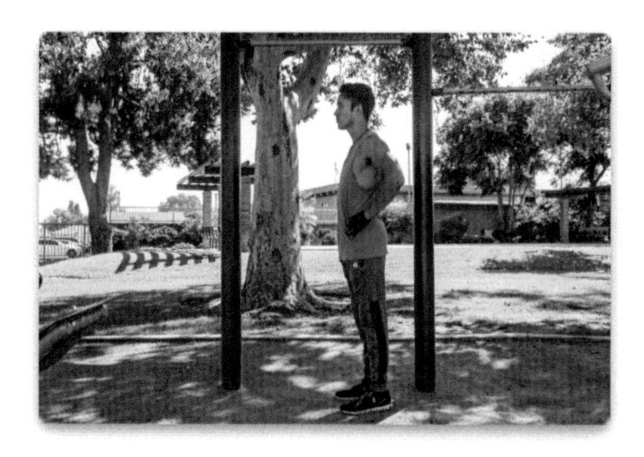
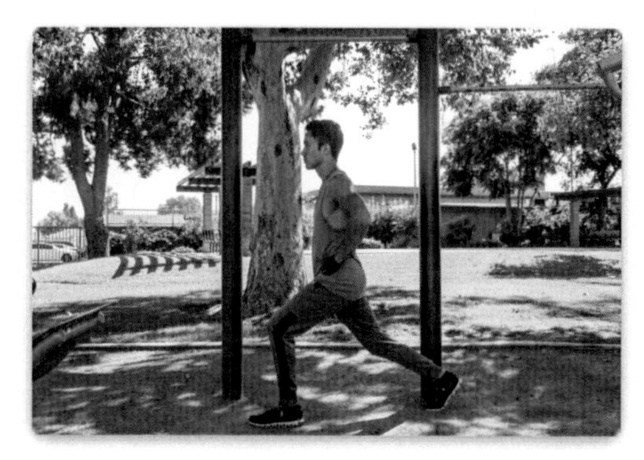
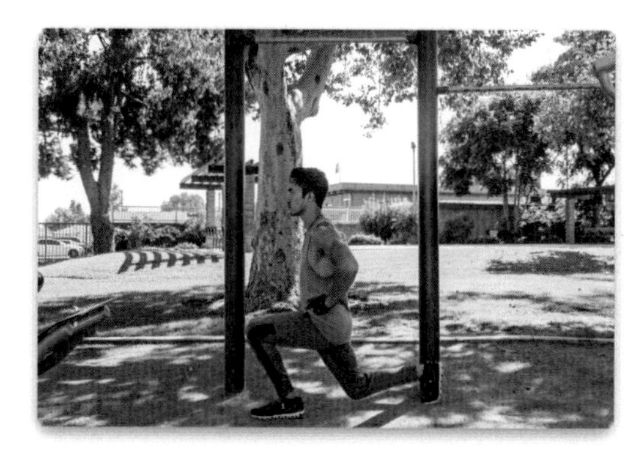

Lunges are another good single leg exercise. Either step forward with the working leg, or backwards with the opposite leg. Try to place all of your weight on the forward leg (the one you are exercising). Squat all the way down until your thigh is parallel with the ground, keeping your chest high. Repeat on the same side all the way to failure (with rest-pause triple set technique if desired), then switch sides.

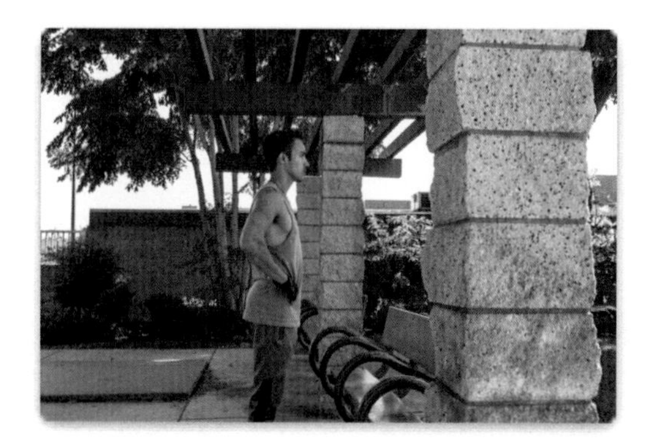
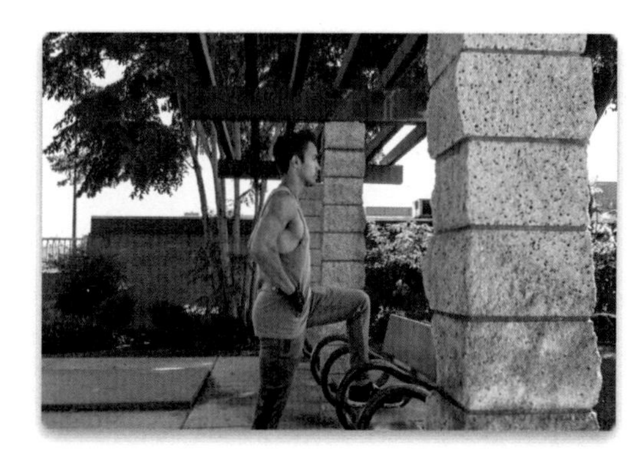
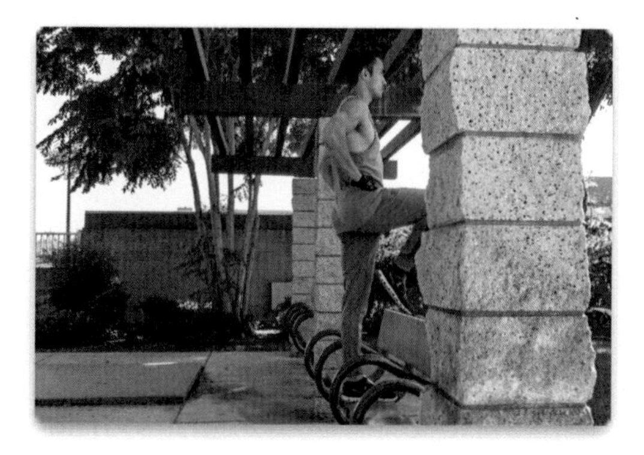

Step-ups are another great single leg exercise, but you do need something to step on (pretty much any safe and stable object will do). Place your foot on an elevated surface and drive upwards with this leg, ending in a standing position, then back down again. Repeat to failure.

ACCESSORY MOVES

In addition to the three primary moves (Push, Pull, and Legs), there are three more accessory moves which add additional value if you have time for them. We would consider the primary moves as the bare minimum for any full-body workout—but if you have the time, throw in these as well!

ACCESSORY MOVEMENTS

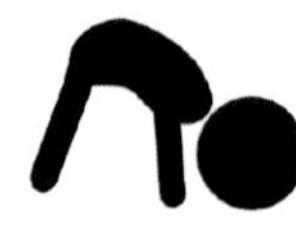

PRESS

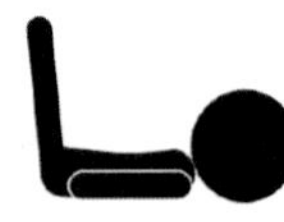

ANTERIOR

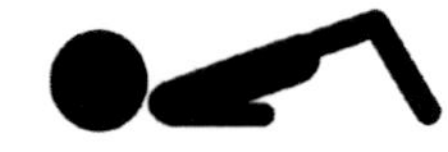

POSTERIOR

PRESS

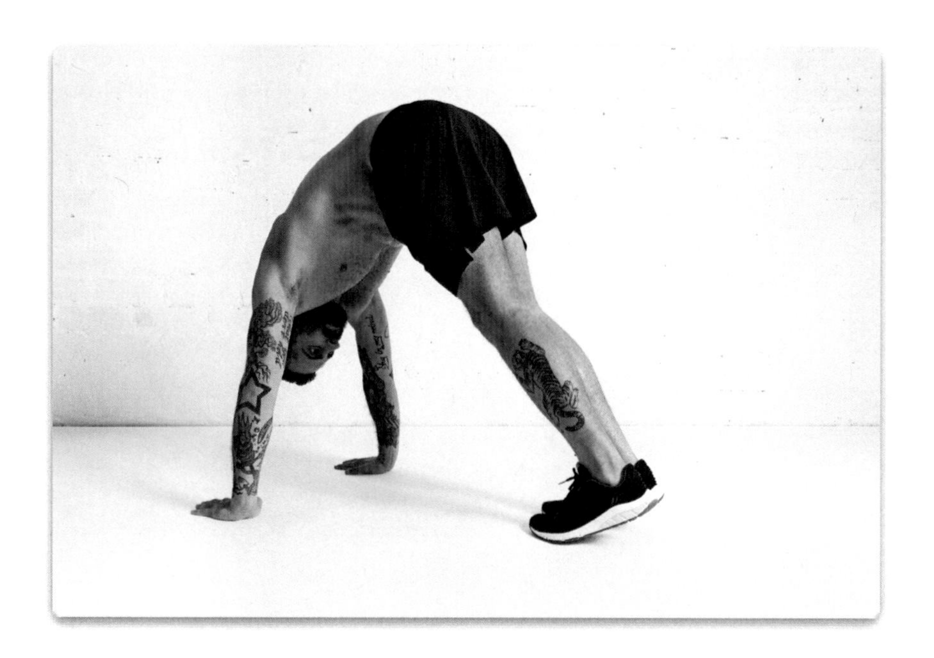

Horizontal pushing movements like the push-up work all of the muscles of your pushing chain including your chest, shoulders, and triceps. Overhead pushing, or 'press' movements, work the same muscles, but place more emphasis on the shoulder muscles and less emphasis on the chest muscles. Adding presses to your pushing exercises is a great way to ensure complete development of your shoulders. You might have to build up some basic pushing strength with push-ups first, but when you are ready to get into pressing, the pike push-up is the place to start. Once you can easily do 10 of these with slow perfect form and highest difficulty, then you can graduate to handstand holds against a wall. Next up is partial range of motion handstand push-ups, followed by handstand push-up 'negatives', or starting at the top of a handstand and lowering down. Eventually the goal is full range of motion handstand push-ups, an advanced move indeed. Because it is dangerous to take these all the way to failure, one strategy is doing a hard set of handstand push-ups just shy of failure, then lowering the difficulty (and danger factor) to a pike push-up and finishing with sets of these to failure.

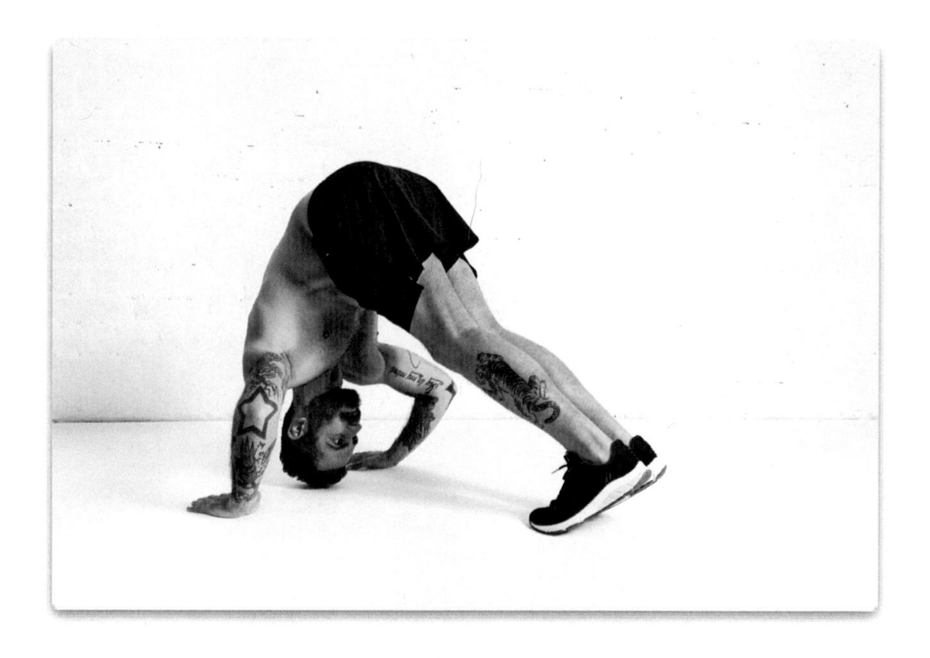

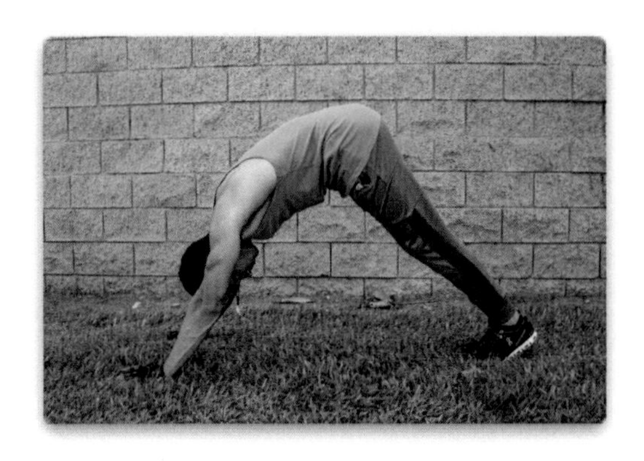

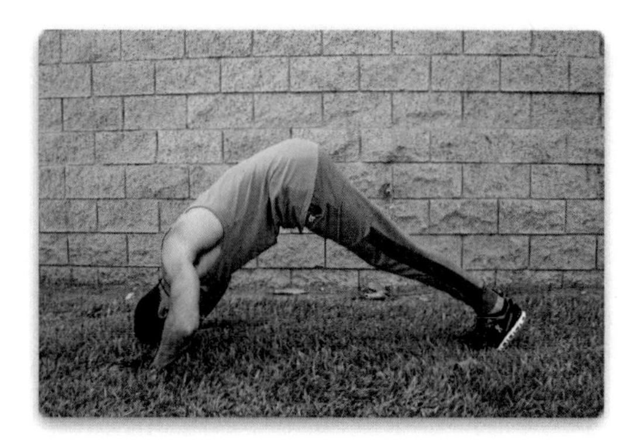

Eventually you will want to add in some overhead pressing movements, for full shoulder development. The best place to start is a pike push-up, shown here.

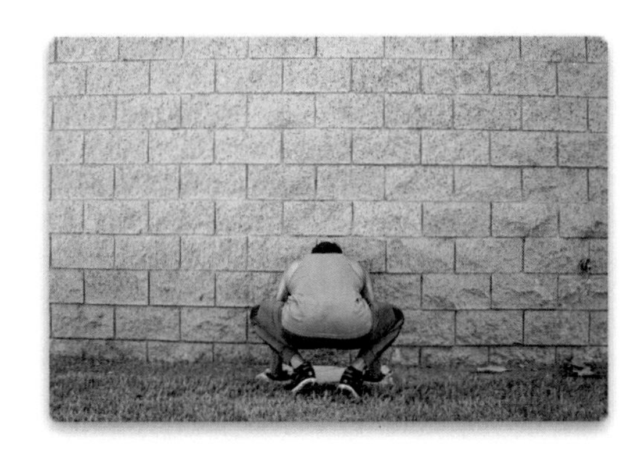

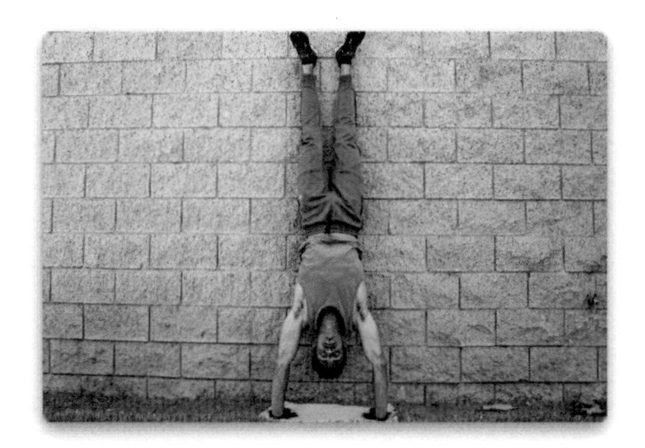

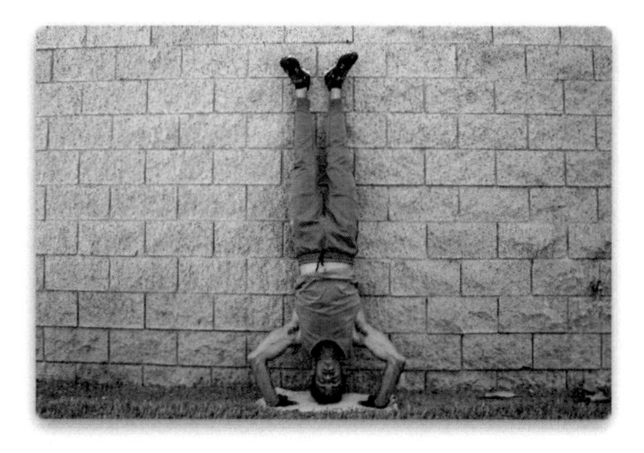

When you can do 10 perfect pike push-ups with no difficulty, you might want to carefully try some handstand holds against a wall. Start by just holding a handstand as long as you can. Don't take these to failure, for obvious reasons! Much safer to hold a handstand until significant fatigue but short of failure, then use a reverse pyramid technique to go to the easier progress — pike push-ups — and do these all the way to failure. The ultimate bodyweight pressing move is a handstand push-up. If you can get to 10 of these, you will have some amazing pressing strength!

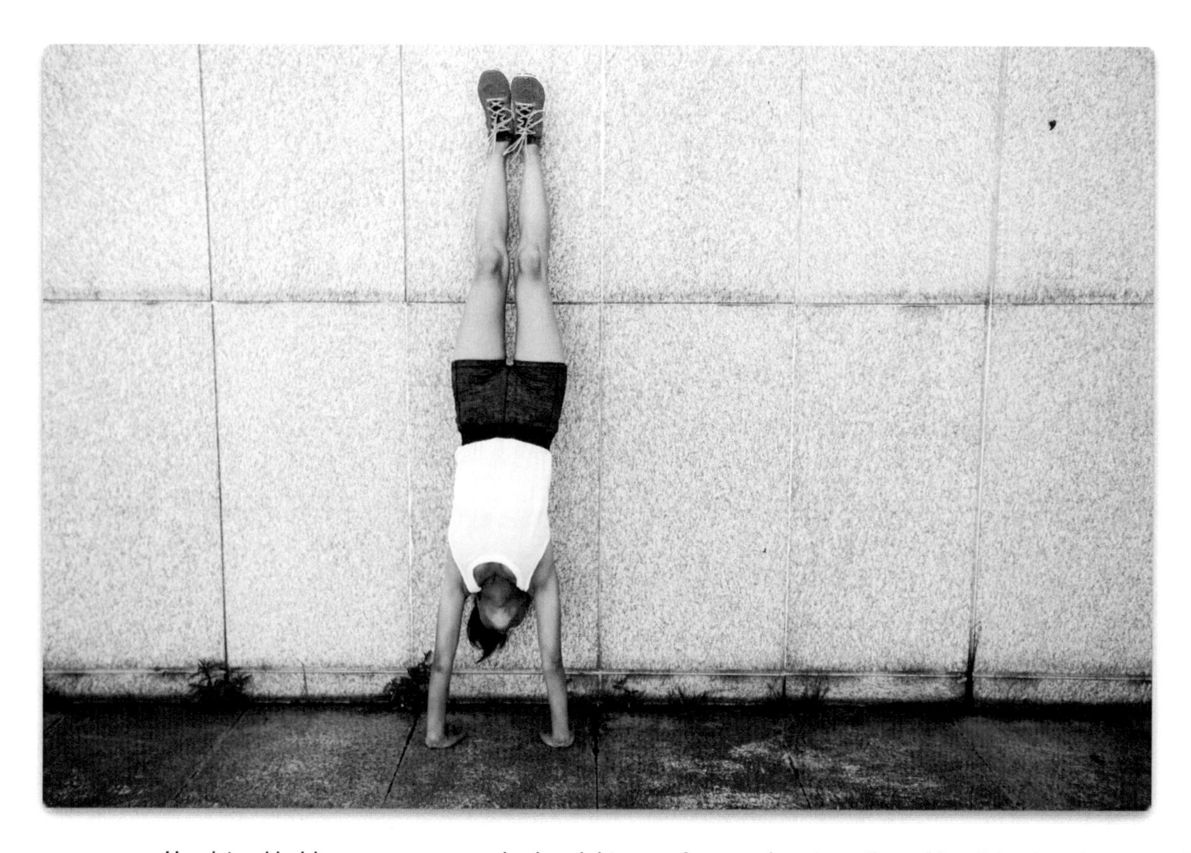

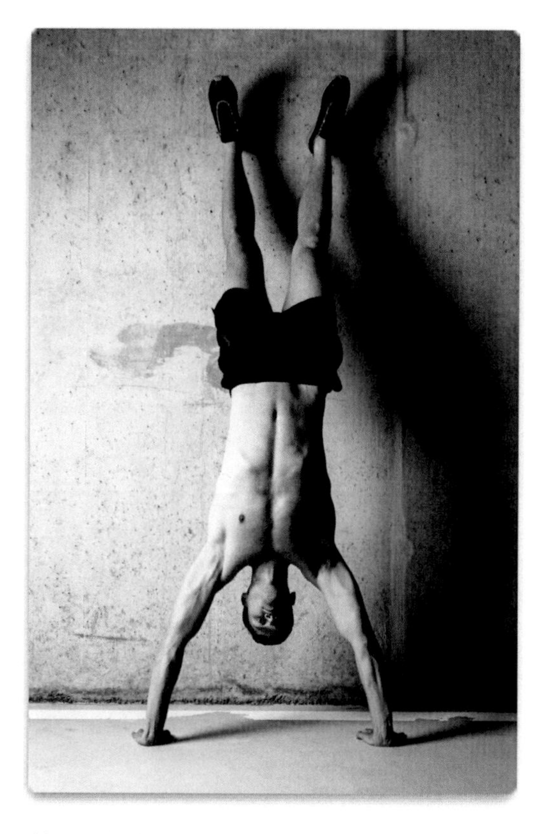

Handstand holds are an awesome bodyweight move for pressing strength, and handstand push-ups are the ultimate bodyweight pressing exercise.

ANTERIOR CHAIN

The anterior chain involves all of the muscles on the front half of the body, especially the core muscles such as the abdominals. The easiest and our favorite is a 'hollow hold'. Lie on your back, with the lumbar part of your back pressed into the ground and your arms outstretched overhead. Use your abdominal muscles to tilt your pelvis up, lifting your feet slightly off the ground. At the same time, lift your arms slightly

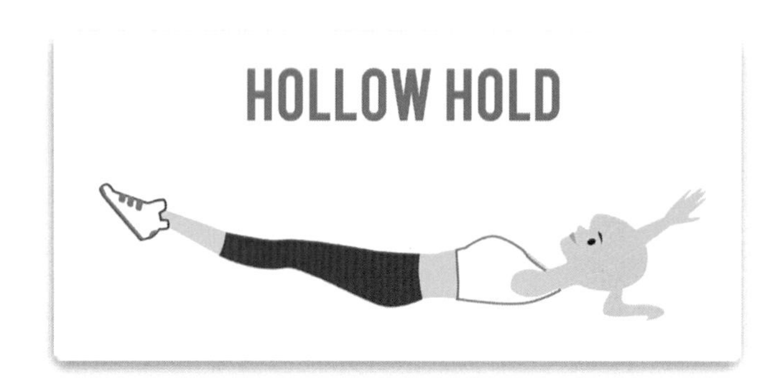

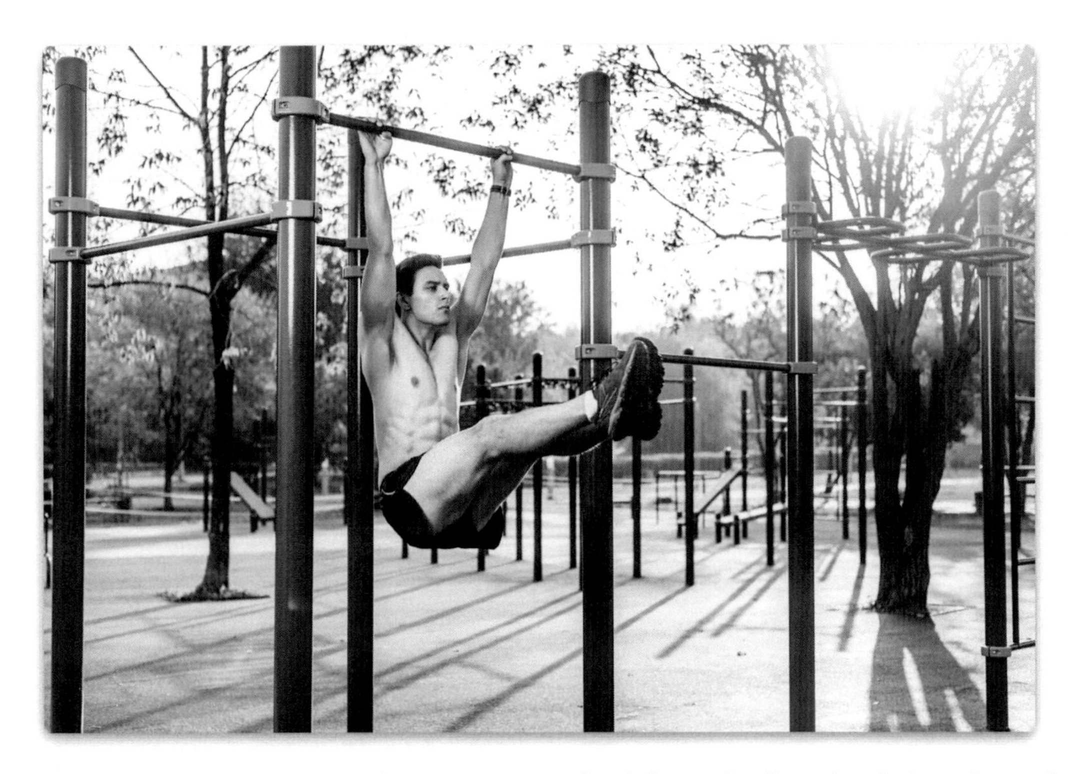

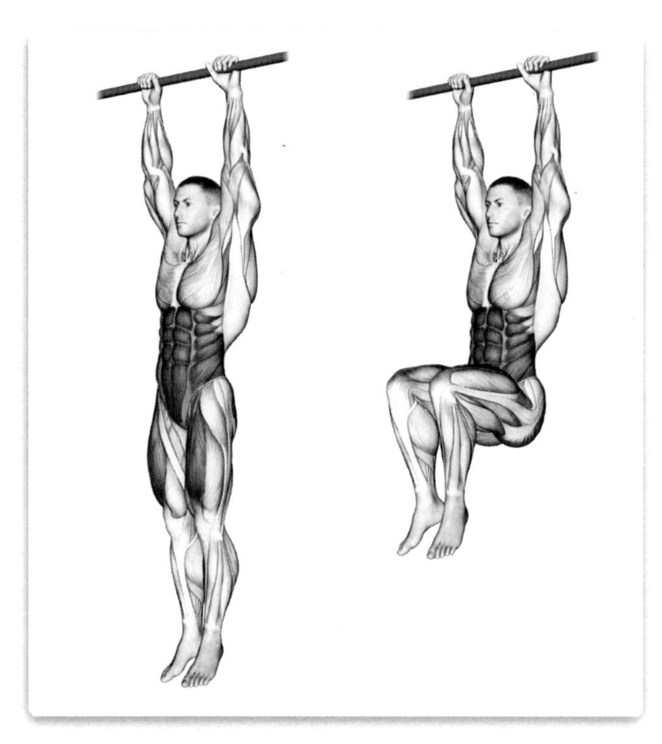

Hanging leg raises are a great anterior chain exercise. Knees bent is the easiest, and try legs straight as a more difficult progression.

off the ground as well, adding even more tension to your abdominal muscles. Hold with the highest ab tension possible, for as long as possible.

If you have a bar available, we love hanging leg raises as well. Try with knees bent to start, and then go to knees straight to add difficulty. The ultimate progression is 'toes to bar', pictured below—good luck!

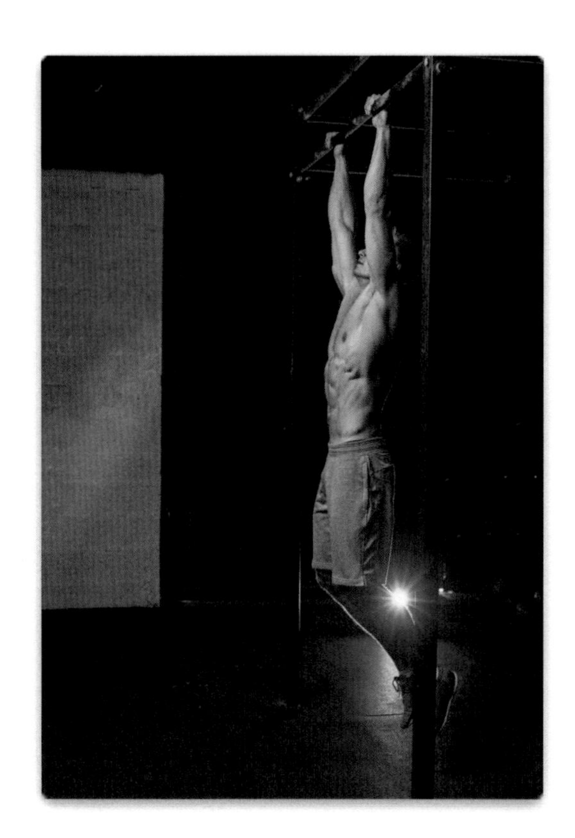

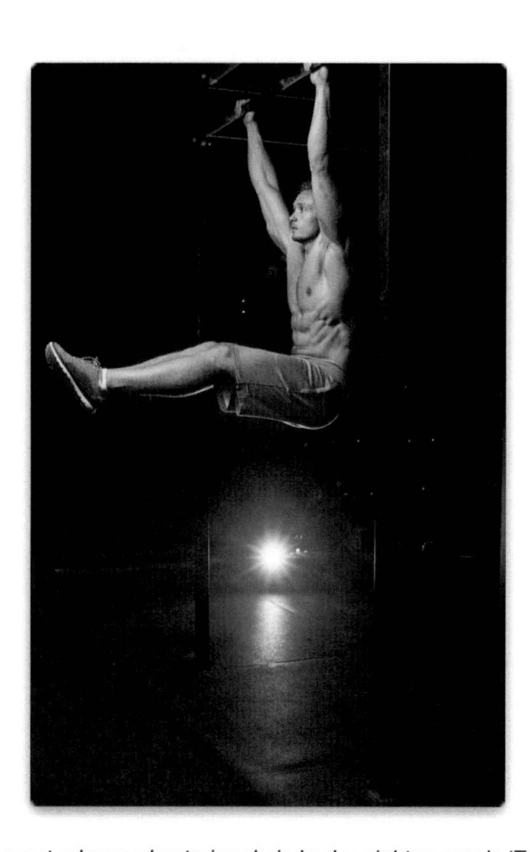

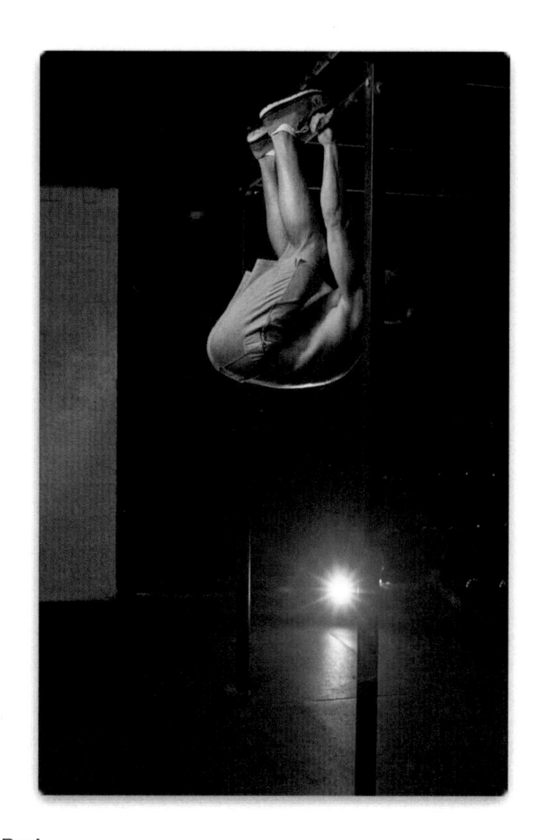

One of the most advanced anterior chain bodyweight moves is 'Toes To Bar'.

POSTERIOR CHAIN

The posterior chain is simultaneously the very most IMPORTANT set of muscles for your general appearance, and also the single most NEGLECTED by absolutely everyone. Why most important? Because these muscles create your posture. And believe us, that is the very first thing anyone notices—consciously or unconsciously—the second you walk into the room.

Stand in front of the mirror and look at yourself. Then try to make your posture as POOR as possible. Slouched shoulders, drooping neck, zero muscle tone in your glutes. Like what you see? We didn't think so. Now do the exact opposite. Stand up as straight and tall as you possibly can. Pull your

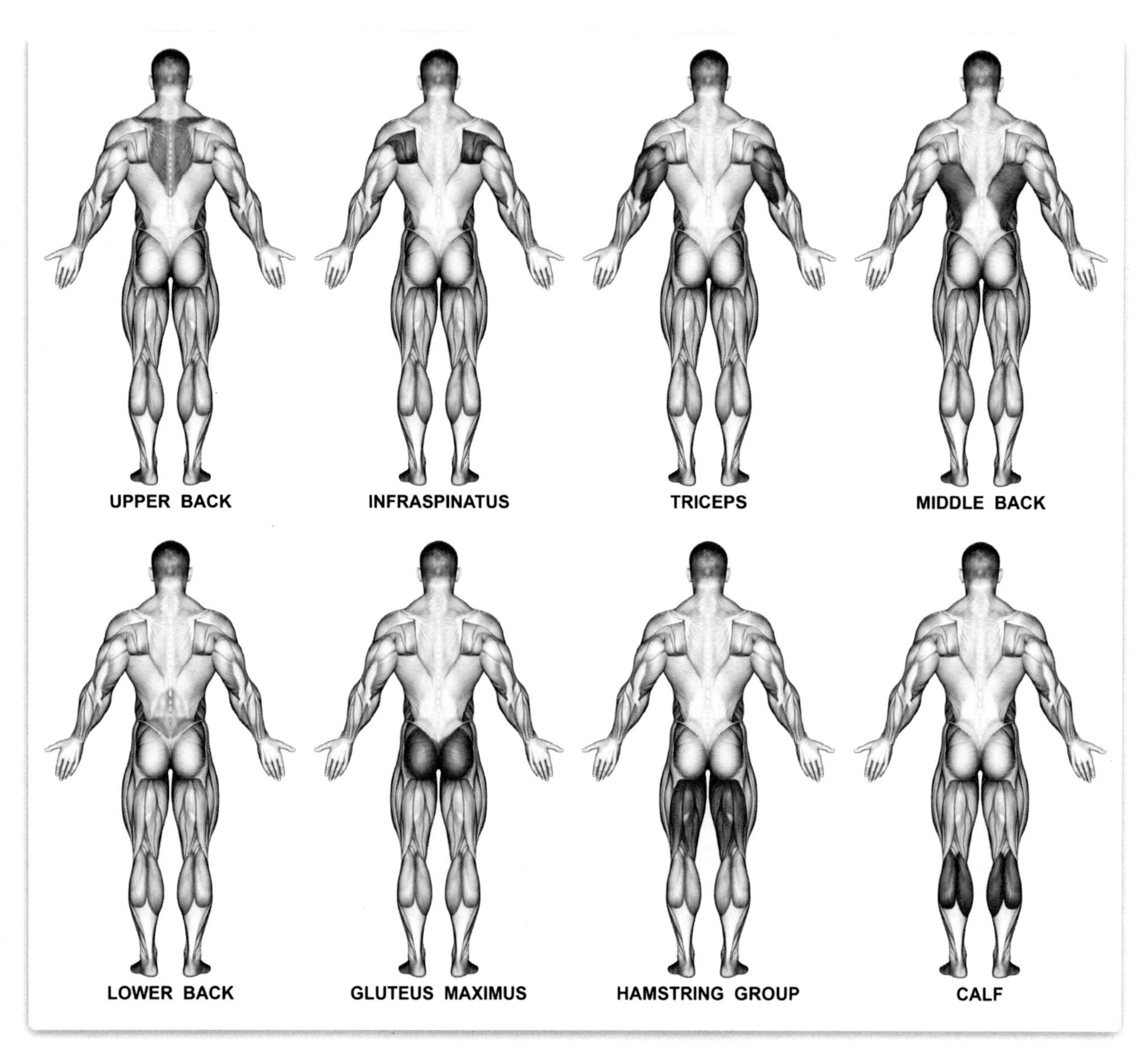

The posterior chain is very important to your overall appearance, as this is what gives you POSTURE — standing up straight and tall.

shoulders down and back as hard as possible. Engage your glutes and spinal erector muscles as hard as you possibly can. See the difference? A tight posterior chain contributes more to your appearance than anything else.

Working the posterior chain with bodyweight is quite easy, and like most of these calisthenics, all you really need is the floor. The best starting point is a 'Superman'. Lie on your stomach, arms outstretched in front of you. Then engage every single muscle on the back half of your body, including the muscles of the lumbar spine, the gluteus, and hamstrings. Once you have placed the highest tension you possibly can in all of these muscles, you hold it for as long as possible.

Next up are glute bridges. Lie on your back with your knees bent, then thrust your pelvis upward as high as possible. Try to engage your glutes and hamstrings and low back as much as possible, and then hold for as long as possible.

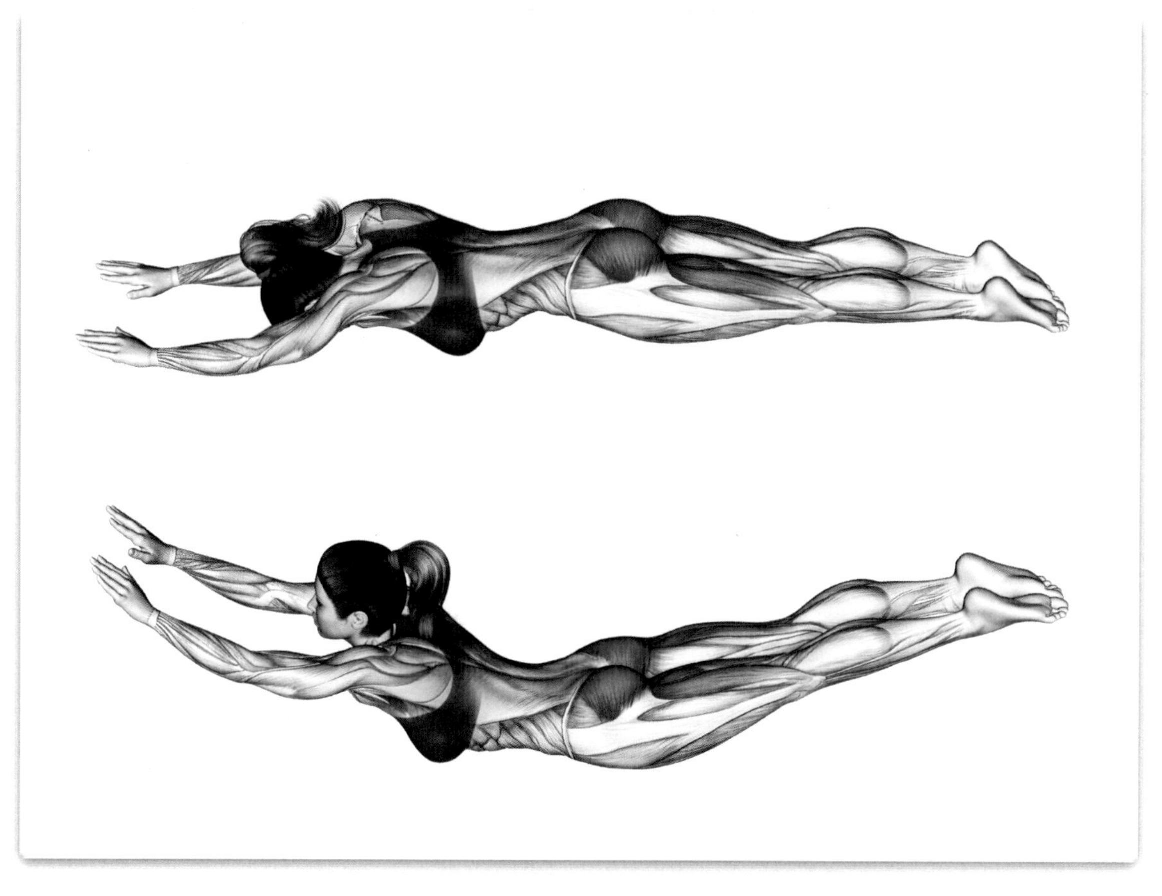

'Supermans' work the entire posterior chain. Hold isometrically with the highest tension you can generate for as long as possible.

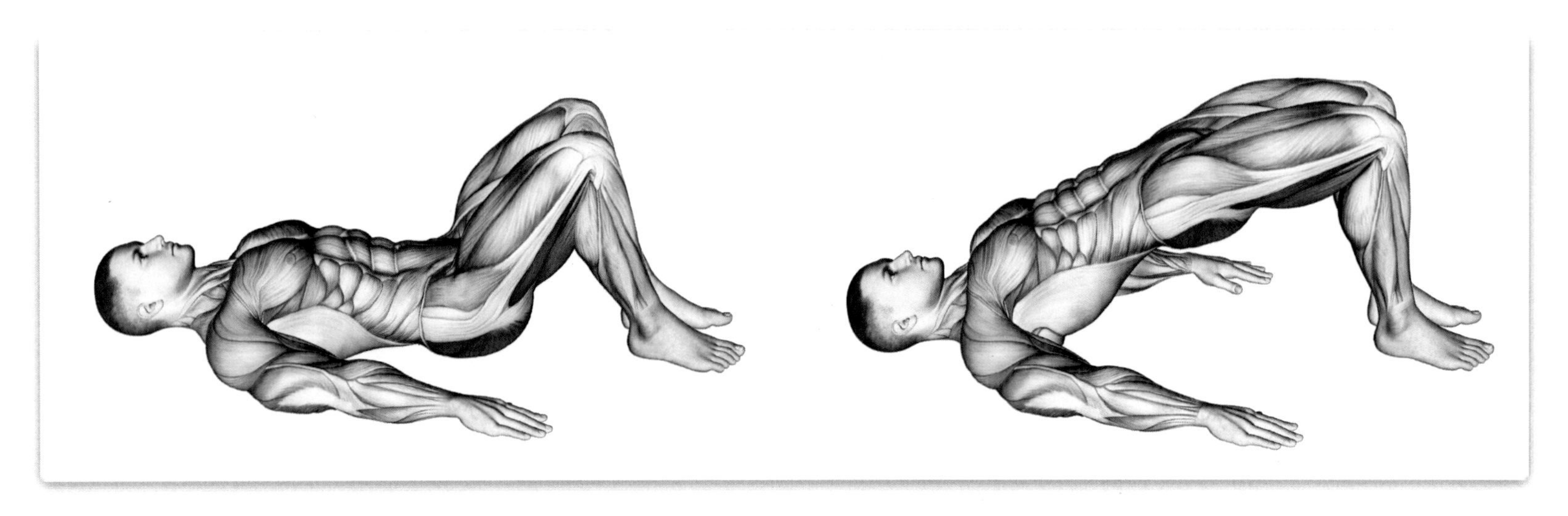

Glute bridges are a great way to work the posterior chain. Try single leg variations to progress the difficulty.

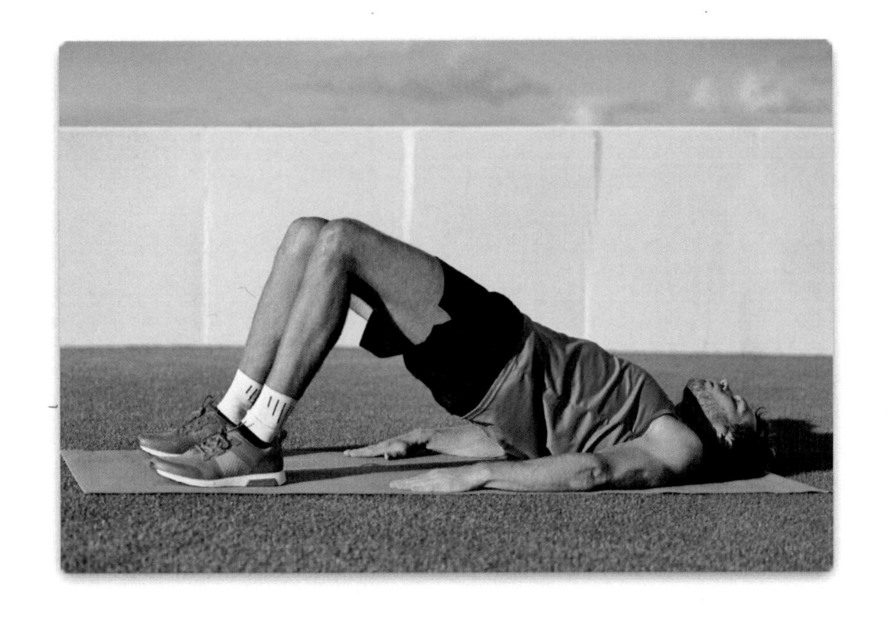

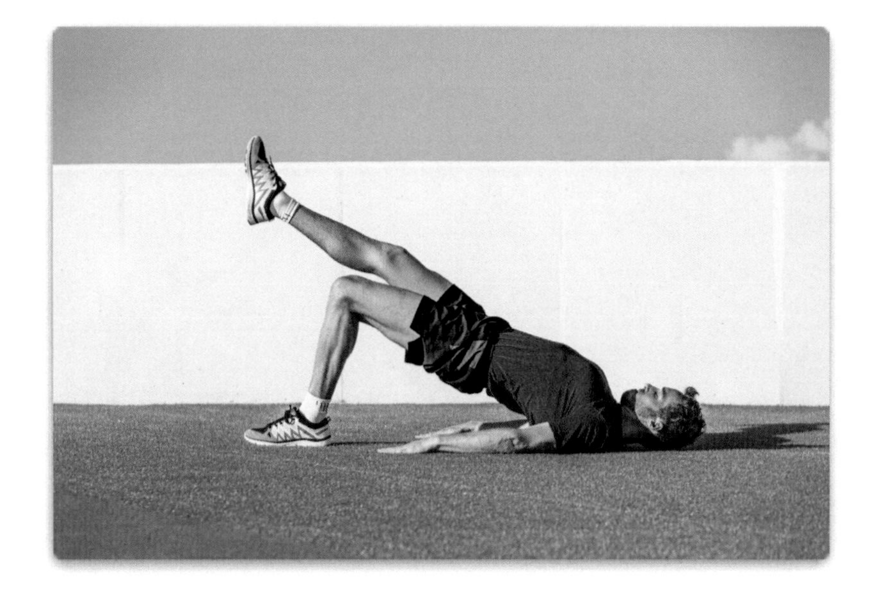

MIND-MUSCLE CONNECTION

We cannot emphasize this strongly enough: putting maximum tension in your muscles comes exclusively from YOUR BRAIN. That's right, your central nervous system is 100% responsible for generating maximum tension in your muscles. And just like everything else on earth, this is something that takes a lot of practice! The ability to squeeze every possible bit of strength out of your muscles is a skill and an art and one that you absolutely have to practice over and over until you master it. And until you can place this maximal tension in your muscles, you won't be able to reach your maximum strength, nor will you be able to progress optimally when it comes to progression and muscle size. When you are performing any exercise, try to concentrate as much as possible, and visualize your brain driving the maximal nerve impulse into the muscles you are targeting—because that is exactly what you are trying to do. The better you are at 'turning on' your muscles, the faster you will progress. This is just one more argument for a high frequency of exercise. If you are only doing pushing movements once a week, you might not be optimally reinforcing the skill of the mind-muscle connection. A daily set, however, gives you plenty of chances to work on the strength of this mental connection.

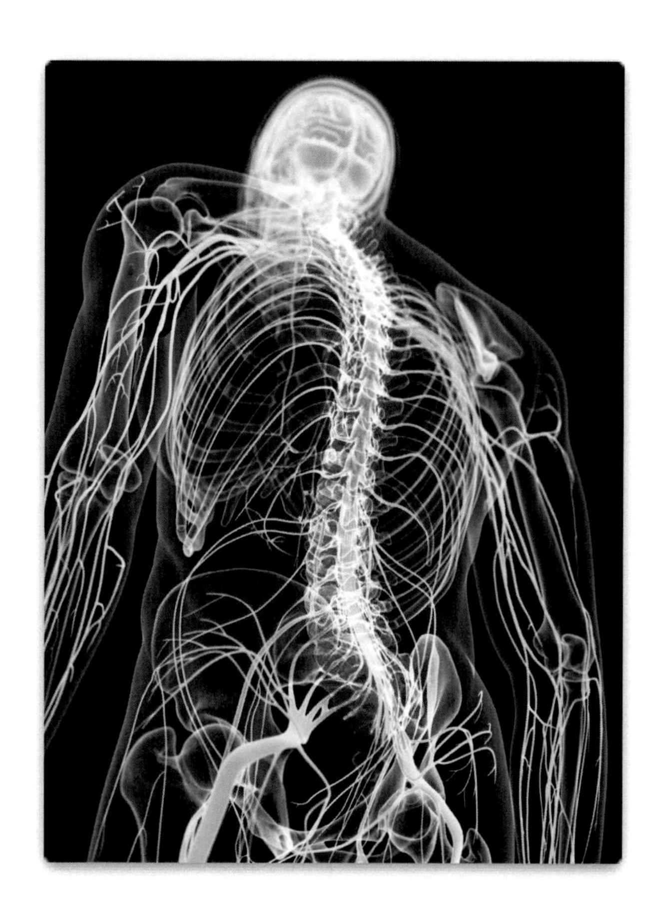

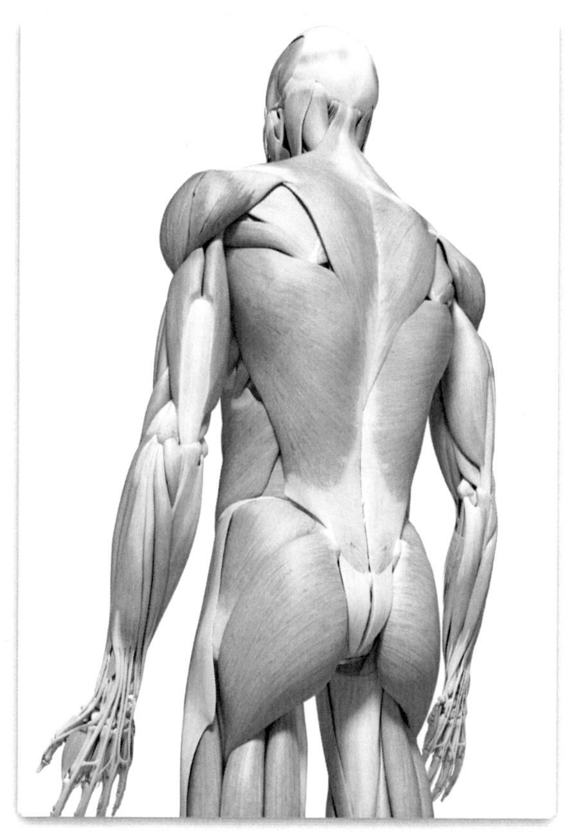

THE CONCEPT OF FAILURE

Back in the intro to Demand Training™, we discussed the concept of failure, and its importance for obtaining the positive adaptations that we are really looking for from exercise. Failure could mean different things to different people. For some, this would mean quitting an exercise the minute things got even a little bit uncomfortable. For others, this would mean continuing until you really can't move another millimeter, no matter how hard you try. And for those who want to wring absolutely every bit of 'demand' out of their 'demand training', there is actually something we like to call 'Triple Failure'. Allow us to explain.

When you are performing an exercise, like a push-up, there are two phases. The CONCENTRIC muscle contraction is the more difficult part of the exercise, when you are moving against gravity. So in the concentric portion of a push-up, you are pushing yourself away from the ground.

The ECCENTRIC muscle contraction is the easier part of the exercise, where you are letting yourself back down towards the ground at a controlled rate of speed, with the help of gravity. So pushing up is concentric, and going back down is eccentric. In 'Triple Failure', you continue the exercise until you hit complete failure at the concentric, or more difficult, part of the exercise. In our push-up example, this would be while you are pushing yourself up away from the ground. But once you reach this concentric failure—where you can't push up even another millimeter —instead of quitting, you try to HOLD YOURSELF RIGHT WHERE YOU ARE FOR AS LONG AS POSSIBLE.

Holding yourself where you are, against gravity, is called an ISOMETRIC EXERCISE. Examples of isometric holds would be a plank or a wall sit. These moves aren't quite as difficult as a concentric exercise, but they are still difficult in and of themselves. So here you are, hitting failure on the concentric part of a push-up, where you are unable to

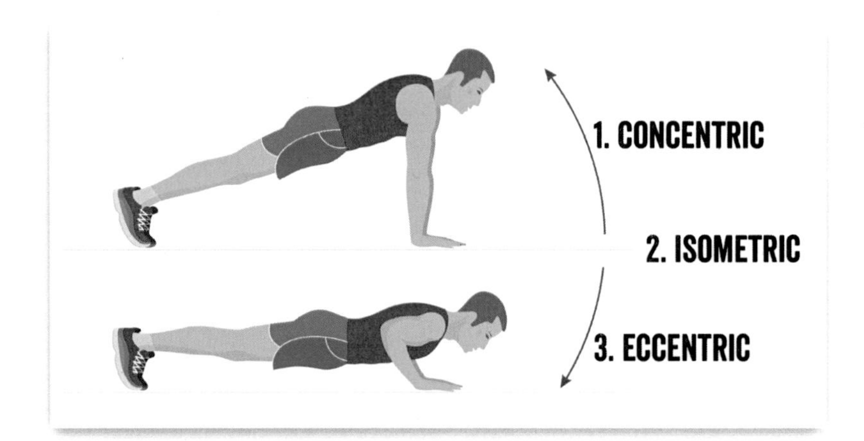

1. ***Concentric***. *This is the most difficult part of the exercise, because you are moving *AWAY* from gravity. You will hit failure here first.*
2. ***Isometric***. *This is a static hold and is the next point of failure.*
3. ***Eccentric***. *This is the easiest portion, because you are moving *with* gravity, and is the last point of failure.*

push yourself up any higher no matter what. That was the first failure of 'Triple Failure'. And now you are holding yourself at that failure part, halfway up the pushing up part of the push-up. Holding yourself isometrically at this point is going to be very very difficult indeed—but holding this until you absolutely can't anymore is the second failure of 'Triple Failure'. And what is the third and final failure of 'Triple Failure'? You guessed it: letting yourself down to the ground, with gravity—the eccentric portion of the exercise—AS SLOWLY AS YOU POSSIBLY CAN. At some point you will be completely unable to prevent yourself from just slumping to the ground in muscular exhaustion. Congratulations—you just hit Triple Failure™. You have sent the loudest message possible to your body that you need a strength and stamina adaptation. This is Demand Training at its finest. If you really want to get the greatest bang for your buck when it comes to resistance training, aim for this kind of failure with every single set. Anything less will feel like a waste of your time.

EFFECTIVE REPS

The single most important resistance exercise variable? Intensity of effort—placing the highest possible tension in your muscles, for the longest possible duration. For this reason, the repetitions closest to failure are the most effective. Imagine that push-ups are fairly easy for you, and you can bang out maybe 30 push-ups without too much trouble, and your all-time max is 40. So how much value are you getting out of the first 10 or 20 push-ups? Pretty much nothing. If you decided to just do 20 push-ups per day, forever, you might prevent yourself from getting WEAKER at pushing movements, but you certainly aren't going to get any stronger. But what about those reps closer to failure? Once you have completed 30 push-ups, and you are trying to beat your all-time record of 40 in a row, things start to change. As you get closer and closer to 40, you struggle more and more. You are placing the highest amount of tension you possibly can, in all of your pushing muscle fibers, for as long as possible. As you approach your 40th push-up, your rep speed gets slower and slower, as you fight and struggle to maintain this muscle tension for as long as possible. Finally, shaking and sweating, you manage to get halfway to 41 before you can't even move another millimeter. You hold there, halfway up, until gravity overtakes you and you slowly sink your chest back onto the ground. Now this was true Demand Training™—your body got the message loud and clear, and you are demanding that it give you more strength and endurance next time.

But what about the first 20 or so push-ups? Turns out, they were really just there to deplete your muscle fibers of energy, to get you closer to failure. What if there was a way to waste less time with the early reps, farther away from failure, and spend more time near the end of the set, where the reps are most difficult—and therefore most effective? Well, there are a couple of ways to accomplish just that. First of all, you can choose a more difficult push-up variation. Someone who can do 40 push-ups can probably do maybe one single-arm push-up on each side (left and right). Why not go straight for the single-arm push-ups and hit failure on the very first rep? You could actually try this. The problem, however, with something so incredibly difficult for you that you can only do it once, is that you have a much higher risk of injury with something like this that you can barely manage. And what is the very first rule of exercise? That's right: DON'T GET INJURED. Ideally, you want to choose a difficulty level where it isn't so hard that you can only do 1 rep, but it isn't so easy that you have to do 40 before things even start to get interesting. Now you actually COULD build muscle successfully, using only a super hard exercise with a 1 rep maximum, and you could also build muscle successfully with a super easy exercise with a 50 rep maximum. But the reality is that the 1 rep max exercise is likely to lead to injury, while the 50 rep max is going to waste a ton of your time. Time is your greatest resource, and injury prevention is your greatest rule of exercise, so neither of these is going to work.

In a perfect world, you would target an exercise that is just easy enough that you can do at least 5 repetitions, with good form—but just hard enough that you fail by the time you get to 10 repetitions (again, with good form). This 5 to 10 rep range is not at all an absolute requirement by any stretch, but it is something to aim towards, as it is a nice compromise between the potential for injury with harder variations and the potential for time-wasting with easier variations.

REST-PAUSE

Now we have established the concept of 'effective reps'—the reps closest to failure. And we have also established the ideal range of 5 to 10 reps per set—a nice compromise between too hard and too easy. Time to discuss the concept of REST-PAUSE. This is basically a way of extending the DEMAND part of your exercise, and making sure that the muscles got the message loud and clear. Rest-pause training is simply taking a set all the way to failure—and ideally to 'Triple Failure'—and then resting for about 20 seconds before trying to do the exercise AGAIN. We know—insanity, right? Well, yes. But because your muscles are so incredibly depleted from your set to failure just 20 seconds ago, you will only be able to do a fraction of the reps you were able to complete originally. For example, if you did 10 push-ups, with perfect form, and hit true 'Triple Failure' on the 10th rep, you would probably only be able to do 4 more after a 20-second rest. All of these reps are already much closer to failure, because you depleted your muscles so much the first time around. And if you were to try one more 20 second rest and one more set, you would probably only get 3 more push-ups before you hit complete failure.

But what you have done here, by taking a set to failure followed by two more rest-pause sets, is massively increased the amount of DEMAND you are sending to your muscles, at only a tiny fraction of the time commitment. And if you are going to go to all the trouble of exercising, and taking a set all the way to failure, it makes a ton of sense (from an efficiency standpoint) to add on a few more reps close to failure, using this failure extension technique.

We highly recommend taking every set to Triple Failure, and then adding on two more rest-pauses to each set. What should we call this concoction? A TRIPLE SET, to TRIPLE FAILURE.

REVERSE PYRAMID

Reverse pyramid is just a way of saying that your second and third subsequent sets are easier, in a descending fashion. In the barbell world, a reverse pyramid set might start out with two plates on each side of the barbell for the first set, and then you take one plate off each side for the second set, making it easier. Using bodyweight calisthenics, instead of lowering external weight we would change to an easier progression of an exercise. Why would we want to do this? Usually if we are doing an exercise with a fairly low rep range to start with, and that rep range is going to be even lower after the first of our three rest pause sets. Let us explain.

Let's say you are kind of new to push-ups and you can only do five of them with perfect form. And let's say you hit triple failure trying to attempt your sixth one. Well, after a 20-second rest, you will probably only be able to do ONE push-up. And if you try to do a third rest-pause set after that, you won't even get one whole push-up. This is not a great rep range. So what do you do instead? You use the concept of 'reverse pyramid', and go to an easier progression—like a knee push-up. So you do your five regular push-ups on your toes, with perfect form, and then hit triple failure on the sixth one. You would immediately go to the easier knee push-up variation, where you can maybe do 8 of these with perfect form (a higher number of reps compared to your first set, because knee push-ups are considerably easier than push-ups on your toes). And then for your third and final rest-pause set of your Triple Set, you can maybe do 5 more knee push-ups. Congratulations, you were able to stay within the fairly reasonable 5 to 10 rep range because you used a Reverse Pyramid technique and switched to an easier exercise.

We highly recommend combining all of these techniques, for each exercise of your workout. So for each exercise you would want a Triple Set (using rest-pause technique) to Triple Failure (concentric, then isometric, then eccentric), using Reverse Pyramid (easier variation) if necessary to keep things roughly in a 5 to 10 rep range. When it comes to time efficiency, nothing is going to beat these sorts of failure extension techniques.

PRACTICAL APPLICATION:

Demand Training is all about communicating to your body that you absolutely must have an adaptation: more strength and stamina. We use failure to send a message, and we want that message to be as loud and clear as possible. So we accentuate failure, in the most time-efficient way possible, by training with high intensity and high frequency. The most efficient protocol is a single Triple Set daily, to Triple Failure, of the Triple Moves: push, pull, and legs.

1. Single full-body set daily.

A full-body workout needs a minimum of three moves: push, pull, and legs.

2. Take each set all the way to Triple Failure.

To really demand adaptation, you want to first fail on the concentric, then hold the isometric all the way to failure, then perform the eccentric as slowly as possible to failure.

3. Add on two additional rest-pause sets to complete your Triple Set.

Because the reps closest to failure are the most valuable, try to maximize the effort of getting all the way to failure by adding on two more rest-pause sets to each exercise.

4. Use Reverse Pyramid technique by switching to an easier exercise if needed.

Try to stay in the 5 to 10 rep range, and use an easier exercise if you need to.

INTENSITY, FREQUENCY, AND VOLUME

When it comes to exercise, you have three basic variables:

1. **Intensity.**

2. **Frequency.**

3. **Volume.**

The P:E Diet approach is based on the fact that intensity of effort is the single most important variable of all. If we do one curl with a one-pound pink weight every minute of our entire day, one thousand curls later we will have NOTHING to show for it. If we do this all day every day, we will STILL have nothing to show for it. For this reason, INTENSITY is the single most important variable.

Next up is frequency. Let's say you are trying to build up a nice tan. You could spend 15 minutes a day lying in the sun.

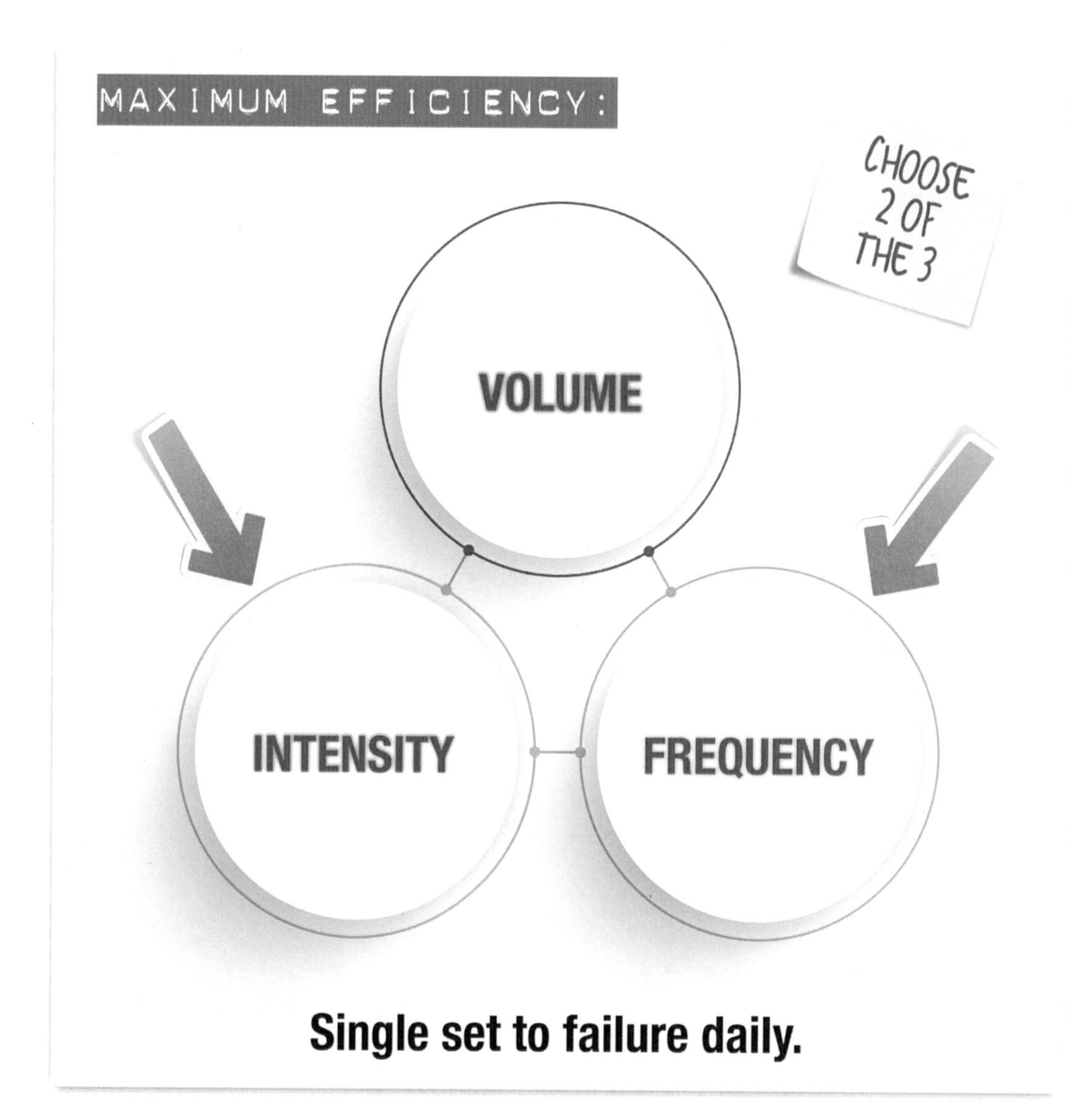

The most time-efficient training strategy of all? Keep intensity and frequency high, but not volume.

Or you could spend an entire 8-hour day lying in the sun once a month. Which makes more sense from a physiological perspective? Because there is only so much sunlight you can recover from in a single day without damaging yourself, it clearly makes the most sense to get a small but adequate dose of sun daily. This will give you the best adaptation (a tan) with the least damage (sunburn).

Muscle is a functional tissue adaptation to environmental stress that is completely analogous to tanning that occurs in response to sun exposure. You want a high enough daily dose to trigger an adaptation, but not enough to damage yourself. For this reason, daily is an excellent frequency for exercise, provided the stimulus is small but effective.

If you are trying to maximize exercise EFFICIENCY—that is, the highest possible return on the very lowest time investment—you clearly want to focus on intensity and frequency, rather than volume. For this reason, we highly recommend a small amount of daily training, such as a single set of push, pull, and leg exercises daily. Believe us when we say that as long as your volume is small, this frequency will not result in 'overtraining' and should be recoverable by most people. Beginners however, who are unfamiliar with exercise with a very high intensity, certainly can and should skip a day if they are severely tired or sore, or if they are having connective tissue joint pains (tennis elbow etc).

Read on for more about these brief daily single set workouts!

PROGRESSION

All of your exercise will have to progress over time if you want them to remain effective. If a particular exercise is difficult right now, that's great—it is this struggle that allows you to place the highest tension in your muscles for the longest amount of time possible. But as your muscles acquire more strength and endurance, the same exercises might become easy for you, and then it's time to make them more difficult somehow.

Luckily it is pretty easy to make any exercise more difficult. First of all, you can simply do the exercise MORE SLOWLY, taking a lot more time to do the exact same move. Look at push-ups for example. Let's say you are pretty good at doing push-ups, and ten push-ups is very easy for you. You can progress this exercise by performing SLOW push-ups: 30 seconds going down, hold for 30 seconds at the bottom of the push-up, then 30 seconds going back up. Just try it! Suddenly, what seemed like a very easy move becomes a maximum effort challenge.

Secondly, you can focus on absolutely perfect form. Try doing push-ups with sloppy form, poor range of motion, elbows wide apart from your body, sagging hips, etc. Takes a LOT less energy than good form. Now try a push-up with PERFECT form. Tighten your body as much as possible. Keep your hands low and close to your chest, elbows in. Make sure you go all the way to the bottom of the push-up, and your nose is kissing the ground with each one. Your entire body should be as rigid as a board. Feel the difference? You can make any exercise ridiculously more difficult by using absolutely perfect form, full range of motion, and slow cadence.

Finally, you can always choose a more difficult exercise variation, like working towards a one-arm push-up (extremely difficult)! And you can combine multiple forms of progression at once as well.

The truth is that it almost doesn't matter, as long as you take each exercise as far as you can, all the way to failure. You could choose regular push-ups and take these to failure, although it might take 50 or more. You could work on one-arm push-ups and hit failure after one rep. Or you could do slow perfect form push-ups and hit failure after 10. In general, you ideally want to keep things somewhere in the 5 to 10 rep ('repetition') range, but to be honest you can make almost any rep range work as long as you max out the intensity of effort and go all the way to failure.

BASIC MOVEMENTS

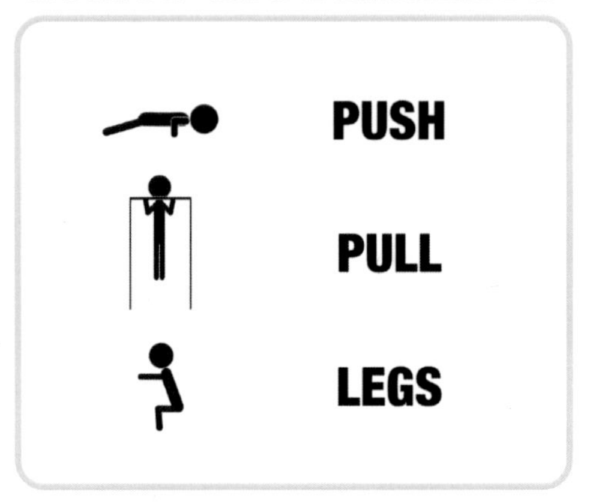

ACCESSORY MOVEMENTS

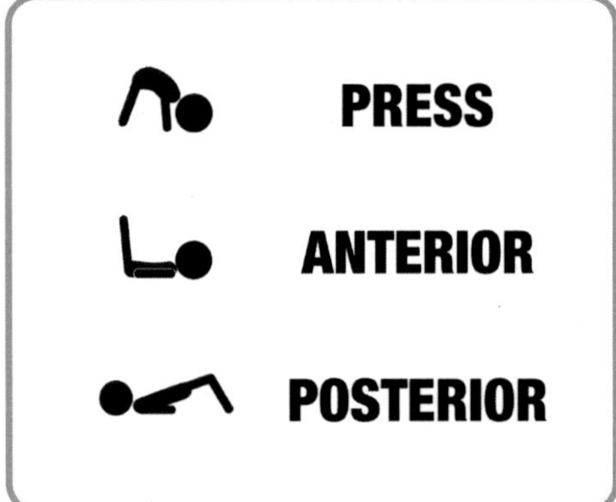

Single set to failure daily on all movements, with two failure extention techniques to increase the number of 'effective reps', or reps closest to failure:

1. REST-PAUSE TRIPLE SET

One set to 'triple failure' (maximum concentric effort followed by maximum time in isometric hold followed by maximum time in eccentric lowering), followed by 15 second rest, then repeating two more times (3 sets total).

Example:

- Maximum standard pull-ups to concentric failure, then isometric hold to muscular failure, then eccentric as slowly as possible to failure → 15 second pause.
- Repeat pull-ups to failure → 15 second pause.
- Final set with easier technique: chin-ups to failure.

2. REVERSE PYRAMID

Most difficult variation first, then progressively less difficult variations on subsequent movements. Goal is to keep failure in the 5-10 rep range.

Example:

- One-arm push-ups to concentric muscular failure, then isometric hold to muscular failure, then eccentric as slowly as possible to failure → 15 second pause.
- Diamond push-ups to failure → 15 second pause.
- Standard push-ups to failure.

Here is a full body resistance workout: push, pull, legs, press, and anterior and posterior chains. Six moves, each done with a triple rest-pause set. Takes about 12-15 minutes.

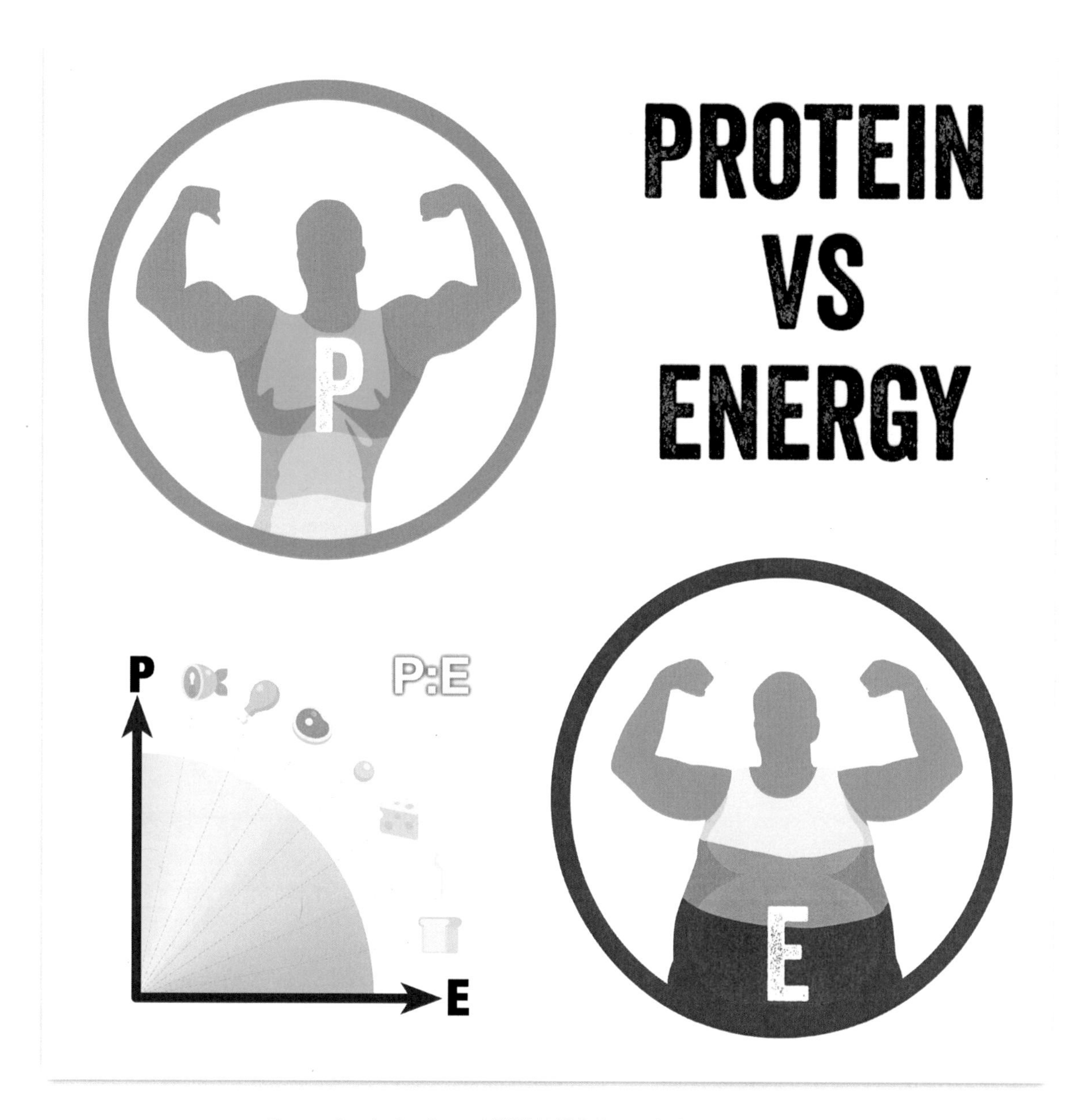

Remember to feed your LEAN MASS, instead of your FAT MASS.

CARDIO

Cardio can provide huge benefits for both health and metabolism. When it comes to cardio, the most important thing to know is this:

<u>You can always trade INTENSITY for DURATION.</u>

What does this mean exactly?

When you are doing light cardio, like a jog or a brisk walk or some other steady pace that isn't terribly demanding, you are increasing your rate of calorie burn in the form of fat oxidation—AND THAT IS PRETTY MUCH IT. You aren't putting a huge demand on your system so you won't get the sort of dramatic positive adaptations that maximum intensity Demand Training™ has to offer. You aren't depleting a ton of glycogen so your metabolism isn't really going to change when you stop exercising. What will happen? You will burn some calories, and cost yourself a lot of time.

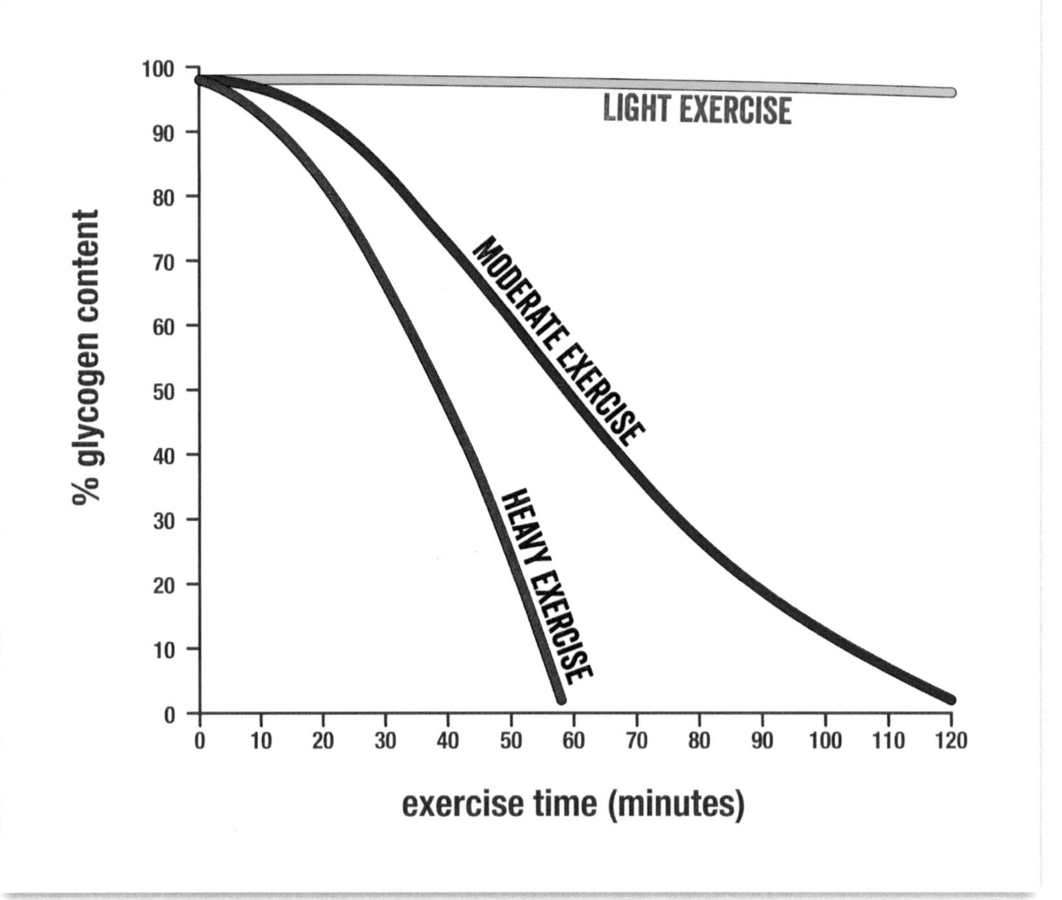

Light exercise burns almost exclusively fat and little to no glycogen, while extremely heavy exercise burns a lot of glycogen. Glycogen depletion has amazing health and metabolic benefits, including increasing fat oxidation and insulin sensitivity.

Let's say you decide that you are going to go on a nice brisk walk for an entire hour. You are going to burn maybe 300 calories—the equivalent of one bagel with cream cheese. Great. And afterwards? No positive adaptations at all. You won't really increase muscle, or stamina, or fat oxidation rate, or anything else. And the worst part? TIME is the most precious resource you have—so you would honestly be way better off just not eating a bagel, and then having your hour back!

Now don't get us wrong—walking is awesome! Everyone should be walking all day long. You should try to keep up a low level of activity all day long, and this is extremely healthy and great for fat loss. PLEASE walk as much as possible. BUT we want you to know that this sort of lower level activity does NOT produce the same positive adaptations as true exercise, with a much higher level of intensity.

As you push the intensity of your exercise higher and higher, the amount of glycogen you burn goes up exponentially. Your overall rate of energy expenditure can go up by one thousand times that of your resting metabolism. You rapidly deplete your muscles of glycogen, and you push your cardiovascular system and your energy production systems all the way to redline. And when you do this, you get a lot of positive adaptations. Maximum intensity cardio workouts will increase your cardiac output, increase the strength and size and endurance of your muscles, increase the number of mitochondria in your body, and increase your overall stamina.

High-intensity cardio workouts have a huge metabolic benefit as well: glycogen depletion raises fat oxidation ALL DAY LONG. That's right. If you deplete a significant amount of muscle glycogen—which can only be done with higher intensities of exercise—your fat oxidation will increase afterwards for hours or even all day, provided you don't eat a ton of carbs immediately after exercise.

Our favorite form of cardio is HIIT: High Intensity Interval Training. HIIT workouts involve doing something with an all-out maximum intensity burst for anywhere from 20 to 60 seconds, then resting (or lightly exercising) for 20 to 60 seconds to recover, followed by another all-out burst and rest pattern. A typical HIIT session will involve a minimum of two all-out sprints but could be higher (usually not more than 10). A classic pattern is 30 seconds of all-out exercise, followed by 30 seconds of rest, and repeated 3 times.

When you are performing Demand Training™ cardio, you could really be doing ANY EXERCISE that involves a good portion of your entire body and that will lead to very rapid fatigue (less than a minute) when performed at a high intensity. These exercises could include simply sprinting on a level surface, or sprinting up a hill, or running up stairs. Non-running exercises could be jumping jacks, jumping rope, jump squats, or burpees. You could also use equipment if you happen to have it handy, such as a spin bike, rowing machine, treadmill, or elliptical machine.

You DO NOT have to have any timers or elaborate timing systems to perform proper HIIT! Our favorite style is simply performing any exercise at the highest intensity you can manage, for the longest time you can manage, until you feel that you absolutely have to stop for a second to catch your breath. This might be as low as 10 or 20 seconds when you first start out, but as you get stronger and improve your cardiovascular fitness, this could be as long as a minute or so.

One of our favorite cardio sprint-type high intensity exercises? Jump squats. Simply drop into a squat (as low as possible), then jump up as high as possible. Repeat as many times as you can (good luck doing more than 30, which takes about 30 seconds). When you absolutely have to stop (highest possible effort), then stop and rest for roughly 30 seconds (you do NOT have to time this of course and it does not have to be exact). Then repeat for another set (you will probably only be able to do 50-75% as many as you did on the first set), again, all the way to failure. Then stop and rest for another ~30 seconds, and finish with one more set of jump squats to failure (again this will probably be 50% or even less of what you accomplished on the first set).

This entire exercise—3 sets of maximum effort jump squats to failure, plus rest breaks in between—is going to take less than three minutes, but believe us when we tell you that it will absolutely leave you exhausted for a few minutes. The next day your legs even might be sore from this effort. But you know what? Your cardio stamina will be like 1% better. Keep doing this daily for a few weeks and you will actually notice that you aren't as short of breath climbing stairs and hills. Keep doing this for months and pretty soon your cardio strength and stamina will be dramatically improved. It

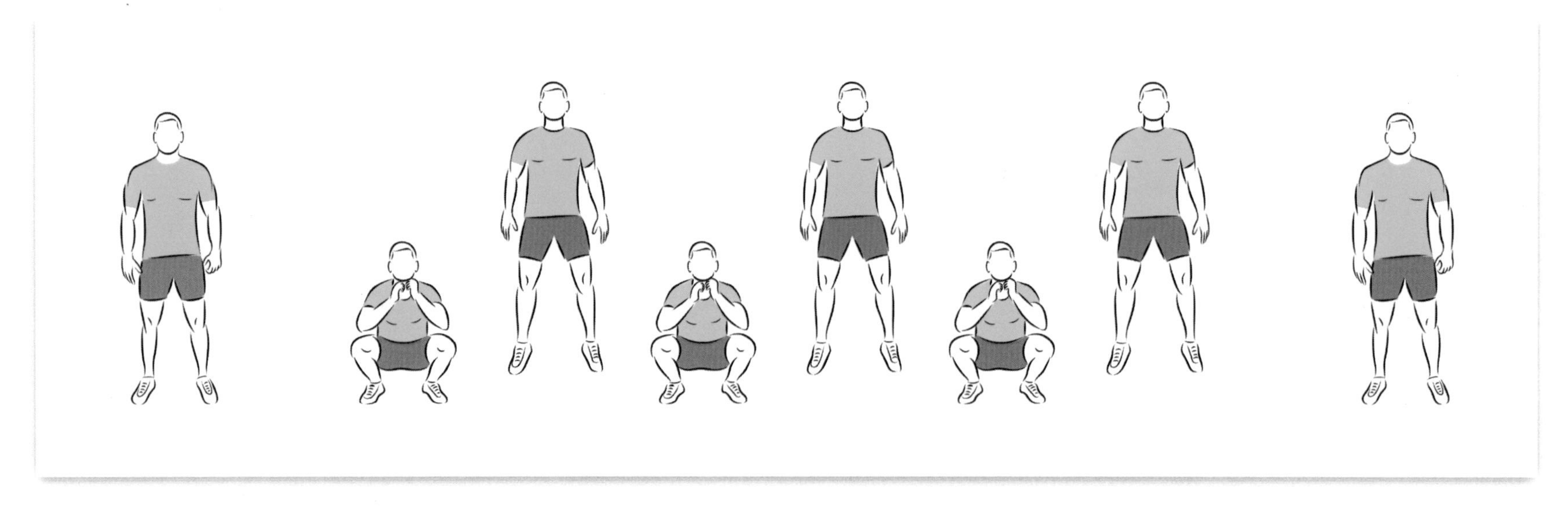

The humble jump squat is an amazing cardio exercise that almost anyone can do anywhere, anytime.

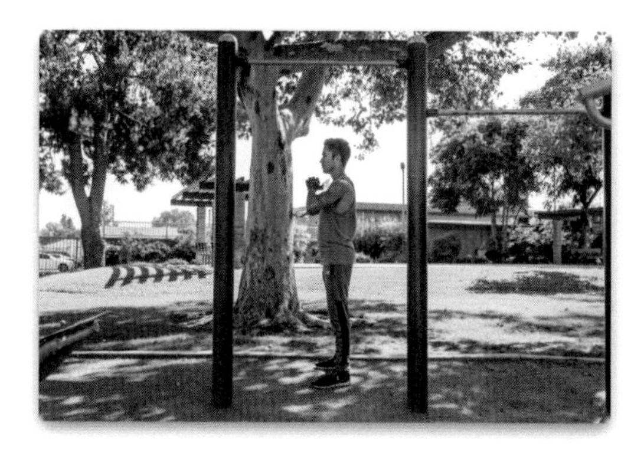

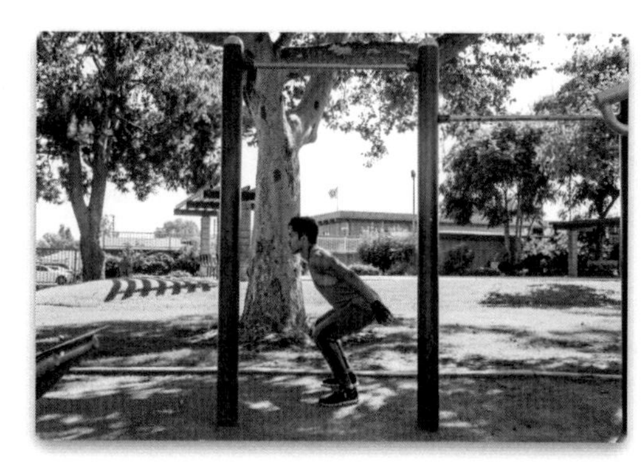

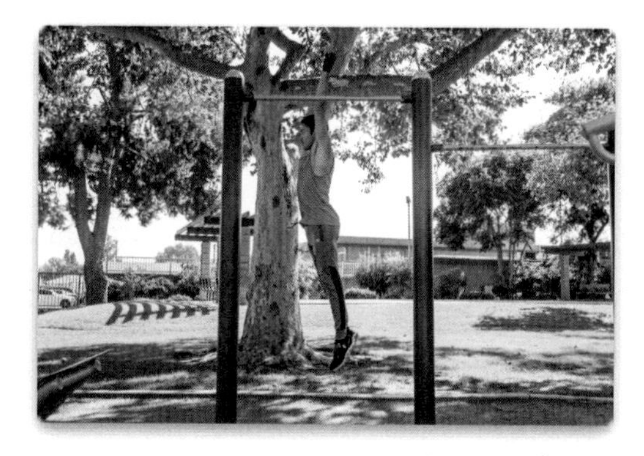

Requiring absolutely zero space or skill or equipment whatsoever, the simple jump squat is one of our favorite bodyweight cardio exercises, and one that can really exercise the hell out of your legs at the same time. Crouch down and then jump up as high as you can, then repeat until you can't do any more.

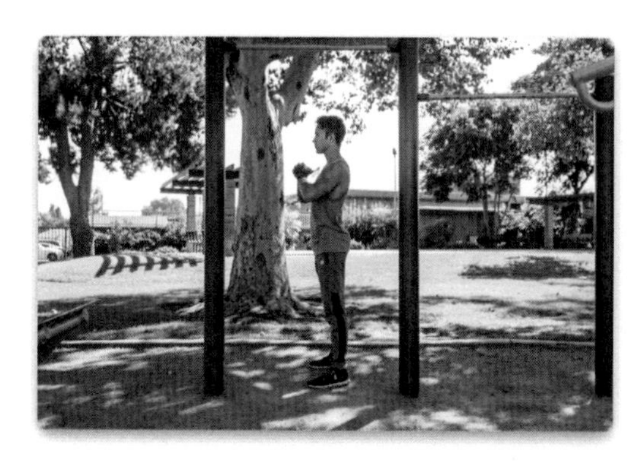

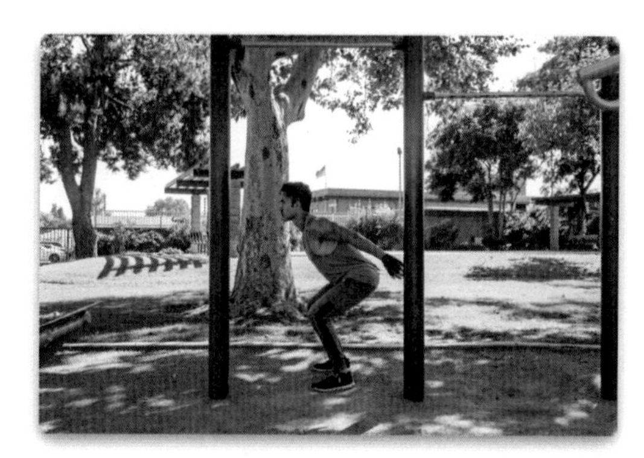

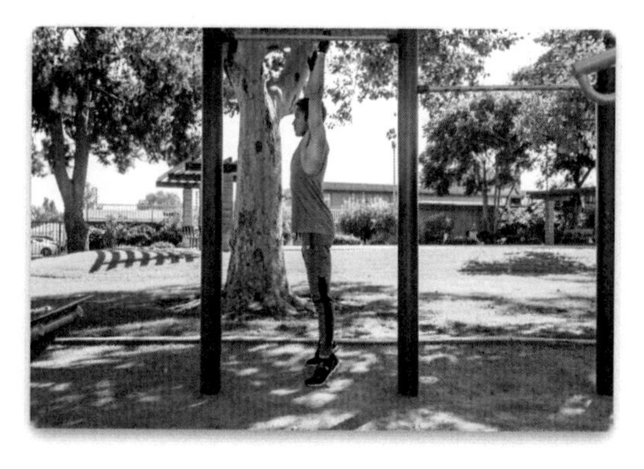

If you have trouble jumping due to orthopedic issues (knee pain, etc), advanced age, lack of physical conditioning, obesity, or any other reason, you should try this non-impact cardio exercise version known as a Full-Body Extension. Crouch down, then drive upwards onto your toes, throwing your arms up in the air while extending your body completely. Immediately drop back down into a crouch, then immediately back into an extension. Try to do these as rapidly and forcefully as possible, until you can't do any more. If done correctly, this is a very safe but very effective non-impact cardio move that can be used by almost anyone!

is all about consistency. The benefits you see come so slowly that most people give up because they don't notice these improvements right away. But as long as you keep going, you are going to reap some huge health and wellness rewards.

If you are really out of shape, you could replace jump squats with just ordinary bodyweight squats. Jumping jacks work as well, and if you are feeling coordinated you can do the same thing with a jump rope. Another great exercise for more coordinated people is stair running. Run up as many flights as you can, then walk back down during your rest breaks.

If jump squats are too easy for you, make them harder by not only jumping as high as you can, but pulling your knees up to your chest with each jump. If you are really feeling masochistic, you can graduate to the dreaded 'burpee' (pictured here). Drop to the ground, kick out into a push-up position (harder variation—actually do a full push-up), then jump up as high as you can with arms overhead. Good luck and try not to die. Pretty easy for the average mortal to hit failure in a short period of time!

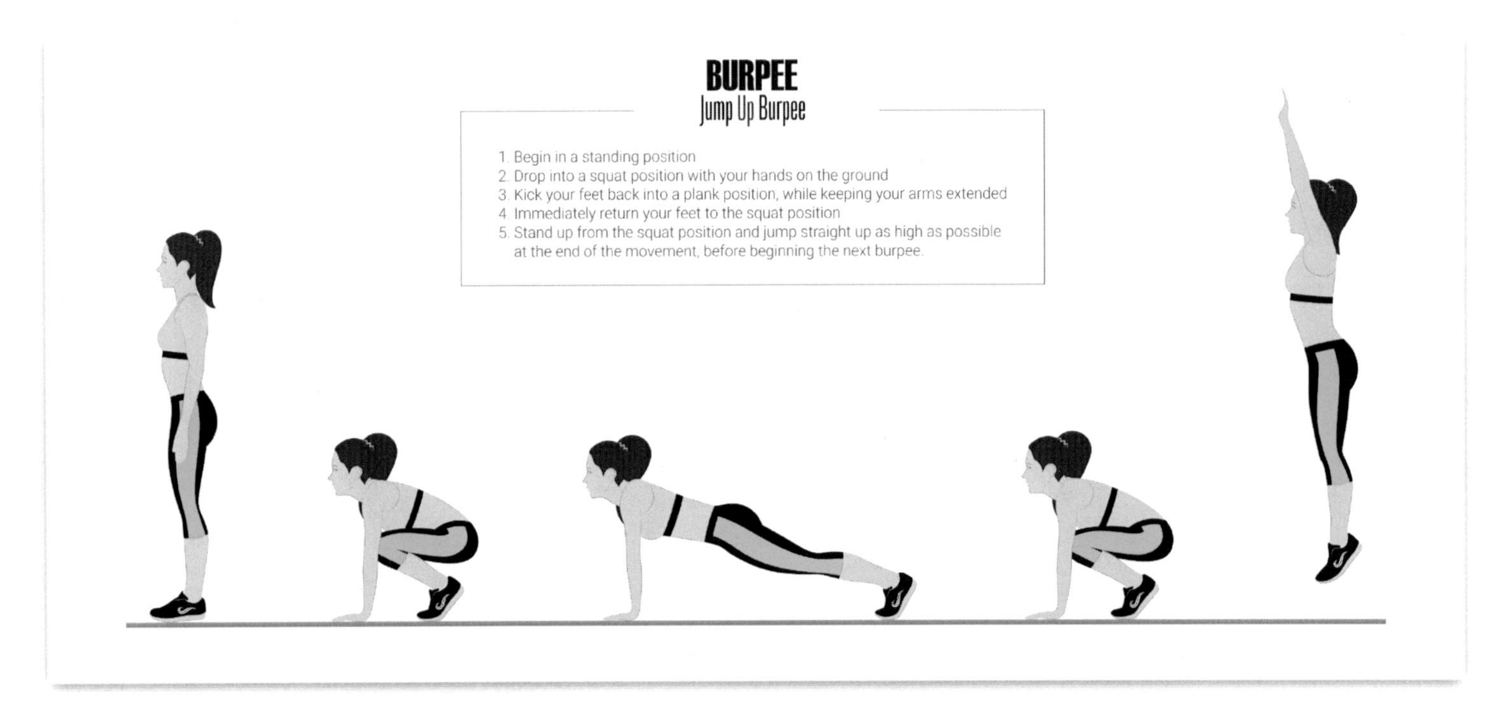

Burpees are hellish but are also a great way to hit maximum intensity cardio in no time at all.

Midlife cardiovascular fitness and dementia

A 44-year longitudinal population study in women

Helena Hörder, PhD, Lena Johansson, PhD, XinXin Guo, MD, PhD, Gunnar Grimby, MD, Silke Kern, MD, PhD, Svante Östling, MD, and Ingmar Skoog, MD

Neurology® 2018;90:e1298-e1305. doi:10.1212/WNL.0000000000005290

MIDLIFE CARDIOVASCULAR FITNESS AND DEMENTIA

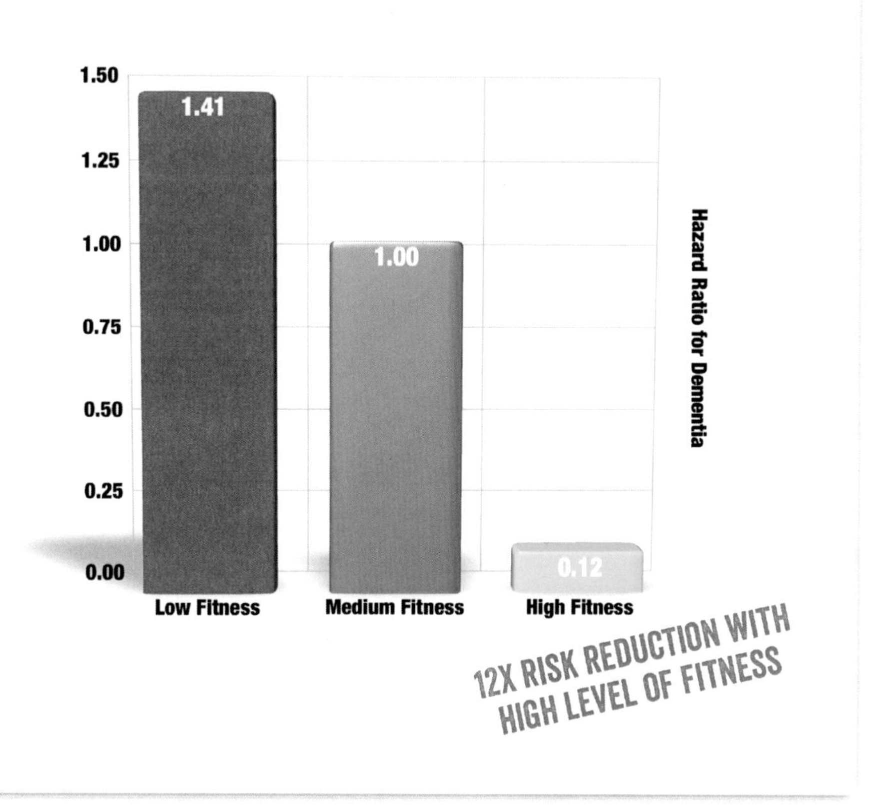

A high level of cardiovascular fitness is associated with a TWELVE-FOLD REDUCTION IN THE RISK FOR ALZHEIMER'S DEMENTIA.

NANO-WORKOUT

Let's face it, the number one barrier to exercise is TIME. Nobody has time to exercise. For your average person, exercise is a huge production. First, you need a gym membership. Then you need a gym class schedule or an appointment with a personal trainer. Next it's time to put on your exercise clothes, lace up your gym shoes, and grab your water bottle and your towel. You drive all the way to the gym, put your stuff in a locker, and spend ten minutes doing some warm-up exercises. Finally you start your routine, which is expected to last about an hour (although a casual observer might notice that only a few minutes of this hour involve serious exercise at the highest intensity). By the time you shower, change, drive home, and destroy your transiently increased fat oxidation with a high-carb smoothie, the entire affair is literally HOURS.

If you have a ton of time and you love the gym, then go for it. For the rest of us, we need an entirely different paradigm. And our answer is the 'nano-workout'.

When you really break it down, any full-body resistance workout only requires three moves: push, pull, and legs. Cardio could be any single movement that is capable of maximally taxing your cardiovascular and energy production systems. You could even combine a leg exercise and a cardio exercise, in the case of jump squats (provided you are jumping as high as possible and maximally taxing your leg muscles). So you could actually accomplish a full-body workout with just these three movements:

1. **Push-ups (to failure).**

2. **Pull-ups (to failure).**

3. **Jump squats (to failure).**

Even adding in a few extra rest-pause failure extension sets to each of these, so you are really doing 3 sets of each, you have a workout that is only 7 minutes in duration.

A triple failure rest-pause set of push-ups, pull-ups, and jump squats is the core nano-workout of The P:E Diet. You could replace push-ups with any pushing move and you could replace pull-ups with any pulling move; you could also replace jump squats with any cardio exercise (as long as you added in a leg resistance exercise such as bodyweight squats). To many people this feels way too brief to be effectual. But as long as the intensity is high enough, and you are consistent with these exercises, you WILL progress and gain both strength and stamina. Doing this nano-workout in a consistent fashion is infinitely better than doing nothing because you don't feel like you have the time for your current vision of 'exercise'.

So we have a full-body cardio and resistance workout that takes easily less than 10 minutes and requires no equipment at all except for something to pull on (TRX or other suspension trainer, pull-up bar, etc). But it gets even better: YOU CAN DO EACH OF THESE MOVES SEPARATELY AT DIFFERENT TIMES

THROUGHOUT YOUR DAY. Let's say you have a spare two minutes, ANYWHERE and ANYTIME. Guess what —you could do your triple set of push-ups RIGHT NOW on the ground. Boom, 2 minutes later, your pushing workout is COMPLETED. You can do your pulling workout later at home, in the park, or wherever you have a spare 2 minutes and something to pull on. And then jump squats could be worked in later, anywhere and anytime. Now you not only have a nano-workout, but you have divided it up into ultra-tiny subsets that take almost no time whatsoever.

By keeping the intensity as high as possible (maximum), and the frequency high (daily), you can get all of the benefits of exercise without the huge time commitment that most people have traditionally associated with exercise. And now that time and equipment are no longer barriers to entry, there is no reason at all why you can't start the exercise part of your health journey RIGHT THIS VERY SECOND.

What is the very best workout? The one you will do consistently, long term.

CONSISTENCY

Is Everything

Consistency.

To get strong, be strong, and stay strong you have to train every single week for your entire life. Period.

Inactivity melts muscle. Pain and injury melts muscle. Taking time off from training melts muscle. You can't NOT train, and you can't stop training.

You need training that is safe, easily accessible, sustainable, and enjoyable because you need to do this FOR THE REST OF YOUR DAMN LIFE.

Consistency is everything.

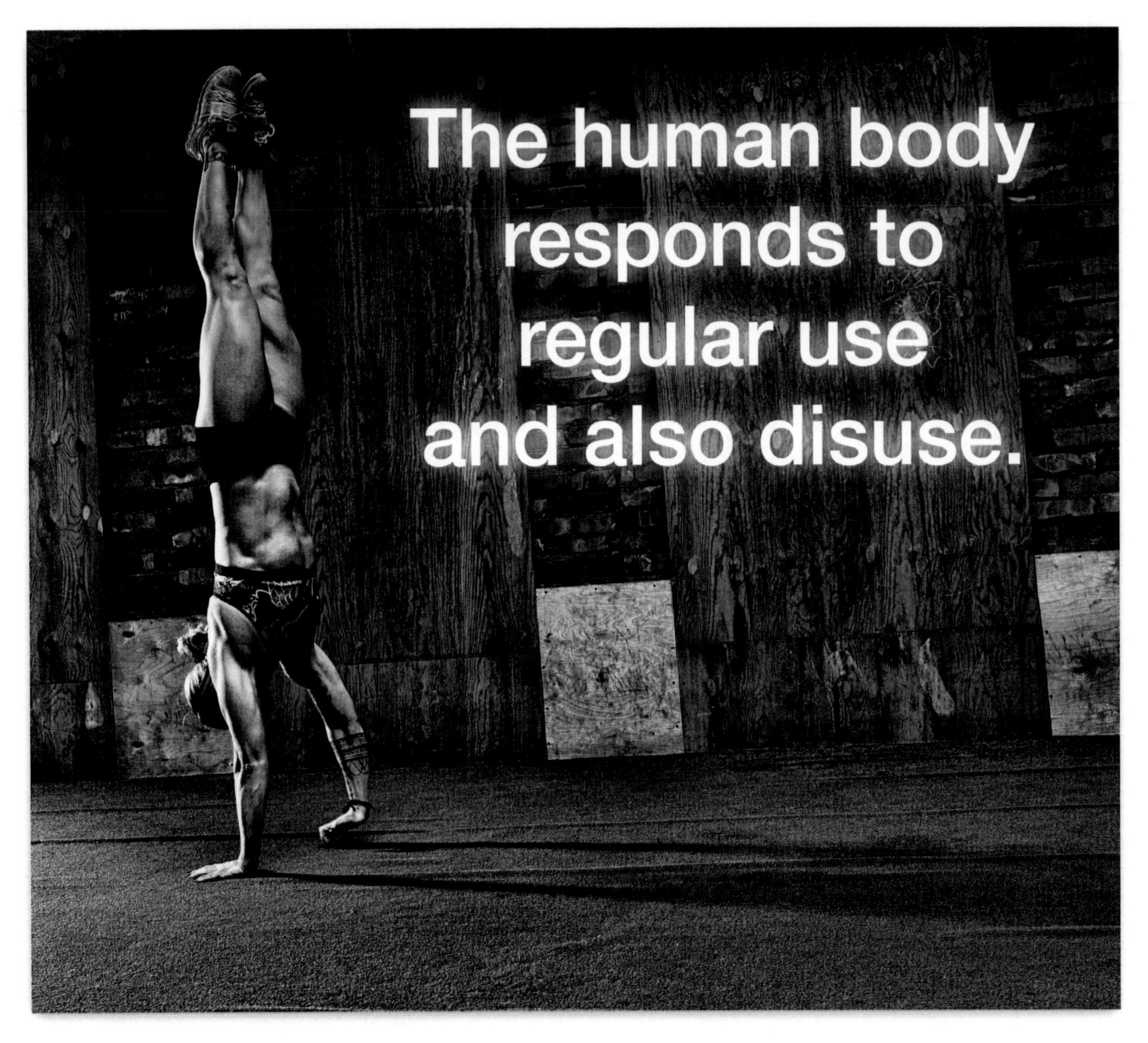

The reality is that you have created your body exactly the way it is with your diet and exercise inputs. Eating more protein than energy and performing resistance exercise builds a lean muscular body, while eating more energy than protein and being sedentary builds a weak and overweight body.

It's often easier to do something EVERY day than to do it SOME days.

IF YOU MAKE THE ACTIVITY A PART OF YOUR DAILY ROUTINE, THERE'S A GREATER CHANCE IT WIL ACTUALLY GET DONE, AND YOU'LL SPEND LESS MENTAL ENERGY WORRYING THAT IT WON'T.

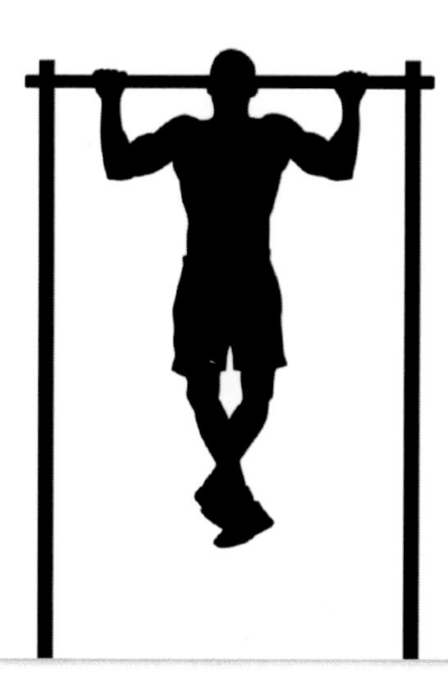

Aim for some sort of workout every day. You could probably get by with every other day, but daily is better. Also this way if you miss a day it really isn't a big deal and you don't have to feel bad about yourself—you can get right back to it tomorrow.

CONSISTENCY

A few final words on consistency.

The benefits of exercise are so tiny and gradual that it is sort of like building a sandcastle one teaspoonful at a time. After the first workout, you have pretty much zero to show for your efforts. Same thing after the second workout. And the third. And the fourth. And maybe the same after the tenth workout. Most people just give up, because this feels like a huge waste of time and effort. We look at those who are further along than us and we just assume that they have something that we don't have, and never will. And so we stop trying.

The reality is that everyone you see who is stronger and more muscular than you started off at the same place you did. In fact, the biggest difference is that they didn't give up. They kept grinding, day after day, even if it felt ineffectual. And now? A thousand teaspoons later, they have a respectable sand castle.

Start today, and never give up.

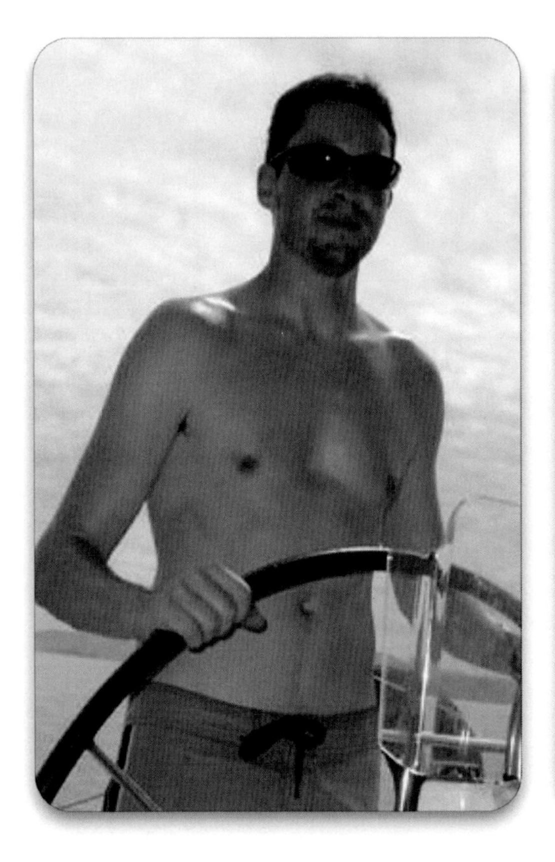

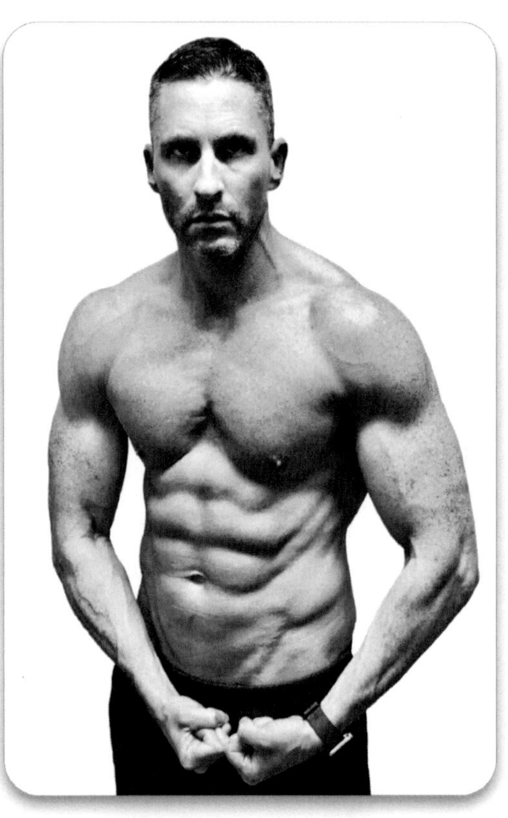

Dr. Naiman built his entire physique using these brief daily high-intensity bodyweight exercises — mostly simple pull-ups, push-ups, and squats. All it takes is a few YEARS of consistency.

Things to do EVERY DAY:

HAVE A FASTING WINDOW	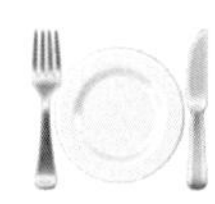	**Bare minimum would be 12 hours overnight**
EAT SOME DAMN PROTEIN	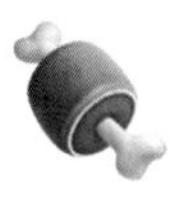	**Everyone could target 1 g/lb of DESIRED weight**
MAX OUT ON MUSCULAR TENSION	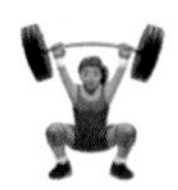	**One set of push, pull, and legs to failure**
MAX OUT ON POWER PRODUCTION	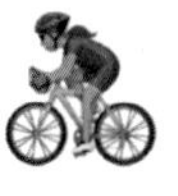	**Brief and high intensity sprint intervals**

FIND YOUR COMFORT ZONE —

THEN GET THE HECK OUT

• feel hunger before eating •
• feel cold from thermal loading •
• feel muscular failure from exercise •

Get comfortable with being uncomfortable. Don't eat until you are actually hungry. Allow yourself to be in a mildly cold environment without reaching for the thermostat — maintaining body temperature used to be a calorie burn that was automatically built into everyone's day. Make sure you are putting a high amount of tension in all of your muscles at least once briefly every day.

BEWARE: UNIFOCAL OVER-RELIANCE

What? Huh? Allow us to explain.

When it comes to optimizing diet and exercise, you have a number of levers that you can pull in order to improve your results. Here are only a few of the possible diet 'levers' you can manipulate in your quest to optimize health by achieving higher lean mass at a lower fat mass:

- Carbohydrate reduction.
- Fat reduction.
- Protein prioritization.
- Micronutrient prioritization.
- Total energy quantity reduction.
- Intermittent fasting.

When it comes to exercise, you have the following, as just a partial list, of weapons at your disposal:

- Resistance exercise.
- Cardio exercise.
- General activity level.

There are also some other lifestyle hacks that can be helpful. Here are just a few, in no particular order:

- Sleep.
- Sunlight.
- Mindfulness.
- Gratitude.
- Relationships.
- Meditation.

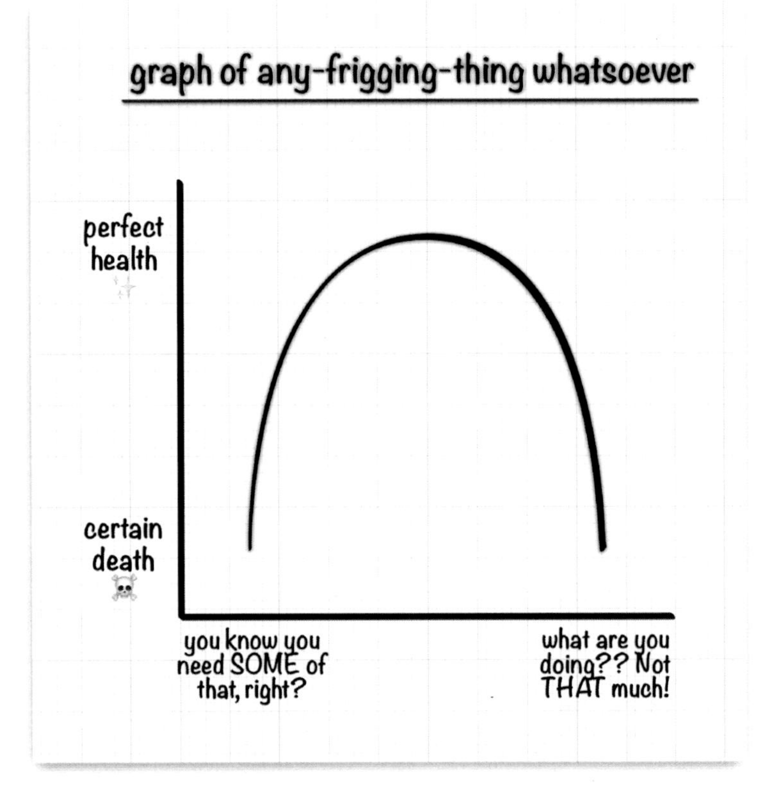

But here comes our point. If you just choose any *ONE* of all of these levers, and fixate on it completely, you might miss out on all of the other levers. What's more, you might even pull that lever so hard that it breaks off in your hand, metaphorically speaking—and your results actually WORSEN.

For an example, let's look at low carb diets. We all know that person who is a rabid low carb fanatic. To be fair, the second that person went on a low carb diet, they did effortlessly lose a bunch of fat and they immediately felt better. But now, if they stall out and reach a plateau on their low carb diet, they might make the mistake of just trying to 'low carb' harder. Maybe they will shave their carbs from 50 total grams daily down to 20 grams daily, by eliminating all green vegetables. Maybe they feel that if they can just get their carb grams all the way down to ABSOLUTE ZERO—with a pure carnivore diet, for example—they will finally get the results they are looking for.

There are two huge problems with this approach. First of all, you are missing out on all of the other levers. And some of those levers are some VERY low-hanging fruit. For example, if you aren't doing any resistance exercise at all, just adding in a set of push-ups and pull-ups and squats daily could be far easier than banishing all trace carbs from your life. Maybe just going for a walk after dinner would be both easier and more efficacious? The second problem is that by pulling this lever until it breaks, you could actually start WORSENING your results. For example, skipping the salad and only eating steak, in order to get your carbs from 20 grams all the way down to zero, could actually lead to poorer satiety and more of a fat loss stall.

We see the same mistakes being made in the plant-based community. Not getting the health results you want? You just need to 'vegan' even harder—there must be some traces of animals in there somewhere. We see the same thing in those who are only using exercise to lose weight. Perhaps one hour of jogging isn't enough and you need to jog for two hours?

In all of the diet and exercise camps, you can find examples of this sort of over-reliance on one facet of health. But you need to be mindful of *ALL* of these if you really want to get the outcome you are looking for. We would encourage everyone to pull each of these levers to a moderate degree, rather than just grabbing one lever with a death grip and leaning on it until it snaps off at the base, leaving you with nothing.

And now it is your turn. Remember, every day gives you a brand new opportunity to progress your diet and exercise. You only get one trip through life, and you owe it to yourself to live it lean, strong, and healthy. No matter where you are at in your progress, always live in the present, and be sure to enjoy the journey!

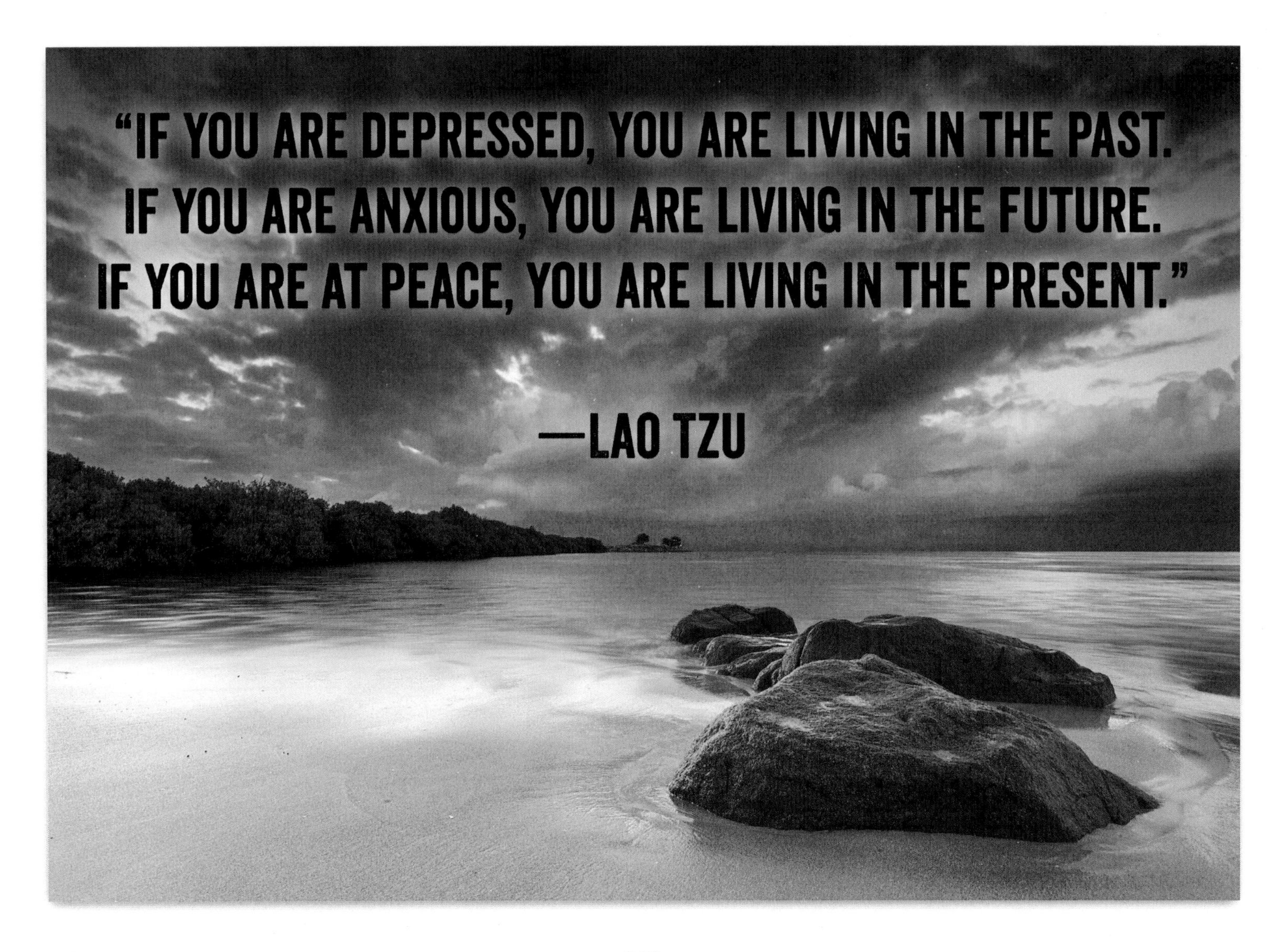

Lightning Source UK Ltd.
Milton Keynes UK
UKRC011215170321
380509UK00001B/3